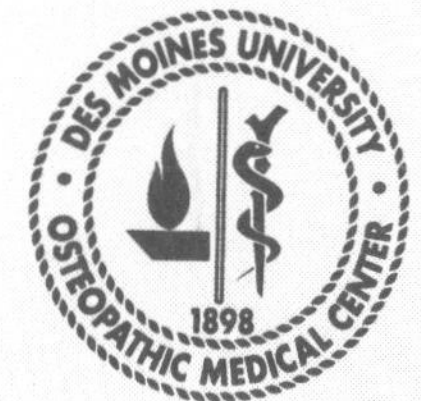

Presented to
DMU Library
by
Gerald J. Cooper, D.O.

Early Osteopathy
in the
Words of A. T. Still

Early Osteopathy *in the* Words *of* A. T. Still

Illustrated

Edited by R. V. Schnucker

KIRKSVILLE, MISSOURI
THE THOMAS JEFFERSON UNIVERSITY PRESS
AT NORTHEAST MISSOURI STATE UNIVERSITY
1991

NMSU LB 115 Kirksville, Missouri 63501 USA

Library of Congress Cataloging-in-Publication Data
Still, A. T. (Andrew Taylor), 1828-1917.
Early Osteopathy in the Words of A. T. Still, / edited by R. V. Schnucker

p. cm.

Contains articles from Dr.Still's writings in the Journal of osteopathy and rare photographs of him.
ISBN 0-943549-11-6
1. Osteopathy. I. Schnucker, Robert V. II. Journal of osteopathy. III. Title.
[DNLM: 1. Osteopathic Medicine—collected works. WB 940 S857e]
RZ 337.s75 1991
615.5'33—dc20
for Library of Congress 91-7097
CIP

Designed and edited by R. V. Schnucker at The Thomas Jefferson University Press of Northeast Missouri State University. Permission to reproduce photographs, illustrations, and copies of printed material courtesy of Kirksville College of Osteopathic Medicine and Still National Museum of Osteopathic Medicine, Kirksville. Printed by Edwards Bros., Inc., Ann Arbor, Michigan.

The paper used in this publication meets the minimum requirements of the American National Standard for Permanence of Paper for Printed Library Materials ANSI Z39.48, 1984.

Kirksville College of Osteopathic Medicine gratefully acknowledges the
generous support of The Thomas Jefferson University Press
at Northeast Missouri State University
in the publication of this book.

Table of Contents

List of Illustrations

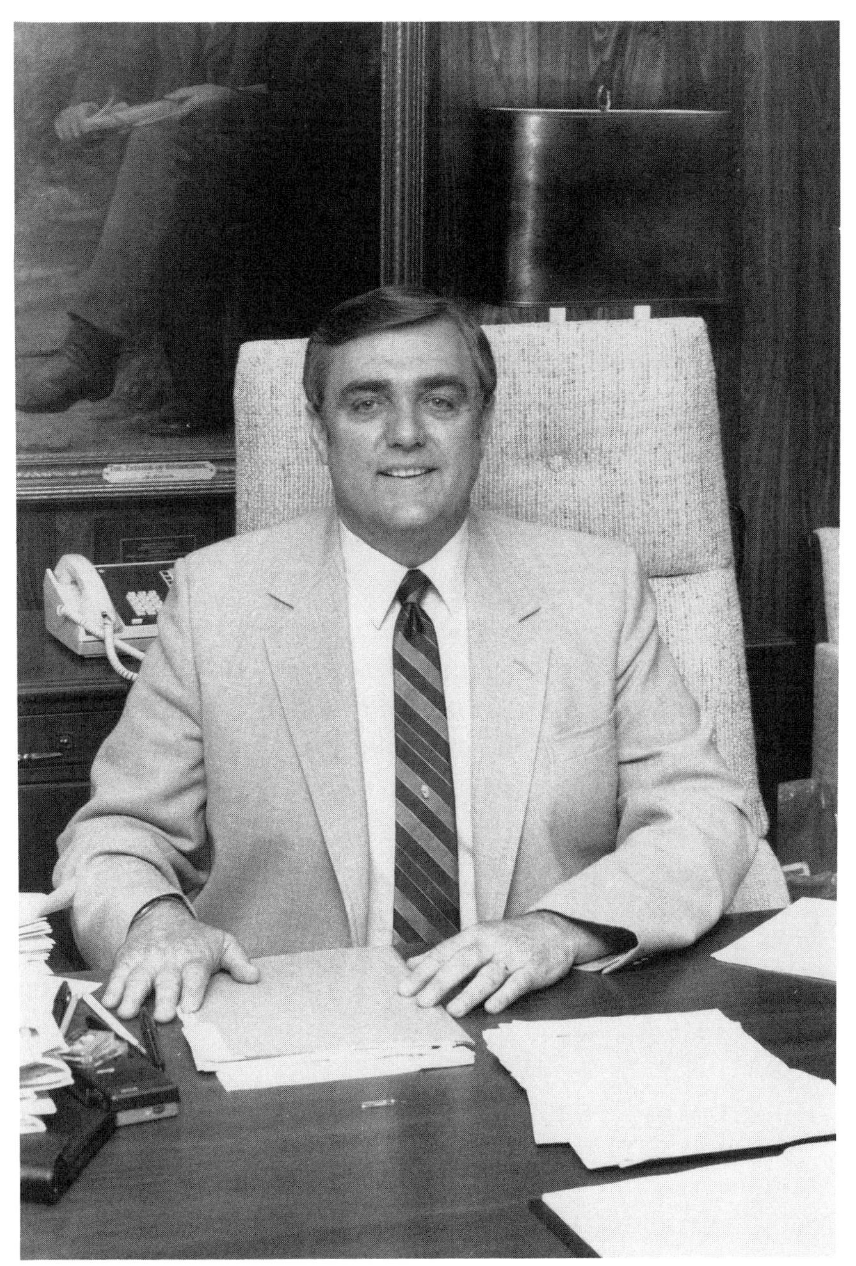

Foreword

ONE HUNDRED YEARS AGO, Andrew Taylor Still, M.D., started the American School of Osteopathy in Kirksville, Missouri. Many in the allopathic medical profession scoffed at his ideas of drugless medicine, prevention, health and wellness, and care for the total family. Nevertheless, Dr. Still began his school with a handful of students, whose ranks have expanded today to more that 31,000 osteopathic physicians internationally.

To spread the word of his revolutionary theory of medicine, Dr. Still founded the *Journal of Osteopathy* in 1894. Through this journal, Dr. Still provided further education and evidence of his significant discovery. This special book contains articles from Dr. Still's writings in the *Journal of Osteopathy* and rare photographs of him. As you read these articles, it is interesting to note how many of Dr. Still's hypotheses of medicine hold true today. Indeed this important compilation of his work underscores the rich heritage that osteopathic medicine holds as we approach our second century of service to mankind.

As president of the Kirksville College of Osteopathic Medicine, it is my honor to dedicate this special Centennial publication in memory of the "Old Doctor." He has left a lasting legacy for the thousands of osteopathic physicians who have followed in his footsteps.

Kirksville, Missouri
March, 1991

Fred C. Tinning

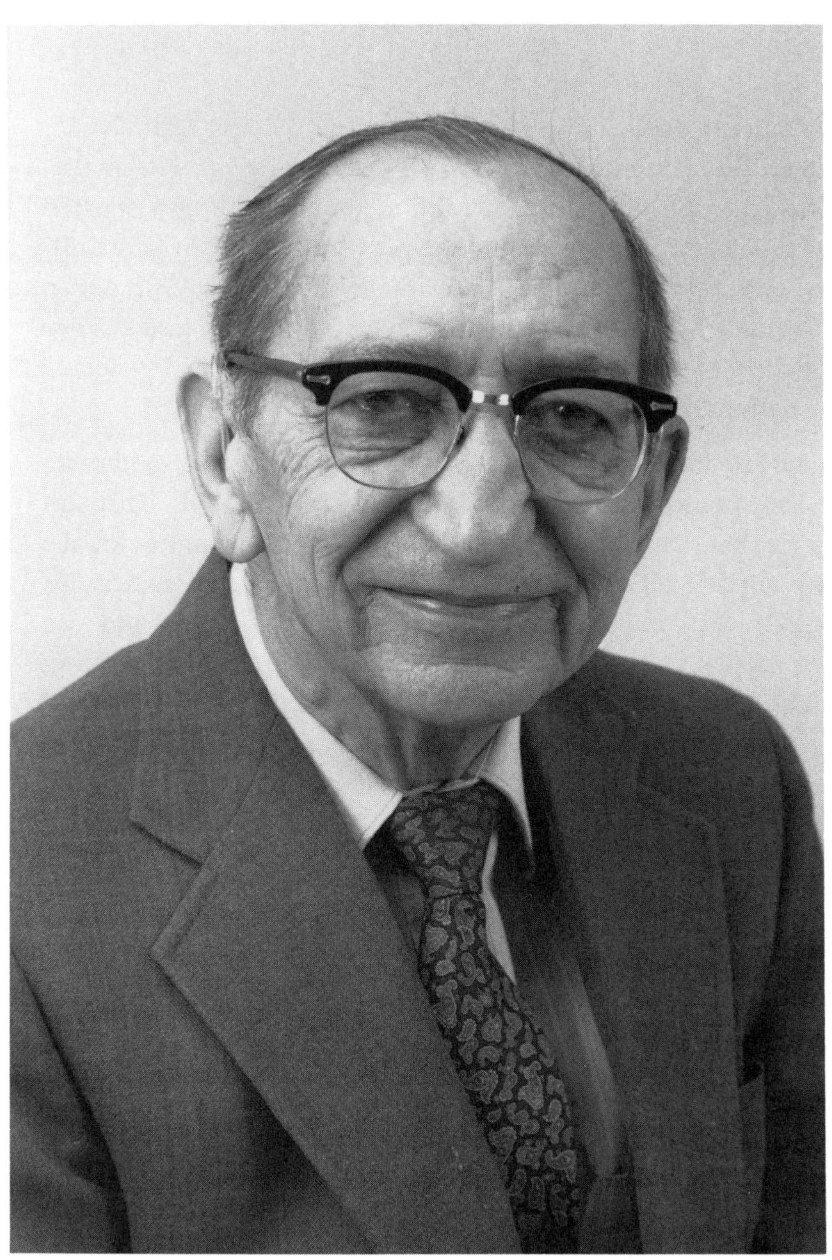

Preface

IN THE WRITINGS OF Dr. Andrew Taylor Still, the founder of the osteopathic philosophy, there is the following statement in the preface of his book *Philosophy of Osteopathy:*

> It is my object in this work to teach principles as I understand them and not rules.

This typifies the teachings of A. T. Still. In his writings you do not find a "cure" for a disease. Rather, he lays down the principle and the procedures that can be followed to alleviate the condition.

There are no rules to follow to heal a disease, but rather, the approach is to first find the area affected and treat this, and then the whole man.

A. T. Still was a pragmatic philosopher in the practice of medicine, far ahead of current methods and thoughts. His contribution was that "man is a unit" and therefore appropriate therapy could follow. He sought to lead a profession toward a method to diagnose and treat the whole man, not just a disease.

Max T. Gutensohn, D. O.

Kirksville, Missouri
March, 1991

Editor's Preface

About the time in life when most of us are either thinking about retiring or have retired, Andrew Taylor Still was beginning his career as the first osteopathic educator by founding his school dedicated to the scientific principles of the new medical theory he had discovered. The first school had a very modest beginning. It was located in a simple building, with a handful of students who didn't always understand what was going on—to the extent that Dr. Still asked some to repeat the course of instruction. The town of Kirksville was curious about the new school but not overly enthusiastic. Yet, in a very short span of time Dr. Still's school proved to be such a success that it soon overshadowed the Normal School that had been in Kirksville since the end of the Civil War. Railroads ran special trains to bring patients and students to the remote northeast Missouri town. In time, Dr. Still's school became the "mother" institution of all Osteopathy. It is fitting that in the one hundredth year of the founding of the first Osteopathic school the many articles and observations of its founder as published in the *Journal of Osteopathy* be gathered into one collection so that a new printed record might exist testifying to the genius and insight of Dr. Andrew Taylor Still; that is the purpose of this book. Included, too, are photographs from Dr. Still's era.

The surviving copies of early editions of the *Journal of Osteopathy* are yellowed and fragile. The pages are easily broken into pieces when handled. Fortunately, the excellent library at Kirksville College of Osteopathic Medicine has rescued those copies by having them de-acidified and preserved for the future. Without the help of KCOM Library Director, Mr. Larry Onsager, and his staff, it would not have been possible to compile this book. In the early efforts to make this book possible, Dr. Patricia Gately went through all the journals and identified those pieces written by Dr. A. T. Still.

In the process of creating this book, a number of problems emerged. First, the early *Journals* used a five column format, then three, then one. This posed a problem in selecting a format for the current book. The most efficient solution was to lay out the first part of the book in vertical columns and the latter part in horizontal columns. Second, printers at the turn of the century used different line spacing within a column and different type sizes within a column, which is reflected in the irregular column lengths found in this reprinting. Third, it was not easy to identify all the pieces written by Dr. Still. Most of the time the pieces were signed, but often they were not. The careful work of Dr. Gately and Mrs. Katrina Davisson has virtually guaranteed that all the pieces have been accurately identified for inclusion here. Finally, some of the pieces were repeated throughout the life of the *Journal*. As a consequence, some of the items that appeared in the journal were not included here; i.e., extracts from Still's autobiography and the long summary of his writings that appeared shortly after his death.

The photographs are from the Still National Osteopathic Museum and the library archives of KCOM. Without their generous help and cooperation, this book would be minus any illustrations. Mrs. Elizabeth Laughlin was helpful and supportive in opening the Museum for use and in making her own personal documents and photographs available. A very special word of thanks must be given to Mrs. Katrina Davisson, who spent many, many hours copying and recopying the *Journals* and searching out documents, needed photographs, and other materials that make this book a reality. Her positive and kind spirit made the task move with efficiency and dispatch. Mr. William Castles, Director of Public Relations at KCOM, played an indispensable role in bringing the book to publication, and none of this would have been possible without the interest and support of Dr. Fred Tinning, president of KCOM.

All of us hope you will appreciate the words of Andrew Taylor Still and the pictures of those early days of Osteopathy.

Robert V. Schnucker
Editor

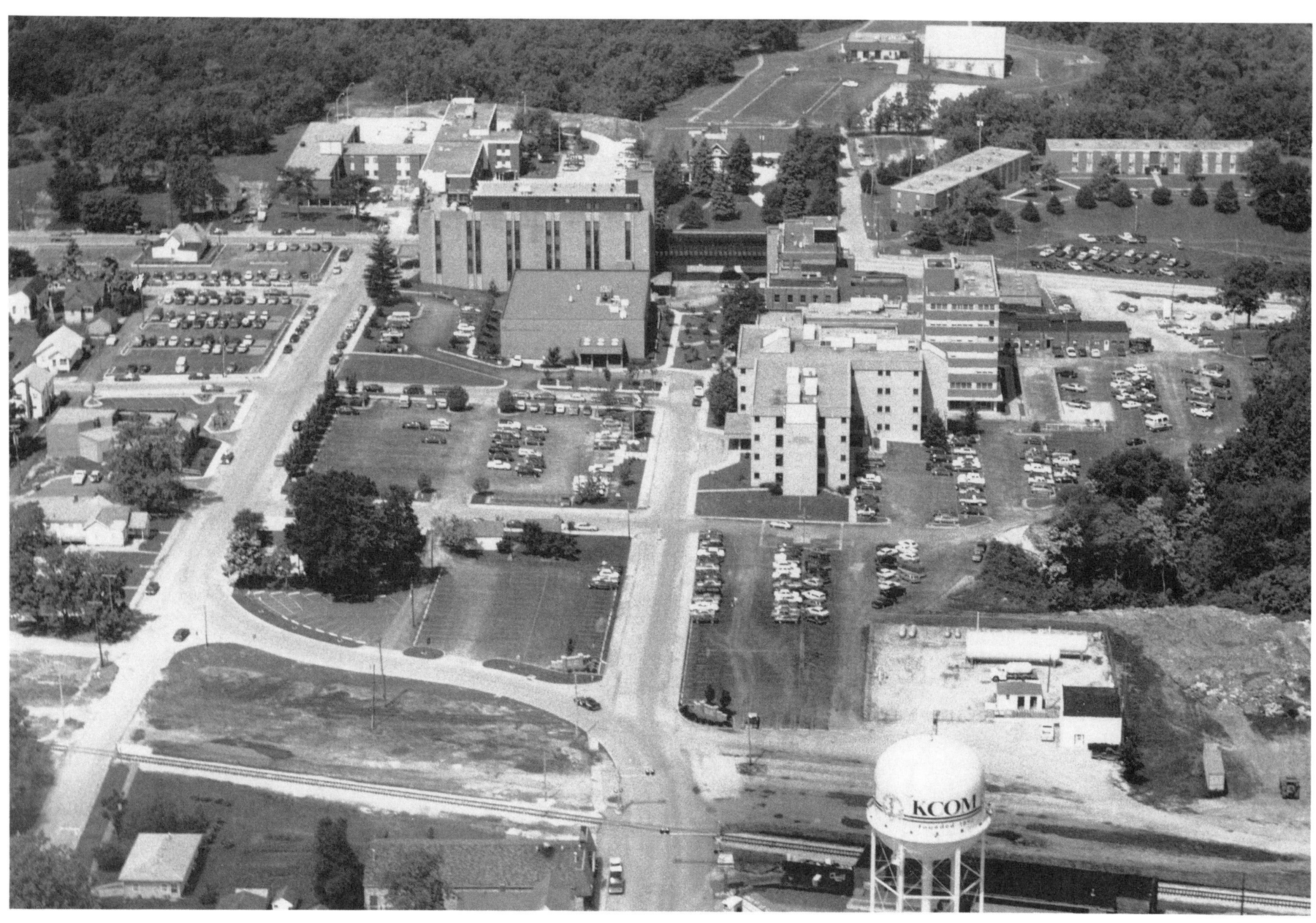
KCOM

May, 1894

ADDRESS

By Dr. A. T. Still to His Students and Diplomates May 7th, 1894.

To the Students and Diplomates in Osteopathy—Greeting: At the threshold of your Osteopathic duties you have the supreme satisfaction of knowing that you are confronted with a science. By a systematic, rigid adherence to its never failing laws you will ever prove an honor to yourself, a blessing to this school and a benefactor to mankind. You should ever remember that Osteopathy adheres strictly to the well defined and immutable laws of nature, and it is an unerring Deity who wills it so. And as such it only remains for the Osteopath to conform to these laws and his efforts in this life will not only be crowned with success, but made rich with the thanks of his fellow-man. You are indeed to be congratulated upon the splendid grades attained at the close of the recent examinations—for an average of 98.7 per cent for the entire session is not to be excelled or even equaled by any institution of learning of whatever nature on the American Continent. The American School of Osteopathy stands to-day the very essence of success. It has reached this successful attitude in spite of vicious schemes invented by designing men to connect our beloved science with antiquated ignorance and modern chicanery, and force us to accept relationship with allopathic drugs, homœopathic pills, electrical shocks, medicated sweat tubs and orificial surgery. We are proud of the fact that our science, so dear to our hearts, is giving more relief to suffering humanity where properly applied, than all the sciences known to human sympathy combined. We pride ourselves on the truth that we are daily giving to suffering souls health and comfort, peace and happiness, relief from pain, and good will toward men. This is the sole object of our school, and we should strive to maintain it in its stainless purity. No system of allopathy, with its fatal drugs, should e'er be permitted to enter our doors. No homœopathic practice, with its sugar-coated pills, must be allowed to stain or pollute our spotless name. No orificial surgery, with its ancient ignorance and modern mendacity can possibly find an abiding place within the mind of the true, tried and qualified Osteopath. Osteopathy asks not the aid of anything else It can "paddle its own canoe" and perform its works within itself when understood. All it asks is a thorough knowledge of the unerring laws that govern its practice, and the rest is yours.

Eminent physicians and surgeons of the "old school," who have attained considerable prominence in their respective localities and who were former instructors in this institution of learning, have cheerfully and freely given us their affidavits as an evidence of the high regard in which they hold the science of Osteopathy. To them, as their sworn statement shows, Osteopathy stands pre-eminently above all things else. They do not link it with various other devices for the relief of suffering humanity, but make it the all absorbing and permanent science of the age. So with pleasure I submit you the following sworn statements.

"Kirksville, Mo., Jan. 13, 1893 —I am a fully qualified physician and surgeon, registered to practice. I have an intimate acquaintance with the methods of treating disease known as Osteopathy, in which no drugs are used.

I solemnly and sincerely swear that I believe and know the above system to be in advance of anything known to the general medical profession in the treatment of disease.

Andrew P. Davis, M. D.,

Registered in Mo., Ill., Colo., Cal., and Texas.

William Smith, Physician and Surgeon. Registered in Scotland and Missouri.

F. S. Davis, M. D. Registered in Texas.

Subscribed and sworn to before me this 14th day of January, A. D., 1893.

My commission expires September 5, 1895.

(SEAL) Wm T. Porter,
Notary Public."

Thus will be seen the position that Osteopathy occupies in the estimation of these gentlemen, who doubtless would blush with shame to see their names affixed to anything inconsistent or contrary to their sworn statements. It will be observed that allopathy, homœopathy, eclecticism and orificial surgery in particular are conspicuously evaded—and surely they would not stoop to belittle our science by mixing or connecting it with these fading sciences of antiquity. You are thus appealed to, to be likewise in the practice of your chosen profession. Remember that all power is powerless except the unerring Deity of your being, to whose unchangeable laws you must conform, if you hope to win the battle of your life. Osteopathy to you should be the guiding, glittering star of your career. In its study you will find room for every thought, a place for every idea, and comfort for every fear. New and difficult cases will be presented to you for adjustment, but stick to Osteopathy. Do not warp your intellect or stain the good name of this school by straying after strange gods. Always bear in mind that Osteopathy will do the work if properly applied, that all else is unnatural, unreasonable, is therefore wrong and should not be entertained by the student or diplomate, who has the brains to grasp in all its fullness the most advanced and most appreciated science of the Nineteenth Century. If Osteopathy is not all within itself, it is nothing. It walks hand in hand with nothing but nature's laws, and for this reason alone it marks the most significant progress in the history of scientific research, and is as plainly understood by the natural mind as the gild at evening tide that decks the golden West. Hear me again! You are the only true and brave soldiers in the great army of freedom, battling for the liberation of fettered bodies. On your conscientious work will rest the thanks of man. Live up to the great cause of Osteopathy and let not the weary one fall by the wayside. Lift in sympathy and love the suffering brother from out the depths of disease and drugs. Let your light so shine before men that the world will know you are an Osteopath pure and simple, and that no prouder title can follow a human name. Stand by the "old flag" of Osteopathy, on whose fluttering folds are emblazoned in letters of glittering gold—"One science, one Lord, one faith and one baptism."

GRADUATING EXERCISES

Of the First Class of the American School of Osteopathy.

The second day of March, 1894 marked the first mile stone in the progress of the American School of Osteopathy and will always be remembered as a red letter day by the students and friends of the new science.

Osteopathy remains no longer in the realms of doubt, but has become a fixed fact in the great field of thought and action. If the doubtful and the skeptical could have faced the magnificent audience that greeted Dr. Still and his graduating class that evening in Smith's opera house, they would have been immediately convinced that Dr. Still's method of treatment and the science of Osteopathy was destined, not only to occupy a most prominent position in the scientific world, but that it would eventually be the accepted method of treating diseases.

The exercises opened with speeches from several of Kirksville's most prominent attorneys and citizens. They were plain and outspoken in their views as to the necessity of Kirksville, arousing herself to united action whereby they might give evidence of their high appreciation of the institution that has grown up among them.

The injustice of the existing laws of the State was deplored—and the people were urged to assist in removing from our statutes, a medical law so obnoxious and offensive to free institutions and a free government.

A law which is designed to shut out a science which has for its object only the benefit of the human family, is certainly a disgrace to Missouri, and a stain upon her fair name. It is a law kept alive only by ignorance, prejudice and self-interest, and to be universally condemned only needs to be known.

After being introduced by the chairman of the meeting, Dr. A. T. Still, President and Founder of the American School of Osteopathy, took the rostrum and delivered one of his characteristic, forceful addresses. The Doctor was at his best, and his remarks bristled with keen, incisive and unanswerable arguments. During his address he held his audience spell bound, and that the address was appreciated was evidenced by round after round of applause at its conclusion. His address was followed by the presentation of diplomas to the graduates by Dr. Still. In his plain, earnest, straight forward way he impressed upon the students the responsibilities and duties which devolve upon them, and impressed them with the importance of the great science they had chosen as their life work.

Some excellent music concluded the exercises at the opera house, after which the class and about fifty invited guests repaired to Pool's Hotel, where an elegant repast was served. Some excellent toasts and responses were listened to, after which good-night was said, and all left feeling it was an evening profitably spent

Below will be found a list of those who graduated and received diplomas: Mrs. Nettie Hubbard Bolles, of Olathe, Kansas; Miss Mamie B. Harter, of Sedalia, Mo.; Mrs. Lou J. Kern, of Springfield, Mo.; Messrs. Joseph H. Osborn, Herman T. Still, Frank B. N. Palmeteer, Arthur G. Hildreth, Miller Machin, all of Kirksville; Elbert G. Rickart, of Quincy, Ill; James D. Hill and Adolph A. Goodman, of Kansas City; Messrs. Arthur A. Bird, E. H. Higbee, Fred Still, A. P. Davis, F. S. Davis, and William Smith.

June, 1894

DR. STILL.

Will the People of Kirksville Persuade Him to Remain or Will They Allow Him to Depart From Our City.

An Enthusiastic Meeting of Our Citizens at the City Hall Monday Night.

From the Kirksville Democrat.

At a meeting of the citizens held Monday night at the city hall, to devise ways and means for making a donation to the American School of Osteopathy in order to retain the School and Dr Still in our city, S. M. Link was chosen chairman and J. O. Gooch secretary.

Several of our enterprising citizens had been working up a scheme to procure the fair grounds site for a location for the school and had met with so much encouragement that they determined upon calling the meeting to further the ends desired.

The project of donating the fair grounds was pretty generally discussed, but it seems that some of the stock holders are loth to give up the fair grounds and that some other grounds will be selected.

S. M. Pickler, in a speech, offered to donate five acres of ground on the west side of town and sell at $100 per acre ten or more acres off the same body of land.

R. M. Brashear proposed to donate ten acres of ground in the eastern part and if Dr. Still decided to locate on same, he thought he could insure a street railway from both railroad depots to the location. Other propositions are being formulated.

A committee was appointed by the chair to receive written propositions from those offering to donate ground, and take subscriptions of money toward buying more ground or making further donations toward securing the location of the institution.

This committee set Tuesday morning as a date for meeting and conferring with those making land propositions and also to secure money donations.

It has been learned that Sedalia has made Dr. Still a substantial proposition to locate in that city and our citizens feel it is high time they were making an effort to retain him here.

The meeting was largely attended and many of our best and wealthiest citizens were present.

At the close of a general discussion of the subject, the following resolutions were unanimously adopted:

We, the citizens of Kirksville, assembled at the Mayor's office this evening, May 28, 1894, to take into consideration the advisability of assisting to erect an Infirmary in conjunction with Dr. A. T. Still for his use and the benefit of humanity beg to express our appreciation of his great ability as the founder and exponent of the School of Osteopathy: That we as citizens feel proud of him as a fellow townsman: That we have the utmost confidence in his skill as a healer, as is evidenced by hundreds of his patients who come halt and lame and depart in a few weeks with light hearts and straightened limbs: That we believe in his integrity as a man; and we feel proud that he has gained a national reputation and made Kirksville known in every State in the Union. And we most earnestly ask Dr. Still to remain with us and we promise him substantial aid, and our most hearty support in holding up his hands, as the greatest healer of modern times.

The law of life is absolute. That wonderful, unknown and incomprehensible force which furnishes the power to move the machinery of all animate bodies is felt but not understood. Of ourselves we are unable to supply any one substance required in the economy of our bodies, yet there is a force within us which can select from the given materials such substances as are needed to form any part of the human system.

A PLEA FOR TEMPERANCE.

A. T. STILL.

Was God ever drunk?

Was Nature ever intoxicated?

If so, do you believe that God was intoxicated when he was formulating the divine image, man?

If not intoxicated, and he was duly sober during this important period of formulating the superstructure of man which is material, motor and mental in its oneness; if it was really necessary that this grand mind of the universe should be duly sober and in full exercise of all that pertains to mind or thought; is it not just as necessary to keep this grand superstructure not only sober, but under sober influences that it may be able to operate all the parts, principles and qualities of the divine law pertaining to human life?

If I must carry you farther, then allow me to say, that he is wholly devoid of reason who would throw the human machine from a normal to an abnormal condition and expect normal results in its execution of the laws of harmony and life.

Then why should a normal brain, normal nerves, normal blood vessels, in locality, form and calibre, be made abnormal by the powerful narcotics, stimulants, astringents or alkaloids and expect in the results, a display of the beauties of life in action, comfort and duration?

Have such minds any claim to recognition as philosophers?

Nay, verily, not even to be called respectable fools.

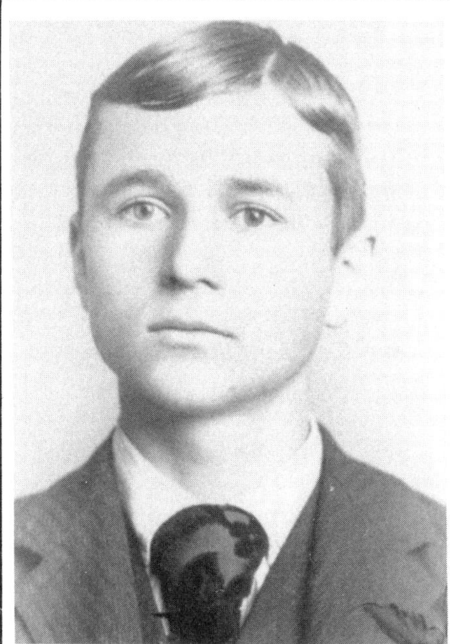

OBITUARY.

Fred Still was born in Baldwin, Kansas, on the 25th dav of January, 1874. As a youth and young man he was quiet and studious, not inclined to the more active and boisterous sports of boyhood, but seemed to find his chief delights in mental activity. He graduated from the city schools at 15 years of age, and was the youngest scholar ever entering the preparatory department of the Normal School. He was a member of the first class of Osteopathy which opened in the fall of 1892. The following summer he was a very successful operator, being devoted heart and soul to the science. The one object toward which he strove, the one hope inspiring his whole being, was that he might be able to take up the banner of Osteopathy when his father laid it down, and carry it to higher planes and more complete development.

Fred's death was caused primarily by being crushed between a horse and the wall of a barn, causing a complete displacement of the heart, inflicting an injury, the adjustment of which was beyond the reach of human power. During his long sickness every comfort that thoughtful heads and loving hearts could devise were given him, but they only served to alleviate his suffering and to briefly prolong his life.

His last waning strength was given to the cause of Osteopathy. While lying on his bed in sunny California, a little girl with a broken wrist was brought to him. While his uncle held the arm, Fred set it and sent the little one away happy, leaving behind her heart-felt thanks.

During his life he was always conscientious, exemplary, and estimable, and no young man in the city was more respected than he.

Although he is gone the influences of such lives as his cannot be lost. His example is worthy of emulation, and to the bereaved family the comfort comes that Fred is "not lost, but gone before."

We live in deeds, not years—in thoughts, not breaths;—
In feelings, not in figures on a dial.
We should count time by heart-throbs.
He most lives, who thinks most,—feels the noblest,—acts the best.

FRED.

We hate the word, "He is dead."
It makes us to cry piteously, that we have lost our best,
As in mind we call the endless roll of our loving dead,
Our souls cry out in anguish, while our loved ones are at rest.

One by one their forms appear: I cry again, "I love my dead."
I view their faces each in turn, father, mother, my dear son Fred.
Tears from my eyes from morn till night, adown my face as rivers flow,
I ask and reason, "If he is not dead, where O, where, then did he go?

"Dead!" "Dead!" "He is dead!"
Why, O, my friends, please tell me why,
When a friend is dead, "He did not die?"
Like a philosopher, when dying, he said—
When this "job" is done, I'll return, not dead."
I hate the word, "He is dead, dead!"
It may be true, but not with Fred.

A. T. Still.

OFFICERS AND FACULTY

OF THE

American School of Osteopathy.

Dr. A. T. Still, ... President.
H. E. Patterson, ... Secretary.
Mrs. Nettie H. Bolles, ... Instructor in Anatomy.

June, 1894

Business Department.

The business management of my affairs is in charge of H. E. Patterson, our well and favorably known fellow-townsman, who has filled many positions of trust and honor, establishing a reputation for honesty, sobriety and justice. He has the entire confidence of the business men of Kirksville and vicinity.

A. T. Still.

To Prospective Patients.

Those coming to us for treatment will save themselves much inconvenience, by preparing for a somewhat longer course of treatment, than is usually done by the average patient. Very few cases can be safely discharged on less than one month's treatment, and longer time should be given in most cases. After the cause of the trouble has been removed the patient should remain under treatment for a time in order to more surely receive lasting benefit. Of course some cases are cured in a few treatments, some in a single treatment, but they are comparatively few. All should make up their minds to take just the course of treatment that may be prescribed at the time of their examination.

August, 1894

TO PATIENTS AND VISITORS.

A. T. STILL.

Upon presenting yourself at our office for examination and treatment, first secure a number from the file of cards which are put up in a conspicuous place in the waiting room. You will receive attention in the order in which the numbers are held. At the time of examination you will be requested to give a short history of your case, how long standing and what treatment you have had. You will will soon find the Osteopaths use no drugs. They will look you over as an engineer would look over his engine, to see if it is in running order. If found out of fix, they adjust the machine and start it to running.

If a wheel, pulley, belt or any part is wrong, he goes to work adjusting, till all is corrected. An engineer who is ignorant, who does not know the use of all the parts of his machine is not a safe person to take charge of the lives behind his engine. Laws are enacted and exacted of him that he may be competent to fulfill the trust reposed in him, and that your lives may be safe when in his care. My students are required to pass a grade of 90 per cent in Anatomy before they are admitted to the operating rooms to take instructions in adjusting the human body for disease. This is no place for empty brag and foolish promises. You will find my operators are all well qualified engineers who know their business. We are not Gods, nor Christian Scientists, or Faith Doctors, nor Spirit Doctors, but simply Anatomical Engineers—we understand the human engine and can put it in running order, subject always to the laws of Nature.

If you come to us for treatment you come of your own free will, and not through any trick or scheme of mine or any of my helpers. Remember that when many of you come to me, you are not the most choice kind of patients. Remember the company you have kept before coming here. You have been with Doctors who blister you, puke you, physic your toe nails loose, fill your sides and limbs with truck from hyperdermic syringes. You come to me with eyes big from belladonna, backs and limbs stiff from plaster paris casts—you come with bodies suffering with all the diseases that flesh is heir to. Remember you have been treated and dismissed as incurable by all kinds of doctors before you come to us, and if we help you at all—we do more than all the others have done. And yet of all the various forms of affliction that have been treated here—75 per cent have been greatly benefitted and 50 per cent are sent home well.

I am not telling this to solicit your patronage. I claim this as the only place where man is looked upon and treated as an engine. Search the annals of history for the truth of what I say. This is no time to brag; let results speak.

My motto is "Help the needy, and deal justly with all." I am not going to "get rich or bust." I have made but one rule in life, "reason first, justice and humanity all the time." All persons claiming to be from my school, who can not show their papers as a student or diplomate in Osteopathy are imposters and are obtaining money under false pretenses.

August, 1894

THE TONGUE OF A BUZZARD.

[In all my reading and inquiry, I have as yet failed to find any description of a buzzard's tongue similar to the one given below. I wish to take no credit from any one, but so far claim this as my own discovery.—A. T. Still.]

I found the skeleton of a buzzard fast in the crotch of tree in which it had had its nest. I think from the appearance of the bones, it had been there at least a year, for they had been well cleaned by the winds and rains.

When I opened the mouth I found the tongue to be a bone as large as a lead pencil—with three lances or arrow points that could move and cut like a pair of scissors. Upon pressing the three blades together it became a dart from one half to three quarters of an inch long. Thus while in the form of a dart it could pierce the tough hide of any animal it wished to eat, then rip it open with the scissor blades.

Those lances are very hard and sharp and are wisely constructed by nature, who never fails to do all her work well.

TIMIDITY.

A. T. STILL.

Timidity takes possession of us only when we are at a loss to judge of the end from the beginning. For instance, we are timid about going under the influence of chloroform because we do not know whether we will perish or survive its use.

The same timidity comes over us in the use of drugs.

In Osteopathic treatment we have no timidity as Osteopathy strengthens us in all cases. In no instance has death ever occurred as the result of the treatment though thousands have received benefit at the hands of the skilled graduates of our school.

I have been engaged in the study and discussion of the Science of Osteopathy for over twenty years, and I have never found a fair minded man, I mean one who could and would reason, who did not say "Yes, Sir" to my reasons why Osteopathy could cure diseases. Osteopathy is the only science of healing that asks no other system to help it. All truth is self-existing and knows no surrender.

Wonders are found by persons who cannot find wisdom.

A. T. S.

October, 1894

In response to the oft repeated inquiry. "Why do you not publish the names of your patients that the world may know what an extensive business you are doing?" We give the following reply:

I am positively opposed to publishing the names of any or all who take treatment at my office. In the first place no lady or gentleman wishes to have their names, ages and diseases spread before the world in a newspaper or almanac. Of course many would allow their names and diseases given to the world, but I do not want them yet. Perhaps I may if my business runs down. Then I may bawl for food as a calf or any other animal would if it was hungry. Another reason for my objection is that no paper in this town can hold the names of the patrons of Osteopathy and get in any politics, even a corner an inch square. My books are open at all times and I have the most gentlemanly Secretary in the world to give you all the information you want.

A. T. Still.

"Life is that calm principle sent forth from Deity which vivifies all nature."—A. T. Still.

The first requirement for an accurate diagnosis is a thorough knowledge of the human engine, all its powers, parts, and principles. Thus armed, you are prepared to decide whether the trouble is in the boiler, steam-chest, wheels, valves, shaft or any other part of the machinery. Without this you cannot give a correct diagnosis, prognosis or treatment. A. T. Still.

December, 1894

HISTORY OF OSTEOPATHY.

It is now something over twenty years since Osteopathy presented itself to the student of mysteries, to the student of facts, to the student of truths. Osteopathy when it first presented itself to its founder did so in a rude shape as all sciences do, and to be sure was not inviting to any marked degree. But its discoverer was not to be discouraged by its homliness. On the contrary he saw in its shapeless form jewels that shone like diamonds in the rough. It then only remained for him to clear away the rubbish, wash the jewels to a brilliant hue, and give to mankind a living, breathing science—a thousand facts that must be admitted, a thousand truths that cannot be successful-

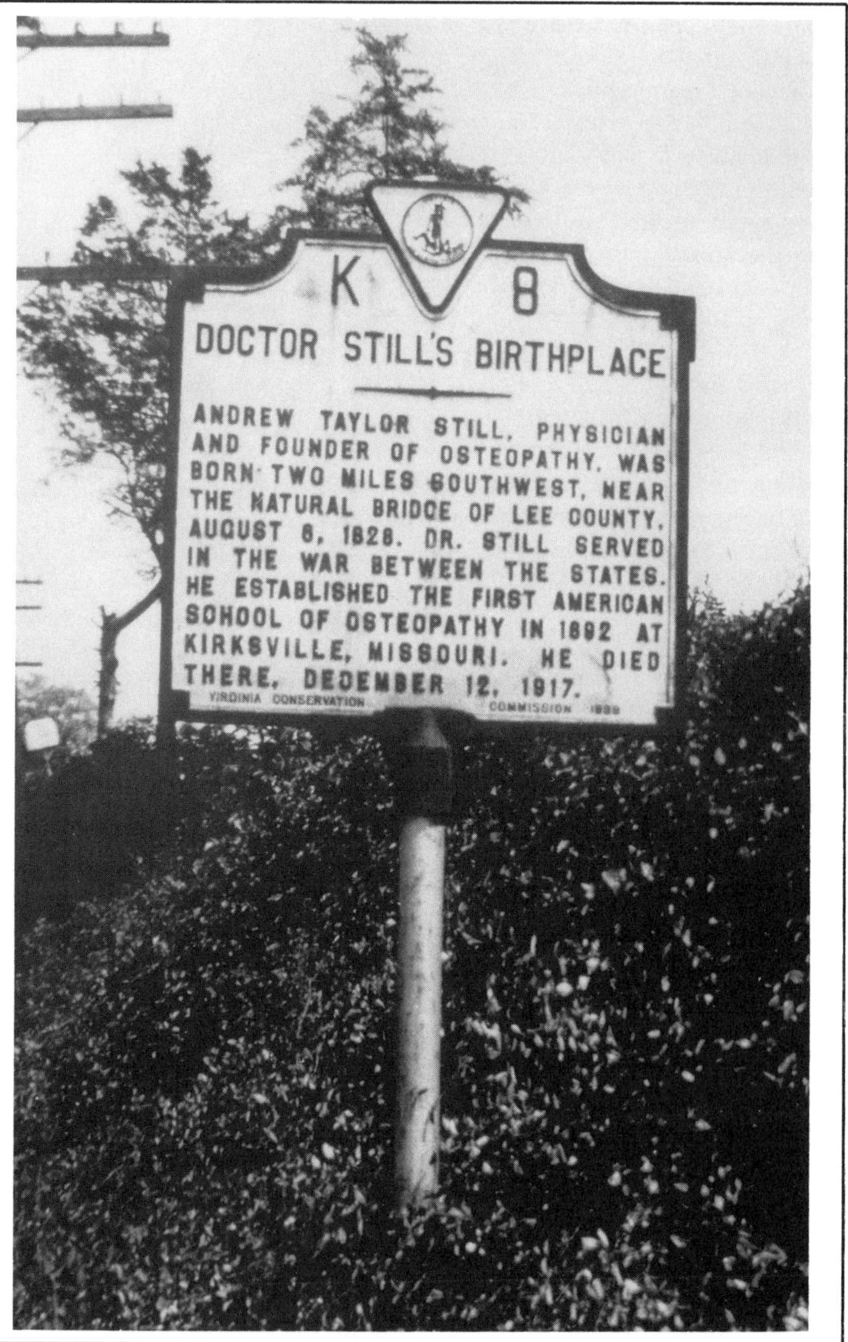

ly denied. In presenting the science of Osteopathy to the impartial, unprejudiced student, its founder, after twenty years of ceaseless toil, feels that another oasis on the desert of life, has been discovered; another fountain on the arid plains throws forth its life-giving waters from which it asks all to come and drink freely. He does not ask this feeling any delicacy as to what the result will be, for after years of successful treatment of all or nearly all diseases human flesh is heir to, he knows whereof he speaks.

Why and how does he know this, you ask? You are answered with another question, why and how does the silversmith of long years' experience in his profession, know when the finest of watches are adjusted to keep perfect time? The student of Osteopathy, who applies himself closely for twenty years to the study of this science, will know what's the matter and what's the remedy, in all the ailments that flesh is heir to. The founder and the truthful students of Osteopathy do not profess to be able to resurrect the dead, neither is it expected to teach to others in three or six months what has taken him years of ceaseless toil to fathom, and lift from its darkest recesses to the sunlight of truth. He who goes forth as a graduate of the American School of Osteopathy should be fully prepared and equipped to successfully battle in public and in private, in the office or on the rostrum with every denier and every defier of the lofty science he has the honor of defending. He should go forth fully prepared to meet the arguments of all comers. If he fails in this, he is false to himself and a sham to the science he represents. Osteopathy at its present stage of development, chalanges the admiration of the student of progress. It unfolds a thousand facts as simple as A B C. But you must understand these facts in order that they may be simple to you. You must, in addition to this, discard the idea that Osteopathy is a special gift to its founder and cannot be taught to others. On the contrary it is placed before the world the same as the science of electricity, and one principle after another has been discovered till an unbroken chain of principles has been formed, strong enough to stand the test of eternity, natural enough to live as long as nature's well defined lines remain unchanged. Who could ask more? Who wants more? All mysteries are hidden in nature, all facts are found in nature, all discoveries are made in nature. Then does it not follow that nature's unchangeable laws must be followed in order to find what you seek? Osteopathy is one of the natural sciences; Osteopathy is found in nature; Osteopathy is founded on nature; Osteopathy is natural; Osteopathy is NATURE. How plain, how simple, how concise! Can you conceive of a simpler way to present this wondrous modern science? A science that has stood the abuse of a failing profession; a science that has been butchered by its recruits; a science that has stood alone in the realm of wonders and put at defiance its harmless slanderers; a science that has had aimed at it a thousand poison ous arrows, all of which have falldn harmless and broken at its feet. Osteopathy stands to-day the marvel of the most progressive age known in the history of the world. It asks no favors; it shrinks from no responsibilities; but it does ask from the incredulous, investigation. It appeals to the intelligent, thoughtful people to court its virtues, to seek its truths, to expose its fallacies, if they can be found, and testify to its deeds of valor nobly done. Osteopathy has taken no backward step and don't intend to. Side by side with the most modern sciences it will be found marching to the wild, grand music of progress, while on its pathway, just in front, will be falling the golden dawning of grander days to come. Out of the darkness it has cut its shining way that's not to be obscured by fraud or fiend. Onward and upward will be its cry till mankind will do homage to its priceless truths and bow in humble submission to facts and figures that cannot lie, to deathless deeds that breathe the breath of human life. A. T. STILL.

KIRKSVILLE, MO., Dec. 24, '93.

December, 1894

OSTEOPATHY.

The first annual address to the pupils of Osteopathy, delivered Jan. 1, 1891, in Kirksville, Mo., by Dr. A. T. Still, discoverer of the New Science of Health.

He said:—

"Despise not the day of small things," was said long ages ago. That is just as good to-day as then. You can be counted on the fingers of one hand. One year ago one thumb was enough, as the writer of this feeble address was all there was of the school and its pupils. Sit still, men, while I tell you some good news! Since you five entered the school of bones, applications have been legion to become pupils of this grand school. Money is offered to establish a Hospital School to treat the sick and teach the philosophy of healing without poisonous drugs, on whose trail at every step you behold death, insanity, idiots, drunkenness, opium eating, morphine habits, chloral eating, whiskey drinking, drug doctors, conjecturers and no conclusions by its advocates. You are now in the pursuit of a study that is as true as mathematics. You can answer yes to all questions as surely as the astronomer can trace the velocity and magnitude of the heavenly bodies, besides you have a truth to argue from and a fact as its voucher. Thus your answer is absolutely yes and no. At at early day you will have to fill the chairs of professors of the greatest institution that ever had a place on earth. Its name is and will be Osteopathy. Now let me say to you in solemn truth, that no gray haired nor youthful physician has ever answered the question, What is the cause and cure of asthma? You can, and prove what you say by your work. Can the M. Ds. do as much? No! not to the present age. The same of goiter, heart, lung and all other diseases except contagions and infections. Have you not cause to be proud of the step you have taken? When you are old and all the world can look over your life and say, "No man, woman or child has been made a drunkard nor addicted to any of the habits of drugs by you," such as morphine eating, pill taking, whisky drinking, or any of the whole list of habits belonging to drugs caused by your school. Can any one of the one hundred and fifty thousand M. Ds. of America say as much? No, but they can safely say, "We have made two each for every year, which makes three hundred thousand sots we, the M. Ds. of America, have made, and seven out of every ten of us are addicted to some drug habit." The big medicine men of America ask legal protection. They ask the legislatures to prohibit and punish by fine and imprisonment any and all treatments of diseases but the Old Bangwell system of pukes, purges, blisters, skin syringes, poor man's plasters, and so on until the money is gone, then advise the mountains or Florida, where buzzards are plenty. You may be laughed at, but the last laugh will be sweetest, which will be yours. Should I live twelve months look for more of the same kind.

December, 1894

ANNUAL TALK

To the Students and Diplomates of Osteopathy
By A. T. Still, Dec. 25, 1894.

Ladies and Gentlemen of the Faculty, Students and Operators:—

Twelve months have passed, twelve golden links have been forged in the chain of Time since last we gathered for a Christmas talk. And when twelve times the moon has waxed and waned again, if the "silver cord of life" be not loosed, I hope to truthfully report even greater progress than to-day.

My heart has been made to rejoice at the success of the rule requiring the students to attain a grade of 90 on the scale of 100 in Anatomy. The past twelve months have fully shown the importance of thoroughness in this science.

This regulation will, with impartial hand, reward the patient toiler and drive the sluggard from the clinics of Osteopathy. Under our new laws each candidate for admission into our ranks must wear the helmet of intelligence and the breast-plate of honor; must bear the shield of morality and be armed with the spear of industry. This science reveals not its treasures lightly and exhibits the full depth of its wealth only to those, who by constant research delve in its mines and gather rare jewels with which to decorate their mental fabric. It is Truth, its laws eminate from the great central heart of the universe and govern man with the divine simplicity that reigns throughout all nature. It has demonstrated to the scrutinizing philosopher that the eternal artisan is fully competent to plan, construct and run the machinery of life, from the Alpha of the cradle to the Omega of the grave, far better without than with the use of drugs—those deadly destroyers of life which have been used ignorantly, but popularly, for ages.

The tree of Osteopathy is of sturdy dimensions and must be protected from parasitic growths, the most prolific of which are members of the medical fraternity who have naught to recommend them to the shelter of its branches save an empty purse and a brain teeming with antiquated ideas: men whose successes have been successful failures—the result of their cut and try methods.

We are democratic in view and do not wish to enter into reciprocity with any of these fossils of science.

You, who as yet have but a slight acquaintance with Osteopathy, know that it has found an abiding place in all earnest, enquiring minds, and though but infants yourselves in the science, you have seen the giant of ignorance felled by the shaft of your intelligence as Goliath went down before the pebbles of David.

Progress is our watch word; rapid have been our strides toward the goal of perfection in the past year.

The Osteopath of to-day—providing he has spent the passing hours in filling his brain instead of his purse—stands as far in advance of the position he occupied twelve months ago, as the white glory of an incandescent light is in advance of the feeble rays emitted by a tallow candle.

Ever remember that the Osteopath is an engineer with his hand upon the lever of nature's unerring law; and if his brain be not "deformed in its utter bareness" and his hand devoid of skill, he will guide his locomotive engine—man—from the dismal swamp of discouragement and disease along the line of improvement to the station of health.

In the mighty warfare that is being waged between health and disease, stand true to your colors; use the tactics of a wise general, marshall your forces with discretion; let your onslaught be fearless and if your brain has not lost its clearness and your hand its cunning, victory will perch upon the banner of health and disease be vanquished.

A year ago our facilities were few, our patients many. To-day—erected at a great cost and under the supervision of a fine architect—there stands, almost ready for use, a building which we trust will meet at least the present requirements. Above it the American eagle—emblem of freedom—rears its head. Its massive oaken doors open wide to you in welcome; its operating rooms invite you to enter and lay aside your pain; its lavatories, where the cool water plashes in marble basins, ask you to be refreshed; its waiting-rooms offer a place for social converse; in its class-room you will be furnished with weapons for the coming conflict, weapons more powerful than sword or battle-axe, ideas 'leaping from awakened intellect—keen-edged and brighter than the sunbeam," burning with indestructible life. These must be your weapons with which to meet the world.

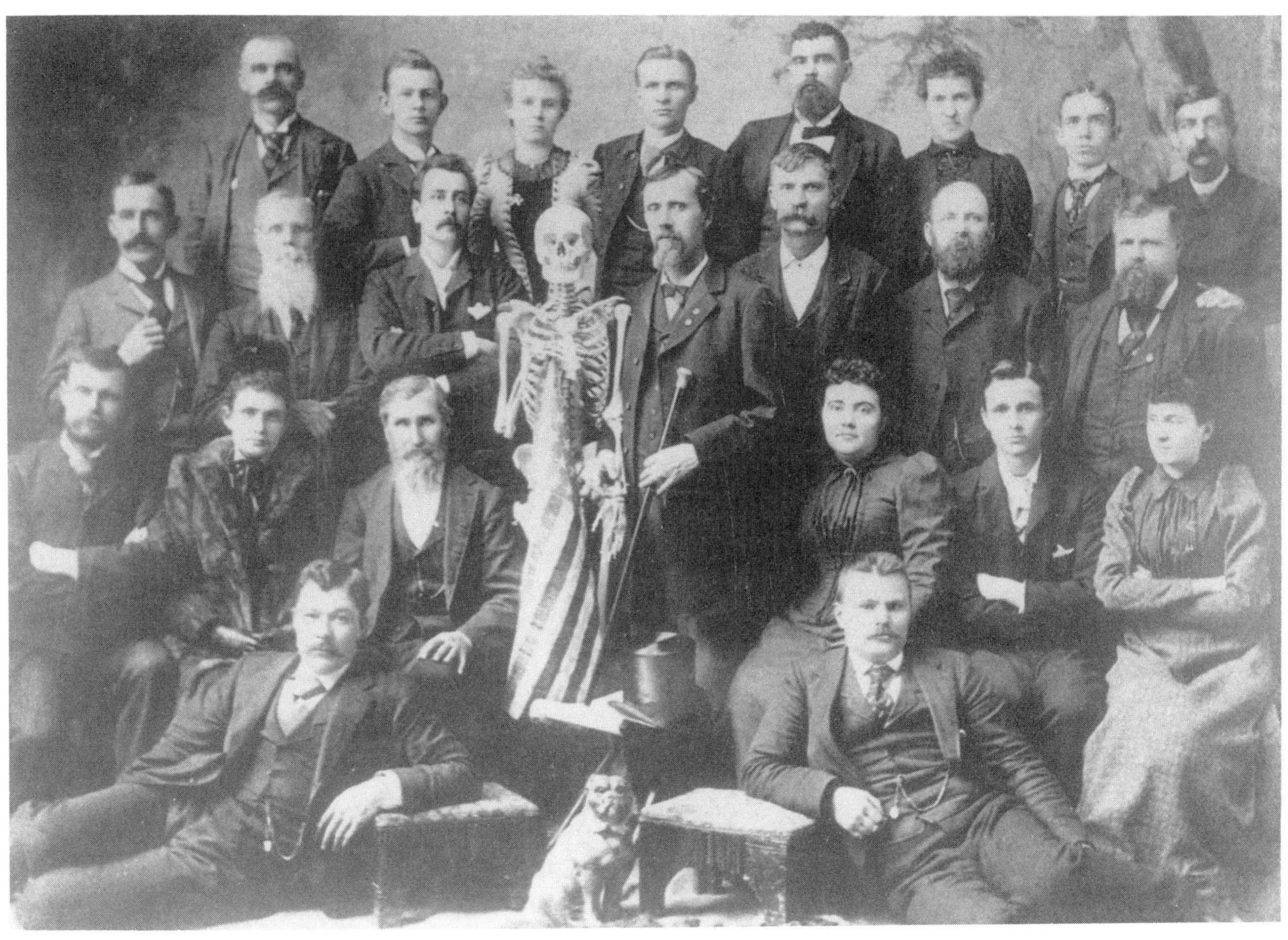

The First Class, Winter 1892

Twenty years ago the craft of Osteopathy was launched upon the stream of Time.

At first its progress was slow, its way shrouded by the gray mists of tradition. But so true was the workmanship in every respect, so strongly and staunchly was the vessel built in every part that it has steered clear of the strands and rocky reefs that have threatened, has successfully combatted with the tempests of ignorance and superstition, and "will sail majestically on and on until the ripples before its prow break on the shores of eternity."

December, 1894

Dr. Still Gives the Students of Osteopathy a Practical Talk.

"As we have just lost one of our mosr learned professors of our Normal by the deadly disease, erysipelas, which is only one of many thousands who fall by it annually, so you set out with the truth that it has met no opposition by drugs from any school of medicine by either large or small doses. But Osteopathy says, Stop, and it obeys. Now allow me to say, it can be cured by you. For example, you take facial erysipelas, it generally begins by sores or wounds in the nose or on the face near facial, superior and labial veins. Now let me tell you those veins become irritated to contraction and refuse to receive and pass arterial blood from the face until the capillary arteries give way and spill the blood in the soft parts, which soon forms matter which is poisonous,and is taken up by the absorbents and continues to compress and poison until death of the whole system is the result. You need not fear defeat if you attack three general ligations: the nerves, veins and arteries. Use your reason and deal with a man as a machine. You are now in the place to put on the life preservers and not the life destroyers, which means no drugs, poultices or local applications. Your philosophy is abundantly able to save life. Carefully guard first the nerves, second the arteries, and lastly open the veins which you know full well how to do. Yours is a philosophy, no guess work, when combating diseases, as you have been carefully trained in all the machinery of life. I trust you will never compromise your dignity by giving drugs any countenance when you are dealing with diseases. I will soon take up pneumonia as my next.

Our philosophy gives you a feast while the philosophy of drugs gives you the nightmare of superstition.

December, 1894

Twelve months ago to-night, all the professors and students of Osteopathy congregated at my house. Had a good time and adjourned with a resolve to push the unfolding of the new and grandest science that was ever given man to solve, and at this place and date report the progress made. As we cannot all meet, it must suffice to report by letter. The faithful student of Osteopathy indeed must see and feel truly proud of the position he occupies to-day compared with that occupied by him a year ago. As I am a Methodist and did speak in class a year ago, I will now speak again.

I have never, during the twelve months just past, allowed a deed, drug or act of any man, woman, child, beast, bird or reptile to move my mind for a single day or hour from the study of the Divine law of life as found in man. I feel that the year has passed me to a much higher knowledge of Osteopathy: of this I am proud. I have been able during the twelve months just past, to avoid the greater part of the exhausting labor, and secure more positive results.

To solve all diseases and cure all the curable, an operator has to know the meaning of the word Asphyxia. True diagnosis and prognosis can be given only by those who understand the law of Asphyxia. This belongs to the new method of solving the mystery of disease and death of a part or the whole of the body. My operators have a full knowledge of this law. They do no guess work. They know the end from the beginning. I do very little of their work over, for they do not "cut and try," as their work is absolute in all cases. The American School of Osteopathy has a corps of Diplomates and students who would be ashamed to place "M. D." after their names instead of "D. O."

Osteopaths are born of women, and not of Colleges. I have found that native ability is the first and all important requirement of the law of God in the forming of Philosophers. Osteopathy can neither be presented nor defended by ignorance. You may sow wheat, but the ground giveth the yield. I find this is true: poor ground, poor wheat. My plow will be set deeper and deeper as the years roll round. Diplomas from this School will live to the glory and honor of all who have had the intellect to grasp this science.

The Osteopath will find much annoyance and may meet with some hardships, in applying the principles of this science to the relief of the afflicted; but this springs from one source only,— Medical men and Schools. Their opposition arises from the fact that Osteopathy can and does cure many diseases by them pronounced incurable. These cures coming before an intelligent people, then the afflicted go en masse to the Osteopath and are cured by him. Then follows the effort to have the healer removed from that place; not for mal practice, but for curing, and demonstrating that Osteopathy is a truth, and drugging is not the law of healing, but the law of killing, and making opium and whiskey sots.

I have had twenty years experience in Osteopathy and have proved, to my own satisfaction, that there is no such thing as failure in treating any disease by this method, when taken in anything like reasonable time, and the subject is not eaten up by drugs, or to enfeebled by age or wasted vitality. Success is the motto of the person who has mastered this science· he does not know what it is to fail. I have found that I must either book a cure for all cases, or book for myself ignorance and stupidity in failing to apply the science at the right places and times, as the law of Osteopathy indicates.

A. T. STILL.

December, 1894

The word Osteopathy means, and is a name given to my discovery, which is a fact, able to prove to any well balanced mind that there is but one true, self-evident law, or way to treat diseases successfully.

It proves that man, or any other animal, is but a machine run by positive laws of animal life. No well informed anatomist, can think otherwise for a moment. We find a machine with all the parts, qualities, and requirements that perfection means, A complete system of nerves from the brain to all parts. A complete system of arteries, plowing from center to surface, feeding all parts with blood in quality, kind and quantity, just enough, no more, no less, to fill the divine law of animal life.

I have no time nor patience to spend in bragging about my wonderful cures; am not asking you to come to me to be healed, nor to have you hound on the street.

I write this for one purpose only. It is this. I invite you to come to headquarters to learn all you wish to know. I have no traveling agents to hunt the afflicted, promise everything and do nothing. Therefore, if you are tired of drugs, medicated baths, Christian Science, Magnetic Healers, or any other system of "cut and try," come and see me, my sons or my operators, judge and be governed accordingly.

This is not written for fools to read, as they cannot reason, but for unprejudiced, progressive minds that have the power and will to reason. We believe Osteopathy will cause you to think, and fill your heart with hope and joy.

I found in my experiments, that bone was not only the frame work of motion, but the protection of the machinery of animal life. Also, that life was a law of itself, over which drugs have no control, or very little, at best. I found that drugging was the cause of much disease, such as fibroid tumors, paralysis, and many others, with the fact of habits fastened upon you. Instance, opium, alcohol and chlorali which is called "Professional."

The question is asked often, "How does Osteopathy compare with Alopathy? Osteopathy cures, Alopathy kills, teaches you

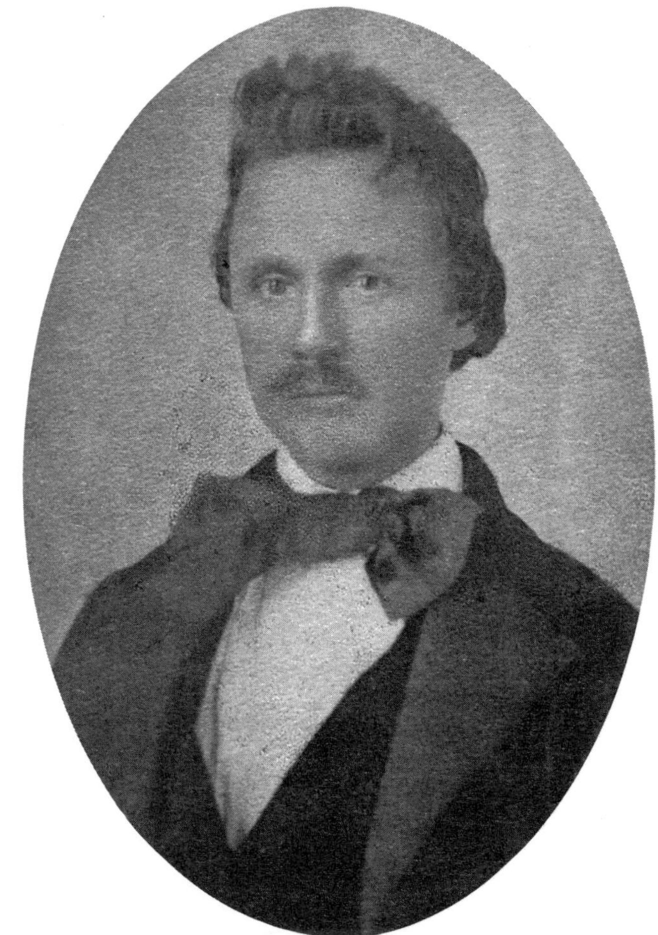

A. T. Still, Age 30

to drink whiskey, eat opium, ruins your whole manhood until you are a total wreck, and makes you ashamed to be in society until you get another dose of morphine; then you are the most pitiable fool, and the biggest liar in the country. All persons know morphine; eaters are liars while using it. Osteopathy cures fevers and all diseases of any climate and sends you home to make a living for yourself and those dependent upon you. That is how a truthful comparison stands. Vote as you see. Osteopathy is a blessing to our race. Alopathy is a curse. Eclecticism is a whopper for "pepper sas" and Tr. Rei. Homeopathy is like the wing of a mosquito, not much music but a strong bill.

A. T. Still, D. O.

December, 1894

ORATION AND PRAYER.

Delivered July 4, 1891, By Dr. A. T. Still.

Our oration is honorable and right, our subject is life and death, slavery and freedom. Our people said over one hundred years ago: All men are free and equall by nature. There was much opposition but we are free. We respect all nations, fear none, extend freedom to all; our laws make no lords nor surfs. Our people move in the front line of all progress. Our society is good or bad, you are free to choose ignorant or wise, sober or sots, philosophers or fools. Osteopathy with science and reason, other pathologies with drink, drugs and their seasonings. Our schools are deep or shallow, our theology is wet or dry, hot or cold, formal or fussy, spiritual or material, conditional or decreed. Our sick use medicine or let it alone according to their knowledge of man's superstructure. One finds diseases come from the liver, the other from the deranged stomach, then the big wise ones say it is microbes; but Osteopathy does not care how disease comes, but how to make it leave and let the suffering human go free, and says, come unto me all ye ends of the earth and I will give you rest.

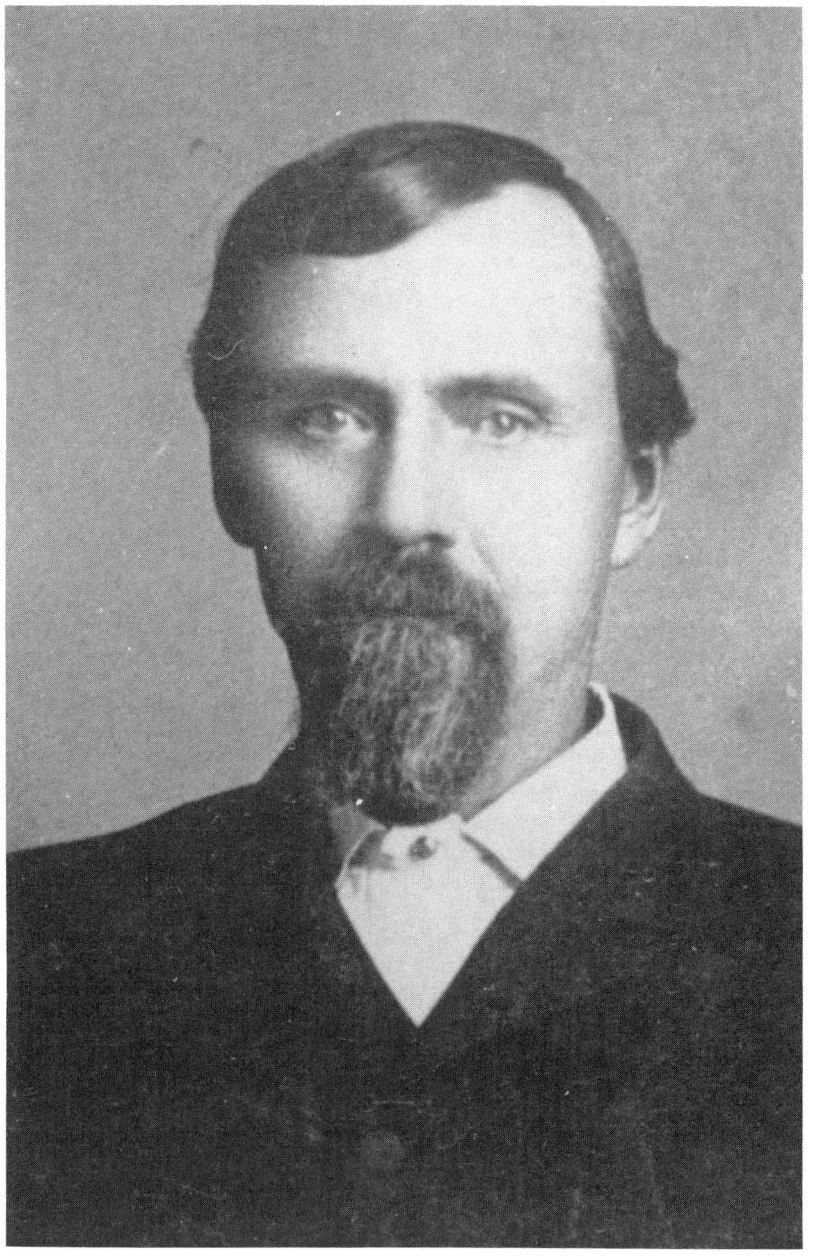

A. T. Still, c. 1890

And the choir sang,

"De year ob jubilee am coming, which was followed by prayer, then the dismissal.

THE PRAYER.

Our Father, who art in Heaven and in Earth and in all things but whiskey and such things as men have no business with, thou hast been asked to take the place of father, by us; give us our daily bread and no whiskey; give us reason and keep snakes out of our boots. Give us good knowledge of our true bodily forms and tell us how to know when a bone has strayed from its true position and how to return them to their natural places. Also lead us not into temptation to get drunk when our limbs are on a strain and make a few pains, but teach us how to cure or stop fevers, mumps, measles, flux and all diseases of the seasons as they roll round. Thou knowest our people do foolish things when they are sick. O, Lord, throw a few lightning bugs of reason on our M. Ds. Thou knowest their eyes can't all open at once like a litter of pups, but light them out one at a time, and if thou failest, open the minds of the people, so they will not be subjects of experiments any longer. And deliver us from all drugs, for thou seest just in front of us a world of maniacs, idiots, criminals, nakedness for the babies and hunger for the mothers. For thine is the kingdom from now on. Amen.

NOTICE

To Applicants for Treatment.

All applicants for treatment, at A. T. Still's Infirmary, are requested to not board at places not friendly disposed to the advancement of our science. If you do not feel able to pay $1 per day for hotel fare, please ask my Secretary, who will direct you to good private places, at from $3 to $5 per week. I do not think patients improve as well in some boarding houses as in others. I do not wish to take patients or their money, simply for the profit there is in it to me.

A. T. STILL.

January, 1895

On Monday morning, January 14th, the students of Osteopathy met in the lecture room of the A. T. Still Infirmary and Dr. Still addressed them in the following characteristic manner:—

Good morning. I'm from Virginia and shall introduce myself by saying —How are you? I am not very well myself but in spite of that little drawback will talk to you for a short time. As I said, I'm from Virginia but I came west at an early day and am practically a Western man.

My father was a minister—in one sense a missionary, and I've said prayers ½ mile long (as long as the longest chapter in the Bible)—said those prayers as I walked between the plow handles that a lapse of memory in that direction might not result in a strapping from my father. Those were the days of small things —my father's salary the first year was the munificent one of $6.00. Think of it ye Beecher's and Spurgeon's and Talmage's with your costly tabernacles and your salaries rising high in the thousands.

Our schools were of a rude western nature, and one paper to a family was a big thing. While I was at school in Tennessee, the editor, of the Holstein Journal—a paper in which my father was interested—came to our house one evening bearing every appearance of a man physically tired out and exclaimed "well after laboring all day I have succeeded in getting out 160 papers.

To-day such is the rapidity with which our giant printing presses work that with ease 680,000 copies are struck off in 12 hours. But so accustomed are we to the magnitude of the results obtained in this day that we fail to appreciate the greatness of our age.

Nothing looks large to us now. In the past a spoonful of castor oil assumed enormous proportions, to-day it does not for it is seldom seen and is in use only among the stupid.

But I will not assail the M. D's, some of them have come and placed themselves among us and when a man sweats in agony over a lost cause (even fears being kicked out of the lunatic asylum) it would be ungenerous to dwell on his defeat.

* * * * * *

Between you and me as far as the lunatic asylum is concerned I would as soon go to a sausage mill as to enter one.

Homeopathy has reduced the dose in drugs and in the same ratio has Allopathy found it possible to get along with less of those deadly articles. Every step that drops even 1 grain of drugs develops mind that sees more deity and less drugs.

It has been said to me—"If you should die even now your children would have much to be proud of." But I say if I die now put on an extra shovel of dirt for the things I have failed to accomplish, but if I die in 18 months from now cast off the added amount for the new discoveries I hope to make in this Science by that time.

This is an informal school taught at my request for your benefit. If you make one subject thoroughly it will take all your brains. This subject is, man. Know yourself, if you do it in 5 years you will do better than I did in 35. Years ago I dug one skeleton after another out of the sand heaps of the Indian burial grounds and studied them until I was familiar with the use and structure of every bone in the human system. From this I went on to the study of muscles, ligaments, tissues, arteries, etc. It has been my lifework and yet there are things for me to learn. You are admitted to the school now as an accommodation because you did not know that this building would fail to be ready for occupancy at the promised time. You see one lie always calls for more to cover it up.

Do not think that your payment of $500.00 will make me happy. Such is not the case, I would far rather have a much needed rest than all your money, but since you are here I will teach you all I can. You will enter upon new fields of learning but do not think for a moment that after 2 or 3 months of class work you will be shoved into the operating rooms. That is a procedure in which I have been bitten. Before entering the operating rooms you must make a grade of 90, on a scale of 100 in Anatomy; To admit you there sooner would be to connive at your ruin, to make you marvelous, to send you out in the world to make money, to make you think that Solomon's head would be too small to fill your hat.

Motion begins in the human foetus at about 4½ months after conception. Activity of the Osteopath begins at about the same date.

After 1 year in school you will arrive at the stage where without proper guidance you are likely to take a hammer to a looking glass. At the end of 18 months provided you have gone out into the world you reach the point where you are anxious to see Pap.

In two years you just learn that steam blows up but do not yet know how to control it.

It is a privilege for you to begin now and not my desire, take heed that you improve your present opportunity, for gaining the bread of Osteopathic knowledge from headquarters. You may be called on to dispense it in Europe, Asia and other distant points of the globe. See to it that your supply is of the right kind. An Osteopath asks no favors of drugs—if you go out to your patient accompanied by a physician and allow him to suggest various medicines as remedies then you have disgraced your diploma.

Either God is God or He is not. Osteopathy is God's law and whoever can improve on God's law is superior to God himself. Osteopathy opens your eyes to see and see truly; it covers all fields of diseases and is the law that keeps life in motion.

As an electrician controls the electric currents, so an Osteopath controls the life currents, and revives natural forces.

To turn on the blaze of an incandescent light, would you make a hypodermic injection into the wire, would you give a dose of belladonna or apply cocaine? A thousand times no, yet such a proceedure would be no more ridiculous than pouring those things into man, who is but a machine. Take the course of wisdom, study to understand bones, muscles, ligaments, nerves, blood supply, and everything pertaining to this human engine, and if your work be well done, you will have it under perfect control. You will find when diptheria is raging and its victims dying, at the rate of 114 per day, as was the case in Red Wing where my son is located, that by playing along the lines of sensation, motion, and nutrition—if you do not play ignorantly—you will win the reward due your intelligence, and lose not a single case. You will also meet that terror to the ordinary physician—Brights disease, let me make an illustration along that line, by comparing the progressions in kidneys disease, to the different stages of milk. Place milk in a pan, it is simply milk and represents the kidneys in natural working order; leave the milk a little longer, until it is old, then it corresponds to diabetes, leave it until it rots, and you have Bright's disease.

Even here you will not experience defeat, for with your accurate knowledge of the human machinery, you will not only know, but meet all its requirements; and so it will be all along the line of surgery, obstetrics, and general diseases. If success does not attend your efforts, it is not the fault of this science; whose every working is exact, but of yourself.

You who make this your life work will go out into the world as representatives of the only exact method of healing. You will be recognized as graduates of a legally incorporated school, and will never know the ridicule, the obloquy, the contempt that were heaped upon me when I first tried to make known this beautiful truth.

No preacher will pray for you, as one possessed of a devil, no innocent child will fly from your presence in fear of one spoken of as a lunatic. No, your fate will not be my fate, for my untiring efforts placed this science, and its exponents upon a footing to command the respect and admiration of the world.

TO PATIENTS AND VISITORS.

Upon presenting yourself at our office for examination and treatment, first secure a number from the file of cards which are put up in a conspicuous place in the waiting room. You will receive attention in the order in which the numbers are held. At the time of examination you will be requested to give a short history of your case, how long standing and what treatment you have had. You will soon find the Osteopaths use no drugs. They will look you over as an engineer would look over his engine, to see if it is in running order. If found out of fix, they adjust the machine and start it to running.

If a wheel, pulley, belt or any part is wrong, he goes to work adjusting, till all is corrected. An engineer who is ignorant, who does not know the use of all the parts of his machine is not a safe person to take charge of the lives behind his engine. Laws are enacted and exacted of him that he may be competent to fulfill the trust reposed in him, and that your lives may be safe when in his care. My students are required to pass a grade of 90 per cent in Anatomy before they are admitted to the operating rooms to take instructions in adjusting the human body for disease. This is no place for empty brag and foolish promises. You will find my operators are all well qualified engineers who know their business. We are not Gods, nor Christian Scientists, or Faith Doctors, nor Spirit Doctors, but simply Anatomical Engineers—we understand the human engine and can put it in running order,

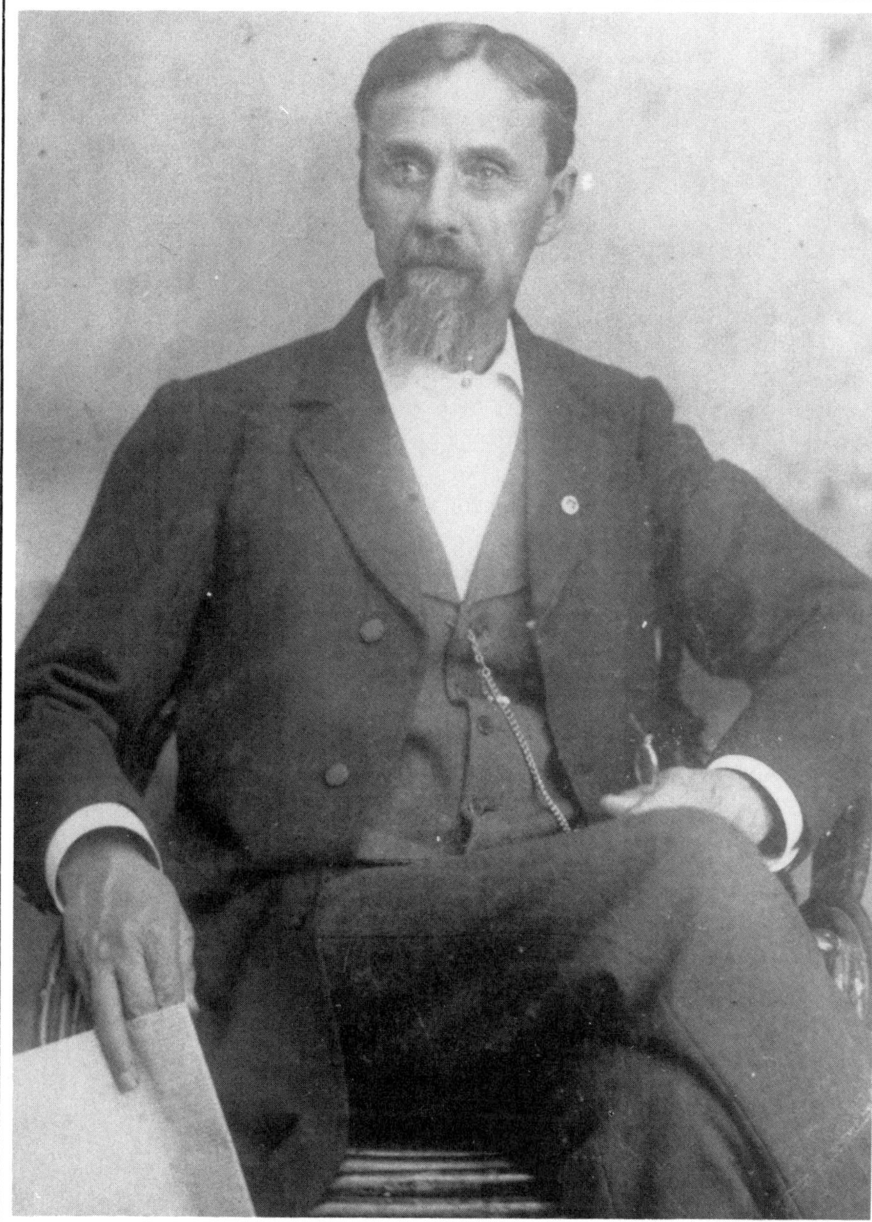

A. T. Still, c. 1894

subject always to the laws of Nature.

If you come to us for treatment you come of your own free will, and not through any trick or scheme of mine or any of my helpers. Remember that when many of you come to me, you are not the most choice kind of patients. Remember the company you have kept before coming here. You have been with Doctors who blister you, puke you, physic your toe nails loose, fill your sides and limbs with truck from hyperdermic syringes. You come to me with eyes big from belladonna, backs and limbs stiff from plaster paris casts– you come with bodies suffering with all the diseases that flesh is heir to. Remember you have been treated and dismissed as incurable by all kinds of doctors before you come to us, and if we help you at all—we do more than all the others have done. And yet all the various forms of affliction that have been treated here—75 per cent have been greatly benefitted and 50 per cent are sent home well.

I am not telling this to solicit your patronage. I claim this as the only place where man is looked upon and treated as an engine. Search the annals of history for the truth of what I say. There is no time to brag; let results speak.

My motto is "Help the needy, and deal justly with all." I am not going to "get rich or bust.", I have made but one rule in life, "reason first, justice and humanity all the time." All persons claiming to be from my school, who can not show their papers as a student or diploma in Osteopathy are imposters and are obtaining money under false pretenses.

Dr. A. T. Still, Pres.
H. E. Patterson, Sec'y.

January, 1895

RECOLLECTIONS OF BALDWIN, KANSAS.

The following lecture was delivered to the class in Anatomy by Dr. A. T. Still on Wednesday morning Jan. 23rd, in Memorial hall of the A. T. Still Infirmary.

Ladies and Gentlemen:—

Tthe faces that greet me this morning, with the exception of those belonging to members of the class, are strange ones. I have no time to make use of adjectives but will speak briefly.

Twenty-one years ago I delivered the first lecture on Osteopathy to a large and attentive audience—more attentive, perhaps, than even this one. My lecture room on that occasion was in the basement story of the Baker University at Baldwin, Kansas. It was full of cobwebs, broken glass, old boots and the accumulated dirt of years. My audience was a man by the name of John Wesley Reynolds, a man who wore a slouch hat and was of uncouth appearance. We shut the doors, pulled off our hats and the talk begun during which I said to my audience of 1 that I was firmly convinced of the fact that either the existing system of medicine was a system of falsehoods or else God had made a failure. If medicine was the best remedial agency He could devise for the relief of humanity then I felt that I could improve on it. At that time it was no more popular to talk against medicine than against religion.

To give you a fair idea of priestcraft in Baldwin in that day let me tell you that from the pulpit of a church which my money had helped to build, a minister denounced me as an apostate of the first water—declaring that I must either change my tactics or land in hell. So strong, in fact, was his denunciation that on the following Tuesday as I passed down the street more than 200 children fled from my path as though I were an unclean leper, a huge serpent or a wild boar from Russia. I had the whole road to myself. All this because I dared to talk upon the streets of a coming philosophy that was to revolutionize the old order of things, to free man from the slavery of drugs and restore to him his inalienable right to heal.

I welcome you here to-day to see the wonderful progress this science has made, to show you something of the fruition of my life work. Osteopathy has fought and fought hard for every step gained, its path has not been strewn with flowers but lined with the stones of opposition.

But you will ever find that before wearing a crown you must expend much effort. Your crown of Intelligence will cost you great labor. Every muscle in your body aids in the winning of this coronet. When you first enter upon life the muscles move before the mind reasons. What is the first thought on looking at a new born babe sucking? That it is a wonderful machine which puts itself in motion for self preservation, by using the facial, gustatory, nutritive and other muscles.

Then, too, it inflates its lungs and yells, making use of other organs, and let me tell you the louder it yells the better stock it is. If it does not squall at a tender age it is sure to be stupid in after years. I would rather my children would pull hair until they were bald headed and strike blows to bring blood from their noses than to be lifeless, inert, putty children.

The craft of Osteopathy has been launched upon the sea of time and like the ironclads that sweep the bosom of earth's oceans it has proved its seaworthiness and commands the respect of other vessels. It has been thoroughly tried in every quarter and not found wanting, its engineers compel the respect of woodcraft which has done its duty and was considered good in times past.

Dungleson tells you that Osteopathy is, bone disease. I tell you that it means all that the M. D's have tried to mean by the word "Remedy" for 400 years. It succeeds where they fail, because it is bound to the motor laws of Deity. Osteopathy is an unerring law but it is not a new law for all law is eternal. You rode into the world on the law of life and you will ride out of it on the law of death and no man knoweth which of these laws is the stronger. How long does an apple exist as a green apple? It passes in swift successive stages from a beautiful blossum to ripe perfection. We would not love God if he left all our apples green, as the apples of ignorance are. Now the apple of intelligence has red streaks upon its sides, showing great advancement towards maturity. Green apples give you stomach ache, so does gamboge and aloes. Ripe apple takes hold of the proper nerves and muscles and removes the aches and ills.

No wonder there has been a great deal said about Eve's apples. Poor woman, I suppose they were the best she had. There is one apple with a red streak on it up in Minnesota; it does not cut off the tonsils in case of so called diphtheria but deals intelligently with the nerves that carry blood to and from the affected parts and destroys the disease. Is it really diphtheria: green apple says, yes—red apple says, no. After a thorough examination of the best known authorties it is decided that red apple is right. This red striped apple, this intelligent Osteopath says, as all Osteopaths do, that diptheria is only sore throat allowed to rot. In the first stage of rot it is like blinky milk, in the second stage it is like clabbered milk, in the 3rd stage it is like milk that is utterly disorganized and under the old method of treatment this 3rd stage of rot results usually in death. But the Osteopath with his thorough knowledge of the laws that govern life loses not a case. You may possibly think rot a strange name for a disease but I want to tell you these truths in words you will not forget. If you want to talk unintelligibly you may as well begin by saying *acene po qua que ta la ma monce*, etc. But if you do so, any one who takes the trouble to open your clamshell with the tongs of reason will find only a fool inside.

At the season of the year when vegetation decays Scarlet fever stalks abroad, it begins with cold and in fair, red haired children is followed by rash and sore throat —as a general thing it touches the little one with dark locks very lightly.

The medical world cannot define fever further than to say it is a peculiar increase above the normal temperature, The Osteopath says it is an increased flow of electricity and in scarlet, and other forms of fever, by the application of scientific law instead of the use of drugs, overcomes the foe with man as with an electric light, the supply force must equal or be greater than the demand or the light will be feeble and the man will be frail. If you have a No. 4 incandescent light fed by a No. 3 battery 1 per cent of the force is wasted on the approaching wires and the light is dim. If you have a No. 4 trouble and a No. 3 battery with which to meet it you will make a failure—in both cases, strengthen the battery and the result will be satisfactory.

Dividing the body at the umbilicus the upper part may be considered an acid, the lower as alkali in property. When an increase or improper distribution of acid causes sore throat, throw up alkali from below and neutralize it and the sore throat will disappear.

Some of you thought you were coming here to a faith doctor. Some of you thought me a Christian Scientist—but if you were a cow and kicked me, you would find the Christian element wanting; neither am I a masseuse, for massage is a combination of ignorance and force.

Some thought to find me with a sort of conjuring machine in my sleeve out of which I squirted a healing fluid. I am often asked by intelligent people—Do you hypnotize? I answer "yes, set 13 hips in one day." Still they are incredulous, wink their eyes, get me off in one corner and implore me in a whisper to really tell them the truth about the matter. Osteopathy is no magical secret, it is a principle old as time, true as Deity, lasting as eternity. This principle runs through the entire universe—in the sky we have constellations of worlds, in the body, constellations of molecules. In the sky we have rain clouds, in the body lying alongside the veins are the lymphatics which prepare water and pass it into the veins thinning the crop of blood. This analogy may be carried out indefinitely.

Once again I will speak to you of fibroid tumors, a repetition of these things is necessary in order to firmly impress them on your memory. Now-a-days a woman cannot be fashionable unless she possesses a fibroid tumor. I tell you that more of these excrescences have been removed in one day in Minnesota than during the years intervening between the presidency of Washington and Jackson. Every effect has its corresponding cause and it behooves you to search for it.

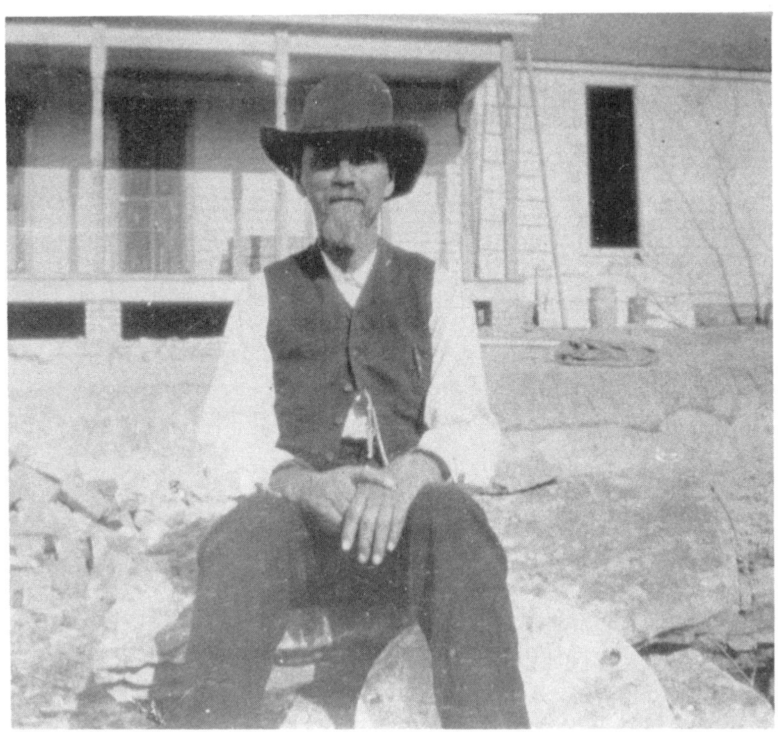

A. T. Still, c. 1894

I remember a Dutch woman came to our house once to sell me some limberger cheese. My first impression was that my feet had gone into the third stage of rot and I wanted to excuse myself before the woman found it out. But when she explained her business I found the odor caused by the cheese.

Now if you hunt for the cause of the alarming increase in fibroid tumors you will find that it lies in quinine, tincture of iron, and belladonna. Here is the place for you to gain a knowledge of this science which will enable you to go out into the world and vanquish all such diseases.

But you must not be like a politician who when called on unexpectedly for a speech, made a failure because he had left his little note-book at home. Carry your little book in your head and be ready to meet any emergency.

You are learning now to harness the horse that pulls the load of life. See to it that your lesson is well learned and no ends left loose.

To-day Osteopathy takes possession of its new building, puts on its own hat, all paid for.

This house is mine. I make it yours on each Wednesday morning and gladly welcome you to its rooms.

February, 1895

OSTEOPATHY DEFINED BY A. T. STILL.

It matters little at what point I commence my talk to you, for the subject of life has no beginning and is equally interesting at all points. I see this morning many strangers, strangers who have come to headquarters to learn something of this science which bears a new and unfamiliar name. You wish to know if its discoverer is possessed of intelligence and if the science itself has merit.

You wonder what Osteopathy is; you look in the medical dictionary and find as its definition, bone disease.

That is a grave mistake. It is compounded of the two words, Osteon, meaning bone, Pathos—Pathine, to suffer. Greek lexicographers say it is a proper name for a science founded on a knowledge of bones. So instead of bone disease it really means bone usage.

The human body is a machine run by the unseen force called life, and that it may be run harmoniously it is necessary that there be liberty of blood, nerves and arteries from generating point to destination.

Suppose in far distant California there is a colony of people dependent upon your coming in person with a load of produce to keep them from starvation. You load your car with everything necessary to sustain life and start off in the right direction. So far, so good. But in case you are side-tracked somewhere so long that on reaching the desired point your stock of provisions is in no fit state to be consumed, if complete starvation is not the result at least your friends will be but poorly nourished.

So if the supply channels of the body be obstructed, and the life giving currents do not reach their destination full freighted then disease sets in.

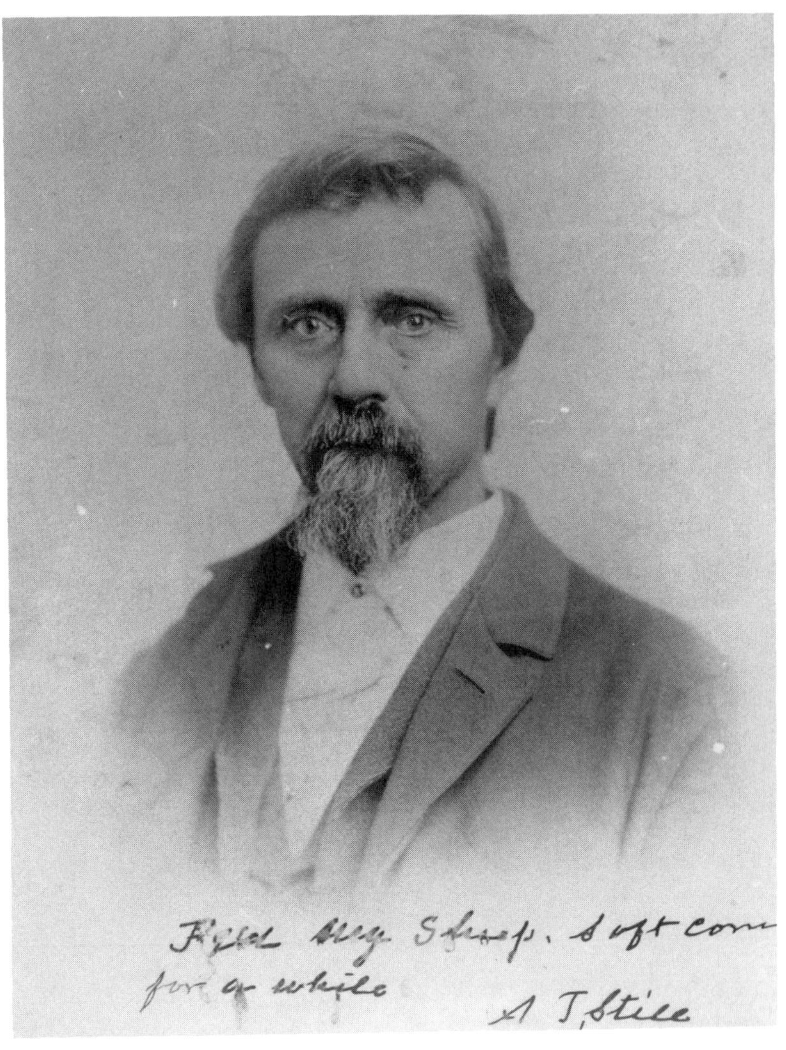

What does an M. D. do in such a case? As a darkey would force a disabled mule to carry him by applying the whip, so a doctor of medicine attempts to use the whips of quinine and other stimulants to drive the blood through the body. By too severe an application of the morphine whip sometimes life is driven into death.

Under like circumstances an Osteopath would remove the obstruction by application of the unerring laws of his science, and ability for doing the necessary work would follow. As a horse needs strength instead of the spur to enable him to carry a heavy load. So a man needs the freedom of all parts of the machinery power that comes from the perfect of his body in order to accomplish the highest work of which he is capable. After the heart receives the blood it sends it on to the brain to take on knowledge.

When you look at a skull you think "What a large cavity; what a quantity of brains I must have!" They say Webster had almost a half bushel. In the center of the brain is the corpus collosium looking like a half moon or a small stomach and here it is that mentality dwells. Of the contents of the skull one ounce is used for thought, the remainder generates power for nerves.

God would not be idiotic enough to send the blood to the brain for wisdom and fail to have a supply there. His intelligence is immeasurable and there is every evidence that mind is imparted to the corpuscles of the blood before it does its work.

Every corpuscle goes like a man in the army with full instructions where to go and with unerring precision it does its work whether it be in the formation of a hair or the throwing of a spot of delicate tinging at certain distances on a peacock's back.

God does not find it necessary to make one of these spots of beauty at a time, he simply endows the corpuscles with mind and in obedience to His law each one of these soldiers of life goes like a man in the army with full instructions as to the duty he is to perform. It travels its beaten line without interfering with the work of others. Now you say I am going to get God into trouble by making a statement claiming that each one of the five million corpuscles contained in a single drop of blood knows just what is expected of it. Is this blasphemy? No. As the troops of Gen. Cook obey his commands unfalteringly so God's infantry imbued by him with mentality go forth to fulfill their appointed mission in unswerving obedience.

You dare not assert that the Deity is inferior in power to a man of His own creation.

While speaking of the army let me say that I served as a surgeon under Fremont and I know what I am talking about when I say that a surgeon's outfit was complete when it contained calomel, quinine, whiskey, opium, rags and a knife. And if a patient had one foot in the grave and a half pint of whiskey in a bottle the doctor would work as hard to get the whiskey out of the bottle as to keep the foot from the grave.

Medical men administer old bourbon innocently for the sake of stimulating the stomach and as a result in the course of time many a man finds himself a drunkard in the ditch. It is the system which is wrong. As a child follows the advise of its mother so the medical student heeds the teachings of his Alma Mater.

From her walls he goes out instructed to give so many drops of a certain liquid to excite the nerves and so many drops of another liquid to quiet them. And so all the way through his path is laid out.

If after diagnosing, prognosing and prescribing the patient goes down, then wine and whiskey are administered to aid in rallying the weakened life forces.

If a council of the same school is called his course is commended. In just this manner the love of strong drink is instilled in many men and I tell you that if our national curse of drunkenness continues for a period of five hundred years God will have to send people in a balloon to repopulate the earth which will have degenerated under the influence of whiskey from a world of beauty to a bald knob.

My father was a progressive farmer and was always ready to lay aside an old plow if he could replace it with one better constructed for its work. All through life I have ever been ready to buy a better plow.

So when I found a way out of the big drunk of ignorance and superstition into which we were born—the belief that God was a poor mechanic and needed the help of medicine—then I was ready to walk in the more enlightened path. I fully realize how tough the old way was when I remember how they used to hold my nose and spank me to get to administer a dose of caster oil. Then they ask God to bless the means used for my recovery and I suppose this petition included both dose and blister.

Osteopathy does not look on man as a criminal before God to be puked purged and made sick and crazy.

It is a science that analyzes man and finds that he partakes of Divine intelligence. It acquaints itself with all his attributes and if the student of it does his work well and goes out with his brain full of its teachings instead of his pocket full of cardamom seed he will find by results that its principle is unerring.

God manifests himself in matter, motion and mind. Study well his manifestations. A. T. STILL.

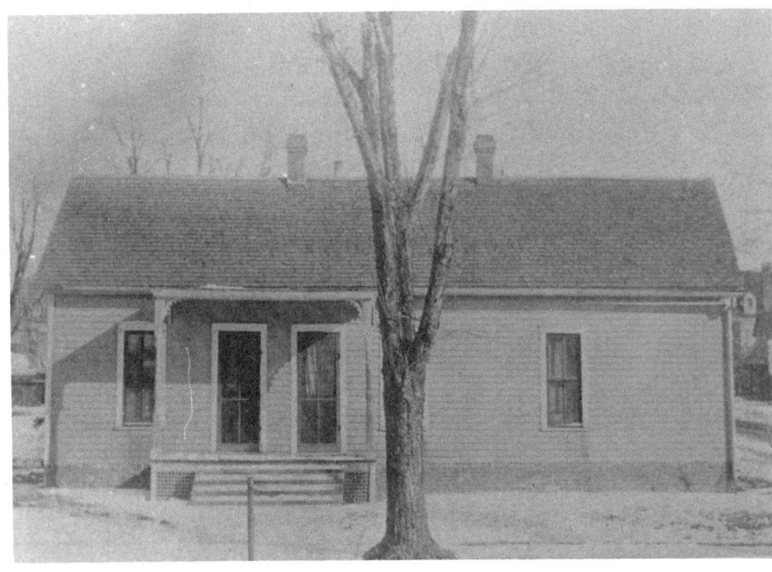

A. T. Still's First Residence
Corner West Jefferson and Main Streets

A HERO.

M. H. S.

Once in long cycling years a giant soul is born
That dwells, in thought, upon the mountain height,
And sees afar the glorious dawn of a new day,
While multitudes below yet walk in night.

Such souls bear deep the impress of the Infinite;
All helmeted with Truth they dauntless stand,
And wage Earth's fiercest battles of the mind and write
True words of guidance with prophetic hand.

Just such a soul of Titan build dwells with us now,
And rears the white flower of a blameless life:
As pure as Galahad, as wise as Merlin, sage;
As brave as Lancelot—his years as rife.

With noble, generous deeds as Arthur's—the good king—
And king he is with loyal objects true,
Crowned with the laurel leaves of Fame and incense of
Sweet praise from grateful hearts for life made new.

All hail to him the eager throngs now cry! thrice hail!
The dumb lips speak, once sightless eyes now see,
The halt and maimed are healed as when in days of old
They followed Truth in far off Galilee.

True benefactor of the world, unto the child
Of thy great brain. Fair Osteopathy,
We bring our incense! Nourished by thy mind
'Twill reach perfection in the days to be.

And tongues from every distant clime will speak its praise,
From sunny Southern vale to towering granite hill,
Its virtues will be sung. And deep, for aye, in loving hearts
Will be enshrined the name of ANDREW STILL.

February, 1895

On Sunday, January 20th, the doors of the A. T. Still Infirmary were thrown open to the colored people of the city, many of whom availed themselves of this opportunity to examine the interesting features of this beautiful new building. When they had gathered in the Memorial Hall Dr. Still gave them a short talk as follows:—I have invited you here because among you there are men who helped to build this house. I wish more had come to stand under the shelter of the roof they helped to make. Doubtless those who are absent had in mind only the dollars to be received for their labor and gave no thought to the mission of the building being erected. This is the great Still house—to instil sobriety instead of drunkenness, to instil principle instead of guess work.

Last Thursday dedicatory exercises were held in this house. It was filled to overflowing and a larger regiment of people returned to their homes unable to gain admittance than I ever met on a battle field.

The room you now occupy is Memorial Hall—as named in honor of my son Fred, whose portrait you see on the wall. He was a bright intelligent boy, a boy known to you all, one who would not wear a ring upon his finger considering the skin which God had placed there is a rarer jewel than money could purchase.

He had hoped to carry the banner of Osteopathy far into the future, but as the result of an accident his health was impaired, and he left us in answer to Nature's summons.

You see these paintings, this flag of our nation—a flag of silken texture and expensive trimmings—these are donations from friends and show the kindly feeling of the people toward us.

Since the days of Magistus the delusion has flourished that man must swallow medicine to rid himself of disease. The people substituted their judgment for God's intelligence and in so doing created drunkards and lunatics.

The great Yankee Inventor of the Universe by the union of mind and matter has constructed the most wonderful of all machines—man—and Osteopathy demonstrates that He is fully capable of running it without the aid of whiskey, opium or kindred poisons.

Since the introduction of quinine 60 years ago fibroid tumors have increased at an alarming rate. This deadly substance enters into the system and causes the formation of an excrescence fed by the blood vessels. When arteries fail to feed it any longer, it begins to exude blood into the abdomen.

What then? The medical world says it must be removed by the surgeon's knife. The result is that 75 per cent of such cases die.

Osteopathy—a drugless science—finds the utero genital nerve made tight by the fastening of certain segments. It proceeds to reverse the order of things, starts the great splanchnic nerve into action, restores vitality and carries away the excrescence.

Take your choice between a system that produces tumors and one that destroys them.

In the days of slavery when you colored people had simple plantation remedies such as horsemint tea in case of sickness you recovered. Death was a rare visitor among your race. Now you play the fool like your white brothers, take strong medicine and die like rats.

Quit your pills and learn from Osteopathy the principle that governs you. Learn that you are a machine, your heart an engine, your lungs a fanning machine and a sieve, your brain with its 2 lobes an electric battery.

When the cerebellum sets this dynamo in motion oxygen is carried through the system and vitalizes the blood, the abdomen, the eye, the entire man. Nature put this battery in you to keep the blood healthy and salts it with oxygen. The corpus collosium is the center of reason.

You do not use more than an ounce of brain for thought, the remainder is used in nourishing the vital forces. Use this ounce of brains to free yourself from the bondage of the old medical laws.

My father was a physician and I followed in his footsteps and was considered very successful in the treatment of cholera, smallpox and like diseases. When that terrible disease meningitis was slaying its victims by the hundreds all schools of medicine united in their efforts to conquer it but without avail. It entered my family and in spite of all medical skill death claimed four victims and our home was desolate.

Then in my grief the thought came to me that instead of asking God to bless the means being used it were far better to search for the right means, knowing if they were once found the results would be sure. * * *

I began to study man and I found no flaw in God's work. The intelligence of Deity is unquestionable, its law unalterable. On this law is the science of Osteopathy founded and after struggling for years under the most adverse circumstances it stands to-day triumphant.

If I were at present called on to give medicine I would be as much afraid of Dovers Powders as a darky is of a skeleton.

If I should give calomel I would do it with my eyes shut and I would want to keep them shut for nine days so uncertain would I be as to results.

If because I denounce drugs you call me a Christian Scientist go home and take half a glass of castor oil to purge yourself of such notions.

If you consider me a mesmerist a big dose of pills may carry the thought away.

I am simply trying to teach you what you are; to get you to realize your right to health and when you see the cures wrought here after all other means have failed you can but know that the foundation of my work is laid on Nature's rock.

What is the nature of the cases that come to us? Do you remember Lazarus? If so you will know that his food was crumbs and well mumbled crumbs at that. Well we are like Lazarus in that respect—we get the leavings of the medical world—their incurable cases.

We get men who have been tanks for the receiving of acid, iron and mercury—mercury which transforms their livers into cinnabar and makes of them rheumatic barometers sensitive to every weather change.

This same mercury in certain forms is a great friend to dentists for when taken into the system it hunts for chalky substances, seizes upon the teeth and oftimes causes the girl of 17 to substitute china store teeth for the pearly incisors bicuspids and molars that nature meant to last a lifetime.

I have a pup at home and when he disobeys my laws I apply a switch to him as a reminder of his short comings. So Nature applies to you the switch of pain when her mandates are disregarded, and when you feel the smarting from this switch do not pour drugs into your stomachs but let a skilfull engineer adjust your human machine so that every part works in accordance with natures requirements.

Think of yourself as an electric battery. Electricity is simply oxygen put in motion—when it plays freely all through your system you are well. Shut it off in one place and congestion may result, in this case an M. D. by dosing you with drugs would increase this congestion until it resulted in decay. He is like the Frenchman who lets his duck rot that it may boil the sooner. Not so does an Osteopath proceed he removes the obstruction, lets the life giving current have free play and the man is restored to health.

The one is man's way and is uncertain, the other is God's method and is infallible. Choose this day whom you will serve:

March, 1895

THE THIGH BONE.

I have something to tell you of a wonderful process of building which, mentally, I have to-day seen going on. Now, do not credit me with too much excitement or weakness of mind, Oh, ye philosophers, astronomers, divines, teachers, and law-makers, but follow me for a few minutes while I draw your minds out to such an extent that you can both see and hear the remarkable work I am to report.

The commander of my store of wisdom has for once called a halt as I view one of the most mysterious and beautiful sights of my life—the working of the Grand Architect and his subordinates on a bone, human in kind, a femer.

Draw your mental microscope, raise it to its greatest power as you read the specifications for this unique building. Now, the order is given by the commanding general to his subordinates, "Attention. officers, infantry and cavalry! Fall into line, you workmen, and proceed to execute with mathematical precision. Every block and every stringer uniting with minute exactness. Let your work be correct, faultless, for the specifications require a construction so careful that though the Infinite Mind became for a time a sub-committeeman to examine your work, it would be found that you have fulfilled the requirements of the specification demanding the building of a thigh bone, perfect in all its material and mental parts.

And ever remember that the word "perfect" means no more, no less than the fiat of the Infinite that His work has been concluded with absolute exactness.

Behold with me the division commanders, each in place, bearing the insignia of his rank; the commander general speaks positively to the ordnance department, "Fill and keep the magazine of force and motion supplied with that which is chemically pure and needful in the building up of this wonderful structure which is only a part of the superstructure commonly called, man."

All orders are given in silence and obeyed without a murmur.

Every subordinate comes with that which is necessary for construction and the masons of the Infinite go forth with pleasure to execute the design of their Superior, knowing their work will be carefully examined and their lives will pay the forfeit in case of failure to fulfill all requirements.

The Commander General says to each subordinate, "Carry your burden and deposit it in workman-like style or death will be the penalty." The well-trained army, knowing this to be the truth, proceed with the atoms as selected by the Divine Critic—and no more care is expended in the selection than is expected to be shown in depositing them in and on the wall according to the place of previous instruction.

The order has gone forth—each workman obeys the command; thousands upon thousands and millions after millions hear and obey this fiat: "Go and labor day and night and night and day until this part is completed, inspected and received.

A part of the constructing force is engaged in repairing all waste and losses that occur during the years of mortal life. Nor do they forget the command of cleanliness, which is the reverse of construction, to carry away all worn out fragments of this wonderful part of the machine. While they are adjusting it to its natural place in the engine, other divisions and commands are fulfilling the order of a like femer to be its helpmate.

Being now held in place to the body and accepted as finished, they wait with anxiety another's higher order: Arise more and forever, house and care for the great in-dweller, the spirit of man, the essence and secret of God, life, the unsolved problem of eternity.

A. T. STILL.

March, 1895

LATEST AND BEST.

Osteopathy is as broad as the universe and is governed by the same unerring law. Within the last thirty days I have discovered and demonstrated that within the laws of this science more can be accomplished in freeing helpless and hopeless females from torture and trouble than all other systems combined. I regard this as the most wonderful revelation yet made in this science. A. T. STILL.

March, 1895

OPPRESSED MANHOOD.

I know a man whose fame for kindly deeds spreads far and wide,
Whose name with tender thoughts enshrined in many hearts doth bide,
He loves all things that dwell beneath the heaven's sunny arch—
He loves all things, save one, and that one pesky thing is starch!
His daily prayer for years has been, "Don't starch my shirts like timber.

But leave the bosoms nice and soft, the
collars also limber."
He says he'd rather have his share made
into bread for dinner
Than in his clothes to tempt him sore to
quarrel like a sinner.
Alas, alas! things often times in this old
world go wrong!
And prayers sometimes unanswered are
though they be loud and long.
His face doth lose its saint-like smile and
take on one of pain,
If by a chance his linen's stiff—in fact, he
raises Cain!
When collars rub his aching neck and
bosoms rasp his chest
He loses his religion quite, he'd like to
swear his best.
The dreadful words I'm sure he thinks,
it would not do to tell,
There's one composed of letters four that
ends in double "l."
He fears he'll fall from grace and lose his
soul in deep perdition
If things continue day by day in such a
stiff condition.
And so, to make his peace with God, he
tells his piteous story
In words so touching I am sure he'll gain
a pass to glory.
Now, listen to his tale of woe and see if
you don't think
St. Peter will ope wide the gate with just
a nod and wink—
"'Tis only my religious birth prevents
continuous wail,
Lord, Lord, just see, my shirt is starched
from collar unto tail!
I dread each Sunday morning, Lord, Thou
knowest I'm no flirt,
But I cannot be good with quarts of
starch upon my shirt!"

A. T. S. and Teddie.

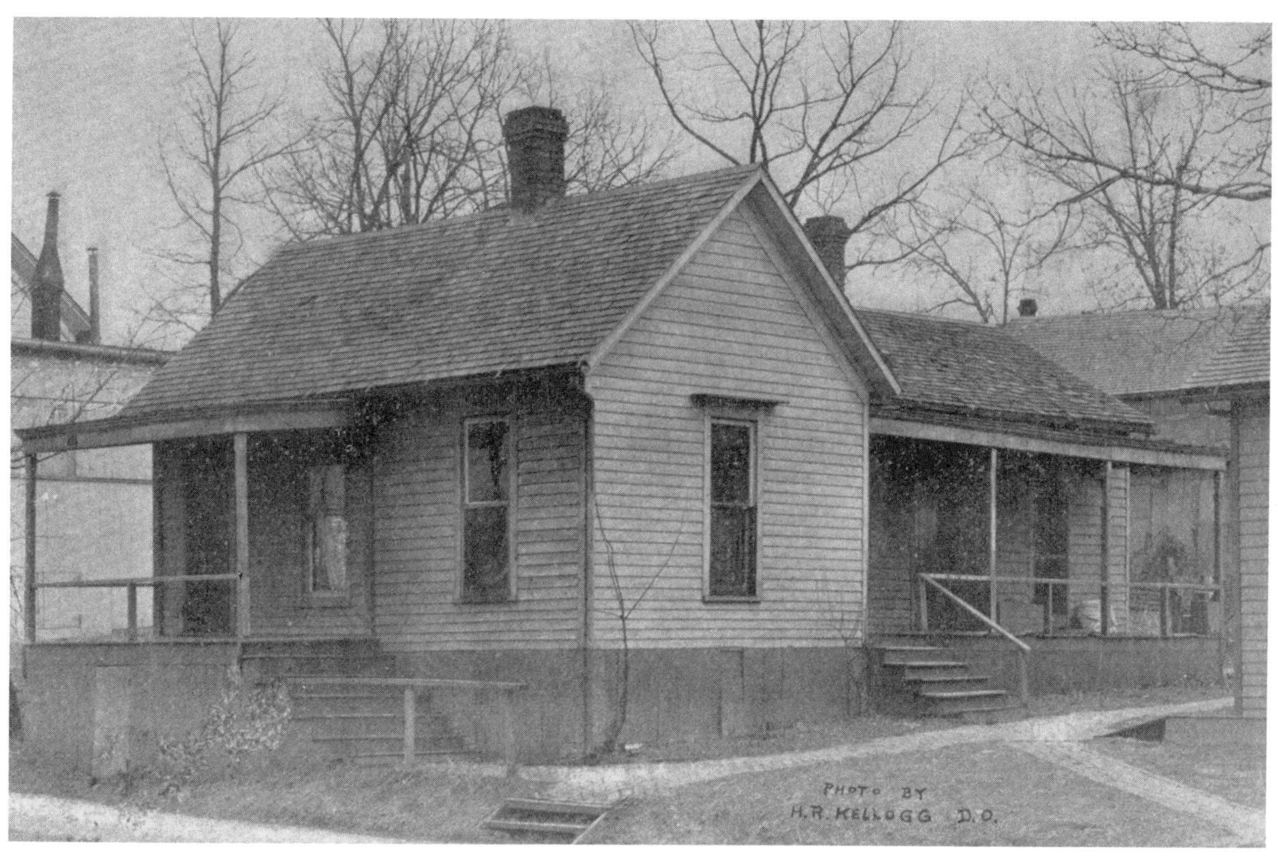

Where Osteopathy Began

April, 1895

DR. STILL'S TALK IN MEMORIAL HALL APRIL 25, 1895.

Wednesday mornings we make it a rule to talk in this hall on Osteopathy. To those persons who have been here for some time, perhaps these talks, like some sermons, may act as a narcotic and induce at least a few moments of slumber; but the strangers present may desire to know what Osteopathy is? The same question is asked, What is medicine, what is Homeopathy? I take great pleasure in telling you what I know about it. Before I pass to that subject allow me to say, some persons think I am an infidel, some that I am a hypnotist, or a mesmerist, or something of that kind or nature. Disabuse your minds of all such stuff as that now, once and forever.

One observation upon our surroundings this morning, of budding trees, growing grass, opening flowers, too plainly tell that intelligence guided, directed and controlled this wonderful creation of all animate and inanimate things. Deity, the greatest of all creators made this mighty universe with such exactness, beauty, and harmony, that no mechanical ingenuity possessed by man, can equal in creation the mechanism of that first and great creation. Botany, Astronomy, Zoology, Philosophy, Anatomy, all natural Sciences, reveal to man these higher, nobler, grander laws and their absolute perfection. Viewed through the most powerful miscroscope or otherwise no defects can be found in the works of Deity.

The mechanism is perfect, the material used is good, the supply sufficient, the antidotes for all frictions, jars, or discords, are found to exist in sufficient quantities in the materials selected, and the processes through which they pass, after the machine is put in motion and is properly adjusted, to maintain active vigorous life. Man the most complex intricate and delicately constructed machine of all creation, is the one with which the Osteopath must become familiar. Business sagacity and sense teach us that in all departments of art, science, philosophy or mechanics you must have skilled and experienced operators. Would you think of taking your gold watch when out of repair, to a skilled blacksmith or to a silversmith's. Certainly to the latter you would go—Why? Because he is a man educated and skilled in adjusting this delicately constructed machine, he knows its construction, the function each wheel ,pivot, or bearing must perform in order that your watch will, with accuracy, register the time. Even then you will not leave your valuable watch with every one who displays a placard—"Watches Repaired." The skilled blacksmith can do good work in his line, he can make a horse shoe to perfection, he uses vice, bellows, anvil and hammer; so does the silversmith. The materials differ in the quantity used by each, more perhaps than in quality. The great difference being in the delicacy of the machinery and the weakness of its parts, the susceptibility of any foreign substance introduced into the machinery of the watch to produce irregular motion, obstruction, wear, decay and finally death. The blacksmith can set the tire on a wagon or carriage wheel, place it upon the spindle properly adjusted and it is ready to roll—The point I wish to have you bear in mind is this, that to be an Osteopath you must study and know the exact construction of the human body—the exact location of every bone, nerve, fiber, muscle and organ the origin, the course and flow of all the fluids of the body, the relation of each to the other, and the functions it is to perform in perpetuating life and health. In addition you must have the skill and ability to enable you to detect the exact location, of any and all obstructions to the regular movements of this grand machinery of life; not only must you be able to locate the obstruction, but you must have the skill to remove it. You

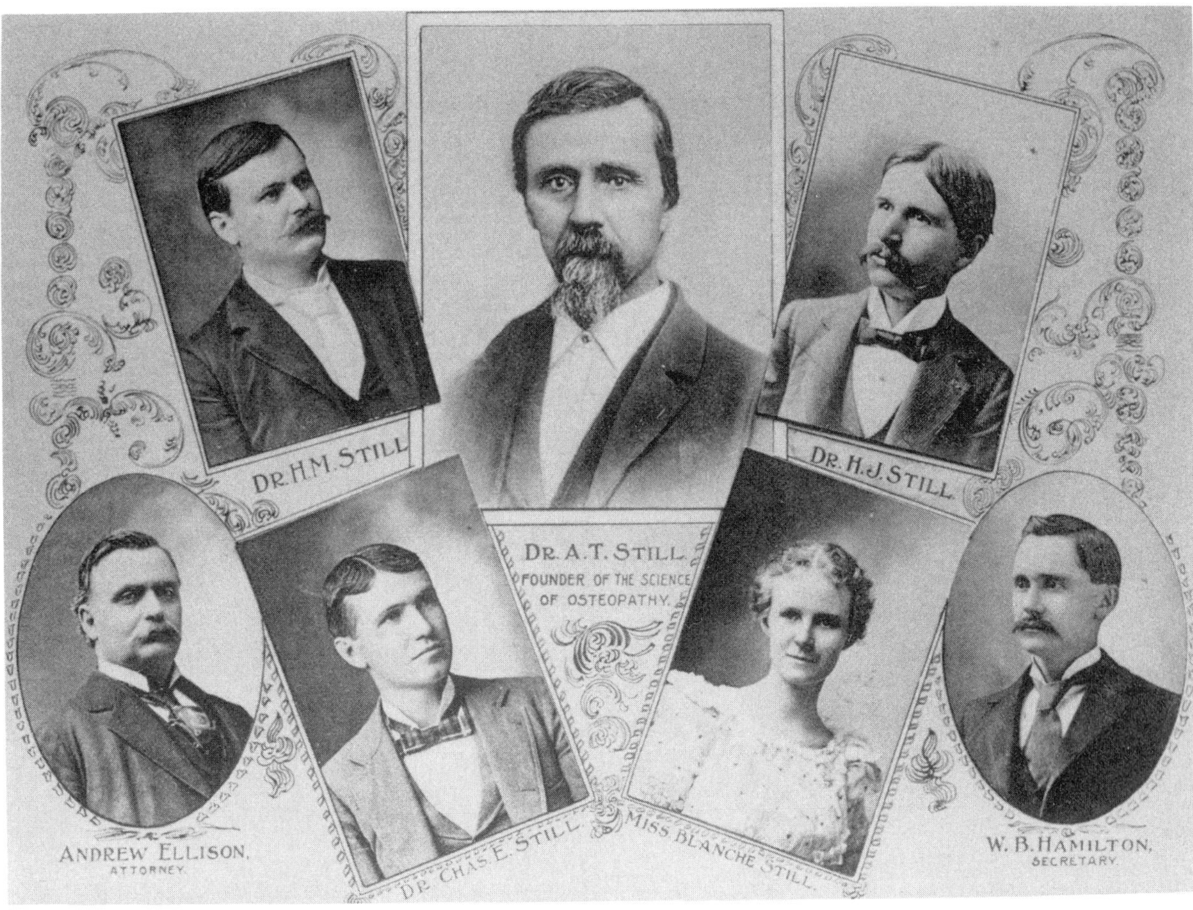

must be able to wield the sledge hammer of the blacksmith, as well as the most delicate drill of the silversmith. The aim of this school is to furnish to the world skilled Osteopaths. Our ability to do that is beyond question.

(Parenthetically allow me to say a few very ordinary blacksmiths, in Osteopathy are springing up, here and there, who in time will demonstrate their failures as did one of their predecessors who started in to make and iron wedge; after pounding the iron a while, he admitted he could not make a wedge but believed that out of the flattened iron he could make a bell, finally he saw he must fail in making a bell—chagrined and mortified at his failure, when in his greatest despair, he triumphantly exclaimed, I know I can make a whiz, as he thrust the hot iron into the slack tub. A whiz is all these blacksmiths will make.) But I am sad at the thought of the impositions thus palmed off on the public, and the association of the word Osteopath with the names of such pretenders. The consoling thought is their days are numbered.

The Hoosier when he meets another says, how are you? The reply invariably is, "moderate." We want no moderate osteopaths, we want and must have all osteopaths, who, when he or she finds Pneumonia, Flux, Scarlet fever, Diphtheria, etc., knows the exact location and cause of the trouble and how to relieve it. He must not be a blacksmith, and only able to hit large bones, muscles, etc., with a heavy hammer, but he must be able to use the most delicate instruments of the silversmith in adjusting the deranged, displaced bones, nerves, muscles, etc., and remove all obstructions, and thereby set the machinery of life moving. To do this is to be an osteopath.

You who are here to-day have only to use your sense of sight, to satisfy you whether I speak truly or not. Medicine as shown by dispensatories has called to its aid 12,000 different potions in its efforts to heal diseases. With all these the most intelligent of the profession are not satisfied with the results. This long list of poisons is an attempt to prove God made a failure in providing a law by which disease might be reached and arrested by a thorough knowledge of that law—I believe God made no mistake. I believe man made the mistake when he undertook to inject poisonous substances into the human system as a remedy for disease, instead of applying the laws of creation to that end. Here is where osteopathy and medicine part company—When I touch the keys on this piano, the effect of the stroke is to produce sound, when in tune the combination of notes produce harmony; the same law is found to exist in the vocal chords.

I see in the audience a lady who came here a few days ago, suffering from Aphonia who had been in that condition for ten weeks, whose voice you can hear now all over this hall, (at the Dr's request, the lady spoke in a distinct audible tone.) This is a restoration of voice brought about by simply adjusting the vocal organs. Deity created the organs and also the law of their adjustment when out of order, neither did he mistake in the creation, nor in the law.

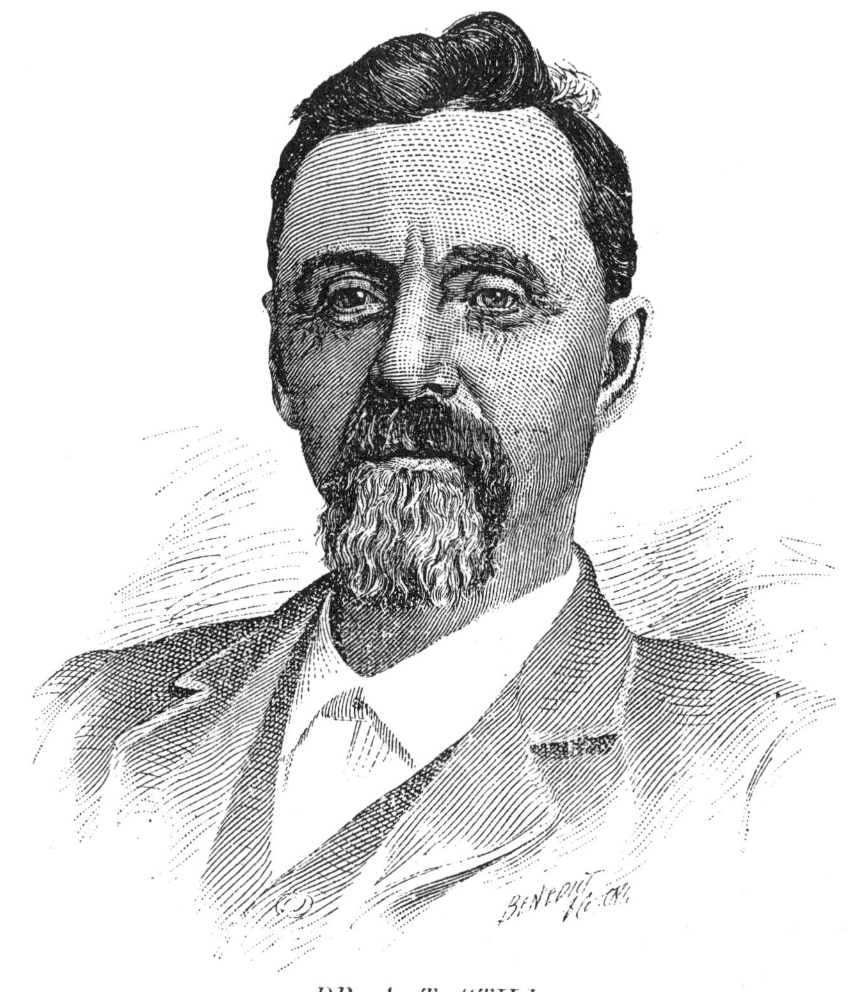

DR. A. T. STILL.

Regarding the evil effects produced by the free use of drugs, much can be said upon that subject, yea! volumns could be used to trace the injuries produced by the use of calomel. This morning I will mention only one or two. About 60 years ago quinine was first used, and then very sparingly but soon on account of its supposed efficacy in malarial fevers, it soon became the great panacea as a febrifuge. Not only the size of the doses was increased but the frequency in doses also. Prior to that time fibroid tumors were as few in the human family as, Governors from Missouri are in Heaven. To-day I verily believe the greater number of Fibroid tumors we find in people are produced from the great quantity of quinine used, together perhaps with belladonna and other poisonous substances. These excrescences, the foundation for which was laid by one generation of Doctors, furnish this generation, with an ample opportunity for the use of the surgeons knife. The attempted removal of them by the knife, usually removes the patient to that other land, about the time the tumor is removed from the body.

Bereaved husband and friends reverentially listen to the minister relate that in God's providence the sister had been called to her eternal home far beyond moving worlds and burning suns. By way of consolation to the bereaved husband, he quotes the scriptural text with an addendum attached, "Whom the Lord loveth he chasteneth" (with another wife.)

April, 1895

The first requirement for an accurate diagnosis is a thorough knowledge of the human engine, all its powers, parts, and principles. Thus armed, you are prepared to decide whether the trouble is in the boiler, steam-chest, wheels, valves, shaft or any other part of the machinery. Without this you cannot give a correct diagnosis, prognosis or treatment. A. T. STILL.

April, 1895

The law of life is absolute. That wonderful, unknown and incomprehensible force which furnishes the power to move the machinery of all animate bodies is felt but not understood. Of ourselves we are unable to supply any one substance required in the economy of our bodies, yet there is a force within us which can select from the given materials such substances as are needed to form any part of the human system.—Dr. Still.

April, 1895

Consumption, croup, hay fever and asthma, the four great cannibals of the world, have never failed to capture their chosen ones or thousands at will in defiance of the skill of all the learned men of the medical profession. They take the babe, mother, father, minister and doctors of all schools, because they are all equally helpless. The doctor's drugs, lymph and all, take the place of seasoning as salt and pepper do, only to give relish to the four eaters of flesh. But you O. P's know, by happy experience, that there is a balm in Gilead for "daughters" and sons, that says to those four cannibals, Stop, and they do. You must not eat of our loved ones till age has marked them with the gray hairs of declining usefulness. Does not the violinist know what notes to touch to cause harmony? Are you not as wise as a fiddler? Are you as dumb as a brute! No! gentlemen, I think better of you. You know what strings to touch to sound the lungs, or any other part of the whole system, or you have slept on your post and should be ashamed of yourselves, and should never be allowed to wear a stove-pipe hat till you have traveled in sack-cloth and ashes till you have attoned for your ignorance and stupidity. Is not God's law absolute? If so, defend the nerves, arteries and veins and look for the results. They will not deceive you as cause and effect are absolute. —A. T. Still, Dec. 24, '91.

April, 1895

Comparison of Alopathy and Osteopathy.

The question is often asked, How does osteopathy compare with alopathy? Osteopathy cures. Alopathy, if it does not kill, teaches you to drink whisky, eat opium, ruins your whole manhood and usefulness, makes you a mental and a moral wreck, causes you to shun society, hate your neighbor, fight your mother and abuse your wife and children. When you are filled with whiskey or opium, then you become a pitiful fool and a monumental liar. All men are liars when under the influence of whisky or opium.

Osteopathy cures fevers and all diseases of any climate and sends you home to make a living for yourself and those dependent upon you.

Osteopathy is a blessing to our race; alopathy a curse. Eclecticism is a whopper for "pepper sass," and Tr. Rei. Homeopathy, like the mosquito, has not a musical wing, but a remarkably long bill. Choose between them.

[From a lecture delivere by A. T. Still in December, 1891.]

April, 1895

PROGRESS OF OSTEOPATHY.

In the March number of the JOURNAL OF OSTEOPATAY the announcement was made by me that within the last thirty days I had discovered that by the laws of this science greater relief to afflicted and suffering females could be afforded than by all other systems of pathology combined. Thirty days additional experience warrants me in saying that I know the key that unlocks the heretofore hidden mysteries of the cause and cure of those diseases peculiar to the female, has been found. That this law of life furnishes an effectual and permanent cure of many, if not all, of those diseases which for centuries have perplexed and baffled the medical practioners of all schools, in every country and clime, and for which no successful cure has been found. For many years this law of life has been my constant thought. I have learned what I know of the human machinery, little by little, but by this mode I have been able to increase my stock of knowledge. To do this I have resorted, under necessity, to rolling poor Indians out of their terrestial resting places, after the immortal part had gone to the happy hunting ground, that I might have before my eyes the exact and perfect structure of man. In this way I began my life work. There is, perhaps, some credit due me in the way of discovery of a mode of treating diseases without using drugs. Yet of this latest discovery, I, at my advanced age and with all my past experience, feel that it is the most important discovery of my life; that in results it will bring more joy, happiness, and comfort to the oppressed, burdened and afflicted mothers and daughters of the land than all discoveries heretofore made. At this time I am fully persuaded, in my own mind, that within the next twelve months nine-tenths of all diseases peculiar to females can be successfully cured by Osteopathy. This discovery only confirms former statements that this science is not fully known and understood. That the law is sufficiently broad to furnish a cure for all diseases. My only object in life is now and for years has been to understand this law of life in all its possibilities. In this desire I may, and doubtless will, fail, yet the consolation is, the pathway has been extended far into the gloom and shadows of darkness, ignorance and superstition, and the sunlight of reason is illuminating that pathway with such powerful rays of light that the entire domain will be thoroughly surveyed and reclaimed from that obscurity in which it has remained since the dawn of creation. The march of this science for twenty years has been marked at each mile-post by victories won. At each advance human suffering has been relieved, and to the list of diseases conquered, new ones, as its trophies of conquest added.

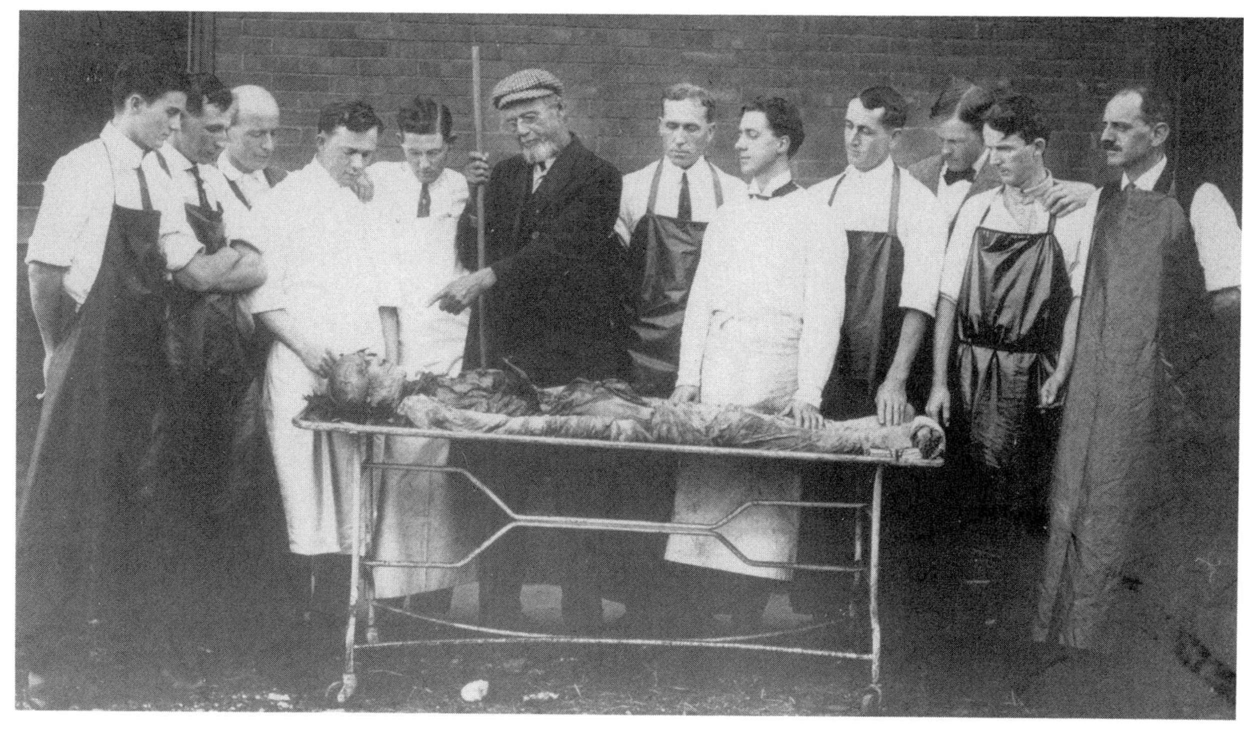

A. T. STILL.

April 25, 1895.

April, 1895

I have found the final resting place for another great failure or nuisance known as Pessary. I am now prepared to say to all ladies, put pessaries of all kinds in the stove. Doctors have kindly endeavored to assist God in his lack of knowledge of how to hold an organ in its normal place, but have failed just in proportion to the measure of their lack of knowledge of the form and design of the delicate muscles and nerves, with their wonderful powers and uses. A married lady who has not had the knife of torture, or the Pessary of ignorance, to annoy her delicate nerves, is too rare a jewel to be anything like a common thing, or daily sight. I believe the key of the science lately found, and spoken of in the last JOURNAL, will give ease, comfort and cure to any lady or anything that has more of the female than the male gender in make or look. I believe I could do Gov. Stone some good. DR. A. T. STILL.

Special Notice.

C. E. Still and Charles Hartupee, of Red Wing, Minn., Mrs. Hunt of Minneapolis, Minn., and H. T. and H. M. Still, of Evanston, Ill., are all graduates of the American School of Osteopathy and are amongst the most successful operators who have left this school. They ask no aid from any drug yet known. They are all successful practitioners and know how to treat disease without the use of drugs. An Osteopath grounded in the faith has no use for drugs, because he is not taught to use them, but to shun and despise their use as he would the deadly nightshade. When he compromises with drugs, he is not entitled to confidence, as then he becomes an apostate.

A. T. STILL, President.

May, 1895

CAUTION.

In various sections of the country unscrupulous persons are claiming to be Osteopathic doctors.

Unless they can show a diploma from the American School of Osteopathy, beware of them. No one is endorsed by this school unless he or she has a regular diploma.

We wish to impress upon the public this fact: no person has the right to claim he is an Osteopath unless he can present you a diploma showing his grade in anatomy is above 90, and issued by the American School of Osteopathy.

We endorse no one excepting those to whom diplomas have been issued.

Remember every graduate from the American School of Osteopathy has won his or her diploma by industry and hard study. The meritorious and deserving receive diplomas at this school. They are not bought and sold as commercial commodities. Trust no one as an Osteopath unless he has a diploma.

Osteopathy is so far ahead of all other systems of treating disease that our janitors and hostlers are taken for Osteopathic doctors. Beware, however, of them; patronize none but those who have a regular diploma from this school.

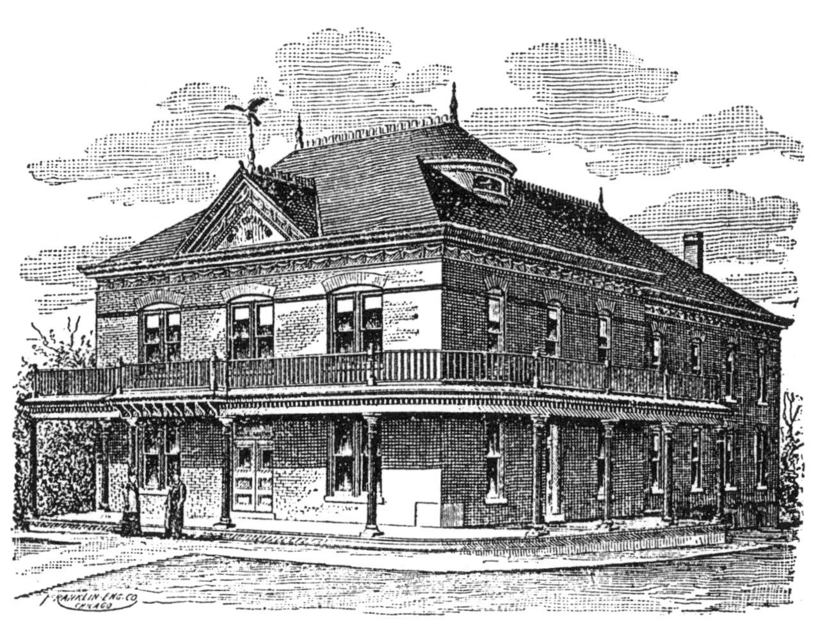

A. T. STILL'S INFIRMARY, ERECTED IN 1894.

May, 1895

LADIES AND GENTLEMEN:

I cannot express myself as an orator; timidity came to me at my birth or may be was waiting for me a week before hand. It is easy for me to use such big words as "I will" or "I wont" and I do not hesitate to say—I will demonstrate that Osteopathy is a science. The purpose of these meetings is to give you an insight into its nature; the average American can't tell whether it is an earthquake, a cyclone or a comet. Even the Governor of our great state thinks it a special gift or a secret. We know that it is a science founded on truth, a science which any man of intelligence who will studiously apply himself may learn, a science which has control of fever, flux, measles and diphtheria and it never goes into line of battle to meet these foes under a flag of truce but waves the black flag of defiance.

In this work I depend upon the absolute laws of Deity; if you object to that, all right; you may take guess-work if you choose, but I will not loose my hold on Deity. If you want to see the result of guess-work methods, look at our grave-yards full of babies, little children, young mothers, men who failed to reach the prime of life. I tell you God never meant to fertilize the earth in that manner. It is the ignorance of man which produces such results.

I remember that in the harvest fields out in wind-swept Kansas while the men wore shirts, the most of them were shirts with holes in them. One day a Dutchman sat down against a bush to rest and something crawled through one of these holes. The Dutchman pulled that something out and found it was a rattlesnake and he said to it, "What's dat? You want to bite?" About that time I found something in my bosom. It was Osteopathy. I pulled it out into view and asked of it as the Dutchman did of the snake, "You want to bite?" The answer came, "No, I want to give to mothers the comfort due them. I want to give ease and quiet to children so that they may eat all that is necessary for life and growth and may sleep, so fulfilling the law of nature and developing from an atom to a full grown being. And in this one form you will find all that heaven and earth contain.

My neighbors said of this strange thing I showed them—it is nonsense, you are crazy, until I grew ashamed to hold it to view even in the great freedom-claiming state of Kansas. And when they spoke so of this science backed by God, I did as the Dutchman did when his wife died, "I got so mad, I bawl."

The nineteenth century triumphed over slavery, but who appreciates true freedom, for there is about one wise man to ninety-nine fools among the people. I tried to explain to them that the brain acted as a common battery, but they thought these secrets belonged to God and reproached me for going against the teachings of my father who, during his life, had been a good physician, using pills, purges, plasters and all the poisons he had been taught were essential to the curing of disease. He lived up to the best light he had, but a fuller, brighter light has broken on us from the intelligence of God that is better than the old guess-work. I shall give all my life to the study of these human engines, these combines of mind and matter, and whenever I find a new truth I will trumpet it to the world.

I want the character of my discoveries to be such that when an inquirer asks whose writing is upon the pages of Osteopathy, the answer may be—"They bear the stenography of the Architect of the universe."

It has been said to me, "Are you not afraid of losing your soul running after this new idea, this strange teaching?"

I have no fear that following a law made by God will lead me from Him.

I do not want to go back to God with less knowledge than when I was born. I want my foot-print to make an impress on the fields of reason. I have no desire to be like a cat, which has the lightest tread of any animal and walks here and there without creating any disturbance. I want my steps to be plainly seen by all book readers. I want to be myself not "them," not "you," not Washington, but just myself, well plowed and cultivated. I expect to continue searching into the construction of this human engine—the body of man. I find much to interest me in the brain with its two lobes, medulla oblongata, spinal cord and various sets of nerves. It is the machine which controls the telegraphy of life.

In the heart I find chambers where blood is stored to pass out through the arteries of the entire system and returns through the veins to the heart in an impoverished condition, there to receive nourishment from the chyles which passes through the thoracic duct to renew the blood. Each vein has a water bucket; God is a great water bucket man. The lymphatics are water supplies; they thin the Jersey milk of the chyme and make it ready for the pulmonary arteries.

Sickness is caused by the shutting off of some supply (here a fine illustration was given by the use of the electric lights.)

In case of paralysis you go from one doctor to another to find one who can throw a current on the spinal cord; finally you come to an Osteopath who touches the button and turns on the light. So in case of diphtheria, you want the Lord to send a man that plays understandingly on the machine He has made. An Osteopath conquers the disease by knowing how to apply the principles and practice of this science along the lines of sensation, motion and nutrition then you are happy and want to kiss the doctor, get drunk or celebrate in some way.

The principle of the electric light is the same as that of Osteopathy; it has two batteries composed of opposite chemicals, bring them together and an explosion or light is produced.

The same principle shows why a bird keeps warm—its heart-beats are quick. The snow-bird has about 360 heart-beats per minute while the elephant has only about one in three minutes and the whale still fewer.

Why is the wind-bag, or lung, placed in the breast? To explode oxygen and sustain life. If the machine is in a healthy state, would you poison and contract it until the battery cannot act?

Oxygen is sent through the entire body and throws a bomb-shell into the camp of death. But some refuse to accept the new and better way. They want the same old whiskey, etc.

All right, no gun can shoot stronger than its construction waraants and they can do no better.

The people have to be educated in this respect; they are like rats in a trap. Their doctor may be a good man but he is practically helpless under the system he advocates. He lets his wife die, lets his child die that he would give worlds to save, dies himself because he travels away from God's instruction.

An Osteopath is a human engineer who should understand all the laws governing his engine and thereby master disease.

When asthma tries to destroy life, when the pulmonary nerves thicken and get stupid, he puts on steam by working on the nerves that control the lungs and harmony is the result.

In case of flux when the bowels are on fire with pain, the Osteopath presses the button of ease and in a few minutes the agony is over and the child is hungry.

Soon I expect to find the button to press that will produce an accumulation or a reduction of flesh as the case demands.

Shame upon the knife that cuts a woman like a Christmas hog. Almost one-half the women of to-day bear a knife-mark, and I tell you God's intelligence is reproached by it.

An Osteopath stands firm in the belief that God knew what to arm the world with and follows His principles. And he who so far forgets His teaching as to use drugs, must forfeit the respect of my school and its followers.

I am the father of Osteopathy and am not ashamed of the child of my brain. A. T. Still.

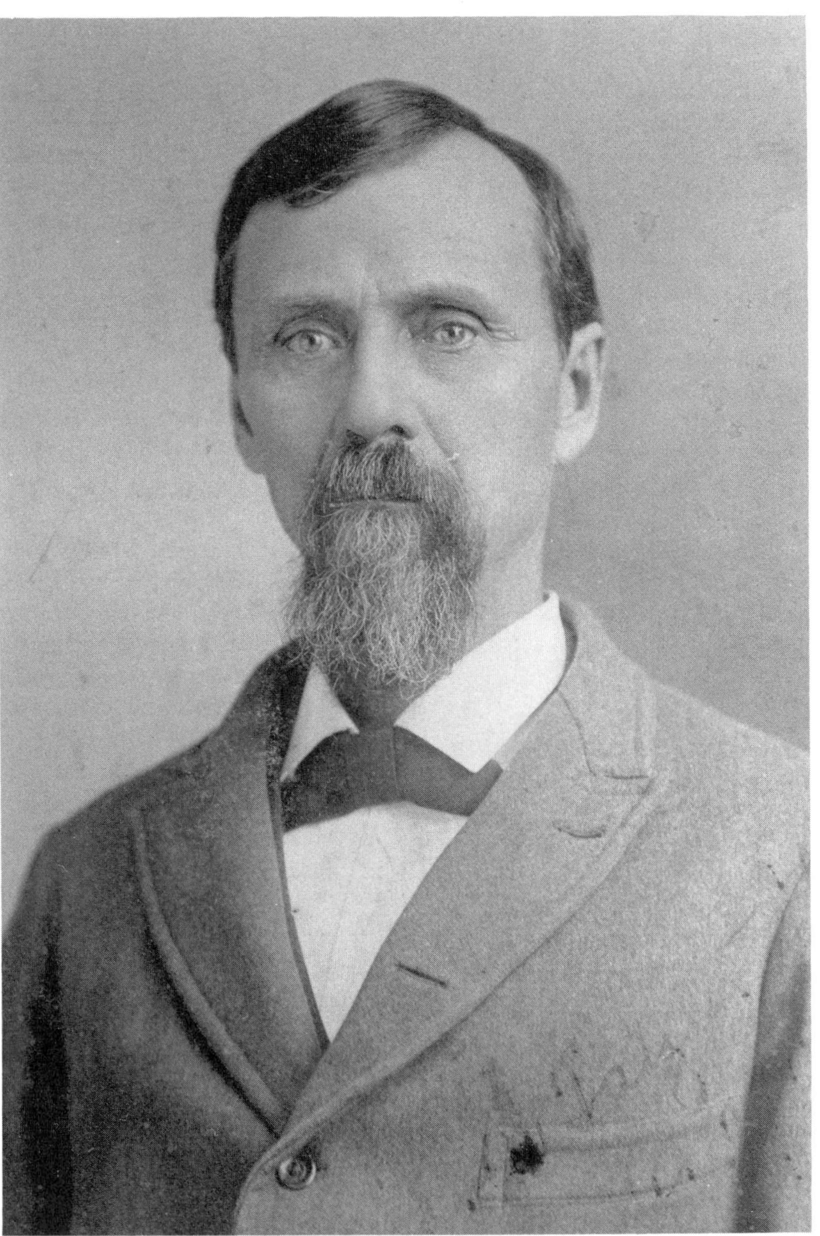

A. T. Still, c. 1900

May, 1895

M. D's.

I have no desire to quarrel with or disturb the M. D's., as many of them are men learned in their profession which they have been deluded to believe is a science which will enable them to successfully vanquish disease in the constant battle that is being waged between life and death.

Personally I am a friend to M. D's.—they are the very men who have made me an Osteopath.

I used to chop wood with an old, worn-out ax and it was of little account; I saw a new one containing more steel, fine in make and shape, fitted to do its work well. I traded my old medical ax for the better ax of Osteopathy made of the sharp steel of reason and it cuts to perfection. A. T. Still.

May, 1895

I Want Riches.

I do not want riches that is given by money alone. I believe daily labor is one of the greatest sources of comfort in any man's life.

No man should have such a large amount of money as will encourage him in being indolent or lazy. He should trim all the useless weights from his mind, review the past, cast out all ideas that have been found erroneous and adopt wiser methods for the future.

A man must labor with both mind and body in order to be happy.

I want all the wealth I can get if knowledge is wealth—dress and show are not objects worthy of attainment to me, they are not ham and onions; no, never! When I hear some poor human engine creaking with pain and can press the button of the door of ease, I am then filling my craving stomach with the oil of joy and the angels food of love.

A. T. Still.

May, 1895

To the Student of Osteopathy.

In searching for causes of disease you began anatomy at the bone. Remember bones are held in place by ligaments, one ligament containing many parts or fibres which cross at all angles, it being a rare thing for any two of these fibres to run the same course for their entire length.

Now if we should begin in the N. W. T. and run S. E. and another and longer one should begin N. of N. W, T. and run S. of S. E. and all be bent from E. to S. E. what would then be the condition of N. W. T. at center or cross line on S. by S. E.? What would happen to the covering of each ligament? Suppose a muscle be fastened at N. and S., then suppose the brace at S. be moved to S. E. what will occur in space between S. and S. E.? All fibrinous cross openings will be shoved N. by E.

Should you move brace back to S. you would still have fibres fast in fibrinous cross spaces. You are now at sea if you fail to obey the law of parallaxes. You must, under such circumstances, trace and adjust all muscles and fibres from origin to insertion, giving S. W. T. more on center of all these muscles and fibres pressing them as far beyond a straight line in this direction as they have been moved in abnormal line in the opposite direction to produce the disease; if you do not pursue such a course you will fail to get the relief sought.

All points in insertion mark a change in vitality. Since you have the fact of all muscles being fibres of a very delicate nature, you treat all first as divisions, then as individuals. Each bone is a summit of attachment. Summits are to keep fibres from pressing on nerves, veins, arteries and facies.

A. T. Still.

May, 1895

WHAT A STUDENT MUST BE.

An operator, in order to be a success, must know the full meaning of the phrase==blood and nerve supply. He must know the exact location of each nerve vein and artery in every part of all the limbs, the head, neck, chest, abdomen and each organ and gland of the whole body.

A student gets word anatomy in the class-room and learns practical anatomy in the clinics of Osteopathy.

A full knowledge of the form and action of all muscles and ligaments must precede the entry into this room for the purpose of receiving instruction in clinics; because here it is the philosopher must dwell if good is to come. Either an Osteopath is a philosopher or he is merely an imitator and cannot progress beyond simple imitation.

He who would enter this school of science must not do so with the expectation of becoming fully qualified to cope with all forms of disease short of eighteen months or two years. Fully this much time is required for becoming an expert operator.

Osteopathy is doubtless the greatest science now before the people, and is being recognized as such by all those who are competent to form a judgment on the subject.

Should any one think of becoming a practitionee of this science simply because he has failed to make a living in other ways, he would better conclude to change his intentions. We want Osteopathy to be proven a success to all the world and such a man is not capable of making such proof. Young Osteopaths are, as a general thing, crazy to get out into the world long before they are ready to be turned loose.

Experience in the past twelve months has taught me that many desire to enter this school for the mere purpose of saying they have been students of the American School of Osteopathy, and if they could get some slips of paper to show they had been students of my school, they would travel from place to place, and under cover of Osteopathy, would deceive people and obtain money by false pretenses.

We now endorse no one as being fully qualified to do the science justice except such as can show diplomas stating that a grade of 90 per cent. on a scale of 100 in anatomy has been obtained.

By way of caution I would say, never hesitate to ask an Osteopath to show his diploma, and in case he is what he represents himself to be, he will gladly show his credentials. Then you will see that by order of the trustees named in the charter granted October 30, 1895, he has been adjudged qualified to practice. The scale of 90 or more on his diploma has been won by hard study of which he may justly be proud. This diploma shows he has a thorough knowledge of the theory of Osteopathy; as to his practice it must be judged by its fruits.

A. T. Still.

State of Missouri } ss. This is to certify
County of Macon }
that A. T. Still is registered in the Roll of Physicians and Surgeons of Macon County Missouri, on Page three Line Number two, Dated Aug 29 1874, under an act passed by the Legislature of Missouri approved March 27" 1874.

In Testimony Whereof I have hereunto set my hand an affixed the Seal of the Macon County Court this 1" day of May 1893.

J. B. Goodding
County Clerk.
by R. E. Goodding. D.C.

Certificate showing A. T. Still as a registered physician in 1874

May, 1895

OUR HOME.

Kirksville is not only a pleasant home for those who can appreciate culture, refinement and moral influences, but it presents an opportunity rarely met for a safe investment in good, paying real estate. Kirksville has at no time in its history enjoyed a more decided and marked degree of prosperity than through the years 1893 and 1894. Our city was not filled with vacant business and dwelling houses through those years. Rents remained unchanged. Landlords were not forced to ask evictions of tenants for non payment of rents. Not a business failure occurred during the year, so prudently and cautiously do our business men manage and guard their affairs. Not an inuendo or whisper about the solvency of our banks, not a run or withdrawal of funds from deposits occurred. During the extreme stringency in the money market last year, when strikes were the rule, and the cry of discontent, want and suffering came from the four corners of the earth, when the inhumanity of the Pullmans and Carnagies was in the Zenith of its oppression, no cry of want was heard here. With a strike within 57 miles of us, in the month of July, our city furnished no recruits to the army of discontents. Upon the contrary, through that time the saw and the hammer of our carpenters could be heard all over the city, as well as the chimes of the anvil and the whistles of the foundry and the mills. From every street and corner you saw the busy laborer engaged upon the city's public works. At the very time the land was dotted from the Atlantic to the Pacific with discontented, tramping millions, not a man in our city was idle because he could not find daily employment. Kirksville supplied its worthy laborers with employment at sufficiently remunerative prices to banish want and gaunt poverty from their doors; this, too, was all done without any steals, by contractors or city officials, or an onerous burden fraudulently saddled upon upon the taxpaying citizens, because all these things were done under the wholesome, benign laws of this, one of the grandest, great states in the entire galaxy; where the citizens recognize the necessity of obedience to law and courts and juries administer its wise provisions alike to the rich and the poor, and that, too, without sale or denial. Humanely and kindly Kirksville provided for its own.

We know of no city, large or small, speaking from the facts as they are, which can challange the wisdom, the foresight, humanity and enlightened philanthropy of the city of Kirksville in providing for the laborer who is worthy of his hire and at the same time guarding so well the interests of the property owners and substantially improving and beautifying a magnificent little city.

Could this picture, this enlightened philanthropy, be engraved upon the minds and hearts of the avaricious oppressor of the worthy poor of our land; could the million heirs, syndicates and officers of corporations be brought face to face with that law of human philanthropy and rise above avarice and greed, by that advanced step more would be accomplished in restoring contentment, happiness and prosperity than all the sermons, discussions of finance, commerce, and politics, can do from now until the end of time. We fear, however, nothing short of that immutable law of rewards and punishments will ever force this desired step forward.

To our own citizens this teaches an instructive lesson—one that we all should "ponder well." The lesson taught by our enlightened actions in 1894 will live on, because it was born of "God's eternal laws" and demonstrates to us that the path of life is along the line of true, fraternal citizenship, and when we, in all our business and social relations with each other, are governed by these laws and realize that within our-

No 28146

This number fixes the order in which you will be waited upon; register with the Clerk and you will be called when your turn comes.

Do not sit or stand in the Hallways.

Do not ask me or any of the Doctors to stop and talk with you in the Hallways or Waiting Rooms; arrange for a consultation.

After your examination, arrange with the Secretary for a "Treatment Card" before you ask to be treated. Make all business arrangements with the Secretary; do not come to me with such matters.

Most of the actual labor of treating patients must necessarily devolve upon my Assistants, under my direction; I have confidence in their ability, and you must accept my judgment in their selection.

Patients are forbidden talking over their ailments with each other.

No work done on the "No Cure, No Pay" plan.

Work begins with payment.

A. T. STILL.

Patient's Card of Instructions used in The Infirmary

selves we have the power to strengthen, build up and support each other, thereby enabling all the living to provide for themselves through life, we shall have learned that life should not be lived for self alone. Let us all look to the interest of the living. God will care for the dead.

Our Journal has now been launched upon its second yearly voyage. It has been commissioned to attend to its own business; as to whether it has succeeded in the accomplishment of its object, its readers best know.

We made a hard fight for legal existence and gained a glorious victory in the two law-making departments of our state—our representatives and senators being wise enough to see the best interests of the people and bold enough to advocate them. But at the last hour in the day a man of great prejudice, who had been exalted to the high office of governor under the mistaken supposition that he was capable of filling it to the honor of our grand state, for the lack of the valuable article known as good business or horse sense, sent in his veto accompanied by false and insufficient excuses.

This unjust act will not be detrimental to us alone. While causing us to wait two more years for the gaining of our vested rights, it will also consign Governor Stone to the filling of a political blank during all the years of his natural life after November, 1896.

The JOURNAL will drive on in the future as in the past. It will labor to get on a higher and more intellectual plane and will endeavor to appear each month in a new suit of original reading gotten up in the latest Osteopathic style.

Its aim is to become one of the leading scientific journals of the day and it knows no such word as fail. It asks naught but equality and sensible readers who are so lucky as to have been born minus prejudice.

A. T. STILL.

May, 1895

I have just been permitted by Mrs. Sol Morris, who has the manuscripts and pencil cuts of 1885, to review Osteopathy as it appeared ten years ago.

I saw then what I now see and know and have proved to be true.

While at the house of Mrs. Morris in the winter of '85 I had experiences which seemed to rivet me to the comet of reason whose brilliant tail crosses the whole universe; its head was God then as now. That comet was not the material comet of Encke but the comet of life, the comet of Osteopathy. In its journeying toward the earth it has grown brighter and more beautiful each day. It is a cloud-lifter, a heart-soothing boon of heaven, a proof of the intelligence and love of God toward man. It came as a cruiser on the sea of Time and signaling the nations of the earth said, Let whosoever will come and see the great and small battles that occur in the workings of life. The fighting occurs between the great generals of health and disease; the one striving to maintain harmony in the unison of life and matter for the longest possible period, the other struggling for their separation at the earliest opportunity.

The poor comet came and went its celestial voyage; it rang its milk-bell at every door, but no cup was brought to be filled save one thimble sized cup that held but a few drops in 1874 in the state of Kansas, and that one poor little cup got "hell" for being filled.

But the man who held the cup was a Methodist and never does as well as when he has a little "hell." The few drops of Osteopathy received at that time have since raised "hell" in our capital and all over the country and there are now many believers in the doctrine taught by the comet. At first it was said the teaching was of the devil but since then people of intelligence and impartiality do not hesitate to say it is of God.

A. T. STILL.

May, 1895

Consumption, croup, hav fever and asthma, the four great cannibals of the world, have never failed to capture their chosen ones or thousands at will in defiance of the skill of all the learned men of the medical profession. They take the babe, mother, father, minister and doctors of all schools, because they are all equally helpless. The doctor's drugs, lymph and all, take the place of seasoning as salt and pepper do, only to give relish to the four eaters of flesh. But you O. P's know, by happy experience, that there is a balm in Gilead for "daughters" and sons, that says to those four cannibals, Stop, and they do. You must not eat of our loved ones till age has marked them with the gray hairs of declining usefulness. Does not the violinist know what notes to touch to cause harmony? Are you not as wise as a fiddler? Are you as dumb as a brute! No! gentlemen, I think better of you. You know what strings to touch to sound the lungs, or any other part of the whole system, or you have slept on your post and should be ashamed of yourselves, and should never be allowed to wear a stove-pipe hat till you have traveled in sack-cloth and ashes till you have attoned for your ignorance and stupidity. Is not God's law absolute? If so, defend the nerves, arteries and veins and look for the results. They will not deceive you as cause and effect are absolute. —A. T. Still, Dec 24, '91.

Comparison of Alopathy and Osteopathy.

The question is often asked, How does osteopathy compare with alopathy? Osteopathy cures. Alopathy, if it does not kill, teaches you to drink whisky, eat opium, ruins your whole manhood and usefulness, makes you a mental and a moral wreck, causes you to shun society, hate your neighbor, fight your mother and abuse your wife and children. When you are filled with whiskey or opium, then you become a pitiful fool and a monumental liar. All men are liars when under the influence of whisky or opium.

Osteopathy cures fevers and all diseases of any climate and sends you home to make a living for yourself and those dependent upon you.

Osteopathy is a blessing to our race; alopathy a curse. Eclecticism is a whopper for "pepper sass," and Tr. Rei. Homeopathy, like the mosquito, has not a musical wing, but a remarkably long bill. Choose between them.

[From a lecture delivere by A. T. Still in December, 1891.]

Kirksville Mo Feb 15 1892.

This is to certify that W. H. Wilderson of Nevada Mo. Is a Student in my School of Osteopathy or School of bones. He is now capable of doing some work in bonesetting to cure some diseases among males but not what is called female diseases. He has taken the first years course in the Study of O.P. To all whom it may concern.

A. T. Still D.O.

PROGRESS OF OSTEOPATHY.

In the March number of the JOURNAL OF OSTEOPATAY the announcement was made by me that within the last thirty days I had discovered that by the laws of this science greater relief to afflicted and suffering females could be afforded than by all other systems of pathology combined. Thirty days additional experience warrants me in saying that I know the key that unlocks the heretofore hidden mysteries of the cause and cure of those diseases peculiar to the female, has been found. That this law of life furnishes an effectual and permanent cure of many, if not all, of those diseases which for centuries have perplexed and baffled the medical practioners of all schools, in every country and clime, and for which no successful cure has been found. For many years this law of life has been my constant thought. I have learned what I know of the human machinery, little by little, but by this mode I have been able to increase my stock of knowledge. To do this I have resorted, under necessity, to rolling poor Indians out of their terrestial resting places, after the immortal part had gone to the happy hunting ground, that I might have before my eyes the exact and perfect structure of man. In this way I began my life work. There is, perhaps, some credit due me in the way of discovery of a mode of treating diseases without using drugs. Yet of this latest discovery, I, at my advanced age and with all my past experience, feel that it is the most important discovery of my life; that in results it will bring more joy, happiness, and comfort to the oppressed, burdened and afflicted mothers and daughters of the land than all discoveries heretofore made. At this time I am fully persuaded, in my own mind, that within the next twelve months nine-tenths of all diseases peculiar to females can be successfully cured by Osteopathy. This discovery only confirms former statements that this science is not fully known and understood. That the law is sufficiently broad to furnish a cure for all diseases. My only object in life is now and for years has been to understand this law of life in all its possibilities. In this desire I may, and doubtless will, fail, yet the consolation is, the pathway has been extended far into the gloom and shadows of darkness, ignorance and superstition, and the sunlight of reason is illuminating that pathway with such powerful rays of light that the entire domain will be thoroughly surveyed and reclaimed from that obscurity in which it has remained since the dawn of creation. The march of this science for twenty years has been marked at each mile-post by victories won. At each advance human suffering has been relieved, and to the list of diseases conquered, new ones, as its trophies of conquest added.

A. T. STILL.

April 25, 1895.

I have found the final resting place for another great failure or nuisance known as Pessary. I am now prepared to say to all ladies, put pessaries of all kinds in the stove. Doctors have kindly endeavored to assist God in his lack of knowledge of how to hold an organ in its normal place, but have failed just in proportion to the measure of their lack of knowledge of the form and design of the delicate muscles and nerves, with their wonderful powers and uses. A married lady who has not had the knife of torture, or the Pessary of ignorance, to annoy her delicate nerves, is too rare a jewel to be anything like a common thing, or daily sight. I believe the key of the science lately found, and spoken of in the last JOURNAL, will give ease, comfort and cure to any lady or anything that has more of the female than the male gender in make or look. I believe I could do Gov. Stone some good.

DR. A. T. STILL.

Teaching.

Report of third year:

It has been my custom in the past to make mention of the progress of the students in the Osteopathic drill-room. There are now six of them who have passed full grade of about 96 on a scale of 100 in the whole of Anotomy. For two months they have been in the clinics for drill. They are advancing rapidly. I find it is an easy thing to give and have an order executed by them. When they entered the school I agreed, if they attained between 90 and 100 on the whole of anatomy, to make expert Osteopaths of them. They completed this part of the work before entering the clinics and now realize that it is the only proper course to pursue. They have done nobly and wherever they may go in the scenes of operative anatomy I trust that both they and I may be proud of the results obtained.

A. T. STILL.

June, 1895

DR. A. T. STILL

Celebrates the Twenty-First Anniversary of the Discovery of Osteopathy, At the Infirmary, Last Saturday, June 22.

Ladies and Gentlemen:—

I believe that is the usual manner of beginning a speech, I am of such a timid nature I hardly know how to commence my talk and will preface it by taking a drink (of water) as I am very dry.

"I am very dry" is a phrase as old as "Hark from the tomb the doleful sound!" and many men have had that for a lullaby.

How often we hear, "I am mighty dry, my teeth are sore, my gums are swelled, my joints ache," and so on ad infinitum. These painful effects have been brought about by the use of gamboge, aloes, castor oil and kindred angles of recovery. Such angels stood around us often in the past and among them was one not always in open view of the neighbors, one which usually dwelt in the cellar, a short necked angel called king—King Alcohol.

God protect us from the guardianship of such angels.

They were stationed around us by the doctors—and here let me say that for physicians as men I have due respect and give them the right hand of fellowship. They belong to my race, have the same general makeup, two eyes, two hands, two feet and go back on them or to refuse to meet them would be to plead the baby act?

We have no intention of conducting ourselves in that way, we are armed with the unerring javlin of truth and are ready to meet all opponents, adherents of medical theories as well as all others.

I have no desire to make war against doctors themselves but against their fallacious theories. What does medicine do for you? By temporarily allaying a disease it often begets a worse thing and fills the system with poison. In adminstering it the physician is never sure of results and can only stand helplessly by and await developments, trying another remedy when one fails.

They battle with death over the bedside of their own loved ones and cry out in anguish of heart, "God give me intelligence and skill to save the angels of my fireside! Lord, help me!"

But so long as their methods are not founded on unerring law so long will their hands be tied and they cannot combat successfully either death or disease. I do not claim to be the author of this science of Osteopathy—no human hand framed its laws—I ask no greater honor than to have discovered it.

Its teachings have convinced me that the Architect of the Universe was wise enough to construct man so he could travel from the Maine of birth to the California of the grave unaided by drugs. In '49, during the gold fever when men traveled the long route overland, what did they do at the outset of their journey?

They made all due preparations in the way of provisions, strong wagons with three inch tires, ox bolts, covers, etc., everything fit to meet the storms of the plains, and neither did they forget their snake medicine. Without these cool, preparatory arrangements and necessary conveniences they would have ended their trip close to home and their desired object would have been unattained.

God, when he starts man out on the journey of life fits him out with even greater care than this.

Nothing is forgotten, heart, brains, muscles, ligaments, nerves, bones, veins, arteries, everything necessary to the successful running of this human machine. But it seems man sometimes doubts that God has loaded his wagon with all needful things and so he sets up numerous drugstores to help out in the matter, why, we have about seven here and they all have plenty to do and will have until the laws of life are more perfectly understood.

Man wants to take the reins of the universe into his own hands. He says in case of fever we must assist nature by administering ipecac and other febrifuges. But by doing this he is accusing God of incapacity—you may be sure the Divine intelligence failed not to put into the machine of man a lever by which to control fever. The Lord never runs out of material, he constructs lawyers, musicians, mechanics, artists, etc., and I suppose fools are made up of the leavings.

In the past I stood and watched four physicians, the best the medical schools could furnish, battle with all their skill against the dread disease of cerebro spinal menengites in my family. I found prayers, tears, medicine all unavailing. The war between life and death was a fierce one but at the close of it three lifeless little bodies lay in my desolate home.

In my grief the thought came to me that Deity did not give life simply for the purpose of so soon destroying it—such a Deity would be nothing short of a murderer. I was convinced there was something surer and stronger with which to fight sickness than drugs and I vowed to search until I had found it.

The result was that in 1874 I raised the flag of Osteopathy claiming that "God is God and the machinery He put in man is perfect."

This created quite a consternation. Three sows among ten goslings would not have made such a fuss. Some of my friends even went so far as to ask the Lord to take me unto Himself because I had gone back on medicine. I had simply climbed higher than medicine to the source of all forms of life. The great Wisdom knows no failure and asks no instruction from inferior man, when He makes a tomato vine He needs no help. He supplies it with lungs, trunk, brachial tubes, etc., and in due time the tomato arrives. The Grand Architect of the Universe builds without sound of hammer, nature is quiet in her work.

Do you ask why the name of Osteopathy was chosen for this science? It is a compound of Osteon, bone and Pathos-Pathine, to suffer. And we think it a proper name for a science which gives man relief from pain by the adjustment of his bones and all the organs of his body.

Man is an interesting study. Think of your three pounds of brain out of which you only use about one ounce, the corpus collosium; you needn't think I am calling you a fool, for it is true that the corpus collosium is the rostrum on which thought dwells. The remainder of the brain is used to generate the principal of force.

I have studied man as a machine, I am an engineer and know something of locomotives. I can tell you how the positive force of steam drives the engine forward and how the steam escapes at the safety valve.

Man's heart is his engine and from this Fulton borrowed his idea of the steamboat and Morse his thought of telegraphy. You will remember that when Morse was ready to make his first experiment he was heaped with ridicule. To the honor of Thomas Benton of Missouri be it said he wished success to the enterprise. But Henry Clay, the great statesman of Kentucky, called Morse a damned fool and told him to go visit the place where gnashing of teeth is carried on.

Did such abuse injure Morse? No, when a man has a truth abuse does him good. I wouldn't take one thousand dollars for the caw, caw of crows that have croaked at me, they simply act as manure to enrich my life work. Some say, "We don't believe Osteopathy can do what is claimed for it." That is all right, for fifteen cents a man can buy a patent right to call anything a humbug.

I never say I can do a thing unless I am very sure of it. When there is a shut off in the nutritive supply, starvation is the result and some part of the body withers away and physicians can only declare their inability to restore it for in such a case medicine is of no avail. When Christ restored the withered arm he knew how to articulate the clavicle with the acromean process, freeing the subclavean artery and veins to perform their functions.

Some people have an idea that this science can be learned in five minutes, they come here and spend about four hours then go out and declare themselves Osteopaths.

That is very much as if a man who had made an utter failure as a doctor, a farmer, a mechanic or a preacher were to meet an attorney on the street and after a few minutes conversation declare himself a lawyer and decide to become circuit judge on the following week. If

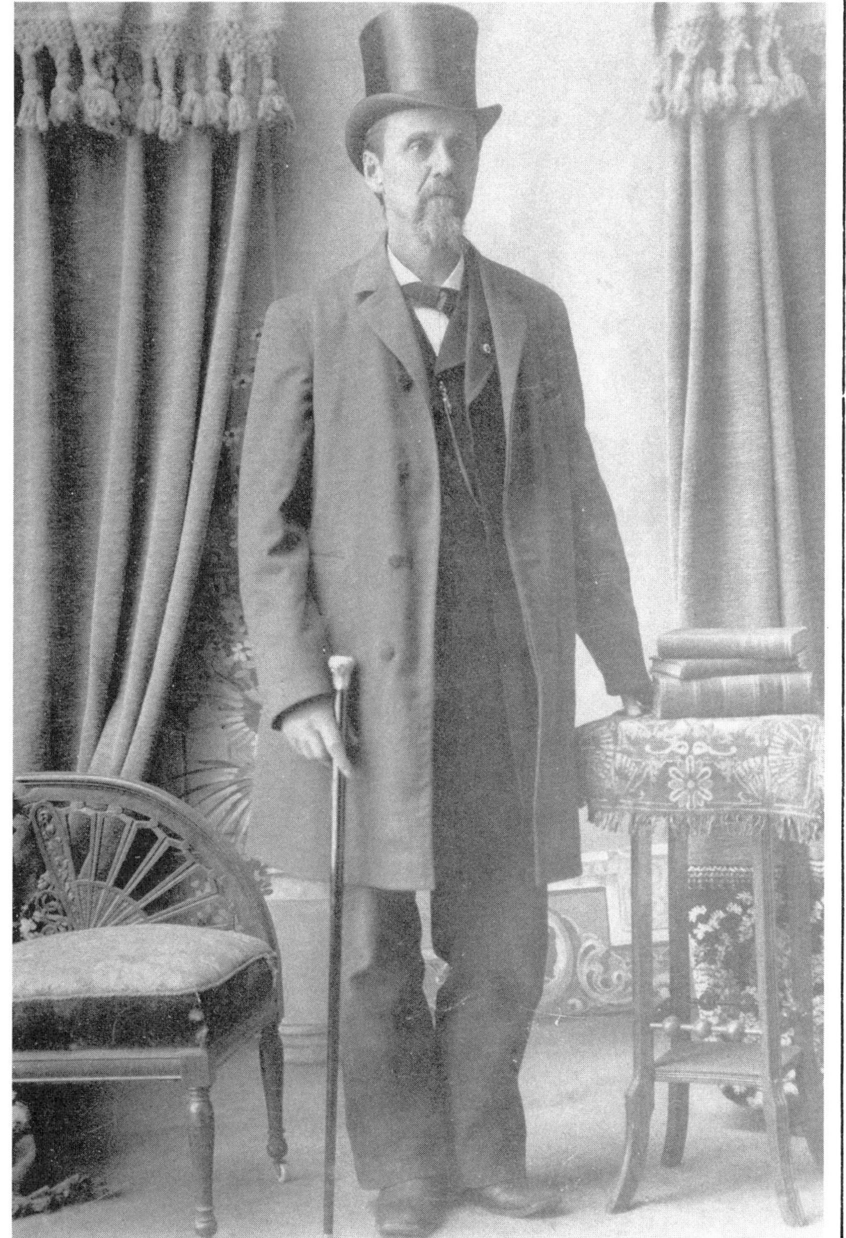

you can learn all of Osteopathy in four years I will buy you a farm and a wife to run it and boss you. A student meets a dangerous point in Osteopathy. Motion begins in the human foetus about four and a half months after conception, after nine months the child is born and becomes subject to the external laws of life. So activity of the Osteopath begins at about four and a half months after entrance into the drill room and at the end of nine months he is just a new born babe and needs constant care. In eighteen months he has reached the point where without proper guidance he is likely to take a hammer to a looking glass and in two years he has just learned that steam blows up but does not yet know how to control it. I have discovered that man is an engine and his supply comes direct from the arterial system. When you understand man you can prove God's perfect work.

I do not understand a preacher's business, I have not made a study of the Bible but the knowledge I have gained of the construction of man convinces me of the supreme wisdom of the Deity.

Now let us ask the Lord a question, and the asking of such questions is right. Can you, Lord, create a man's internal system so he can drink all kinds of water and not have bladder stones? The answer would be yes. God has forgotten nothing and we find a supply of uric acid for destroying stone in bladder or gall stones. I have no fear to investigate along this line for I always find that God has done his work perfectly. Just see how he has regulated the heart beats to supply the proper amount of electricity or warmth requisite in various forms of life, The elephant's heart beats but once in three minutes, while it requires 75 or 80 pulsations in one minute to keep man warm and the snow bird needs 360.

For 21 years I have worked in Osteopathy yet I keep my throat ever ready for the swalling of new things that constantly appear in it. I expect to live and die fighting for principle and shall pay no attention to the twaddle of opposition, merely regarding it as manure furnished my work by ignorance. The Osteopath who keeps his eye on the science and not on the almighty dollar will be able to control all forms of disease.

If such work had been carried on in Massachusetts 100 years ago all those participating in it would have been drowned or burned at the stake. For to those ignorant of the laws of life such wonderful results seem only obtained by necromancy. This, the 22nd day of June, is the anniversary of the child Osteopathy, the child of which I am justly proud. And to-day on its coming of age I am happy and welcome you gladly. And on each successive year that I live I hope to meet you here and tell of even greater advancement along these lines.

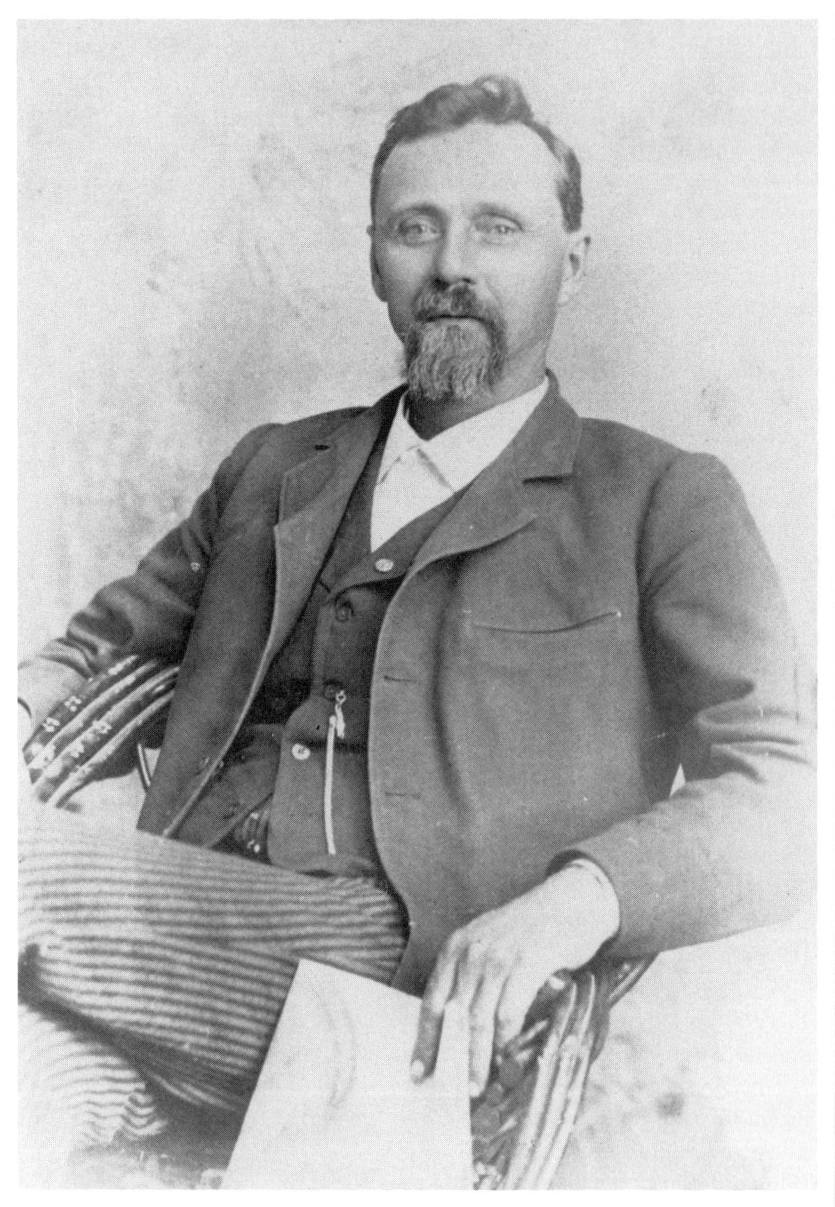

A. T. Still, 1895

June, 1895

REPORT OF PRESIDENT FOR THE 21ST ANNIVERSARY OF OSTEOPATHY.

Since last we met to honor the birthday of our child Osteopathy we have much to report to you. A year ago we were in six small rooms, treating and teaching as best we could.

The work under such unfavorable conditions was very laborious, in fact I found that I could not do justice to either students or patients without a building suitable for the developing of the science and healing of the sick.

I found the work at that time was double that of twelve months before, also I had come to know that the verdict of all intelligent investigators was:—"Osteopathy is the science of life and truth and must be taught." The demand was so great I saw preparations must be made to treat and teach on a large scale or else I must abandon the work altogether.

So I concluded on August 6th, my birthday, to begin the building of the house we now occupy. I think it an honor to the science, to the architect, to the town, the state, the nation and the world. And with due reverence I may say to the Architect of all forms of motion, mind and matter. Its object is the accomplishment of good for both the mind and body of our race and its intention is to fill a place that has been tenantless since history was first formulated on stone or on paper. An effort has been made to occupy this place by the bigotry and ignorance known as schools of medicine. Under this medical system the patient must take the dose measured out by the arbiter of his destiny whether it be harmless or a rank poison.

Neither are you allowed to ask what quantity of whisky or morphine the doctor has in his stomach when he prescribes for you or yours. When the law says we shall have help from no source but such a one as this the following of whose orders often results in death to our loved ones we feel like crying—"Oh liberty, what blood brought you!"

Dr. A. T. Still.

September, 1895

EXPERIENCES ALONG THE ROAD.

In his labors which resulted in the founding at Kirksville of The American School of Osteopathy, Dr. Still's life was one continuous struggle with all manner of difficulties, and had he not been endowed with indomitable courage and iron will, the new science would have "died a bornin',"

Outside of poverty, the greatest difficulty with which he had to contend was the deep-seated ignorance and prejudice of the people which never fails to plant itself square in front of every scheme for the advancement of the human race. From the first, Osteopathy was met by the merciless ridicule and vile slanders of an ignorant people, whose prejudice was caused by the long use of older and legally established systems built upon the vain hope that cures might result from the eternal "cut and try" method of drugs.

True to the experience of nearly all reformers, the journey was a hard and unpleasant one, and it was difficult for him to gain an audience with any but the lower order of intellect. "I could only reach those who fished for their stomach's sake," says Dr. Still. "and I soon found most of them to be untrustworthy blarneys, their heads powerless to reason, and their hearts devoid of justice. Their greatest desire was to steal the science I had labored years to perfect. Bt one time I made a great mistake by setting aside the warning of Masonic friends and allowing two men to accompany me and take instructions in Osteopathy. At the expiration of one or two years they both went back to the use of drugs. One was a salve pile doctor when he came to me, and the last I heard of him he was attending a medical school. I suppose he is marching with the salve brigade at present. The other was a lightning-rod peddler, and soon made me determine never to feed, trust nor shelter under his wing of love anyone of whom my neighbors told me to beware. Their contact with Osteopathy was like the contact of pigs with diamonds—they failed to see its brilliance."

Later on the intellectual masses began to say, "Dr. Still, you are the discoverer of the greatest truth of all ages! You have found that the Deity when he made man failed not to provide the human machine with all that was necessary to run it from the cradle to the grave,' and further insisted that he should teach it for the good of future generations

"This thought," says Dr. Still, "'Osteopathy for future generations,' haunted my mind for months, and in 1893 I opened a school for making Osteopathic doctors, with Wm. Smith, M. D., just from seven years' drill in Edinburg, Scotland, as instructor in Anatomy. He came from St. Louis to laugh at me and carry back to his medical friends the report of his fun with the only thoroughbred ass on earth. But after talking Osteopathy with me a while, he changed his mind and said, 'Dr. Still, you may laugh—I will pray. Allow me to congratulate you on having discovered the greatest science on earth. For two thousand years the medical profession have sought in vain for something better than they had, but always returned to their unreliable system of whiskey and drugs.' I found Dr. Smith a master of Anatomy, a gentleman and a scholar.

"Osteopathy is all in Anatomy and its governing laws. At eight o'clock a. m. Anatomy was taught, and at nine o'clock the students were admitted into the operating rooms. This method was continued for four months, and at the close of the school I found that I had nothing left but sixteen bunglers. No Anatomy—no Osteopathy—a year lost and nothing produced but imitators. There was not a single man or woman who could render service as an operator. I tried all the following summer to get them to reason, but could not because of their lack of knowledge of Anatomy. Two terms were a full course, and when term number two opened in the fall, the brainy members of the old class were on hand to complete their knowledge of Anatomy and to become masters of the philosophy which cannot be given to any save a thorough Anatomist.

"In 1894 I reached the conclusion that it was best to close the doors of the operating rooms to all students until they had made a grade of 90 on a scale of 100 in the whole of Anatomy. Those of the first class who have their grade of 90 or more on their diplomas can reason if they have their native ability. I can put chalk in a boy's hand, and he will make a mark just as big as God has made his head. See what he does with the chalk, not what he says. Look in the pockets of an Osteopath and see if you find drugs, or notice if he runs with an M. D. If he does either his faith in Osteopathy is very weak and his head is soft beyond redemption. A fully equipped Osteopath has no place for drugs.

"My third effort at teaching was more successful. In the fall of 1894 my school opened with about thirty students. Their heads are generally well balanced, none have used intoxicants, and their word have kept inviolate. When I began the class I gave notice that they must reach a grade of 90 on a scale of 100 in Anatomy before being allowed to enter the treating rooms. It required five months to complete the course in Anatomy. Most of them passed 98— some of them 100. Since the members of that class have entered the clinics I find there is no trouble in philosophizing with them. They are at all times and under all circumstances ready to act quickly. Their future will be a brilliant one if they use industry.

"An occasional social drunk will and should kill any man, and I hope that any Osteopath who is fool enough to get drunk may be shunned by all intelligent people. We want no drunken buzzard's money in our school."

September, 1895

WOMEN IN OSTEOPATHY

A New Field That is Peculiarly Adopted to Her Intuition.

I would like to say a few words in regard to women who have been students in my school. I have had experience with them since '93, and find that they learn anatomy easily, retain it well, and soon learn to apply their knowledge in the rooms of our clinics, the only place where a knowledge of the science of Osteopathy can be obtained. They have shown their ability to easily detect the abnormal at any and all parts of the body, in nerves, veins, arteries, muscles, ligaments, or bones. They are a success, and I think no woman is now qualified to marry while in ignorance of the laws God has made her subject to. Ignorant women are slaughtered by the knife of fools. No Osteopathic woman will allow knifing in her flesh. The time is coming, and close at hand, when mothers will have, in the birth of their children, at least a reasonably easy time, and will no longer dread it as worse than death. The horrible agony endured at such times has caused many a woman to risk her life in the hands of a brute skilled in abortion rather than endure it again. So far Ostsopathy has made all mothers happy and all births easy. I think the results in cases of midwifery treated by diplomates of Osteopathy warrant me in saying to the champions of obstetrics, "line yourselves for battle, for Osteopathy has a Gatling gun loaded for the fight and trained on your musty forts." The first shot will be fired against the use of forceps in cases of confinement. If you could see the pitiable looking children who are brought to my office entirely helpless, with heads and necks pulled apart by some ignorant doctor, you would say, "Away with forceps!" Ninety-nine times out of one hundred they are used unnecessarily.

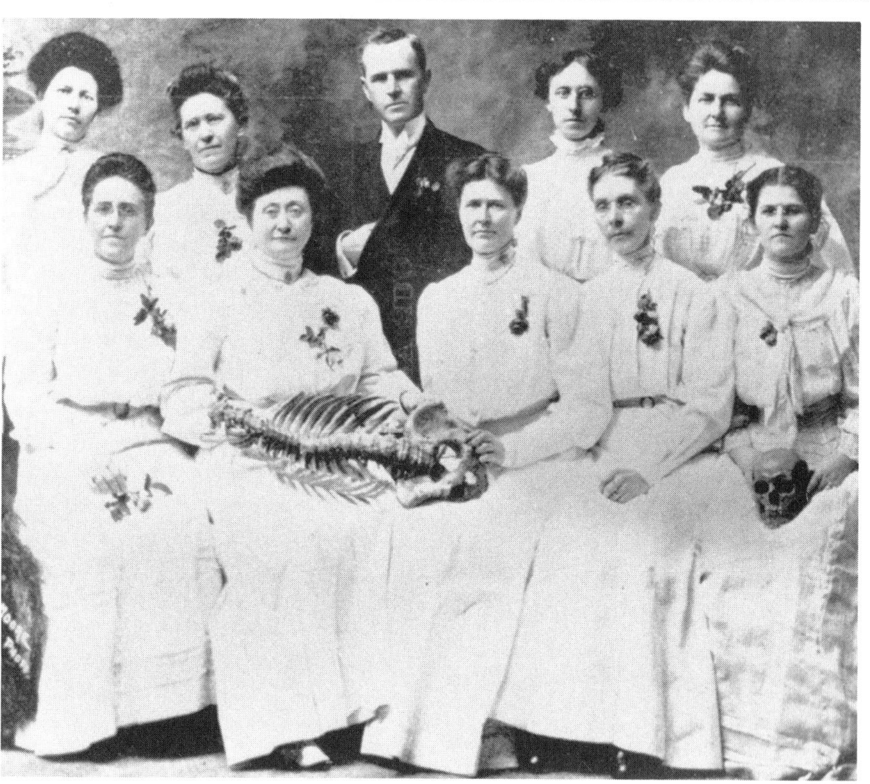

Women Members of Early A.S.O. Class

In normal cases the muscles of nature will do the work, and in about ninety-five per cent. of the cases without the aid of instruments. Dr. Wm. Smith, of Edinburg, Scotland, affirms that three times in four, in Scotland, the forceps are used, and that, as a consequence, laceration is very common. This calls for the needle as a part of the closing torture.

An Osteopath, who is master of the science, has no such results. I have lady graduates in my room who have handled such cases and have proven the efficacy of Osteopathy. They have fitted themselves so thoroughly that they are ready to handle all diseases in a philosophical and scientific manner. They now realize that medicine and midwifery are very uncertain in their results.

In closing allow me to say that I believe if I had five hundred brainy lady diplomates, all would get work and be enabled to make a comfortable living. My school opens October 1, 1895. For information in regard to it, address H. E. Patterson, Secretary, Kirksville, Mo.

A. T. STILL.

August, 1895

SCRAPS OF THE NEW PHILOSOPHY.

BY A. T. STILL.

Since I began to study man as an engine—and especially during the twenty-one years devoted entirely to Osteopathy—my experiences under the tutorship of Nature have been much more satisfying and complete than were the limited schools in which I had formerly been a student. I found that God had made but one law for life and health, and that all law governing man and beast was the everlasting, unchangeable edict of an uncompromising mind. This immutable law of health requires all animals to follow and obey the demands of hunger, thirst, rest, sleep, motion and knowledge, and to keep and maintain the machinery of life as prepared by Nature for life's journey in perfect order and adjustment. God knew full well how to build all parts of the superstructure designed by himself for the tenant soul, and he provided native forces that, unimpeded, will keep man or beast ready for duty during the entire time for which the machine was constructed.

***

A man has good or bad luck—just as he makes it. He is the arbiter of all that comes or goes his way. An imitator is a failure at all times. To succeed as an imitator your work must be the same as that of the original. Therefore you must use your own way even though you adopt the same profession of he who is successful. Borrow no man's brains—they will wither away in your keeping, and you will lose the use of your own natural powers. If often done, you will neither have courage nor manly judgment. Be kind to your own gifts. God sized you up; cultivate your talents or you fail.

***

In Kansas during the hot summer of '74, when I began to show my dislike for drugs I gave as my reason for doubting the efficacy of medicine as a science, that too many deaths occurred under its administration. Infants, youths and middle-aged of both sexes were swept away ruthlessly when medicine had done its best to succor. I believed God made us for a purpose, and wanted us to live to an old age, and so I sought higher for instructions. I did not believe our young and loved ones were born to enrich the earth with their youth and beauty. At one time sickness struck my household a fearful blow, and in spite of the generalship of the best physicians, it laid low the forms of four of my loved ones. Then came the preachers to tell me that this was brought about by the mysterious providence of God. I had then, as I have now, a kindly feeling for preachers, but I did not believe God wanted the preaching of funerals to be necessary until the machinery of life was well nigh worn out. I felt then, as now, that God made all things for good and long use before storing them in the barns as superannuated machinery.

Nor do I think I am the only only one who so believes. Ask any of the ministers who have stood over the pale, lifeless forms of the dead trying to speak words of comfort to the living if questions and doubts ever entered their minds. At such times, friends, have your thoughts not been like this: "Have these lifeless bodies lived out their time or does God make a human being and endow him with hope, beauty and all that is lovely just to feed the ground with tender flesh?" No, no, destruction is not the wish of God. Such results arise from the fact that mankind has not a true knowledge of the channels of the river of life, and by passing its ruffles wrecks occur.

August, 1895

Frauds and Pretenders.

At an early day I expect to visit the capitol, principal cities and many lesser towns of the State, for the purpose of giving the people reliable information on the new science. We are aware that scoundrels and imitators are in the field, and the next issue of the JOURNAL will contain a list of those who are graduates and competent Osteopaths. If in doubt regarding the genuineness of any one who pretends to practice Osteopathy, address the Secretary at Kirksville, who will give you any desired information.

A. T. STILL.

August, 1895

A REQUEST.

We are working to obtain as complete a record as may be possible, of the results secured by Osteopathy in combatting disease and affliction, and ask all who have been treated in the past to write statements of their cases, giving their condition before treatment, the time treated, and the results. We ask all of our friends to help us to reach many patients of former years of whom we have no record. We will not publish any statement without being requested to do so by the person making it.

A. T. STILL.

December, 1895

IMPORTANT TO PATIENTS.

All patients who come here for treatment MUST abstain from the use of intoxicating liquors of every kind while under our care. We do not wish to treat habitual whiskey tubs.

This rule must be strictly obeyed by all patients, and those who feel that they cannot conform to it had better stay away.

We have no counselmen on the street. Patients should become acquainted with the regulations through the secretary, and obey them to the letter for our mutual good.

A. T. STILL.

December, 1895

PROSPECTUS OF A. S. O. FOR 1894 BEGINNING OCT. 1, 1895.

QUALIFICATIONS REQUIRED OF STUDENTS ON ENTRY TO THE CLASS.

Age—No student will be admitted under 18 or over 45 years of age unless by special order of the Trustees. We are not seeking non-age or dotage but good sound material for making creditable Osteopaths. Experience has taught us that after the age of 45 has been reached there is little chance of making a good reasoner in this science,

Education—A good English education or at least a thorough knowledge of business branches will be required.

Character—All applicants for admission must give satisfactory proof to the board that they are of good moral character and total abstainers from drugs or liquors of an intoxicating nature. We will be very exacting on this point as we want no material to be worked up into sots.

A. T. STILL.

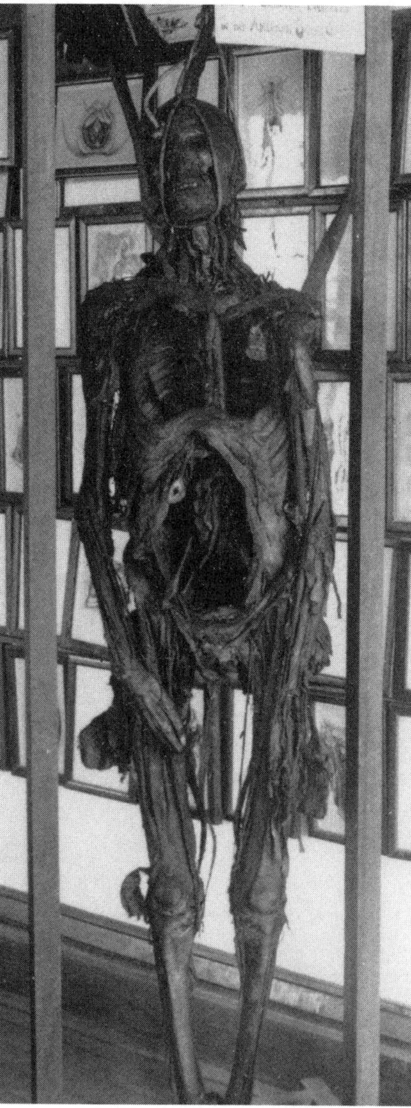

Mike, First Cadaver at A.S.O.

Notice.

All parties keeping or desiring to keep Infirmary boarders will please hand in their cards for publication in the next JOURNAL which will be issued soon. We want to publish a list of all reputable boarding places for the guidance of patients.

A. T. STILL.

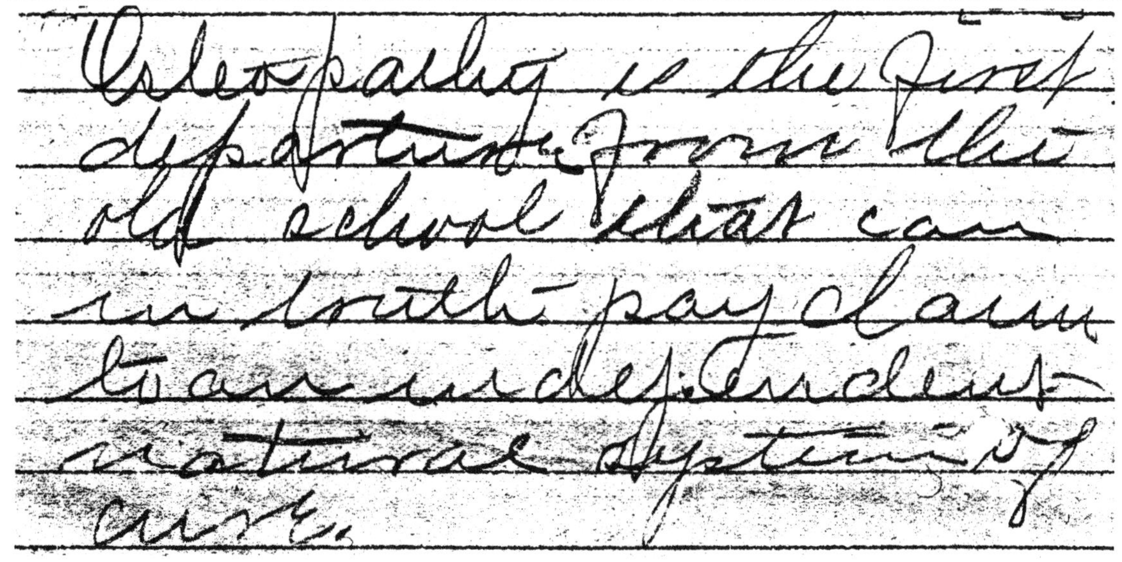

Osteopathy is the first departure from the old school that can in truth pay claim to an independent natural system of cure.

December, 1895

ANNUAL ADDRESS.

Dr. A. T. Still, President and Founder, Talks to the Operators, Students and Patients.

To the Students, Operators and Patients of the American School of Osteopathy:

Our School is now beginning to talk like a grown man, and home is no longer the only place our science spends its days. Even the crowned heads of Europe have paused to inquire about the "heads that wear crowns greater than their own."

From Kansas in 1874, a child entered the field with a sling, a muscle and a bone. It cried aloud; its mouth was wide, its throat was deep and its lungs strong. It loved its mother (nature) and kissed her as only a child that loves its mother can kiss. She said: "My son, go on that boat; it is the Ironclad of Truth; a fight is ahead and you are under marching orders. You will have to pass under the heaviest mounted forts, you will be in seas full of torpedoes, and will have great and small shot fired at your boat. On land geese will hiss at you, and from their dark roosts, old and musty owls will hoot at you. Even governors will be hired to bray at you. The press will look wise for a time and say "amen, good Lord, good Devil! let me ride on that boat if it has plenty of cash." You will pass all these things on your journey; but they will only prove to you that your boat is good and strong. On the ocean it will split the surging waves and on land it is a locomotive engine that makes its own tracks, tries all rails and never fails to be on time. It loads at the great tank of truth and dispenses the water of life to all who may be thirsty—not for money nor vain glory, but for a drop of the yeast and oil of reason that will raise the machinery of mind high enough to see the light house of the city of Philosophy, the green pastures of the Infinite, and confidence in the truth of all truths, which defy and defend one truth by all other truths.

In my report of '94, I gave you some history of the growth of the science during the preceding year; and was pleased to report the progress made by the school, which, although taught in a bungling manner with only a small dwelling for class rooms, made very satisfactory results. So great was the demand for Osteopathy that we were compelled to teach even against great odds. But I am pleased to report the work now up to the very highest standard both in anatomy and clinics. Our house is admirably suited to the work, and equipped with every modern convenience. In place of the old crowded dwelling rooms, we now have a recitation room 50x36, with seating capacity of 300, sixteen of the most complete and comfortable rooms for treating the afflicted, large waiting rooms for ladies and gentlemen. A look through the building will convince anyone that it is a model of comfort from base to dome.

Our graduates of this year are bound to be of very superior qualifications, as they have had all the advantages money and experience can provide.

It has taken very little beer to run our school during the past year. We have had but two or three parched tongues to cool; and will never have another, as our treatment now is to kick out on first drunk. Not even a "moderate drinker" will be tolerated in our class to disgrace our school and science. If the Lord will forgive me for the "swigs" who are now out claiming to be Osteopaths, I will never allow another whom I even suspicion to go out with my name on his papers. I am happy to say if there have been any drunks among students during the past year I have not heard of them.

In concluding I wish to make personal mention of our efficient corps of assistants, to whom is due not a little of the praise for our success of the past year:

Our Secretary, Dr. H. E. Patterson, who is a graduate with the highest honors of our School has been constantly at his post. The business of his laborious department has been conducted in the most thorough and perfect manner.

Dr. C. E. Still, examiner in chief and instructor in the Philosophy, stands at the front with high honors and many scalps of victory dangling from his belt.

Mrs. H. E. Patterson, chief instructor of Osteopathy in the ladies department, is a smiling success, with a head full of useful knowledge which is all devoted to the cause. She is entitled to the love and esteem of the whole institution "in bushels—not in mole skins full."

Dr. Sam'l Landes, a fully qualified diplomate, is one of our very best operators. He does not smile much, but if you enter his room with an ache or pain, he will make you smile if not shout; for he will wipe your weeping eyes with the handkerchief of ease.

I cannot refrain from mentioning our noble senior class, who will all receive their diplomas in the early months of '96. Male and female, the adjective "good" applies to all of them.

I will also speak of the junior class of thirty pupils. Place yourself in front of them, look them square in the face; and if you do not see good hard sense predominant everywhere, I will give you two weeks holidays.

Even John Colbert, our faithful janitor and his wife, our matron, are the pick of the flock.

I think by all the rules of prophecy, I am safe in saying that the future of Osteopathy will be all the most sanguine could ask. It now has a prominent place in the literature of Europe and North America. It has made man study the laws of life as found in the mechanism of his own person as he never studied before. It is our hope of civilization, builded on the rock of life.

In closing these remarks we must not forget

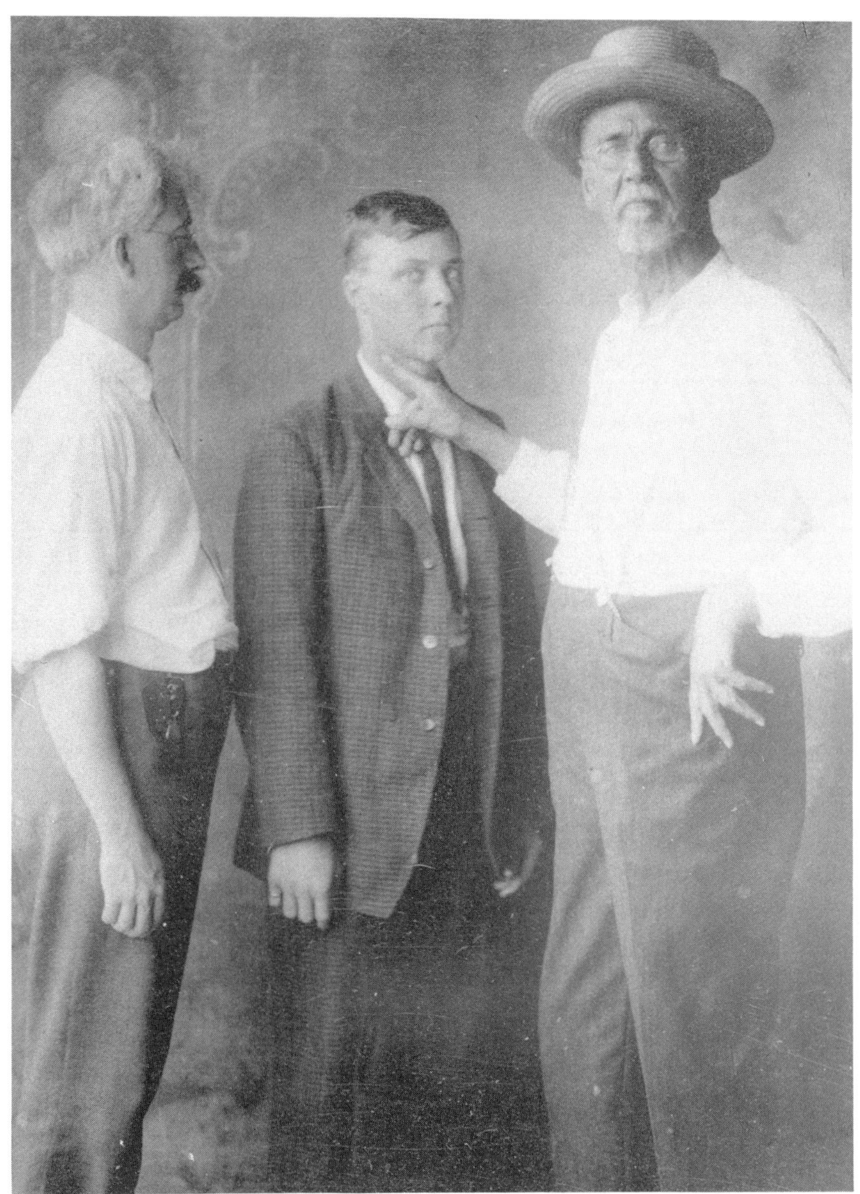

A. T. Still, *right,* with James Waddell Lloyd, *left,* and unknown patient, *center*

our absent friends—those who have been associated with us in our work here. Although scattered far and wide, we hope the good news will continue to come that they are still fighting under the flag of Osteopathy, and will keep it pure and unspotted.

December, 1895

THE CITY OF KIRKSVILLE.

One of the Prettiest, Healthiest and Thriftiest Towns in North Missouri.

Kirksville, the home of Osteopathy, is one of the prettiest, healthiest, and thriftiest little cities in Missouri. It is located on the Wabash railway, 205 miles north of St. Louis, and on the Q. O. & K. C. route, 70 miles west of Quincy. It now has a population of about 6,000 and is growing every day.

The city is clean and healthy. It was originally laid out upon an open plain, but its thoroughfares now penetrate a grove of maples, many giant specimens of which bear the rings of half a century. The business portion of the city occupies a square built up solidly of two and three story bricks and extends from one to two blocks in each direction upon the side streets. The residence portion of the city extends in all directions from the square. The principal streets are well macadamized, and the city abounds in beautiful drive ways. West of Kirksville are the Chariton hills, a dense forest through which winds the Chariton river and several smaller streams, affording a most perfect drainage for the city. The hills and forest extend many miles from the city limits, and abound in pleasant retreats for those who enjoy an occasional day in the woods.

Kirksville, while an old town, is just now enjoying a very prosperous second growth. Since the announcement by Dr. Still of the discovery of Osteopathy and the founding of his Infirmary, the population of the city has about doubled, and a vacant house would be almost a curiosity. During the last three years the city has built 4½ miles of macadamized streets, 20 miles of granitoid and brick sidewalks, put in a first-class system of water-works, a telephone system, and grown from a third-class to a second-class international money order postoffice. It has six schools, including the First District State Normal, the Kirksville Mercantile College, and two public school buildings second to none in North Missouri.

The First District State Normal is known as one of the foremost educational institutions in Missouri. It was established here twenty-five years ago, and has annually from 600 to 700 students. The Normal building is the property of the state, and was erected at a cost of nearly $200,000.

The Mercantile College is open all the year round and is a credit to the city. The Richard Wagner Conservatory of Music and Languages is a recent addition to Kirksville's educational institutions.

There are eleven churches and no saloons in the city. The society and morals are of the highest order.

Kirksville is a city of pretty homes, and a busy, contented people—an admirable and interesting resort for invalids.

In addition to its other attractions, Kirksville has a long list of business advantages, which home-seekers and capitalists should investigate. Seven coal mines are operated in the county, and good bituminous coal is delivered in the city at $1.55 a ton. Among other industries, Kirksville has a wagon and carriage factory, handle factory, barrel factory, 3 brick factories —dry pressed, paving and building—vinegar and cider factory, fruit evaporator, 2 steam planing mills, 2 steam laundries, 1 candy factory, marble and granite works, soda pop factory, foundry and stove works.

December, 1895

OSTEOPATHIC OBSTETRICS.

I have now partly written and will soon have completed a full treatise on Obstetrics. It will be ready for the printer early in the spring. It is Osteopathic from start to finish; and by the methods clearly set forth in its pages the "seasons of torture" will be forced to stand aside. The book will easily go into your vest pocket.

A. T. Still.

Hog Congress.

Evidently the past two years ought to be denominated the "Hog Era" in American politics. The Fifty-Third congress is notable for having tried to hog everything in sight. In the last annual report of the clerk of the House, revealed the fact that seven-eighths of the members of that celebrated body hogged the hundred dollars a month allowed them for clerk-hire, and put it down in their breeches pocket through a system of blood relationship. Taking it all in all it ought to go down in history as the "Hog Congress," for the title befits it better than any other.—St. Joe Herald.

February, 1896

Dr. Still's Address.

[Extracts from an anniversary address delivered by Dr. Andrew T. Still, in Memorial Hall Jan. 10, 1895.]

OSTEOPATHY today in a greater or less degree is the subject for discussion in all North America, in all English speaking nations, and all nations that speak their own tongue as intelligent people. When Europe thinks she has discovered a new remedy for disease—say of the lungs, brain, or any other part of the human body—all North America knows it just as quick as scientific electricity can bring the news to us. When North America has made a discovery the European nations know all about its merits because we are of their blood. And to be an Englishman, a German, Scotchman, Frenchman, or of any other educated nation, means intellectual progress is looked for. It may be that the whole masses are not Galileos, Washingtons nor Lincolns, but now and then a Fulton, a Clay, a Grant, an Edison arises, or some unchained mind moves against tradition with unerring philosophy.

It is our fortune at this time to raise our heads above the muddy water far enough to have a glimpse of a law that we choose to call the Divine Law. That law we use in healing. We have traced it by reason, by philosophy, under the microscope, in the light and in the dark; and we hear a response. That response is so intelligent, its answer is so correct that a man is forced to believe there is knowledge behind it. We have houses much larger than this all over the civilized world. People congregate there every seventh day in the week for some purpose. Ask them what they are collecting there every Sabbath for. Their answer is, "To speak of or give a token of respect to the Creator of all things, that Intelligence commonly known as God."

Now since I have given you the size of Osteopathy at the present day on the globe, I will give you a contrast. If I am a speaker at all I want to prove it by comparison. I want to show you just how large Osteopathy was in the world twenty-two years ago. One man who has the reputation of being the finest mechanic, possibly in the whole State of Missouri, said to me then, "I wish you would go and see my wife." I went with the gentleman. I felt very timid, because I didn't know how little sense he had, nor how much. I had seen a glimpse of what I considered the very candle of God himself, lighted and sustained by the oil of reason.

The speaker said: "Now, Mr. Harris if you will arise I will show this people just the size of Osteopathy then." (Mr. Harris appeared on the platform.) If you examine this man, and are any philosopher at all, you will see in him a mechanic. And if you are a doubting Thomas, just take your old shot gun to him, and he will put it in order and prove his skill. This is the gentleman who first said, "Plant that truth right here." He was Osteopathy's advocate in Kirksville. I said, after a long conversation with him,

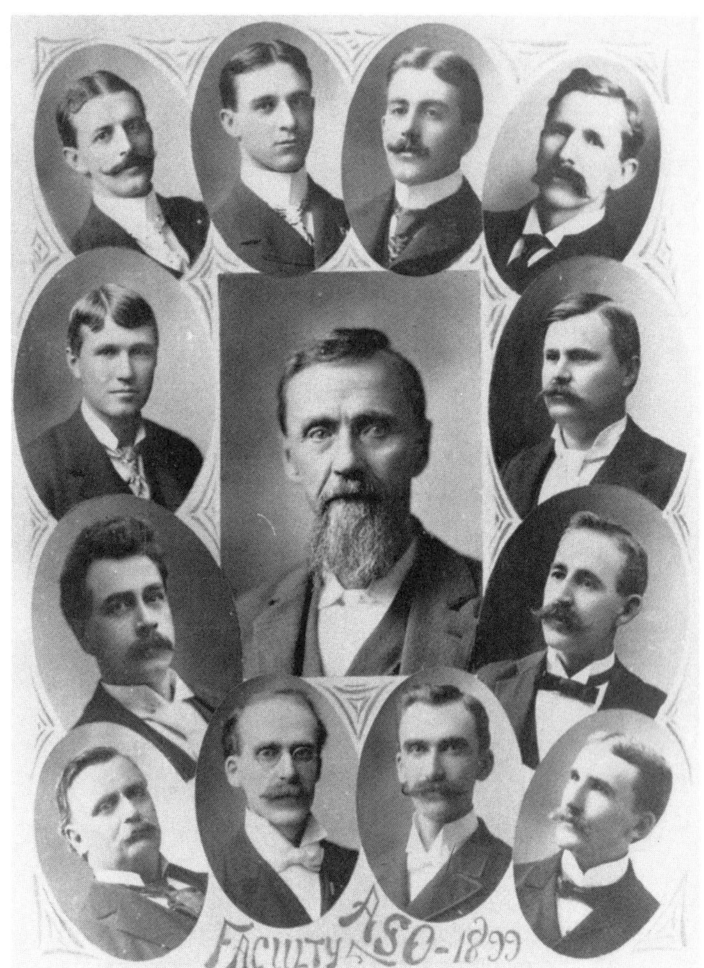

"Mr. Harris, let me ask you a question: Why is it, in your judgment that people are so loathe to believe a truth?" He said, "Dr. Still, in my opinion a man dreads that which he doesn't understand." That was the answer twenty-two years ago, and that is the reason why Osteopathy is not accepted by the masses and is not adopted by every man and woman of intelligence today. A man dreads to give up his old boots for fear the new ones will pinch his feet. We have gone on from generation to generation imitating the habits of our ancestors.

I am as independent as a wolf when he knows the dog got the strychnine. The reason why I am independent is that when I see the deltoid muscle that God himself has placed on your shoulder formed and attached as it is and working as it does with his intelligence, I feel able through Osteopathy to look at Saturn as a small corpuscle of blood in the body of the great universe. When I look at the earth, and the moon, and take the solar system, I find that the Directing mind has numbered every corpuscle in the solar system, and each one of them comes on time—no mistakes.

Whenever you see a man who is afraid of a comet, you find a man who is ignorant on that very point. Do you suppose God himself is going to allow one of his planets to get drunk and butt its brains out against this earth? Hasn't he counted the space for every planet to sail in? Are we following the old Grecian ideas of five thousand years ago—that the sun is making noodle soup out of comets for its supper? I want to tell you that I worship a respectable, intelligent and mathematical God. He knows whether the earth is going too fast or not. He didn't ask your papers to publish that he had better push the earth a little faster to let that comet go by. None of his children disobey, get drunk or lose their minds. I make this assertion from the confidence I have in the absolute mathematical power of the Universal Architect. I have the same confidence in His exactness and ability to make, arm and equip the human machine so that it will run from the cradle to the grave. He armed and equipped it with every thing necessary for the whole journey of life—to man three score and ten years.

The minister said, "And it pleased God to take the dear little child—." It didn't do any such thing. It pleases God when he makes the child that it dies in the service he made him for. When he creates a man he doesn't create him to fertilize the ground when he is a babe. He made him to live on and on, and gave him sense enough to take care of himself if he will use it well.

We take up Osteopathy. How old is it? Give me the age of God and I will give you the age of Osteopathy. It is the law of mind, matter and motion.

When four of my family were attacked with that dreaded disease, cerebro spinal meningitis, I called in four of the most learned M. D.'s of the land, gave them full power to fight the enemy as they chose; to use any and every means to capture the enemy's flag and put him to open shame. When the M. D.'s gave the command to "charge," I looked to see the white flag run up, but the smoke was dense, and the cannons ceased to fire on both sides. When the smoke cleared away the enemy had all our flags and all the children captives; and the doctors joined the procession of mourners, and said: "Death is the rule and recovery the exception."

At the close of that memorable combat between sickness and health, life and death, I gave to the generals of drugs a belt of my purest love. If ever men fought honestly and earnestly 'till all fell into the ditches, I believe they did. They wept not as Alexander did, that he had conquered all and had no more to do; but they had met an enemy whose steel was far superior to any they had ever met before. With me they wept, and said, "We have no steel worthy of this or any great or small engagements."

From that hour until the present time, I have seen the ability of Nature to do her work, if we do our part in conformity with the laws of life.

Since we stacked arms to the relentless weapons of disease, a new thought has been my companion for years, by day and by night, and has been after this manner: That disease is the culmination of effect, and its cause lies in the choice of birth. If to be a child of misery, it sought conception from the womb of the sensory nerves; if to be of great stupidity, its conception and birth must be of the motor nerves. The first child is Neuralgia of all forms, and cries with pain. The second child is Paralysis of all forms; it is stupidity and death. To produce the death of either child, you must disgorge the womb before motion developes the child to maturity; if not it may be a deadly enemy to life and motion. All of which you diplomates of Osteopathy know full well how to do, and give Nature the ascendency.

February, 1896

THE FIGHT FOR TRUTH.

Osteopathy's Battle Against Legalized Ignorance and Stupidity.

Written by "Pap."

The JOURNAL is not enrolled under the banner of a theologian. It is now traveling over the plains and mountains as an explorer, and will report only the truth, and never that until it finds the fact standing right behind the truth, as its endorser.

As an explorer the JOURNAL is now ready to report that much of the richest bottom land which is capable of the highest cultivation, now stands open, while vast extended plains lie spread out before us without even the tent of the squatter soverign to be seen. This vast country has not yet been surveyed, no corner stones are set, the range lines have not been run, and there is no land office opened; but upon this boundless plain we raise and throw to the breezes the banner of Osteopathy. In close range, and directly in view of the most ordinary field glass, stands the Mountain of Reason, rolling down in our presence the greatest nuggets of gold that the human mind ever saw, rolling down from the very bosom of God himself. All this fertility we believe is intended for the human race and the benefit of man. With the power of production found in this soil, with the beauteous scenery and the mountain heights, and in every stone, you will find the exactness with which the Divine Mind constructs.

I see nations climbing up and falling, and rising up and climbing again, to attain that height which would enable them to have a glimpse and an intimate acquaintance with that superstructure that stands upon the highest pinnacle. which superstructure has been explored to a limited extent by only a very few. That superstructure is the master-work of God himself, and its name is man. Ten thousand rooms of this temple have never been explored by any human intelligence; neither can it be explored without a perfect knowledge of anatomy—an acquaintance with all the parts and principles of the machinery of life.

Under this banner we have enlisted. Under it we expect to march, and to go into a fight that will cover more territory than was covered by Alexander, Napoleon, Grant, Lee and Blucher; and to conquer by facts a greater physical enemy than has been heretofore conquered by the world's greatest generals; waging a contest of greater moment to the human race than any human effort ever put forth for the establishment of a political, religious, or scientific principle.

Not like children do we expect to pay attention to the Howitsers of vulgarity that are loaded to the very muzzle with the nightmare of habit and legalized ignorance and stupidity. We will heed not the belching forth of the many guns trained on our flag unless they are the very best of steel rifles, Gatlins, mortars, ironclads or torpedoes, all loaded or charged with the dynamite of uncompromising TRUTH itself. We have no eternity to spend in the useless effort of trying to bring men to the fountain of reason and force them to drink that which is absolutely unpalatable to them. While a man is bound with his habits and is satisfied with fishing forever without getting a nibble of truth, he can, like Bunyon, bring the four corners of his old sheet together, take up his load and toddle along. We will not debate with him; if he is satisfied, he is not the man we are looking for.

A word to the soldiers: This war has been raging hot and heavy for 22 years, and not a single soldier, from privates to generals, has received a wound from the enemy that has drawn one drop of blood, or sent a rigor of fear up or down the back or legs. Their best amunition and greatest guns when fired in our midst has never moved a muscle nor made a widow. We laugh by note, which is our music, and we desire congress to give us the full benefits of free trade, as we have more scalps for sale now than any one market is able to purchase.

Our secretary of war has reported to us that every soldier's wife and the soldier himself has more to eat and more to drink than ever before, even in the physical world, saying nothing of the fountain of love and intelligence that keeps his canteen forever running full.

In our great army of recruits we want no man or woman whose mind is so small and mental vision so dim that it cannot see victory perched upon our banner. Peace and good will to all mankind now and forever more. "PAP."

February, 1896

OSTEOPATHY DEFINED BY DR. STILL.

An Iowa Newspaper Sends a Reporter to Interview the Founder of the Science.

Des Moines Daily (Ia.) News, Feb 4th.

Some weeks ago the News sent a representative to Kirksville, Mo., to make a report on the workings of Osteopathy, a science developed after long and patient study by Dr. Andrew T. Still. The investigation was eminently satisfactory. Scores were interviewed who had gone thither hopeless invalids and in a short time found themselves either fully restored to health or on the high way to recovery. So speedily were some helped that it would seem almost miraculous, yet in every instance the methods employed were explainable on purely scientific principles.

When the venerable Dr. Still was asked how he explained his science, he answered: The world has asked the question till I am tired. The answer lies in this: "A man is a machine with over 200 bones. You can call them braces, supports, or what you please. Muscles, nerves, blood vessels and tendons are distributed all over and through this frame work. There is an engine, and pipes run from that engine to all parts of the body and from all parts blood is carried back to the place it started from by the veins or blood tubes. The force that I have described is the engine of blood fluids. Now, I will draw attention to the engine of force, the brain, which supplies all the nerves in the body. It has its motor that forces blood from the heart to all parts of the human body. There is another class and principle that conveys the exhausted blood and nutriment to the heart. Health is that condition that we are in when all of the wheels of life are in their center and move without any obstruction, great or small. Disease is the creaking of the eccentricities of any or all parts of the machinery. These facts I have proven for thirty years past."

"In all fevers," the doctor continued, "of all seasons of the year—typhus, typhoid, billious, congestive, pneumonia, flux, dysentery, mumps, measles, diptheria, whooping-cough, sore breast and tongue of the mother, milk leg—through the whole of diseases thitherto treated by drugs, successfully or unsuccessfully for twenty-five years, with or without council, I found nothing that I could say was a cure of any case or cases, had I been sworn. My family, friends and patients died, just as quick, if not quicker, with all the skill that friendship and money could rally. They died and we couldn't help it, which proved to my mind then that medicine was not a science. Every day since has proven to me that medicine is farther from a science than Uranus has ever traveled from the sun. The results that I have obtained over disease I have secured when I have handled the engine of life as an engineer handles his engine. So long as I conform to the laws governing an engine, the human locomotive obeys, just as well as any locomotive will obey its engineer when he treats it as the machinist has indicated by the form of any and all parts of the engine. If he should ignore and set aside the laws that govern an engine, that engine will stand still, and the engineer will also sit still. With this permit me abruptly to quit."

There is really no end to the testimony of the efficacy of Osteopathy, in cases of stomach, kidney and heart troubles, gall-stones, spinal affections, prostrate nerves, insomnia, rheumatism, etc. The institution is attracting people from all over the country, and many are rising up to call those blessed who administer this new science.

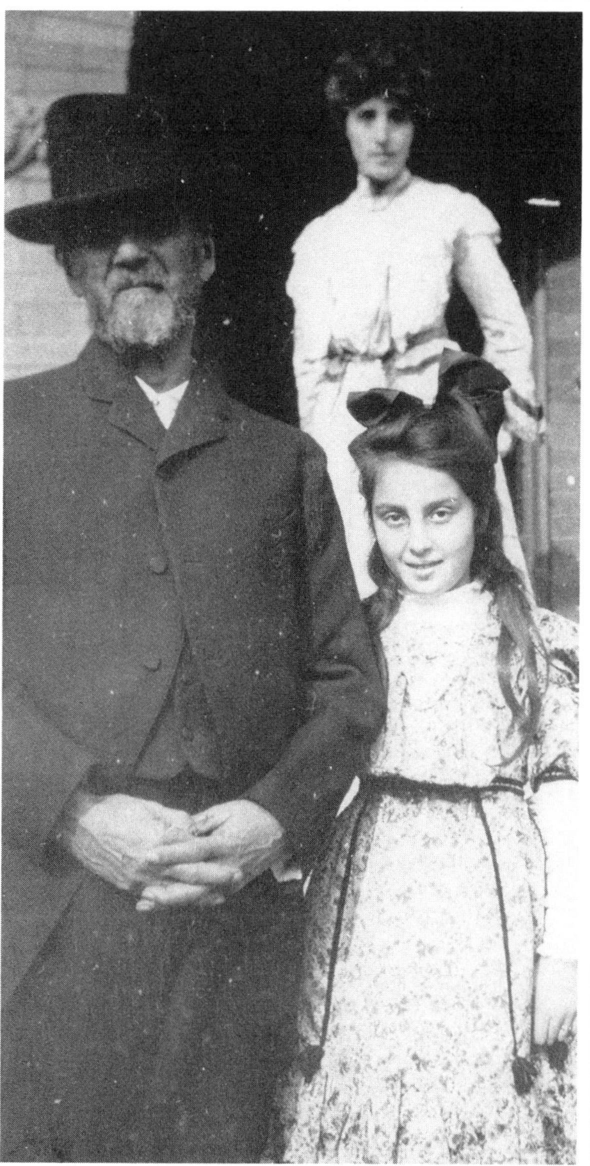

A. T. Still with two patients of the Orschel family from Chicago, 1900

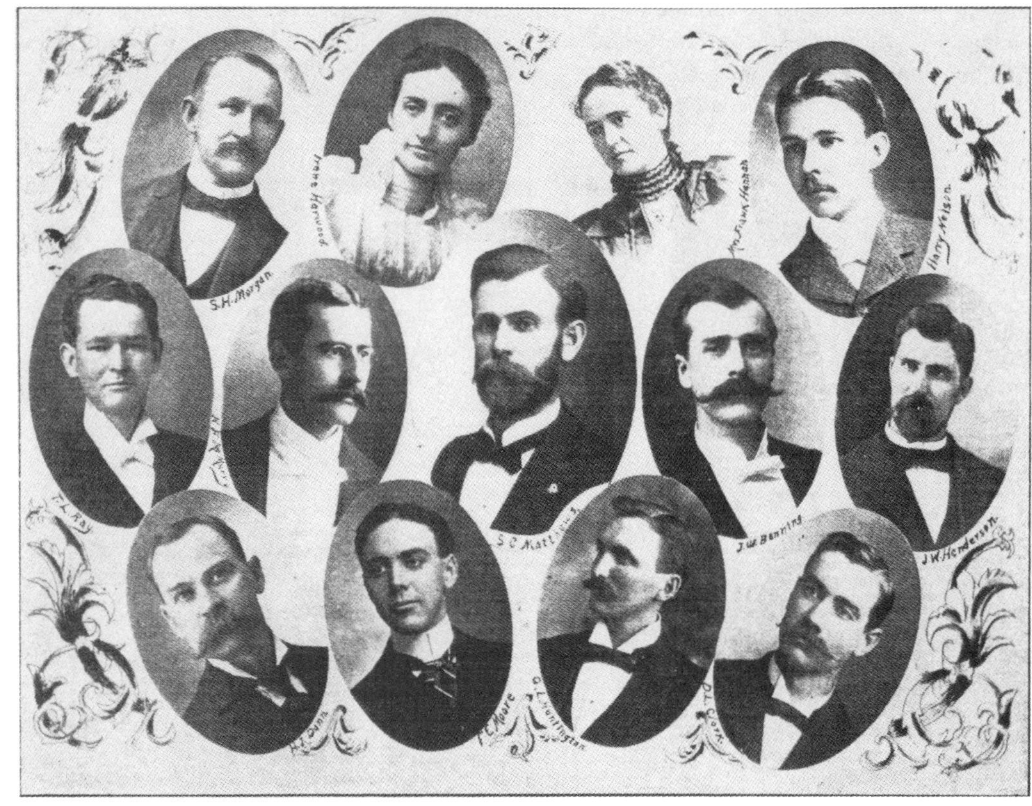

OFFICERS OF THE AMERICAN ASSOCIATION FOR THE ADVANCEMENT OF OSTEOPATHY.

1898

April, 1896

A LECTURE BY DR. A. T. STILL.

Delivered before an Audience of Students and Patients in Memorial Hall, March 12.

LADIES AND GENTLEMEN:—I am here to-night by your request. I am here to answer before the court that tries a man and gives a just decision; where each man is a juror and decides for himself; where each lady sits as a jurist, and conclusions are filed away for herself, family and all her friends. A woman can live an active life until she is forty-five or fifty years old. Then she is looked upon now as a mature woman, and her neighbors come to her for counsel; and at that period of life they can get it. She will go to church, to state houses, political and national holiday gatherings for the purpose of picking up a few crumbs of knowledge which she can bring back and impart to her children, grand-children, their husbands, neighbors and friends.

Now, allow me in the introduction of the subject of Osteopathy to tell you I am proud all over. I don't know why nature or nature's God opened one of my eyes to see a small corner of his work. Over twenty years I have stood in the courts of God as an attorney. I have questioned and cross-questioned, and directed my questions positively on any and all parts of this subject that I desired to investigate. The questions that I asked myself were about the following: if I have any mind at all capable of comprehending or solving by my force of philosophy, the great question "What is man?" You remember that I spoke then, as a man whose mouth begins in front and surrounds the whole head and connects upon the other side. That question "What is man?" covers all the questions embraced in the universe—all questions, none left, none excepted. The question itself says, "Who is God?" "What is life?" "What is death?" "What is sound?" "What is love?" "What is hatred?" What is any individual one of these wonders found in that great combination, Man? Anything left? Nothing at all. Do you find in man's make-up any principle in heaven, on earth, in mind, in matter or in motion, that is not represented by kind and quality in his make-up? You find them all there. You find the representation of the planets of heaven in man. You find the action of those heavenly bodies represented in yours. You find in minature there the mind that controls this power in motion. You find in reason that it is the result of a conclusion backed by the ability to reason, the ability known as the power of knowledge. And when the machine was constructed it was given the power of locomotion, self preservation, all the passions of all the beasts of the field, and all the aspirations of God himself. These qualities you find in man. These qualities you find in a more refined condition in woman, she being the sensitive part of the whole make-up of the human race. She is a finer principle than man.

Let me suggest to you, in the human make-up we find the motor nerves driving the blood from the heart. In association with that the sensory nerves, or a set of nerves peculiar to the veins, carrying the blood back that is carried out by the heart and by the arteries throughout the body to all its extremities, and is returned through what? Through the veins. Therefore, when you find in the make-up of man the motor, or the father principle, you will also find the other or mother part, in the return of the blood to the heart, where it is sent out again for the battle of life.

I am talking to you as though you were Osteopaths of many years' experience, many days of experimenting, and have placed your hand on the side of Christ and found the scar, and have no further doubts. I am placed in a little embarrassed condition, whether to throw a bomb-shell at you, or to just simply fire a smaller ball; or, like the Baptist preacher, fire a shot gun and hit more places. But you needn't look for a Howitzer from me tonight.

When I looked up the subject and tried to acquaint myself with the works of God, or the unknowable, as some call him, Jehovah, another class say, or as the Shawnee Indian calls him, the Great Illinoywa Tapa mala qua, which signifies the life of the living God himself. When I took up the subject first I wanted some part that my mind could comprehend. I began to study what part I would take up to begin the investigations of the truths of God, to place them down as a scientific system of facts, based upon facts themselves. What will I take? That is the question. Where will I begin? Which is the best way? Soon I found that one of my hands was enough for me all the days of my life. Take the hand of a man, the heart, the lung, or the whole combination, and how it runs is the unknowable. I began to want to be one of the Knowables.

The first discovery that I made was this: every single individual stroke that he made came to me as the unknowable. The stroke of death —what do you know about this? I don't know anything. Therefore, it is unknowable. I begin to study and experiment. By accident I got started. I removed growths from the human neck, called goitre. That goitre disappeared in a few hours. The philosophy to me was doubtful or unknowable. A great deal of it is yet. Soon I tried flux. It stopped. I thought I commanded it to stop, and it did stop. I made a certain move there, and it stopped itself, and that law is absolutely unknowable to me yet. I found headache. What is headache? That was also to me unknowable. I found fevers; I found the reverse of that. I did not know what it was. I will show you the same question. You take hold of this incandescent as it stands now at about 80 degrees. As I turn the battery on you have then about 160 degrees. You turn it off and it is dead. We have the motor principle, or the positive, coming forward and bringing the elements necessary to life. We will destroy that—the positive, and let the mother principle take charge of it. What does she do? She clears up the rubbish in the house every morning when the man goes out. She takes the dirt out in less time than her husband brings it in. So the temperature is brought back to its original 80—a change of 80 degrees. How that result is obtained leaves me again in the unknowables.

What is electricity? I don't know anything about it. I simply can show you what it will do. In the human make-up you have one of the most absolute and thoroughly constructed systems, wired from the very ground you stand on to the top of your head. Every department has its wires and telegraph poles, and it has millions of them over your body, each and every one being just where they should be, one for the heart, one for the eye, one for the quilts that cover the eye. Old mother says, "spread a quilt there," and down goes your eyelid. There is your quilt. You see in there the mother standing. You see the philosophy of the father and mother principles of the veins and arteries. When we take up principles—we get down to nature. It is ever willing, and self-caring, self-feeding and self-protecting.

What does all this signify? Why are you making such a fuss? Why are you talking about those divine laws? Are you going to baptize us? Are you going to pass the hat around? What do you mean by talking about those higher laws?

We have made a mistake and kept it up for a thousand years, according to history. We have tried to meet and ward off effects which we call disease by the effect of something we do not comprehend. When we are sick we take poisons, and a plenty of them; the kind and quality of poisons that are deadly in their tendency, and not only that but they are durable. It is said that a dose of sulphur taken to-day is found by analysis in the body sixty days afterwards. How long do their effects last? They may stay sixty or seventy years. When I was a boy I had some poison put in my arm. It made a goose bump, and it got bigger than the goose itself; and they called that vaccination. How long has that been in my body. It has been there through several sieges of small-pox; therefore the effect is endless. When I was about fourteen years old I was ptyalized. Most persons further south know what that signifies. I took several doses of calomel. It loosened my teeth. To-day I am using part of a set of store teeth because I lived in a day and generation when people had no more intelligence than to make cinnabar of my jaw bone.

I see the most of you here are strangers, and a great many would like me to get down to minutia. What is your Osteopathy good for? It has proven itself good to stop croup. Put that on your thumb. In fevers, in measles, never loses a case of flux. When a patient is dead we don't treat him. Take it in any reasonable time, in any case of flux, and it has proven itself absolutely certain. It has not lost a case of diphtheria when it commenced within a few hours of its beginning. It has never lost a single case of whooping cough. Neither has it wrestled with it over three days. Is that of any account to you people who sit up eight or ten weeks watching your children whoop and cough? I believe it has absolute control over the nervous system of the lungs, and if there is no pocket hole made in them, I believe the law is absolute, because it opens the veins carrying the refuse away, and the arteries build it up again, and your cough stops. Headache —that is very little bother to you people that have it just two or three days at a time, and throw up everything you see or hear of. Who but an Osteopath can tell you what a head ache is? "Mr. Dunglison, will you please explain to the people what head ache is?" "Headache is a peculiar condition, either with cold or hot temperature of the head, with an increased or diminished flow of blood. I would suggest a copious vomit." Here is your definition of headache by Dunglison. How much wiser are you now? Go to an Osteopath, "What makes that brain hurt." He will answer you, "What makes a pig squeal, a calf bawl, or a child cry when it is hungry?" You have a cold condition of the head. The cerebral arteries are not supplying the brain with nutriment. Therefore, it gets very hungry, and miserably hungry too. When the veins, backed by the motor nerves, or those that carry the circulation around, circulation of the blood, then they are obstructed; pain follows. There is your stagnation—your headache.

"Dr. Sullivan, you have been a plumber for many years; suppose you would find that at some point the water was not conducted on to the next wash bowl. You would say there was a break or dent in the pipe; wouldn't you? How would you like it if I were to call you up and say, Sullivan, what is the matter with the pipe, it won't let the water pass through; I can't get any water out of it?" If you would say, and stand back with the dignity of a man, "There is something peculiarly wrong. It is probably organic disease of the valves of the heart." However, I would think that an injection of morphine possibly at that time would be of some benefit. That is about the sense that you are answered with when you pay your money and ask the doctor for advice.

The finer the plumber the better he is prepared to judge of the business. So it is with the Osteopath. Let me ask you one thing more, Dr. Sullivan. "Isn't Osteopathy, after years acquaintance with both, is it not a system parallel and high above and on the same principle as the plumber's work?" "Yes, sir."

Nature's God, in constructing that house, proved himself to be the finest plumber known by any person, or by any philosopher. What do you think of it? Are the wires all in place and ready to do their duty? I know what your answer will be. You will say, if you will look you will find every nerve there; you will find nerves, veins and arteries between each and every rib, between each bone of the back. You will find that every bone that is in the human body has a bump to hold up some muscle. You will find every muscle is provided with veins, arteries and nerves. You will find there a cause for a man to reason, that when they are in their normal position, and that a Normal God has declared it is in proper condition for health.

I have been called a crank. Who cares for such names as that? I have been called an ungodly fellow. Who cares for that? I can give you two names where you give me one. I am a long-tongued Scotchman, born with an Irishman's mouth, and I think I have something of an average eye of observation. I have observed for thirty years the workings of a long protected system of stupendous, unpardonable ignorance, criminal ignorance, called Allopathy, Homeopathy, and eclecticism, etc., any and all of them that use drugs, without exception. Why are they criminal? Instance: When I was absent from home one of my children was attacked with fever. An Allopath came in with medicine. He believed in tonics, sedatives, and many other little things. What does the eclectic do? He believes in his purgatives, his sweats, his pukes and his burns; he believes in his hypodermic syringe. He uses it; so does the Homeopath. The Allopath comes in and says, "I believe in both of them, only a little more heroically," being the highest of the trinity of experimenters. I want to tell you that I mean all of that, with no qualifications. I mean it unreservedly! When I came back my twelve year old boy was taking quinine and whiskey. I asked him, "What is that you have in your hand?" "O, a little quinine." "What is in that bottle?" "A little whiskey; I am going to make a little quinine-whiskey." How long does it take that boy to learn that the whiskey tastes better without the quinine? Who learned him to take whiskey? Who started that shower of water from his mother's eyes? That criminal who prescribed that first drink of whiskey.

I call it criminal in any man. You can get drunk and call it holy if you want to.

Here comes up colic. A young fellow goes to see his girl. He is too lazy to make the fire for his mother to fill him up once a week. And he goes out and his Polly fills him up with pie and cake. He comes home with colic. Goes to the pill doctor, and he pops the syringe into the region of the solar-gastric nerve—should I have said pneumogastric? That makes him easy. He fills up with crab apples next time, and he needs another hypodermic. The first you know he uses his own syringe—you see them out in San Francisco, and all of America. "Come along, Tom, let's go and punch our arms." They are not going to be worked in that way anymore, and pay for it. Those hypodermic syringes are almost as common as grasshoppers when you go west or east. What are we tending to? I saw some dogs fifty years ago, and I never forgot those dogs. They were above a mill dam and the water was running very fast, and their tails kept going down, down, down. A man said, "Look at those d—— dogs." Well, I thought if they were not d——they soon would be, and it was but a second until they were over the dam, and were dead dogs. That shows if they try to swim across the current so close to the dam, something happens to the dogs. Something happens to your boy—something happens to your husband.

An Osteopath walks out single handed and alone. And what does he place his confidence in? First, on his confidence in the intelligence and immutibility of God himself, that the strokes of the smoothing planes of God, the steam boilers, constructed by the divine being and placed in man here, when unobstructed, act in harmony. What is harmony but health? It takes perfect harmony of every nerve, vein and artery in all parts of the body. Every muscle that moves has something to make it go. Instance, what is it that constructs the heart that pushes the blood to all parts of the body? Why, an Osteopath will tell you it is the system of coronary arteries, which he must know before he treats your hearts.

When I look upon the work of nature it doesn't work for a dollar and a half a day; I see only for truth. God himself takes as his pay for labor and time, truth and truth only. If it takes him a million years to maka a stone as large as a bean, the time and labor are freely given and the work honestly done. No persuasion whatever will cause that mechanic to swerve from the line of exactness in any case. Therefore, I can trust the principles that I believe are found in the human body, all inside of the skin. I find what is necessary for the health, comfort and happiness of man, the passions, and all else. Nothing is needed but plain ordinary nourishment. We do find all the machinery, qualities and principles that the divine mind intended should be in man for life and all his comforts. Therefore, let me work with that body, from the brain to the foot. It is all finished work, and is trustworthy in all its parts.

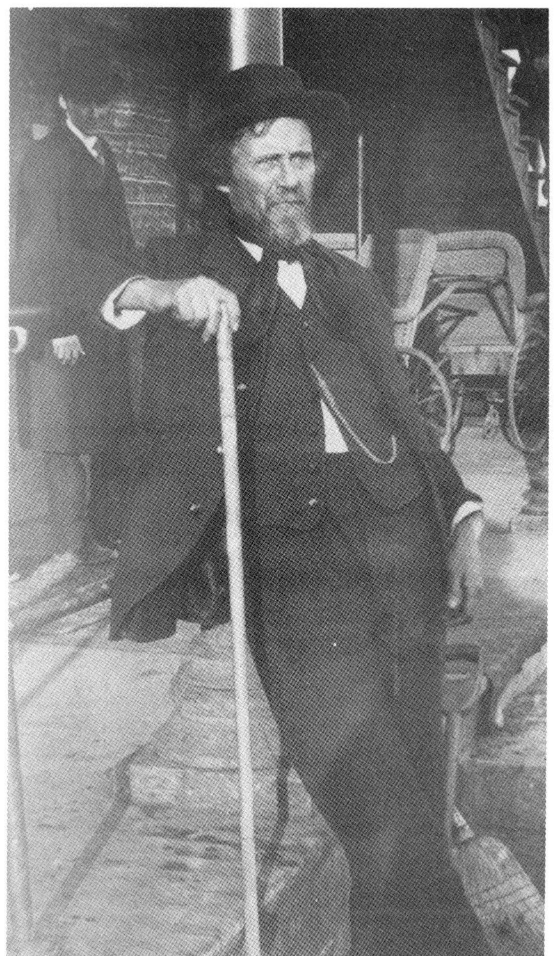

A. T. Still in front of Infirmary

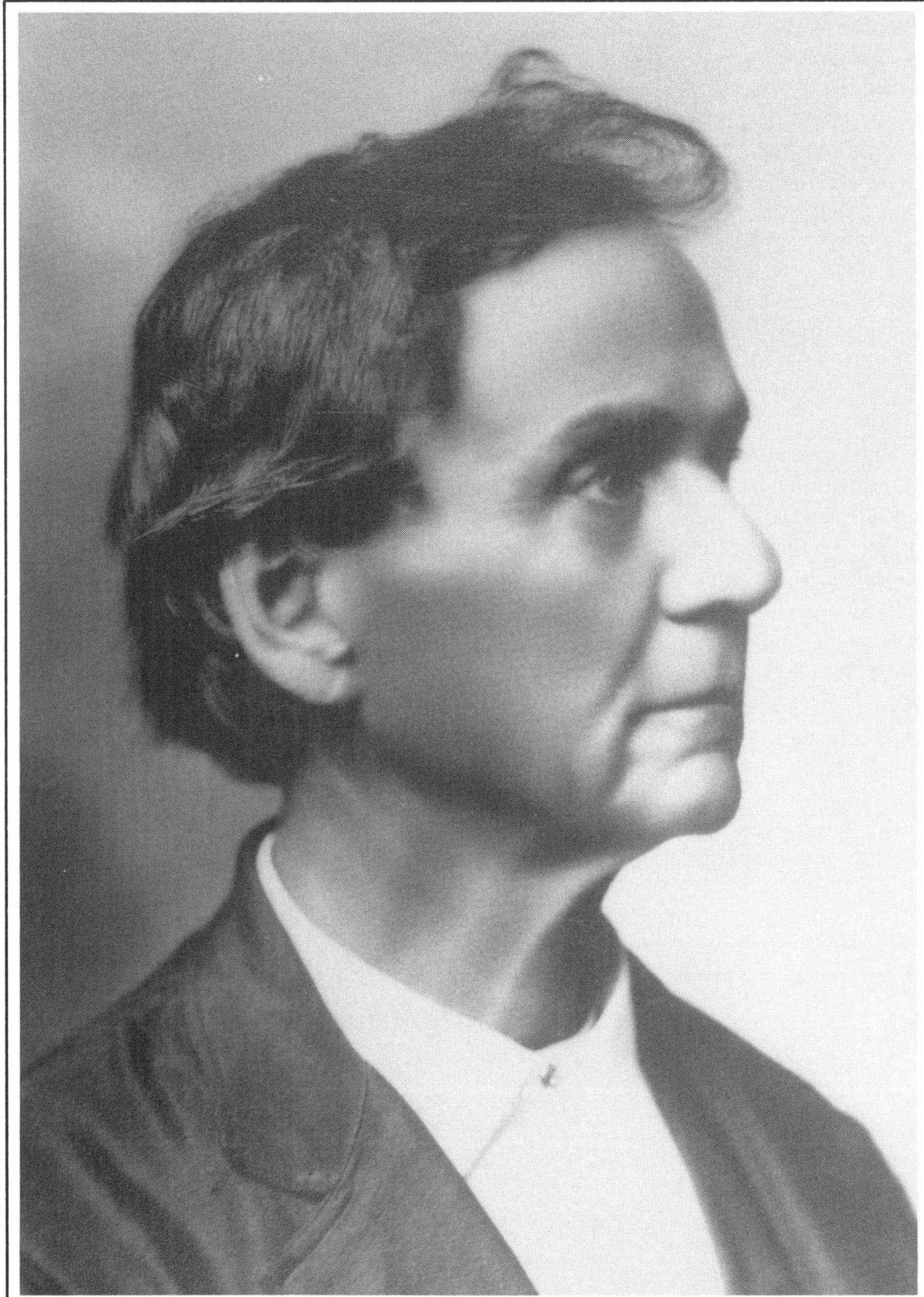

Many thought A. T. Still bore a striking resemblance to Abraham Lincoln; thus the photo of Still minus his beard, c. 1900.

April, 1896

OSTEOPATHIC NOTES.

BY DR. A. T. STILL.

Each student, before entering our school, must show that he is duly sober. We will not countenance alcoholic drinks in any form. Each has entered our school on these conditions. The school will do all it can to advance sober diplomats who stand on Osteopathy alone. They must not be tied to any M. D.'s dog collar. Remember that this school was chartered October 30, 1894, under the laws and seal of the great State of Missouri. The grade you have earned by hard study is on the face of your diploma. You know your business. What use have you for a drug doctor with you, when he knows nothing of Osteopathy at all? He is hungry and tired and wants to ride a mule a few miles till he gets out of the mud. Then he kicks the good old donkey and goes along. Keep sober and your names will not appear in the whiskey columns of the JOURNAL; disgrace the science and it will get there. The people must have sober Osteopaths. You have promised and we expect you to fulfil it.

* * *

With the new year we have introduced into all departments the inductive system of teaching the principles and philosophy of Osteopathy, Anatomy, Physiology, and Clinics. All our older operators know that induction is the gem of our school, and are with the class every morning. They all agree that clinics as taught now enforces anatomy on the mind beyond forgetfulness, and out of the books into their heads; which is the foundation on which one can learn Osteopathy, which means all that is meant by the word remedy.

* * *

Our school will ever fight on the line of qualification, not quantity of books or time, but with an eye to make qualified engineers of the engine equalled by none. Nature has given us the problem of life to solve, and a lifetime in which to solve it, which is the truth of life in all its parts, powers and principles in motion. The anatomy of man, with its life, laws and action, is not the anatomy of quinine, or any drug, whose anatomy has no muscle, nerve or vessel, or principle that would fill the place, or be able to perform any duty as given by the divine hand, to the least atom or place found in all the make-up of man. This school has found, in its few years' teaching, that no superficial knowledge of the anatomy of man, is able to grasp even the border fruits of the inner workings of the machinery of animal life; nor can he or she ever hope to enter the interior of the philosophy of this great law, which has been to man in all the great past, wholly unknown. It is a fact to every person of good mental balance, that the less a person knows of true anatomy, the more lavish he is of his drugs, ignorance and bigotry. If to mix drugs with the human make-up, with the great intelligence shown with its constructed parts, relations and principles in one grand and beautiful whole, is the conclusion of a philosopher, what objections could such minds be able to offer to the proposition of the great question, which is as follows:

"Mr. Philosopher, allow me to ask you, what would you think of a cross between a buzzard and an ape, between a toad and an elephant, a bee and a boaconstrictor? Do you think such an association would be compatible? Do you think it would be profitable to a man's stock, to mix fire with his hay? By the destruction would you expect life and health as a result? Let me ask you another question, Mr. Philosopher: Would you expect to strengthen your horse by putting in his flesh the wolves and vultures of destruction? If you cannot see philosophy in these questions, I am sure you cannot give a reason why any man of intelligence can afford to jeopardize the safety of his philosophy by word or deed, inwardly or outwardly, by giving any poison or poisonous substances not natural to the sustenance of human life. The results would in all reason be the ruin of the bee, buzzard and ape industry, would it not?

Now go back to the thought and object of this writing, which is written to enforce on the minds of the people that Osteopathy is a truth of Nature, put into practice. When fully understood, results follow as sure as nature's law is trustworthy, and the mind and law of God as given, is true, immutable, and ever the same. What use has a student of Osteopathy to spend one, two, or seven years in trying to learn the use and nature of drugs when he never expects to use them? What would you think of a graduate of a Mexican mule ranch, in whose school he had spent three to seven years, to learn how to lariet, saddle and ride mules and broncos, taking command of a ship with his mule knowledge? Would his knowledge of mule riding be of any use to him as a sea captain? None at all. Just so with a "D. O." He has no more use for these three or seven years wasted in drugs and poisons than the ocean captain has for seven years among the broncos, as a useful part of how to ride the bucking waves of the ocean. He can do much better without the cowboy at the head of command; he needs none of his lariets, spurs, pistols or "carahoos."

* * *

I have to report today that we are out of the woods. Columns all in line, arms and amunition all of the latest and best make; officers and men all at their posts. The fight is hot and heavy; blood runs in great rivers from it. An armistice is called for. A proposition is made in writing on the walls. The generals of drugs ask us to be tails to their kites, and to be friends. They are sent back with this announcement, that this war is waged for principle, and no quarter will ever be asked or given until they concede to give us equity in all that is honorable, granting to us all the rights of progress without restraint; and further, that M. D.'s cease to plead the "baby act" before any legislature, or ask for legalized limits to progress, which we think is to ask the legislatures of all the states to feed and prop a falling institution. From now on the shot and shell will be followed by the spears of reason and truth. We have all to lose by such "kiting," and nothing to gain. So, as general in command, I say, "Jerk the lanyard and let her boom." Why not? Have we ever lost a battle, a flag, or a man? No! And we have never had in our school more than six whose necks have been tied to a kite string. They are genuine boobys, at home and abroad—paid nothing for their education, and are too lazy to keep pace with the school. A dollar and a bit of paper to show that they have been in the school are all they see or want. Let me say to you once for all, since October 30, 1894, we have made none such. At that time the school was incorporated by process of law. The school is always willingly opened to all its students who have not lowered the dignity of an Osteopath by being tied to the tail of a medical kite, of which they were duly warned before leaving the school. Our secretary informs us in his report that he has kept posted as to the whereabouts and success of the diplomats of Osteopathy during the past year, and has found no failures to report in their treatment of disease by this science. So far they have all proven their ability and skill, have given perfect satisfaction to their patients, and are making a financial success. And to all such we bid welcome, at all times, as a continuation of our confidence in them. Their works speak more for them than we can.

***

THIS JOURNAL is the only advocate of the philosophy of life and health without the use of drugs, water or grease. This philosophy has never before been known or written; therefore no quotations will appear in its columns. It started alone, and fights alone. It has made its blunders. Who has not? Washington made some; Jeff. Davis made a few. All taught them something. Watts improved as he experimented. In all philosophy you will find wisdom and ignorance side by side: wisdom to reason and ignorance to apply the knowledge. One may reason wisely from cause and effect, force and resistence, but be totally ignorant of what kinds of material to use in the construction of the machines of his discovery. That has been true of Osteopathy to the fullest extent. In the first efforts to construct operating philosophers, I looked at the trunks of the trees only. I did not examine the top to see if they were suitable to go into the building I wished to construct. I now see that was a great mistake. Father Ryan, a C. P., called my attention to that, and said: "But few heads in your first class will ever be able to do honor to your great discovery, and you must raise the standard of intelligence in your school or such heads will ruin the science and disgust the people before the world knows the merit of your discovery." Since then I have taken his wise counsel and gotten all but the very best men and minds out of all the departments. No ignorant man or woman can get into our school, even though they roll in wealth. All future applicants must give full evidence first of at least a good English education, and that they do not use beer, old cider, wine, or alcohol, in any form whatever, or opium or any other drug as a habit. On this foundation of principles the School of Osteopathy will ever stand, regardless of race, birth or color.

Monday, March 30, was the "banner day" at the A T Still Infirmary, the number of patients being the greatest ever treated in one day. The preceeding Monday was the largest to that date—March 23,

---

A gang of workmen are now busy preparing the ground for a large addition to the A T Still Infirmary. Architects are also at work, preparing the plans, and building will begin soon. The business of the Infirmary has outgrown the present quarters, and is increasing every day,

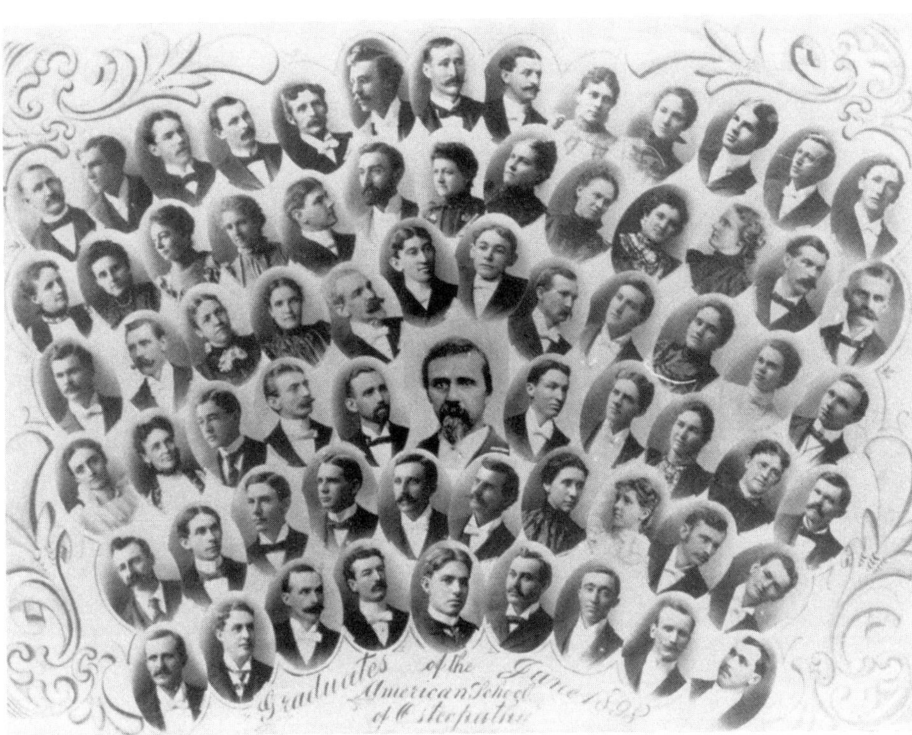

Graduates of the 1898 Class

April, 1896

"HOPELESSLY INSANE."

Has been an expression—a common assertion—before all people of the civilized world, from time whose date is not known. A man or woman may be pronounced insane, taken away from his or her family, and placed in the undesirable prisons, away from home, away from all the loving care of relatives and friends, and placed in charge and under subjection to those who work for money only, there to be treated, good or bad; all of which we have been taught to reverently respect as the best that can be done for their good and the public safety. As you are sane now and out of that prison life, where friendship and kind treatment are extremely doubtful, will you please allow me to ask you this one question, as you and I both may at a very early day be adjudged insane and unsafe to run at large. Did it ever occur to your mind that an expert anatomist possibly would find a partial dislocation of the neck or spine equal to the cause of that mental disturbance, and that nine-tenths of the cases could be traced to that as a cause of the so-called insanity? Several patients who have been brought to me for treatment from different asylums while in that condition, have, to all appearances, gone home mentally sound, whose treatment has been on the line just indicated. I am not bidding for a position at an asylum constructed for mental repairs. I am telling you that I am fully convinced, from reason and experiments, that the old stereotyped phrase "hopelessly insane" ought not to hang over the heads of all the inmates of our asylums. I think these questions should bear with great interest on the minds of the whole world. I believe there is too much truth right along in the line I have indicated, to be carelessly laid down and given no further thought.

A. T. S.

April, 1896

THE DEFINITION OF OSTEOPATHY.

BY A. T. S.

It means very little to a person who does not understand anatomy, and who has not been well drilled in our clinics for one or two years, and in the philosophy that is indispensible to a knowledge of what is meant by Osteopathy. No man or woman can tell you what it means more than to say it is a system of engineering the whole machinery of life harmoniously by keeping open all the communications with the brain and overcoming all stoppages of blood from the heart, and of other fluids. Sensation, motion and nutrition must all work at once, no minus or plus can exist in health, any more than four can go into three twice. With all parts in their nnrmal condition, health is yours. We cannot even give you the outer edge of this philosophy unless you take the steps necessary to obtain that knowledge. You are to blame for your ignorance; we are not. We have the remedy; will you take the medicine?

April, 1896

Our Court House Vote

Is yes. And the reason why is, we believe it will be a wise and paying financial move. If we put up a fifty or one hundred thousand dollar court house and jail, it is our property, as much as a Dutchman's barn, stock and machinery are his. He built his barn because his reason told him he needed it badly. And if he did not have a barn he would lose more than ten per cent interest on one thousand dollars each year; which proved to be good solid Dutch sense. Our county stock is all suffering loss because there is no barn to keep it in.

The next reason why we should improve onr county is, that all our property will be worth at least ten per cent more than it is now. The advanced value on Kirksville property above what it is now without the court house would almost pay the fifty thousand dollars necessary to build it. Every hen, horse, hog and cow would be worth one per cent more. Every acre of land in the county would be worth fifty cents more, as it would bring the money men here to locate. In a word, we look on a vote for a court house as a good move, it makes no difference in which part of town it is located.

The last reason, but not the least, is, that when the people show pluck and business brains hundreds of thousands of money will be invested in this county that is just waiting to see if Adair has any get up and business sense.

A. T. S.

IMPORTANT TO PATIENTS.

All patients who come here for treatment must abstain from the use of intoxicating liquors of every kind while under our care. We do not wish to treat habitual whiskey tubs.

This rule must be strictly obeyed by all patients, and those who feel that they cannot conform to it had better stay away.

We have no counselmen on the street. Patients should become acquainted with the regulations through the Secretary, and obey them to the letter for our mutual good.

A. T. STILL.

June, 1896

DR. STILL'S TALK.

THE following address was delivered by Dr. A. T. Still, in Memorial hall, Thursday evening, June 4th. The hall was well filled with patients from a distance, nearly every state in the union being represented. Dr. Still said:

Osteopathy is twenty-two years old. I have examined encyclopedias and histories, but have never found anything in them about Osteopathy. Twenty-two years ago this month I realized for the first time in my life that the word "God" meant perfection in every particular. Previous to that time I thought He was perfection all but a little, and that the imperfection could be filled out by a little or a great deal of drugs. I saw that the ignorance of drugs was absolute and contradictory to every principle of philosophy as a healing principle, and the so-called science of medicine being a principle with no foundation, I began then and there, on the 22nd day of June, 1874, to place the mind of God as debtor and creditor. When I find any flaw I put it on the debtor side. I charge it up to God as failure. I go to work and look it over to see if I cannot place that, then, on the credit side. I commence then to see how I will go about it. What is your subject? What are you talking and thinking about? I am thinking about that intelligently constructed, self-adjusting, self-firing and self-propelling machine called the human engine. That is what I am talking about, what I am trying with my ability to reason about. I commence and say on the debtor side, "You are a failure so far as fever is concerned, because a majority vote has said, 'You are a failure, O, Lord.'" Don't get excited any of you people because I say this; I will call in a witness which is a very strong one to prove it. When a man is burning up with fever the acts of a majority of the people on the face of the earth say of God, "You are a failure, and we must give him quinine, lobelia, hypodermic syringe, and all such." The "cuts and the trys" and the drugs of all Africa are brought there to put that fire out. Now, Lord, if You can't sustain yourself and put that fire out, we have one against you. "Here is a burning process going on; this man has been out in the rain, re-action is set up, his temperature rises, it continues, and you call it fever. It stops awhile, and then comes on again. What do you call that? Intermittent fever. After awhile it continues without intermission; we have then fixed and established fever. "Now, Lord, there is your machine, get him out if you can. If you do not, down goes an epicac, and there is a failure put against you. Your character as an inventor is at stake before the intellectual and thinking world." And God says to the philosopher, "Examine and see if you don't find a button there that can govern cold and heat?" We will all agree at once that heat is electricity in motion, the greater the velocity the higher the temperature. When we examine, if we find in the makeup of this machine, which is offered to you as a machine of perfection, that it has the power within itself to create heat and not the power to destroy it or suspend it, you have found an imperfection in the machine, which proves an imperfection in the maker. The man who uses drugs and the hypodermic syringe says that You do not know Your business. Take some of these things home with you. This is the first school which ever raised the flag on the globe, as far as history says, that God is truth, and this can be proven. I can take His works and prove His perfection, and he who takes his good old whiskey and drugs and says He is perfection is a liar. He who has lung fever, pneumonia, flux or any fever, and drinks his whiskey denies the whole idea of the perfection of God. He slaps it in the face, and not only that, but does what in my mind says that God is a failure.

I have been called a fanatic. Why? Because I have asserted that the divine mind had plenty of intelligence and a great deal to spare; and you better be taking some of it in and make a practical and sensible use of it for yourself and your families. Without that confidence in the powers found in that machine what will your old earth be doing? She will be sparking the moon that revolves around it, without a living human soul on it in a few thousand years. Our digitalis, our whiskey, our opium, and other foolish things that are called remedies, are fast driving from the face of the earth the human family. 280,000 morphine sots in the city of New York by the census of ten years ago. Chloral hydrates world without end. Nearly 70,000 have had their arms punched by Keeley to knock out, what? The whiskey habit.

Dr. Smith, I wish you would come up here. This is Dr. Smith, our professor of Physiology. I want to know if you do not believe, from your own observation, that the so-called science of medicine, with its stimulents and its other poisons, is doing more harm than good? "Undoubtedly."

She is filling the insane asylums, loading the gallows, and supplying the Keeley Institutes with their thousands annually. That is what your school is doing.

Dr. Smith: "I am not of that school now, doctor; I am of your school."

Where does this thing start? A man goes down to the creek after some fish, and somebody tells him to take a jug of whiskey along for fear he might get wet. He fishes and catches a few cat fish and other kinds of fish; he hasn't many fish, but he is going to make it up out of that whiskey. After a while he has what we call fever. The doctor says, "You need a dose of calomel; however, I would suggest that you follow it up with a few sharp doses of quinine, and it would not be amiss to take a little whiskey." That is our medical science. The result is drunkeness, insanity, death, and showers of tears from families that should have had that man's intelligent services.

Seeing the condition that we were in, I set about to find out whether the God of the whole universe had been foolish enough to construct a machine and throw it into space without any rudders on it or brakes to stop it when it goes down hill; without any claws to hold it when it goes up; or without any remedy placed in that machine called "perfection." The book says, "And the Lord said, let us make man." I suppose there must have been a council, and it must have been a mighty poor council which made a man that wouldn't work.

Let us examine man, and the Maker of man, and see if we can find where He made a failure, and until that is done keep your epicac, with its music, in your pocket.

Some people think Osteopathy is a system of massage, others that it is a "faith" cure. I have no "faith" myself, I only want the truth to stand on. Another class think it is a kind of magnetic pow wow. It is none of these, but is based upon a scientific principle. If these electric lights are based upon a scientific principle, it must be borrowed capital. From what was it borrowed? What machine was it borrowed from? I think that we can find that the first thought in regard to that machine came from looking over the human brain, finding there two lobes containing sensation and motion. That when those two lobes were brought together v e found the positive and negative parts of electricity. On that principle Dr. Morse began his researches and gave us the first principles of telegraphy. Other eminent electricians have followed up the same thought. They also have discovered that the batteries supplying the electricity must be of opposite elements. They must be brought together, the parts contained in the opposing poles. Where do they get these principles? They are suggest by the human brain, the two lobes. That is where they find their point. He finds t e electricity conducted throughout the whole system. If the spinal cord is destroyed motion comes to a stand still. Now, suppose we would call these lights in the center of this room the spinal cord. Here, by turning off the lights, we represent a stroke of paralysis, and that stroke of paralysis to a reasoning man, an Osteopath who is not too anxious to go out before he knows anything, suggests a principle, a reason, a foundation on which to build. I will demonstrate to you that the spinal cord supplies all other parts. It is that which supplies life to the whole machine.

(Demonstrations with electric lights. Lights in the center turned off.)

While these lights are off suppose you try to make them burn by digging around the corners of the building, pouring things into the chimneys or any other available place. Would that help matters? Would an intelligent electrician that knew the A. B. C's of his business expect to renew the lights by any such process? If I had a son and he was thirty-five years old and didn't know more than that in adjusting the human engine, I would have a guardian appointed for him and tell him to use the hypodermic syringe on both sides of his head. There is only one principle by which that paralysis can be cured, and that is to open up from the battery the electric wires on which it will travel, which are now obstructed. An Osteopath says he can do that, and there it is. (Lights turned on.)

Where is the philosopher who will stand up and show so little sense at this age of electricity, as to come in here and say that this is the most stupendous humbug now on the face of the earth? The right hand of the God of the universe is with us, and we are sending the light more and more over the world. I expect when I am gone that I will come back every week or so to see what Osteopathy is doing; I want to see if it is run off of the face of the earth. In the earlier ages the people didn't know anything of medicine, and they lived a long time. The less they knew about it the more good food they ate and the longer they lived.

Our work here is to overcome the effects of medicine. Nine-tenths of the cases that come here, while they are wrenched and strained in many places in the body, we have to treat them first by turning on the nerves of the excretory organs of the system, for the purpose of cleaning up the dirty house in which the human soul dwells. What do we find? We find the liver not acting right, we find some lungs affect d; we find stones in the gall bladder. We go a little farther down to the renal nerves, vei is, arteries, those of the kidneys; they are out of order. We go down to the water bladder, and there find some more specimens. Specimens of what? Of the thoughtless stupidity of man, who, by taking medicine, has converted the liver into a bank of cinnabar. A few doses of calomel and out goes your teeth. Any person in the audience has the privilege of raising his hand and saying I am wrong, if I state anything that is not correct. I am fighting for God, and am going to hit them square in the face. While I am here I expect to tell the straight, unvarnished truth. In order that a man shall be able to comprehend he has to do something. The patient can comprehend enough to know whether he has the back ache or not. He can omprehend enough to know that he has the back ache one hour and the next he does not have it, and that will make him happy. An Osteopath has to know the shape and position of every bone in the body, that part to which every ligament and muscle is attached. He has to know the blood and the nerve supply. He has to comprehend the human system as an anatomist, and also from a physiological standpoint. He must understand the form of that body and the workings of it. That is the short way to tell what an Osteopath must know. Of course you can have a little knowledge of Osteopathy and do some things, but not know how it is done. Before you can walk upon the stage and fight the fight you must master human anatomy and physical laws. Dr. Smith has been practicing Osteopathy for four years, and if he were out half a mile from here I would say that his qualifications are surpassed by nothing I have met with in my travels over America. He can tell you anything you want to know about anatomy or physiology, and give you the authority for it. He has stuck to it; that is the reason he knows it; it is not because he is smarter than any other man, but he has stuck to it until he knows the construction of the human machine and its workings. I do not believe any man knows all about it; there is plenty for any one to learn. If a man comes here to take a course in this science it is a serious matter, unless he is a trickster, and comes here with the intention of getting a little knowledge and then skipping out to fool a lot of suffering people. But if he means to stand by it and get all there is in it, it is a serious matter, and should be considered as seriously as the subject of picking out a girl for a wife; or as seriously as he would say his prayers if he were going to be hung. If he goes into it in this way he will not go far until he finds that there are ten thousand chambers in the human body that have never been explored intelligently. He can jump over a great deal if he wants to. A man can learn his A. B. C's in the morning and he can finish with Greek Lexicon at night, but he has jumped what lies between his A. B. C's and the winding up of the Greek verb. He has jumped. Just so in studying anatomy a man can jump, and when he comes out here and tells you that he thoroughly understands all of the science of Osteopathy, even a respectable quantity, in less than two years, he jumps a little.

We have been placed in a peculiar position—so many people are suffering, and there is nothing at home but drugs and blisters, and they are begging for our juveniles; they will make them great offers, and want us to let them go. Previous to the commencement of this class we tried to accommodate the people the best we could. But I tell you the philosopher is born after twelve months—no nine months' gestation will give you an Osteopath. It must be after a gestation of two years, and then they are only beginners. Even here, where, as Prof. Blitz says, we have the greatest clinical advantages on the face of the earth, the greatest facilities for comprehending anatomy, even though that is the case, at the end of two years our best and most competent operators would like for me to carry the load, like the young man who gives Dad the heaviest end of the log because the skin on his shoulder is a little bit the toughest..

We control all of the fevers of this or any other climate, all of the contagious diseases, such as mumps, chicken pox, scarlet fever, measles, diphtheria or whooping cough; also flux, constipation, diseases of the kidneys and of the spine, etc. We deal with the brain, the liver, lungs and the heart. In short, every division of the whole human body, with all its parts.

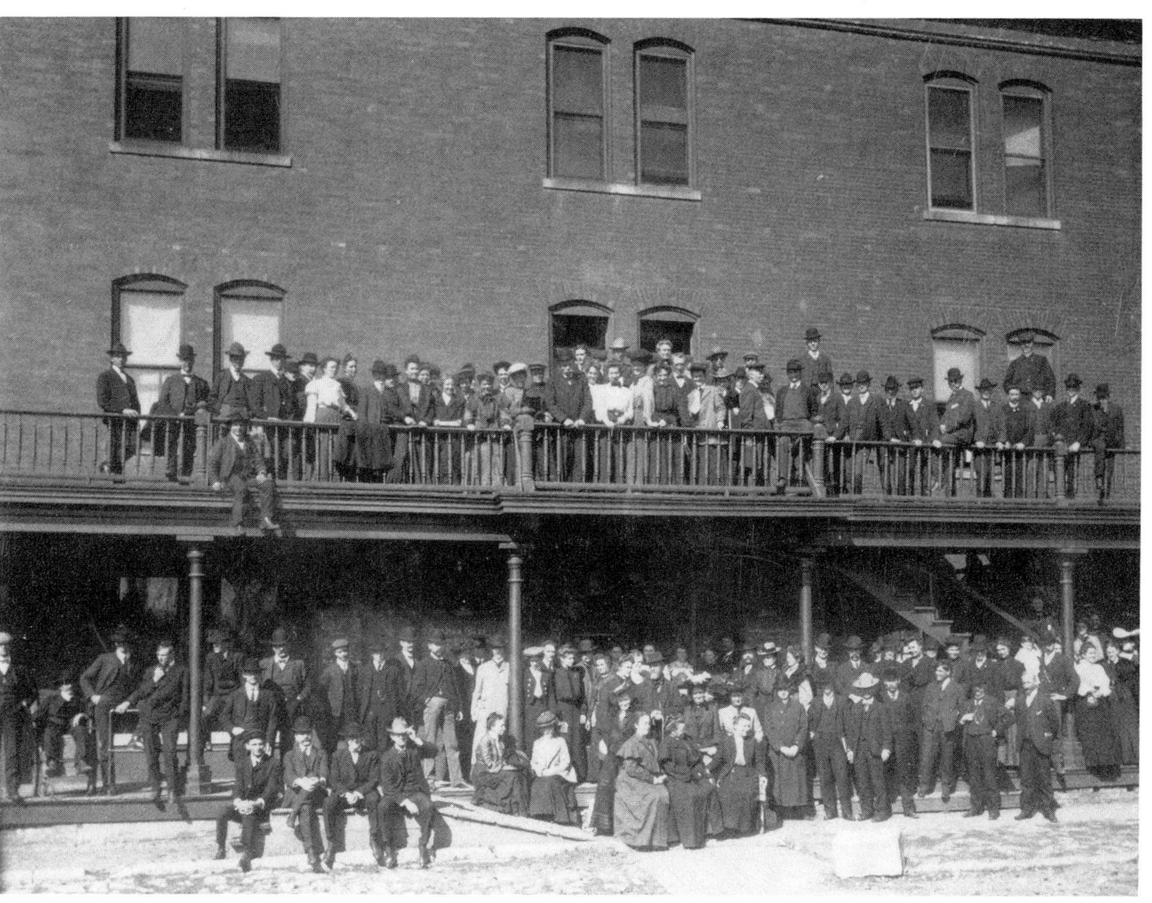

Freshman Class of 1904

I can take a young man in here for a little while and make an imitator of him, and send him out so he can handle diphtheria, croup, in seven cases out of ten; and he can handle some headache. What is he in that condition? He is like my Polly. "Polly wants a cracker," and he don't know what he is saying or doing. You ask him where the glosso-pharyngeal nerve is, and he will say he don't remember; he will look in his book for it, that he did know it but had forgotten. We want you to thoroughly understand anatomy so that it will come to you as quick as "ouches" to a Dutchman's mouth when he gets his finger hurt. It ought to be second nature. It should be be as indellibly fixed as passing the hat is on the minister's mind and as a duty that must not be ommitted before he closes.

Since the school was incorporated we have established such rules as we think necessary to the attainment of a thorough knowledge of anatomy. First you have anatomy, and that is a great book; after you have mastered that you take physiology, and that is just twice as big as anatomy. Then we have what we call symptomatology. We take up the different symptoms or a combination of symptoms. One symptom indicated tooth ache, another one something else. Suppose there has been a stoppage of the blood supply of the stomach, what is the result? What we call cancer. Another symptom would indicate pneumonia. What is pneumonia? You take an Osteopath that knows his business thoroughly and he can give you the diagnosis and never use a single term of the old schools. Take scrofula, consumption, flux, eczema, every one of them. There is a broken current, an unfriendly relation existing between the capillaries of the veins and arteries.

What is flux? An abortive effort of the artery to feed the vein. The vein contracts and the artery spills the blood at the nearest place, passes through the bowels, and death results. The doctor gives his quinine, kino, his gourd-seed tea, and other poisons; he gives his mustard plasters. The child dies. It is a Baptist child, and they bring it to Brother Morgan, and he says, "Whereas, it pleased God to take that child—" I don't believe Brother Morgan would say that. He would say "I believe this death is through the ignorance of the doctor; that child should have lived and worked, as THAT was the will of God."

I came here tonight to tell you that the science of Osteopathy, as little as is known, bids fair in a very few years to penetrate the minds of the philosophers of the whole earth, whether they speak English or not. Today it is known not only by the English speaking nations of the world, but it is known in Germany, it is known in France. Possibly not so well known as the cyclone in St. Louis. But like that cyclone, commencing there and working all over the country, this cyclone will show itself in the legislatures inside of a very few years. Intelligent men that are competent to investigate a science, and honest enough to tell the truth when they have investigated it, cannot fail to see the results of Osteopathy. They see Osteopathy coming home with the scalps of measles under its arm,—and plenty of them—mumps, flux, diphtheria, scarlet fever, whooping-cough and croup. The Osteopath does this. The philosopher has found out that nature had the ability to construct a machine that is trustworthy under all climates. Here is a man living at New Orleans. It does not take much for him to breathe down there; he breathes once in a while and gets along alright. He goes further north and finds himself at 72 or 73 degrees N. latitude. What does he find? He breathes faster, his lungs are stronger. The heart dispenses a larger quantity of electricity, so the lungs breathe faster. That throws the electric current much faster, and it keeps him warmer in the colder weather. Pick the man up and drop him in New Orleans and you would haveto put him in water to keep him cool. He would be warmer because the lungs are increasing the action of the electricity, and he would burn up. How does a snow bird live in cold weather? I picked up a chicken to-day that had not a feather on its back. It was just ready for a preacher to eat. Not a feather on that chicken's back. What was the motion of that chicken's heart? It must have been 180, maybe 280. Why was that heart running at such a velocity as that? To keep that chicken warm until the feathers come out. At every stroke of the Master Architect of the universe you will see the proof of intelligence, and his work is absolute.

I wish to speak to you of the ability of our operators to judge as to your case. They have studied anatomy and physiology to completion; then they were placed in the operating rooms, after having passed through training in the clinics. They are skilled operators and know by experience when they are turning a button on or off, and have handled their thousands and tens of thousands of cases, for 15,000 to 20,000 is about the number of patients that visit here annually. If there is anything one of them does not comprehend, it goes right to the next one above, and if they all get puzzled they come and ask me, and I go to guessing. When you come here go in there and call out an investigation before the operators and talk to them as though you considered they had some intelligence and some sense, and don't stand there and complain and say you want to see the "old doctor." The old doctor is not going to do this work if you pick up and go home. When a man has worked and built up a science like this and has spent twenty years in doing it, if he has failed to impart that knowledge, he should quit. I have men to examine here who know their business, and I simply ask you to treat them with respect until they shall have examined your case. Once in a while there is a very dangerous case, where a person is between life and death, and they come to me about it, and I look at it. I can't set every toe, elbow, etc., of the thousands who come here. When you are talking to a graduate of this school, you are talking to a man who knows a great deal about the body, and his conclusions are correct. There are some who think they know more about our business after they have been in the house five minutes than those who have been here five years. I am within a few days of sixty-eight, and I am going to put in the rest of my days preaching here. I am glad to meet you on the street and have a friendly chat, but when you want to talk about your case go in and see the Secretary. I believe that I can teach this science to others, or I should quit it. I dragged ten years' miserable existence working too hard, when there was no use of it. I have put in tens of thousands of dollars here to demonstrate to you that I can teach it and that men do know it. I do not go over town at the birth of every child, or any thing of that kind. The people send for one of the operators, expect results, and they get it. I don't want people tapping on every window for me to stop and exam- them, after such men as Dr. Hildreth or Dr. Patterson and others have passed on their cases. I am willing to stop on the poarches and talk with you and have a good time, but I don't want to examine you. I know you can have it done better here. You come here with an old skeleton with a little bit of meat on it, and you sneak in here because you are ashamed to come. You are ashamed to come, and you don't let your husband know you have come here, lots of you. That is your side of it. What have you had? You have had the surgeons knife lacerate your body; some of the leading nerves of the body cut out. You come here and you expect of us, what? To make a man or woman out of you after you have been slashed up as if you had had a fight in Russia with three wild boars. The ham strings are cut; can you make a leg of it? Can you make an arm when the sub-clavian artery is cut? Nine out of ten of the cases that come here have tried everything else. They say they are hopeless; but I don't believe a word of that or they would not come here. Many times they have been operated upon, they say. They have goitre and have been treated by the knife, the thyroid artery cut, the hypodermic syringe, acids, poisons, etc. We don't want that kind of a case here because the arteries that supply the parts have been destroyed; we have less material to work with than we want. You come here loaded with digitalis. 'What for? Why, on account of heart trouble. What do we find? We find a heart probably longer than it ought to be, or too wide. I caution my operators in such a case not to deal with that set of nerves so as to throw too great a force on the heart, but

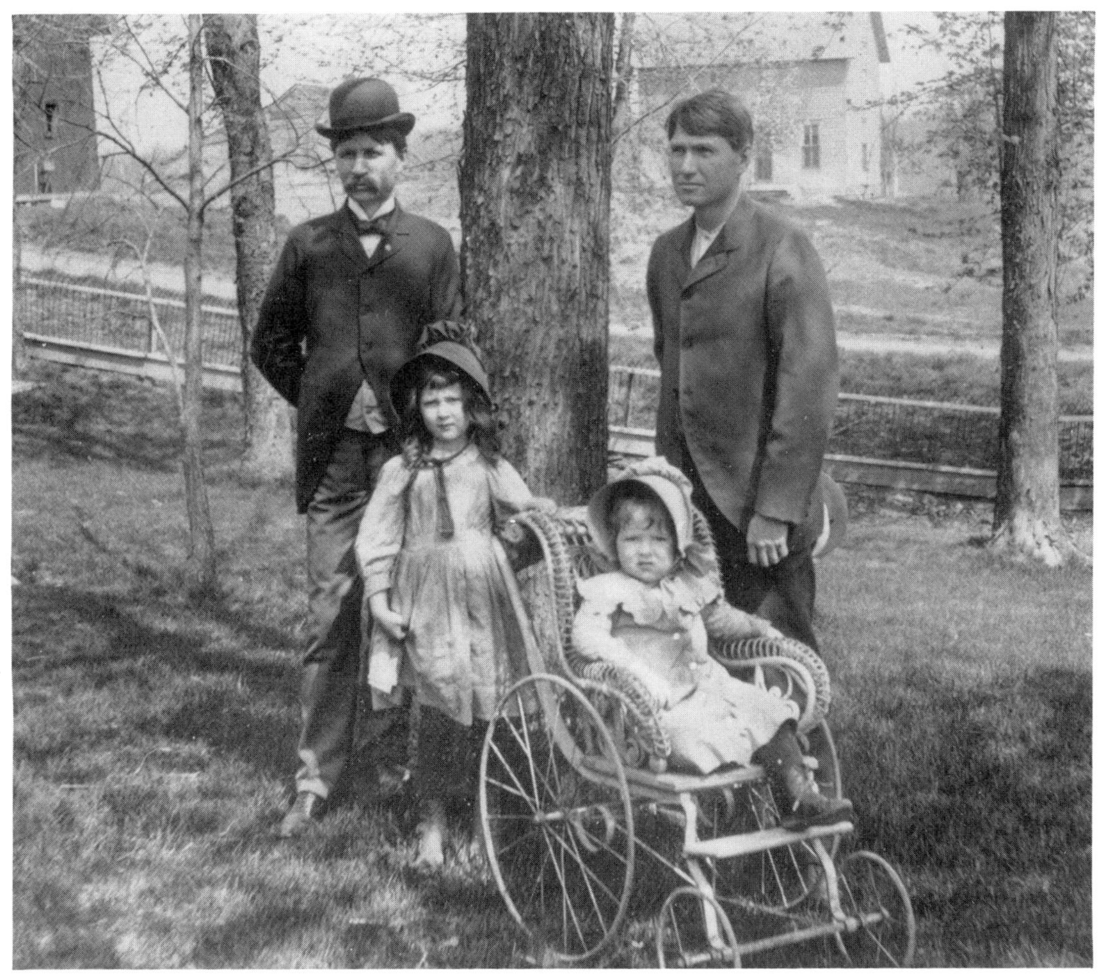

Left to right, Herman, Gladys, Elizabeth and Charles Still, c. 1900

to let it on easy. I say to them, "Boys don't flatter any man, woman or child who comes here; you tell them there is some hope. Two to four weeks will show what chance there is for you." I don't want the patients to say, "Dr. Landes would not give me any flattery, any hope about it." He is not going to do it and stay with me. Dr. Patterson, or Dr. Charley, my son, will not give you any flattery. If they can give you a ray of hope they will say so. You come here with what you call aneurism of any great vessel leading from the heart. Suppose Dr. Charley examines that heart, he hears a rasping sound. He asks you who said it was aneurism. You answer, Dr. Neeley, or else say Dr. Mudge or Fudge, of St. Louis, or some other place. There is the rasping, roaring sound. You can easily hear it. Aneurism—what is that? Dr. Charley Still, what do you find there? He says, Mister, when did you first notice that? "A horse, scared by a pig, threw me off, and then my heart made that noise." "How long afterwards!" "Two minutes." Dr. Smith, how long does it take to make an aneuism on an artery? Ans. "Weeks or months." And his heart made that noise in two minutes afterward. "I myself was thrown from a horse and got a little jolt, and that set my heart tooting, and they told me it was a valvular disturbance. That noise indicates that the phrenic nerve and some muscles are not acting right, and every time the bow or artery is drawn across it makes that noise. They go back to Kentucky cured of so-called aneurism.

I think it is useless to talk any further, as the night is hot, and it takes a great deal of patience to be patient such an evening as this, so I will bid you good night.

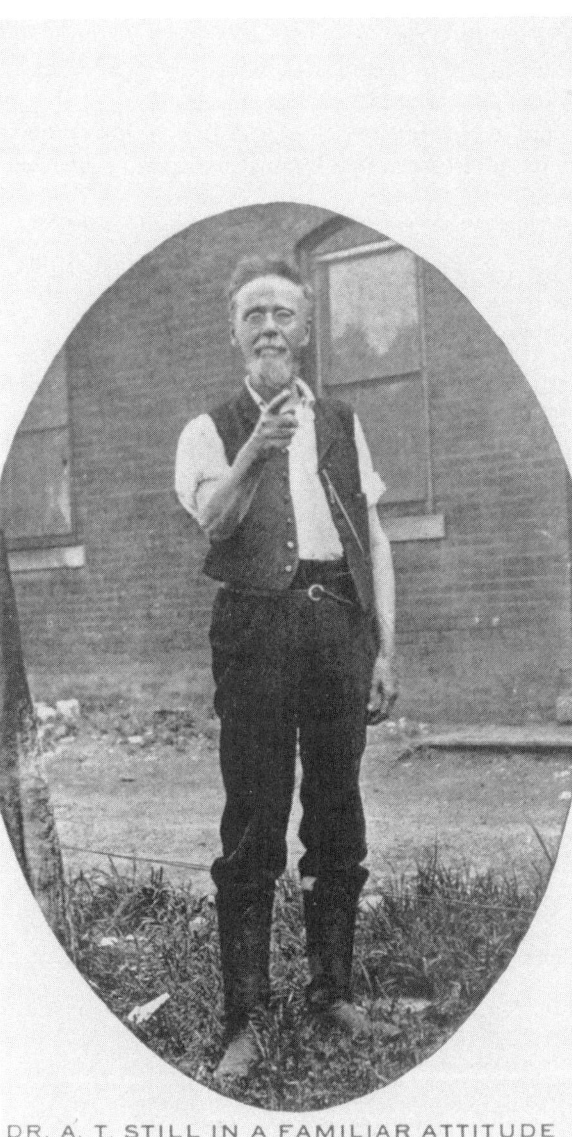

DR. A. T. STILL IN A FAMILIAR ATTITUDE

A. T. Still, c. 1900

May, 1896

"THE FLAG OF TRUCE."

BY A. T. S.

For twenty-five years that sacred emblem of peace has been withheld from view. Our flag for truth has ever given music to the breezes. Strong mortars have thrown shells of great size, loaded with that which had done deadly execution and taken down the flags of all opposition, until 1874, when little Osteopathy planted a single gun in open field in the powerful state of Missouri. Shells have fallen all around our flag for twenty-two years, and on review at roll call not a thread is found to be torn or missing. Each thread is stronger, and calls legions to its defense. Anthems are sung to its praise. Its victories multiply—come in quick succession. The brainy are among its captives. It never records a victors if it has not conquered a general of renown. The scalps of fools and children are never counted, as we do not wish to be tried for infanticide. It must not be the scalp of a bald headed general. We want no toy ladies' man's scalp. It must be a rooster with full comb and spur, or we will never exhibit him as a trophy. This is a war not for conquest, popularity, or power. It is an aggressive campaign for love, truth, and humanity. We love every man, woman and child of our race; so much so that we enlisted and placed our lives in front of the enemy for their good and the good of all coming generations, and asked the Lord who stayed the knife that was in the hands of Abraham of old for the destruction of his own son, to please aid and assist by all honorable means to stop the useless butchery of our mothers, wives, sisters, and daughters; to teach our people better sense than to use any drugs which would cause gall stones, bladder stones, diseased livers, heart and lungs, fibroid tumors, piles, appendicitis, or any other disease or habit which may be traced directly to the unphilosophical use of drugs, which is given by one and produces tumifaction of any or all parts of the body, leaving the subject in such a condition that there is no relief short of the deadly knife of the next experimenter. This war has raged hot and heavy for nearly a quarter of a century. Its position as a witness has been before the judge of love, truth, justice and humanity.

May, 1896

WHAT IS LEFT?

A. T. S.

Go into the A. T. Still Infirmary, stay a few weeks, and you will know something of the meaning of the above heading. From morning until night human forms move in quick succession, some on rolling chairs, crutches and in the arms of their friends, faces pale and puffed with arsenic, eyes bulged out with bellidonna, hips set and stiff with mercury, heel and ham strings cut off, jaws set by calomel, half their teeth hammered out to get the bread of life, others with abdomen ripped open and nothing but the skin united with a gallon of the bowels in a pitable protrusion sticking out front as large as a man's head to help drag out life. Others have an inch or more of the lower bowels cut off, ripped out to one side, destroying all control of the bowels. Right here I will stop, as I see when I shake my memory, the book would not end until you grow old in reading the story of "what is left." Legions come and go all the time; they are living monuments of the malpractice of the M. D.'s who are graduates of legally chartered schools of medicine, and they are the men who say Osteopathy shall not go to Kentucky, Nebraska and other states, and these are what is left of the human forms. They have been haggled and kicked out with empty purses to die.

PROSPECTUS

— OF —

The American School of Osteopathy.

KIRKSVILLE, MO,

From this date the course of study in the American School of Osteopathy will be divided into four terms of six months each. These terms will begin in November and May of each year. At those dates (and at no other time) students will be admitted to the school. The studies will be as follows:

FIRST SIX MOMTHS.

Anatomy—in class only.

SECOND SIX MONTHS.

Anatomy, (demonstrations on the cadaver) Physiology and Principles of Osteopathy.

THIRD SIX MONTHS.

Anatomy, (demonstrations on the cadaver,) Physiology, Use of the Microscope (in recognizing the tissues of the body, deposits in urine, etc.) Diagnosis and Symptomatology, Use of the Stethescope, Analysis of Urine, etc., Clinical instruction in Osteopathic Practice.

FOURTH SIX MONTHS.

Anatomy and Physiology as in third term, (optional for those who have passed the first examination) Diagnosis, Symptomatology, Surgery' (accidents and injuries: their diagnosis and treatment,) Treatment of Poisoning by Noxious Drugs, Midwifery and Diseases of Women. During this term students will act as assistants to the operators in the treating rooms of the Infirmary and thus acquire full knowledge of Osteopathic work.

CLASS EXAMINATIONS

will be conducted every month on all subjects in the curriculum. Their object is merely to let the student himself see how he is progressing. Professional examinations will be held twice yearly, the first after the completion of 18 months of study, (Anatomy, Physiology, Microscopic Work and Urinary Analysis) the other at the close of 24 months of regular attendance. The latter examination will cover all ground not included in the first examination. The "First" must be passed before appearing for the "Final."

The American School of Osteopathy is open to both sexes, with certain restrictions as to character, habits, etc. The special qualifications, which will be rigidly insisted upon in every student, are: Must be over 20 and under 45 years of age, strictly temperate, of good moral character, good native ability and at least a good common school education.

The tuition for the full course of two years is $500. No one will be received for less than full course, and the full tuition in cash or its equivalent must be arranged for in advance.

The cost of living in Kirksville is about the average in cities of 5,000. Good board costs from $3 a week up.

The next term will begin in November, 1896; no students will be admitted to the school until then.

A. T. Still, Pres't.
H. E. Patterson, Sec'y.

We cannot afford to lose any of our institutions of learning—keep up the record of Kirksville for enterprise and liberality.

July, 1896

ANNIVERSARY CELEBRATION OF THE FOUNDING OF OSTEOPATHY.

[Address of Andrew T. Still, delivered in Memorial Hall of the American School of Osteopathy Monday evening, June 22, 1896, at the celebration of the 22d anniversary of the founding of Osteopathy.

Ladies and Gentlemen:—Twenty-two years ago today about noon I was shot; not in the heart, but in the dome of reason. That dome was in a very poor condition to be penetrated by an arrow charged with the principles of philosophy. Since that eventful day I have sacredly remembered and kept it. Not all the time before as intelligent, nor as great an audience as this, but a part of the time withdrawing from the presence of man to meditate upon that event, upon that day wherein I saw by the force of reason that the word "God" signified perfection in all things and in all places. I began at that day to carefully investigate with the microscope of mind to prove an assertion that is often made in your presence, that the perfection of Deity can be proven by his works. When I resolved that I would take up the subject, and find out by investigation whether that work would stand the test, whether it could be proved that, as stated by the gray headed sages of the pulpit that the works of God would prove his perfection. Not all the roads that men travel are smooth. We never have a positive but what we are met with the negative. I am convinced that as far as I comprehend, and I cannot assert beyond that, that the works of God do prove His perfection in all places, at all times, and under all circumstances. I drew a line of debtor and creditor. On the one side I placed the works of God and the acts of man, who is claimed to be the handiwork of God. The intelligence of an association of mind, matter and spirit, the child of God who is the author and constructor of all worlds and all things therein. All patterns for the mechanic to imitate in all his inventions are found in man. You remember that all patterns are borrowed from this one place, be it God, be it the devil or be it man, who is the originator of all things. All patterns for all things are imitations of what is found in that constructed being, man. We see in man, as we comprehend it, the attributes of Deity. We see mind and the action of mind; therefore, there is a representation of the mind of all minds. We find in the universe the solar system; we find there motion, without which no universe can exist. The very thought of mind itself presupposes action. The motions of all the planets of the universe indicate and prove action and force. On time those planets pass and re-pass, to the hour and the minute they run, and pass before you and other globes, indicating to a man of reason the ability of that mind to mathematically calculate the length of every piece used in the whole universe and to arm and equip it with a velocity that is exactly true, and that will run to the thousandth part of a second. Should one quarter of a second's time be lost in the velocity of Jupiter, what might be the result? Increase the electric force of the whole system and fever will be the result in the whole planetary and solar systems. If Jupiter in his rounds should lose one quarter of a second's time on his circuit, what effect would that have on the whole planetary system? You would see such planets as Mercury, Venus and the earth dancing a jig. Then, if we had a medical doctor turned lose there, he would give it an injection of a whooping big dose of morphia. Just on that ground exactly is where he is incompetent to comprehend the revolutions and the time exacted by the Divine moon-maker. We find the same thing exactly in the solar system of man. Suppose the heart fails to make its time. A confusion is started by a retention of the blood at the base of the brain; perhaps the base of the heart, or the base of the bowels, or the base of the foot, or the side or top of any division of the body, and you may expect until Jupiter takes his regular time, gets in line with that star, you will want to go to the Hot Springs to get warmed up.

A great many of you have come here to-night, and what have you come for? A very few have come here to see what nonsense is going on. Between your eyes there are too many miles of reason to call any mathematical fact a humbug. Some heads have less than a quarter of an inch between the bases of reason, or their eyes. You must not be too hard upon those whose eyes take in so little of a mile; you must not be to hard on them, but allow them the great privilege of calling you a philosopher or a fool, because one is just as well understood by them as the other.

My grand-mother was a Dutch woman. She told me she believed a great deal in signs, and all that, —when you set hens, kill chickens, and butcher hogs, and so on. When you see one of those little heads that knows it all, with a little book under his arm, an almanac or something of that sort, claim in a week or ten days to be a great Osteopath, you remember what I tell you. That child was weaned when the sign was in the feet. The next place the sign was in the abdomen, and he is ready to go into the world and make his boasts that he is an Osteopath, that he comprehends it. He is ready to go before the world, and with false statements lie just enough to get more money than he can get by straight-forward, honest dealing before his fellow men. We have such births here; having worked at dentistry, selling drugs, etc., and developed in a few days ready to go out into the world and raise his flag of "Osteopathy."

Twenty-two years ago today I took up the matter solemnly and seriously. Since that time I have not lost a single hour without my mind being upon the work and construction of man, to see if I could detect one single flaw or defect in it; either under the microscope or with the anatomists knife or the rules of philosophy, either my own or the mind of others. I have never yet been able to detect the least shadow of confusion. The Jupiter of life is absolutely and mathematically correct. My investigation has been for the honest purpose of finding out whether or not when the great God of the universe constructed man there was one single defect in the work that has been detected by all the combined intelligence of the sons and daughters of man from the birth of man up to the present time. I had to give the wholesale credit mark and make the vote unanimous for God. And if you cannot make it unanimous, do as they did in St. Louis, a few of you go out. If you can't swallow it, go out and stay.

Why did I become interested in this great question of the intelligence of God? His ability to give us the seasons, cold and hot, wet and dry, the different kinds of fowls and animals and fish of the seas and running waters? The reason why I investigated this was: I believed that man was woefully and wonderfully benighted, from the fact that when he was sick he guessed what was the matter, and guessed he would go for a doctor. And then the guessing commenced in earnest. The doctor guessed what was the matter; he guessed what he would give him, and he guessed when to return, guessed he would get well or when he would die. He entered the grand chamber of guessing then and there, and when the last breath was drawn the guess work was not through with until the preacher guessed where he would go. I said to myself that God knew more than I did, and more than Mr. Michael, or Dick Roberts, or all the men I could think of; more than General Jackson, or Jeff Davis, Abe Lincoln, or even Horace Greely. I concluded that if he did know all things He has certainly placed that machinery on the track of life armed and equipped, with boilers full, plenty of oil, and all the bearings of the running gear of the whole engine in good condition. I began to look at man. What did I find? I found myself in the presence of an engine, the greatest engine that mind could conceive of. Having spent seven or eight years with a stationary engine acquainting myself with all its parts, from boiler to saw, I began to investigate man as an engine. In running my saw I found that if I squeezed it the blade would wobble. I soon found that the hum was gone, having passed to a warbling sound. It was hardly a warble, because when a saw gets hot and begins to wobble the pressure is very light, and it wobbles just before it warbles. I soon found that the harmonious sound of the saw was produced when it was running exactly as it should, keeping the line, and all that pertained to the lumber cutting. I found that wobbling in there, and that was what drew my attention, and I inquired as to what was the matter with the saw of life. found it was out of line, and the friction against the timber produced the heat and what they call buckling. It wobbled to one side like a blubber under a pan cake. That wobble will spoil your saw and stop its work. How many blubbers did I find in the human engine? I found the blubber of erysipelas, of flux, of diphtheria. It is the bursting of the bubble of the wobbling saw; one of the saws of life

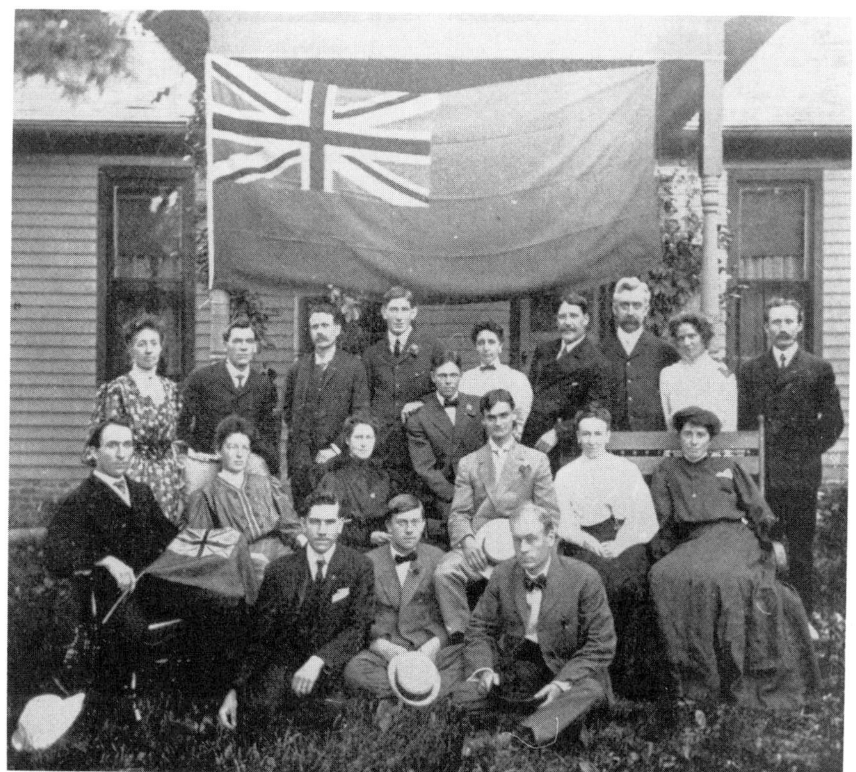

Canadian and English Students at the A.S.O.

just off the track a little. I defy the oldest sages of philosophy to show me the difference between flux and no flux; to show me the time when flux was not there. He must take the number of hours in which this milk soured and began to curdle. It first commenced by being in a stationary position and under a curdling temperature; then the milk sours, in a common pan, and it would sour just the same in the pans of the bowels or the mesentary arteries, veins or muscles. Therefore, you have simply an effect, and you call that effect a disease, a particular disease. Just the same as you call your brother Jim and your sister Sarah Ann. They are effects only. And ninety-nine times out of every hundred that same machine has a wobbling saw; it has left the line; it is not tracking on the course of life by nature given, thus things are not harmonious.

Why should I prosecute this for years? Because I could count as much as an old mathematician could, in small addition anyhow. I could make a mark for Tom Smith, died, under the doctor's treatment; and Jim Smith also is dead, and John Henry Smith likewise is dead. However, I ommited to say that the father and mother were both dead with flux. I began to see during the civil war in that part of the states of Missouri and Kansas where the doctors were shut out the children did not die. I began to reason as to why it was. Our ministers say the birds are provided for, and I just thought if God took care of them he took care of those children too. There is the same ability there to sustain them through the summer and winter. Nature has provided for a great many emergencies. When a mule has worked hard all day and his multifidus spinæ is pulled out like a shoe string, what does he do? He finds a good place to roll, kicks up his heels, kicks another mule or two, and he has gone through his Osteopathic manipulation. He shows a little sense. An old hen when she gets a little of what you call microbes in her feathers, does what? She gets out her microscope and looks through it and concludes they are microbes, and she hunts up a dust heap, and leaves them there. Watch the hog. He knows more than his master; when he gets the fever he goes into the mud and stays there until the fever leaves. Some years ago a man had a time with the cholera and his friends concluded they would help the old fellow cover himself up in the sand and let him die. They went off up the river and left him, and the next morning he was up there ready for his breakfast. They left him down there to die, but he got well.

I have a very kindly feeling for this day. On the 22nd day of June, 1874, at ten o'clock, was the first time I ever saw the gravy of liberty, and I have been sopping my bread in it ever since, and, like eating olives, it was a little difficult at the start, but now they all want olives. The whole of North America is beginning to say, "I will take some olives, if you please." The Irishman took some, but said "Begobs, who spoiled the plums." Our students who have gone out from here, our early diplomats, have withstood the howlitzers in every engagement and have come out victorious. That poor little Ammerman, who is about as big as a little piece of chewing gum after the Sunday services are over, went down into Kentucky, and swung a little Osteopathic flag to the breeze there.

They brought the laws of the great state of Kentucky to bear upon that poor little banty, poor little Osteopath, of little experience, less than a year, on his back. His works followed him into the court and the grand jury of the great state of Kentucky says, "Not guilty."

One of my poor, feeble minded sons, who has been a follower of mine, went up to Minnesota. He was arrested. For what? For not seeing diphtheria where there was none. There is a law there that quarantines against diphtheria, measles, scarlet fever, etc. Well, my boy is just like his father, he knows so little that he is not afraid of it. He has more grit than brains, I suppose. He walked into those houses, as I am told by Senator Nelson of that State. He went into twenty-eight houses in one single day, and the next day took down all of those card boards.

* . . . . *

KEEP OUT!
BY ORDER OF THE STATE
BOARD OF HEALTH.
CONTAGIOUS! DIPHTHERIA!

* . . . . *

It looked like there were dress-makers in every house until you looked a little closer. They were put up there to keep the people from spreading diphtheria. There were hundreds of them in the little town of Red Wing. Senator Nelson said he went into those houses with my son Charles. The children's tongues were sticking out of their mouths their throats were red; but he said Charles never lost a case. He also told me that previous to that time 114 children died with diphtheria in one day, but that Osteopathy did not lose a single case. And for saving the lives of those children he was arrested and brought before the court. And what was the result? The fathers and mothers came out by the hundreds. and the prosecuting doctors and attorneys concluded to "git." Those Swedes and Norwegians said that if Still was found guilty they would hang the doctors. The people declared that from the center to the circumference of Minnesota Osteopathy should live. They also came over from Wisconsin en masse with their revolvers to set at liberty that boy the very instant he was put in jail for violating the laws by saving the children. They declared that the people were the law, and the statute the tool. The statute is a money making provision, and when the people arise they are the law of the country. In Louisville, Kentucky, the people are the law; in the state of Missouri the people are the law; also in Kansas; and also in any part of the United States. Americans will not have their liberty abridged. Neither are they going to take the doctor of their choice through the kitchen any more. Twenty-two years ago I had to crawl in through the kitchen to see a child that had the croup. The child's uncle, John Tibbs, of Macon City, sent me a telegram to come and see Jim Tibbs' child who was dying with croup. They had had a consultation of five or six doctors, who said the child couldn't live. One of them was a good old English doctor who would get drunk occasionally, and he said the child would soon be in the "harms of the Great Hi Ham." The child's uncle and Mr. McCaw met me at the depot, took me to the house and succeeded in taking me through the kitchen; wouldn't let me go in the front way for fear we would meet some of the doctors coming out. In five minutes time the child began to breathe, and the next morning was playing around the house. Since that time there has been an Osteopathic home at that place. Since that time Osteopathy has become known throughout the whole state, and the intelligent man has confidence in it. The philosopher also has confidence in its ability to cure. The fathers and mothers call in the Osteopaths and pay for their services now.

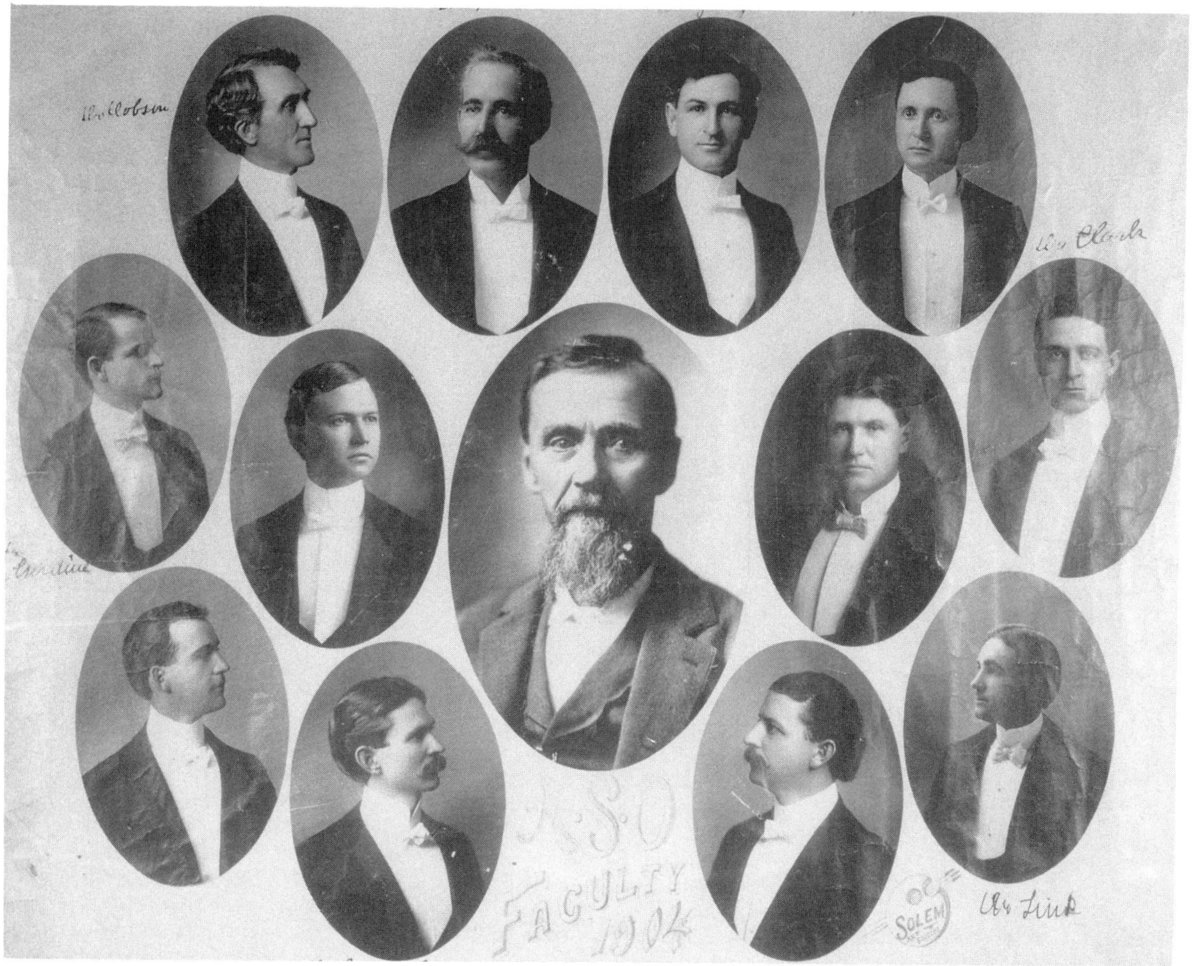

One objection to Osteopathy is that it may make thieves and scoundrels. Men will come here for a little while and go away and say, "I have been to Kirksville; I am an Osteopath," and so on. They will steal from the people wherever they can until they are found out. They are drunken scoundrels, the very trash of your town. So far it is dangerous. The M. D.'s have said it is dangerous, because with a few little cures in a neighborhood, Osteopathy is liable to become the grandest system of robbery in the world. Men will stand up and curse this science to the very last, and then get on the train and go off 300 or 400 miles and say they are from the city of Jerusalem, commonly called Kirksville; that they are right from the rivers of life, and thoroughly understand this science. They are men who have never done anything but curse it as the lowest conception of foolishness and ignorance. Another dangerous point I want to speak of is, that as soon as our students begin to know a little something about it, some one will come in and offer to pay their expenses to foreign parts if they will only go. They say to one of my baby students that they will pay him well if he will only go and practice Osteopathy, when he is no more fit to go than a donkey is to go into a jewelry shop. Men come here and ask me what to do for sore throat, and so on, and say they will pay so much for it. They tell our young students that they have plenty of money and will pay their expenses and $200 a month if they will go with them; and that is a great temptation to a young man who had not has fifteen cents with which to buy his girl chewing gum. Some of them know of this condition, and they will stand around among the patients and strangers and tell them of this and that qualification, and say, "Don't you go to the old doctor, he is jealous of us," and so on. They keep this up until they get him to go off with them, and away they go, like any other deceiver or thief, to pick pockets.

I have followed this science for twenty-two years, fully convinced that the God of nature has done his work completey. I am satisfied that a revolution stands before you today, a healing revolution, a revolution in the human mind that will result in the study of anatomy in our district schools and in our colleges. It is one of the most important studies for all of the schools. When I commenced this study I took the human bones and handled them week in and out, month in and out, and never laid them down while I was awake for twelve months. There is a great danger to the student of Osteopathy, that he may conclude that he ought to be out as quick as some hostler or some fellow that has been around here for a little while, and is out stealing from the people today. You ask when you come here how long it takes a man to become competent to go into a community and withstand the howlitzers that will be thrown against him. We tell you, from long experience in this science, that it will require twice twelve months. I can take you up as a herd of sheep, comb you and grease you, and send you out in the market, and the best judge can't tell whether you are good or bad sheep, but I will not do it. You ask me for truth, I will give it to you. If you send your son or daughter here, you do not want them to go out incompetent. Those who have been with us a year, a number of them are out, and they do some good. Previous to the time we got our institution so we could handle it, we did the best we could. Just like the preacher's wife who borrowed cloth to patch her husband's shirt, she did the best she could; and she stayed home because she had no shoes, and that was the best she could do. We have got to the time now that we can prepare better.

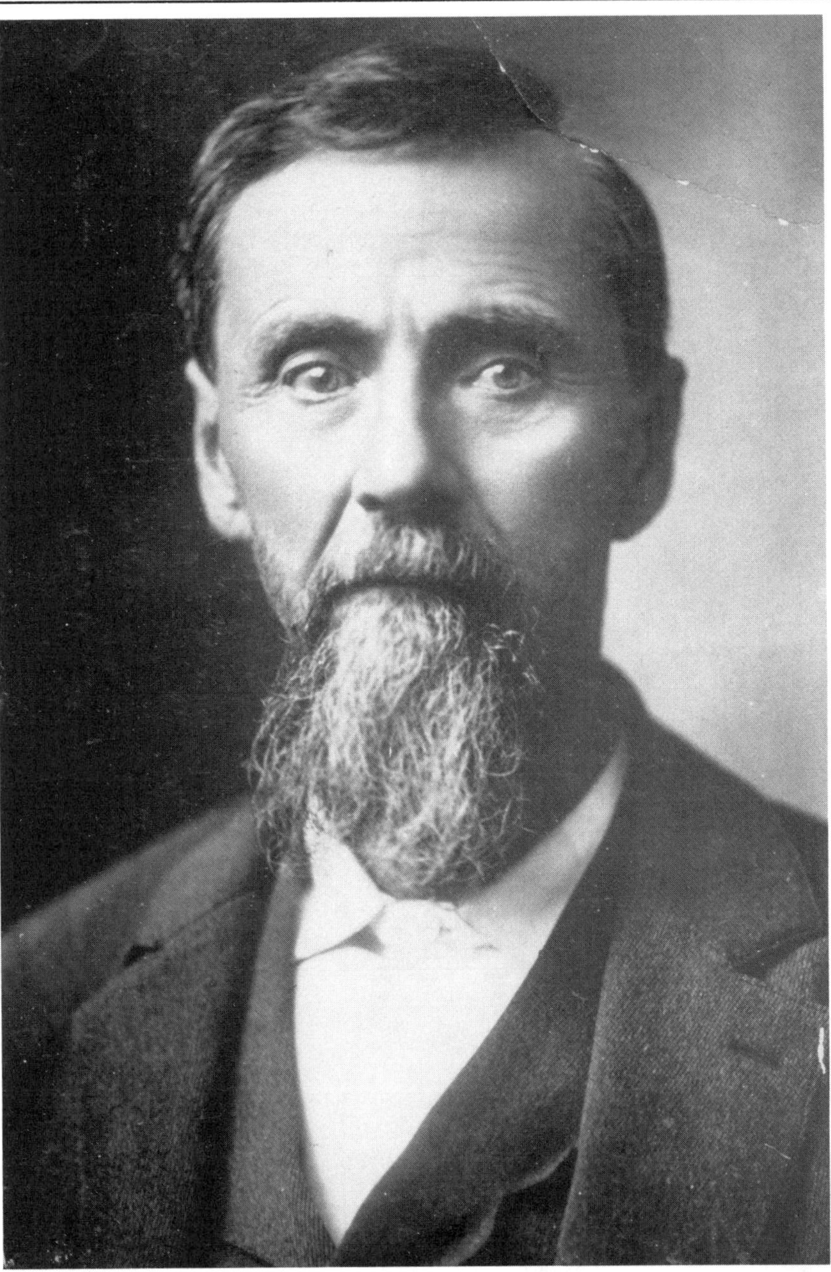

A. T. Still, 1895

Two years ago when I commenced this building, 50x90, hall, ten rooms, etc., the people said, "What is that old fool doing down there putting up a house of that size; he is crazy." Do you know the condition that fellow is in now? He finds that he needs another building 40x60, ten more rooms, in order to accommodate the people who are coming here. Do you see how the work has grown? One person speaks to another and another, and reports what is being done. That is all the advertising that has been done. We print our JOURNAL to answer your questions concerning the science.

For twenty-two years I have been looking at the parts of the human engine, and I find it the most wonderfully constructed engine, with the intelligence of mind and the spirit of God, from the crown of the head to the sole of the foot. I believe that it is God's own medical drug store. The medicine of God is the mind of intelligence applied to the place of need.

If I were to take up this subject and discuss it as a philosophy, no one hot night would be sufficient for an introduction to it. I do not think I could tell it in six months or six years. It is as inexhaustible as the works of the whole universe.

If I live twelve months longer I expect to reverently respect the 22nd day of June, 1897, the anniversary of Osteopathy's discovery.

September, 1896

DR. STILL'S ADDRESS.

Following is a verbatim report of the address delivered in Memorial Hall by Dr. A. T. Still, on the evening of Aug. 6th, the occasion of his 68th birthday:

Ladies and gentlemen: Those of you who have received the light, and those who are in partial darkness:

I am glad to meet you here tonight, this being the second anniversary of the beginning of this unfinished house. We began to build it two years ago, and it has done great good; but without the completion of the whole body it is very difficult for us to execute in order the quantity of business that is now on hand, which seems to double itself every few months. This is also the anniversary of my birth. Sixty-eight times the earth has made her circuit around the sun, and every time she gets around she says: "One circle more is made and added to the number." We are conscious of the fact that but a few more revolutions around the sun —which constitutes one year for this globe— we are conscious of the fact that a few more rides will throw us off. A wild mule will throw a man off at some time, as a general thing. So will this life buck at the right time and you will mark a wreck. After a man has reached the age that I have, one ought not to be surprised to hear of a wreck at any time. Still, I feel sound. I have no back ache, no leg ache or no head ache; but my tongue and throat sometimes do ache. I try to answer all inquiries. People seem to be surprised, as much so as if they should see two suns rise in the morning horizon; they seem to be as much surprised to see a science and truth of God developed that applies to all men and that is without either taste or odor

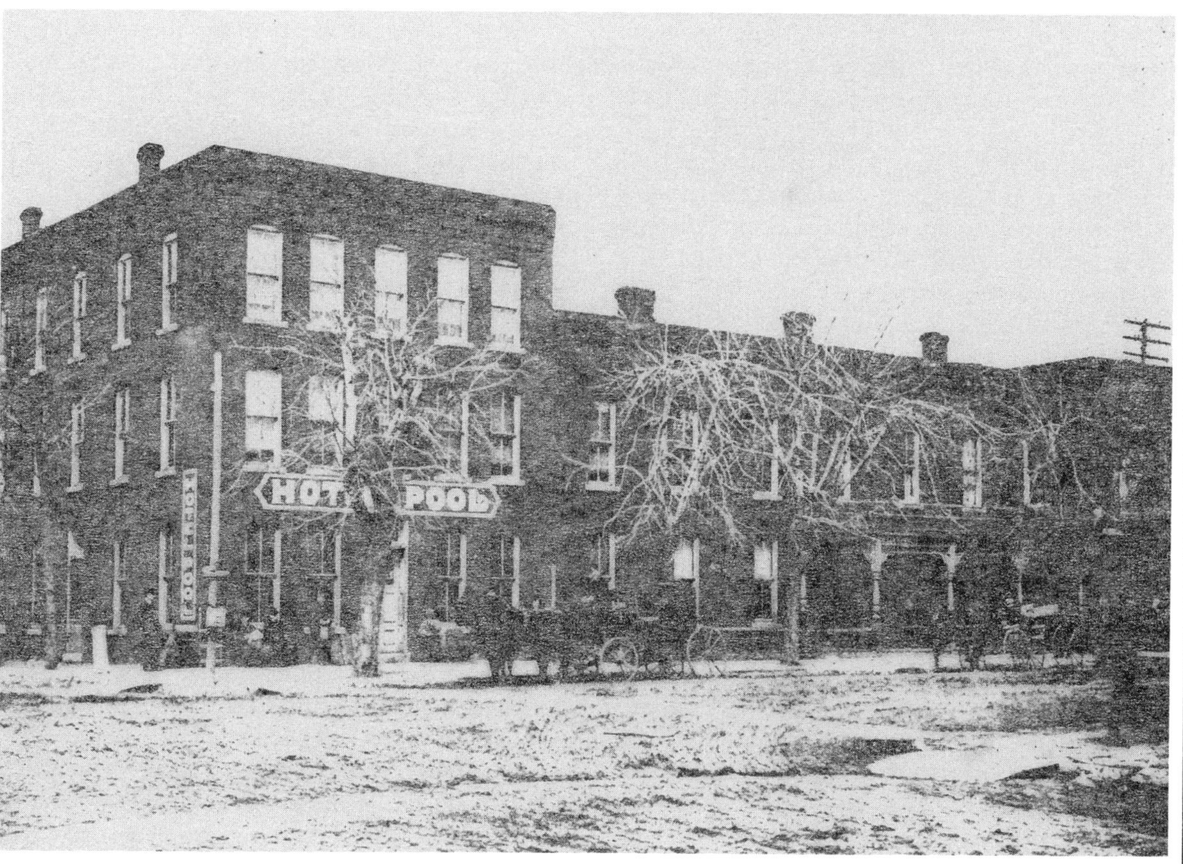

—a science grafted into man's make-up and his very life. They are surprised to find that the Great Architect has put in their places within man all the processes of life. He has placed all the engines of life, and all the electricity for the duties of life. Nature's God has been thoughtful enough to place in man all that the word "remedy" means. It is a difficult matter for a man raised to believe in the use of drugs to realize this fact. In all our diseases, from birth to death, they seem to have been satisfied with the results of drugs when given wisely or given by our wisest men, our fathers, mothers, or whoever may have administered them. Man is surprised to find God to be God. He is surprised to find that man is made by the eternal, unerring Architect. He is surprised from the rising of the sun to the setting of the same to find the eternal truths of Deity permeating his whole make-up. He is surprised to find that the machinery is competent to warm itself and cool itself, select its food, and satisfy its highest anticipations. We see this most wonderful sun standing before us where we never imagined a star to exist. It is the sun of eternal light. The thoughts of God himself are found in every drop of your blood. When a man begins to see what we are doing here he is anxious to ask questions of anyone who knows anything about it, a world of questions. I can answer from morning until night; and when I have answered all that I can on this subject it is but a beginning. Take chronic diseases, contagious, epidemics, all diseases of the seasons, when I say we can handle them and demonstrate it to you, here stands a man who never saw it done, his mind is full of questions. They must be answered. The very instant that you disappoint him by answering that which he thinks cannot be done except by the works of God in the hands of God, that very instant you have answered his question. He will pass on, and on the next corner when he meets you he has a question for you to answer containing a greater per cent of sublimity than the first. He asks that question; then, if you are not a philosopher in the science, well acquainted with it, you have come to a resting place for your mind. No, it does not rest there when you cannot answer the questions that confront you from time to time. You take up the philosophy and learn all you can about it, for you know the questions will come. I am satisfied and pleased to have the people ask questions and receive all the answers they can get. And after I have answered all I can through the papers or with my own mouth, I cannot even answer a moiety of the questions. To answer all the questions that are suggested by a human thigh bone would open and close an eternity. Therefore you must not expect me to answer all of them. Neither must you expect this school to do that for you. You can get enough demonstrations to put you on the track to become a self-generating philosopher. It is as full of suggestions as the rising of the sun, the opening of the mouths of vegetation when the evening shades appear, moon flowers, night flowers, and all others opening their mouths to draw life from the bosom of God. The most sublime thought that I have ever had in my life is concerning the machinery and the works as I have found them in the human construction, faithfully executing all of the known duties and the beauties of life. When I go out in the morning among my friends and one says he wants a certain class of diet, how glad I am that I have that. I make each man, woman or child exactly fill my place when the questions are asked. When she says, "My child has a sore throat," what is she hungry for? She is hungry for a longer lease on that child's days. Can I find that? Can I attack in the proper place to stop the downward tendency, the downward road to death in which that child is being propelled? If I can I say "Yes ma'am. The throat of that child can be relieved and it can be done by one of the simple laws which is as wise as the Infinite can construct it, but lying exposed there for the purpose of the relief of your child," that sole goes away happy. The throat has returned to its normal size. But another person appears coming down across the road that I walk. "I have lost into the ground one of my children with flux and the other is bleeding." What is she hungry for She is hungry for the word that will relieve that child and continue it in life. Do I know what buttons will bring relief? If I know that I do it, and there is No. 2 happy. I do it; my operators do it, and do it daily. This science, as little as they and I know about it, is capable of handling flux, fevers, chills, coughs, colds, and in fact the whole system or systems of disease that prey upon the human make-up.

To-night I am proud to tell you that after all these years—it is forty-one years since Major Abbott and I talked upon this very subject—I am proud to say that after all these years I can hand it to you as a science that can be as plainly demonstrated as the science of electricity. I find in man a minature univers; I find matter, motion and mind. When the elder prays he speaks to God; he can conceive of nothing higher than mind, motion and matter; the attributes of mind, comprising love, and all that pertains to it. In man we find a complete universe, we find a solar system; we find a world, we find a Venus, a Jupiter, a Mars, a Herschel, a Satrun, a Uranus. We find all of the parts of the whole solar system and the universe repeated in man. In the heart we have the solar center; the little toe will be Uranus. What is the road that is traveled to Uranus? It is from the heart through the great thoracic aorta, abdominal aorta, which divides into the iliacs, and from there on down to the Popliteal, etc., until you get to the planter arteries.

When Major Abbott spoke of clarivoyance, he spoke of it as we talked of it as a curiosity that day. My father was of an intuitive mind. He was a sensitive man and had an intuitive mind causing him to worry to such an extent that he would turn his compas around and go across fifty or seventy miles, to what? Because the intuitive law, or the law of Providence, sent him home. Because something worried him, something about a horse; and when he got home old Jim was dead. When he was preaching on a certain occasion in the Chariton hills here, he came to a halt. He says, "I must bring these exercises to a close, I am wanted at another place." By the intuitive law he said "I am needed and we will bring these exercises to an immediate close." He stopped right in the center of his sermon, and picked up his saddle bags (he was a physician), and when he got to the door there was Jim Bosarth telling him to come and set Ed's thigh. There were fifty living witnesses to that then, and I suppose ten or twenty of them are still alive. They wondered how old Dr. Still knew when to take up his saddle bags. That is one of the attributes that God puts in man.

In our school we have decided to have a rest until the first Monday in September. We have stuck to our work here for three or four years without a single week's intermission at any time. We are tired and the weather is hot and the school will have a rest until the first Monday in September. If a man should plow corn all the time from the month of May, all through June, July, August, and all the rest of the year, he would get pretty tired and want some rest. We expect in October a very large class, and in order to have things more convenient we have made this addition to the building, which we hope to have finished in three or four weeks. We will have it well seated and lighted and make it as convenient as possible.

I thank you ladies and gentlemen for your presence here tonight on this occasion. I was still-born, I want to tell you, and possibly the only child that was still-born that ever lived; but when I did kick it was in a great hurry, and I have been kicking for twenty-five years to bring forward the light, to open up and show you the possibility of the science of Osteopathy.

Again thanking you for your attention on this hot evening, I bid you good-by for another twelve months to come.

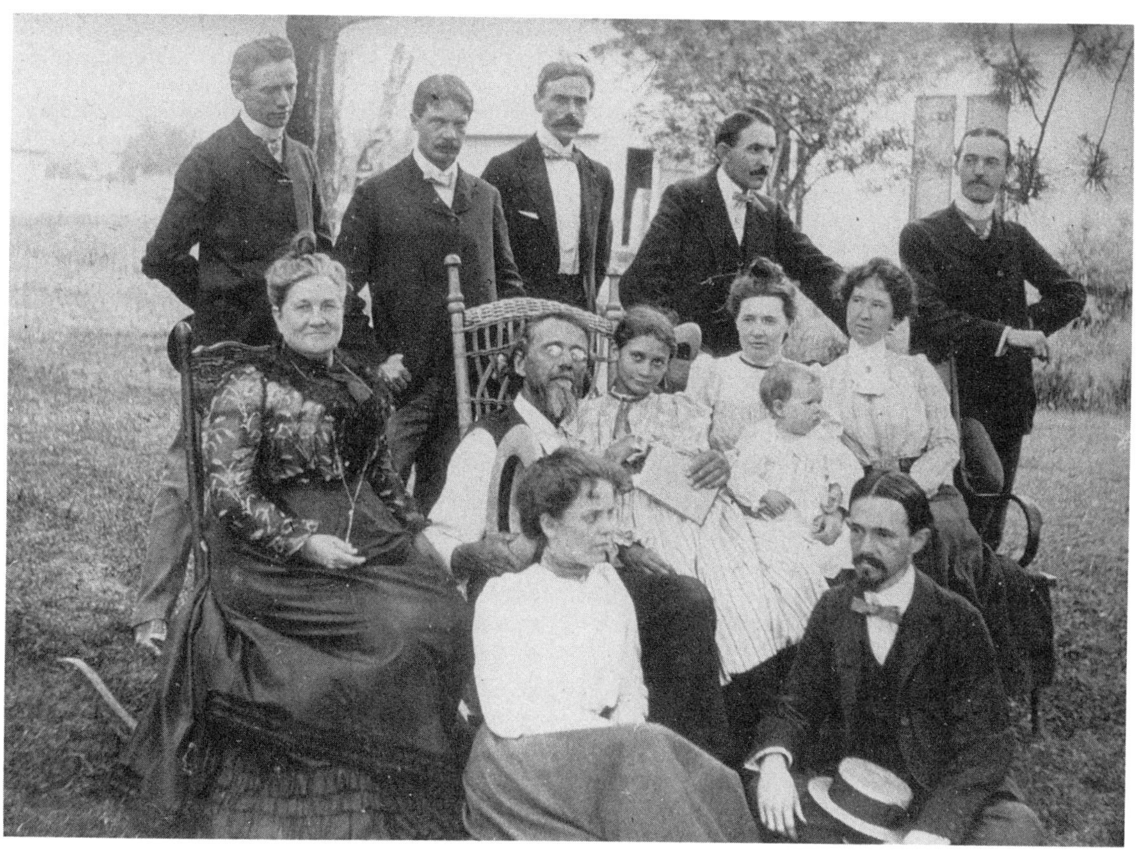

Group of students visiting Dr. and Mrs. Still, 1899

September, 1896

DR. STILL'S BIRTHDAY.

Patients and Citizens Unite to Commemorate the 68th Anniversary of Osteopathy's Founder.

On the evening of August 6th the A. T. Still Infirmary was the scene of a very pleasant gathering, composed of the friends of Dr. A. T. Still in particular and the friends of Osteopathy in general. Besides those from Kirksville there were present many of Dr. Still's associates of years ago from other localities of Missouri and other states. The object of the gathering was to celebrate the Doctor's 68th birthday anniversary. It was also the second anniversary of the ground-breaking for the Infirmary building, and also to dedicate the new addition to the Infirmary now nearly completed. This latter part of the program, however, was postponed as the addition is not yet finished.

About 7:30 the program opened with music by the Kirksville Cornet band from its elevated position in the observatory on top of the new addition. The exercises of the evening were conducted in Memorial Hall. The first was the reading of a poem, entitled, "To Osteopathy," by the author, Mrs. Helen Steadley, of Carthage, Mo., which appears elsewhere in this issue.

Dr. Wm. Smith then took the floor in behalf of Mr. Wm. Sippy, of St. Louis, and in the following brief talk presented Dr. Still a large American flag:

Mr. Chairman, Dr. Still, Ladies and Gentlemen: It may possibly strike you as strange that a Scotchman, not yet an American citizen, should perform the duty which this evening devolves upon me, but a student of this school, who deservedly has the respect of all, Dr. Alvin Sippy, a regular graduate in medicine who has satisfied himself that there is something in Osteopathy and who wishes to learn it, feeling himself devoid of a quality which he believes me to possess in excess, gall, has requested me, on behalf of his father, Mr. William Sippy, of St. Louis, to say to you, Dr. Still, a few words and to ask your acceptance of that which I hold in my hand. More than a hundred years have gone by since the stars and stripes became the emblems of a free people; over thirty years have elapsed since the same flag, altered by additions to its parts, first waved over a united country, the emblem of freedom, in thought, word and deed. It is justly fitted to wave over a progressive school. Dr. Sippy and his father, I, and I think I may truly say everyone in this large audience, has for you, Sir, a profound feeling of respect. We respect you as a man, an American and a good, honest fellow; we wish you all success in your great work, many years of happiness and comfort after the toils and labors of the earlier years of your work. May you be spared for many years to view the results of your boldness and uphill fighting; may this flag, for which in the past you fought, ever wave above the institution which your reason, your "stick-to-itiveness" and your grit have made a reality. Accept this flag, Doctor, with all the good wishes of the donor, an old patient; post it on the topmost point of your building, an American flag where it ought to be, on the top of an American school of learning; and when the breezes have played havoc with it, when it is tattered and torn, put another one there and let it ever wave, the emblem of freedom, over men and women free in thought and progress. What I have said could have been better said, but there is no one who wishes you well more truly, or could have done with more feeling. In the name of Mr. Sippy I have much pleasure in handing into your possession this flag.

With the stars and stripes wrapped about him, Dr. Still accepted the token in the following manner:

Ladies and Gentlemen: Allow me, in the name of Osteopathy, to thank Mr. Sippy, the father of our Dr. Sippy, and all his friends, for this token of his confidence in Osteopathy. This emblem that you bring here tonight is around the bodies of many men who have fallen in the field of battle that this flag might forever wave over the whole of the United States between all her rivers and oceans. I am proud to receive this. No higher emblem could be offered to me; nothing more inspiring. I have seen men fall under it—fall for it. I believe this nation would rise as a unit, even those who pierced it with angry bullets, to protect it. Even that man who fired his gun into it in days that are past and gone, when he comes into port and sees this flag again, will say, "Home again." That is the flag that his father, my father, and yours, have loved as an eternal emblem. Defense if necessary—peace if possible.

In behalf of the American School of Osteopathy I thank Dr. Sippy and his father for this token. It shall ever float in the breezes of Osteopathy, and as it floats on the breeze in all directions, so I hope Osteopathy will spread to all points of the compass. Osteopathy is just as honorable as this flag. Therefore she is sailing over this country of ours, just as this flag is. This flag is floating over our universities and schools throughout the land. We are one nation, one flag. We may differ in a great many other things, but are as a unit in regard to this flag.

I promise you, ladies and gentlemen, that you shall see this flag floating in the air from the top of this building, and when she is gone we will get another.

Judge J. C. Abbott, of Desoto, Kansas, was called on for remarks, and responded by telling something of his associations with Dr. Still during the early history of Kansas while that state was struggling for free statehood. He referred to many characteristic incidents of their long acquaintance, and how in even those early days of '55—'60 the Dr. had expressed a lack of belief in the efficacy of the indiscriminate use of drugs. In closing the Judge presented to Dr. Still, as President of the American School of Osteopathy, as a slight token of esteem, a gavel with which he might call his meetings to order; also a minature tripod from which swings a kettle, in memory of their early experiences of camp life. While both bear the finest finish, and are beautifully designed, they are prized the more highly for being the Judge's own handiwork.

The remainder of the evening was occupied by Dr. Still, whose address appears in full in another part of this issue.

The evening is one long to be remembered by Dr. Still, and all friends who were privileged to attend. The Doctor is very grateful for the many expressions of confidence and friendship, and the tokens of esteem received as he passes this his 68th mile-stone in the journey of life.

September, 1896

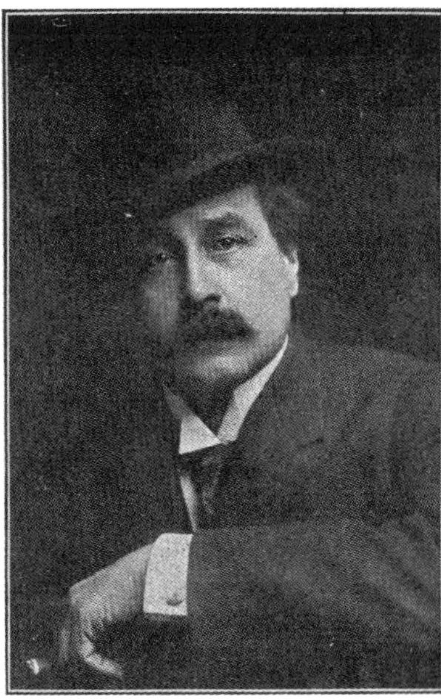

Wm. Smith, First Anatomy Teacher of the A.S.O.

FOUR YEARS AGO.

Dr. Wm. Smith Gives an Account of His First Visit to Dr. Still.

Four years elapsed between my first visit to Kirksville and my return. In that time great changes have occurred; the weakling infant Osteopathy has grown into a stout and stalwart young giant, a power for good in the length and breadth of the land; many old faces have disappeared; many new ones come upon the scene. A brief account of what I found in 1892, followed by what exists in 1896, may be of interest to the many readers of this JOURNAL.

I never heard of Osteopathy or Dr. Still until I arrived in Kirksville. Then from all, save doctors, I heard good reports of him and of his work; but from them nothing but evil. The discrepancy in the reports interested me. I judged that in him there must be something out of the common. To hear a man spoken of by laymen as a "second Christ" and by physicians as a "d——d old quack," convinced me that there was a man living ahead of his time, a man of views so advanced that he was misunderstood. I determined to meet him. As soon as I could do so I called at his office—a one-story frame building, uncarpeted and with many broken windows, the wasps building tiny nests in secluded corners. Here I found about a dozen persons waiting to see him, all talking of the wonders he was daily doing. The mention of the fact that I wished to see Dr. Still provoked a chorus to the effect that I must "wait my turn."

My turn came, and I found myself in the presence of a tall, athletic man apparently about 50 years of age (actually 64). I explained that I had heard so much abuse of him in some quarters and so much good in others that my curiosity was aroused and incidentally, mentioned that my right arm was to a slight degree affected; that I had imperfect use of my elbow. Without saying a word he grabbed (that is the only word available) hold of it, gave it a quick turn, and then said "How is that?" To my intense surprise I found that I had perfect command of what had been impaired in motion for six months. To my request that he would tell me of his work he readily acquiesced, and for two hours I listened to a man in perfect love with his vocation discoursing upon it. What he told me seemed so foreign to all I had been taught in medical schools, so utterly nonsensical and chimerical, that I asked for proof of his statements. The proof was readily given by about sixteen patients who gave me their statements as to their condition when they came to Kirksville and what had befallen them under the treatment. My one desire then was to learn of this man who had the power of life and death, so to speak, so largely in his hands; who could do what all the medical world declared to be impossible.

Right here let me say that when Osteopathy is to be investigated it must be with a clear and unprejudiced mind. If a man, a physician, comes to Kirksville and hears what he will hear and then tries to reason it out on the basis of what he learned in a medical school, there is only one conclusion to which he can come: that Osteopathy is a fraud and a delusion, a gigantic humbug which is taking from the pockets of the sick and afflicted thousands of dollars monthly. BUT, if the enquirer will just approach the matter as though he knew nothing (and after four years experience of Osteopathy let me tell ANY doctor that he knows very little), take nothing for granted, accept no statement for or against Osteopathy; but just interview a dozen patients and accept them as reasonable men and women and not as hysterical persons, half-fitted for a lunatic asylum, nor utter and gratuitous liars, he is BOUND as an honest man to come to the conclusion, as I did, that there are still some things in the healing art which are not known to the medical profession. Let him examine further and he will find results obtained quite impossible under treatment with medicines. Then let him inquire of the patients who tell him in their stories, how many doctors had declared their recovery impossible, and then, and not till then, let him make up his mind as to whether or not Osteopathy is a fraud, its practitioners humbugs and its supporters liars. If all these persons claiming to be benefitted are liars where can the profit come in from running the business? To pay such an army of liars would consume the capital of a state. If they are hysterical, why did not their doctors cure them?

An obscure medical sheet in St. Louis started out this summer with the statement that it was "going to expose Still if it took all summer." We are waiting calmly for the exposure, but in making the statement the editor (who seemed to be suffering from an attack of humor and smartness) undertook a task much beyond his strength, being quite unaware that several of his confreres in the medical profession in St. Louis and all over the country had started out with the same intentions, but had finished up by sending patients to Kirksville, patients whom they could not cure, but "Still" could and did.

For four years Osteopathy has had bitter persecution (aye, for fourteen) at the hands of the medical profession. No lie was to mean to tell, no means to undermine it too low for the hands of certain of its members; but to the honor of the profession let it be said that dozens of others have stated that they regret their past actions; had they only taken the care to investigate before acting, their conduct would have been different.

Of course this opposition has hindered the work; Osteopathy has fallen back. From the little four-roomed one-story frame building has grown an institution of three stories with 17 treating rooms, a printing office for the issuance of the JOURNAL OF OSTEOPATHY, large retiring and bath rooms, two large halls for lectures, etc., one with a seating capacity of 400 the other 1100, class-room accomodation for 500 students, with all the requirements for a thorough education in this special work. While four years ago Dr. Still and two of his sons could do all the work in the treating of patients, there is now a corps of 20 operators in this one institution, and all with their hands filled with work. My first class had 14 members; now there are over 100 students, and a class of about 60 will start in the fall. What we want is more opposition; we wish to be exposed; we wish all to know that Osteopathy is worth opposing, and that it is in exposure that it gets advertisement. There is nothing that we are ashamed of—except the few mean-minded, ignorant, jealous, one-horse little doctors who come around trying to get six months' tuition and a diploma for nothing, and who, when they are told that they must put up their money like other people and take the full course of instruction, run away and cry out "Fraud," "Humbug," "Swindle," "Robbing the people," and so forth, or else put out a big advertisement saying that "Having now completed a full course of instruction under the great Dr. Still, we beg to state that we are now prepared to treat all cases in a superior manner to what he does."

Osteopathy goes right along with an even tread, trying to give better and better instruction to its students to fit them for the battle with disease, death and doctors. It has tried to do it all the time, but now it looks as though the seas of oppression were getting more feeble in their force, the beacon light of prosperity and peace shines out on the horizon. The day is fast approaching when EVERY honest physician in the world will recognize its value. The dishonest individual members of an honorable profession may then, as now, be disregarded.

WILLIAM SMITH, M. D., D. O.

October, 1896

A FEW WORDS FROM DR. STILL.

A Life's Story.

Listen to a life story told in five minutes or more. I was born on this globe sixty-eight years ago. I had the luck, good or bad, to be born in a house of drugs. Father was an M. D., also a D. D. And at the end of thirty-five years I began to reason how a doctor of divinity could blend with the foolish teaching of medicine. Questions arose with me, how can man harmonize the idea that all God's work is perfect, and never in running order? His finest machine, man, never in running condition. Has the God of all wisdom failed in this one superstructure, man, and why did he say it was good if he knew it would not work as he thought it would when he made it, and why should a D. D. who with uplifted hands say, "his works prove his perfection," and take a dose of quinine and whiskey to assist nature's machine to run the race and do the duties of life? If so, where is the proof of his faith in God's perfection, and why should he eat and drink of all that is deadly in effect? I did not wish to think or speak irreverently of our divines nor our M D.'s, who follow just behind God to fix his machines for the harvest of life. But why follow his work, if good and wisely made, by the hand and mind of all intelligence? I began to reason about on this line: Would God get offended at man, if he would say to him, you have failed in enough places to admit of a few suggestions? When man in his wisdom or lack of wisdom, would say by word or deed, "Thou hast failed to make this and that part or principle to adjust itself to suit the seasons, and climates of the globe on which it was placed, and your machine must have additions and be oiled by drugs and drinks or it will be forever a failure on the field of battle between life and death now raging all over the world." Such questions arose and stood before me for years. I found to my mind that there was a great mistake in God's work or man's conclusions if drugs were not in absolute demand when man is sick. Now I was in a close place, and saw at once that if I voted to use drugs I would by that vote set aside the ability of God to provide for his man under all conditions, and he had not the mind and intelligence claimed for him, and if I voted for God, I would soon find 75 per cent of the human race in line to oppose that conclusion. To defend and maintain that the works of nature had been able to prove perfection at every point of observation or under our most crucial test of philosophy. I soon found to be popular I would have to enter a life of deception, and at that time I determined to run up the white emblem of truth with the red sword of eternal war for that flag, and by it I would stand until I was dead; dead, and folded in it to begin the common rest of all human forms which is as natural to the body of man as the love of a mother is to her babe.

Gems.

IF God knew a man would not use his mind, why did he not put horns on him and call him a mutton-head?

WHAT is the value of a mind when placed on the back of a coward? If mind is a gift of God to man for his use why not let him use it? A mind is not in use when doing no good.

JOY is the reward which all beings strive to obtain. Joy is that feeling that comes to a contented mind. Its effect is rest to soul and body. When a person is in possession of that precious gem, all is peace and love to man and beast, friend and foe. Joy comes often in a small way; it lasts but a short time, then gives way to cares.

PROPHECY is what can be seen by a cloudless mind, either the past or future. The events of the past and coming days must all be in sight of the eye of the mind. To prophesy well, you must see through the two veils, one of the past and one of the future. If an event is to arise tomorrow, where is it now? Memory calls up the past; reason sees the future.

OSTEOPATHY in meaning is equal to a well known mechanical science called plumbing. The plumber adjusts his pipes so all parts of the house are supplied with just enough pure water for all demands for health and cleanliness. An Osteopath goes farther and adjusts the battery and all nerves thereunto belonging. An Osteopath is a plumber and an electrician combined.

WE all have visions occasionally, even though it should take a yellow jacket's nest to bring them out of the brain. The more stupid seldom get to the altitude of joy found in visions. Now let me give you a few of the apple pies of the night. My cat dreams, my dog dreams; so can you, if the brain has not been soaked too long in the morning hours of "sit on the sweet roost pole of human stupidity." No dream, no good dog, no good sense.

"I Want to See the Old Doctor,"

Is a common expression and has been for four months, while I was building. I am now prepared to meet you, and make your acquaintance. I will now give you the reason why I have been as you have thought, hard to find. In May I saw at a glance that I had no house to suit the business that was demanding attention. My house was not one third large enough for the work. I closed my eyes and ears to all business but to build and that in the shortest time possible. I stepped out of all office business and left it in the hands of the vice president and secretary to manage the sick. I knew they could and would and they have done the work to perfection, and can do it at all times, whether I am there or not. I will be in the building much and often. I will talk to you, have you taken to all parts of the house, in school and dissection rooms, and try and give you a chance to know that thorough qualification is in all our branches from furnace to flag. Don't stop me in the halls or upon the streets to tell a long tale of woe. I will listen to you after you have been to the Secretary, who is a thorough diplomate in the science. Go to him first and do as he directs. He will come to me with your case if there is anything uncommon in it whether you ask him or not.

Question?

"Would you advise me to study Osteopathy?" is a question asked almost daily. The mail is loaded with such questions as follows:

"Do you think I ought to study Osteopathy, send my son, daughter, or advise some well informed lady or gentleman to study the new science?"

To all these questions I will say: yes, if they want to. I do not want a student to come and tell me he or she was persuaded to come by some one. If they cooly decide to make it a profession for life, I would say, send them by all means. We will send them back prepared to do honor and good and make you proud that you had advised them to go and learn the machinery of man and the laws of life.

Staking Out My Calves.

I will not stake out any this year. I will have some nice yearlings for market next year. Some nice Herefords, Durhams, Jerseys, Muleys, and some nice black Polled Angus. I have sent out one pedigreed two-year old to Vermont. He has torn up jack with the medical law. I have a Polled Angus and Durham in Chicago. I tell you they roar loud. I have three Jerseys in Kentucky. They paw and scrape and look well on dress parade. I sent three to Denver. They are sixteen to one in any market. I have a Texas ranger in Ohio and a few others out, all pedigreed.

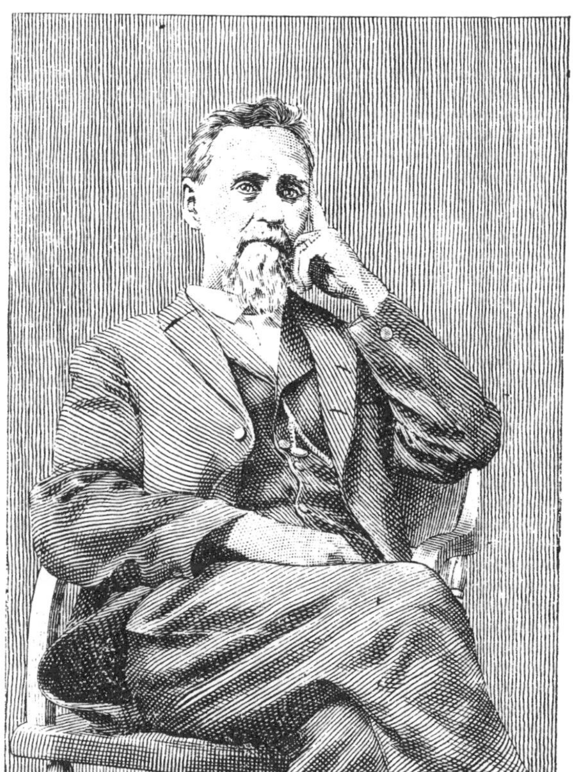

A. T. Still.

December, 1896

CLASS MEETINGS.

I was raised a Methodist. I found the idea of class meetings was a very good thing. The class leader would ask us how we had prepared and what arrangements we had made to die, and so on all along the road to heaven; if we had read the bible, been to Sunday School, visited the sick, fed the hungry, clothed the naked, paid our quarterage, and fed the Lord's horse which the preacher had ridden, and so on, and all was pronounced good and marked "O. K."

I was drilled so long, much and often in class that I got so well posted that I could examine myself quite well, and when the time came that the people wanted and urged me to establish a school, and teach the science of Osteopathy, I opened a class meeting to examine myself as to my qualifications for the great task of conducting a college of such dimensions as would be required for the purpose desired. I had seen enough of life to know that no man could be a success in any enterprise, and be ignorant of anything pertaining to the duties from start to completion of all that would be required in a first class college of learning. First a good and practical knowledge of the principles to be taught, then a knowledge of building—must be of much experience to plan and construct a building to suit the work. That would require much thought and originality to harmonize the needs of such a house. There was no book or plans that could instruct the builder. Inventive genius must be the guiding star from base to dome. Then the most important question of all came: "Have I the $75,000 cash to pay for all of a four story house, 60x176 feet long, with 68 rooms, steam heating, water and electric lights, all with a finish to date?" Answer must be, "Yes."

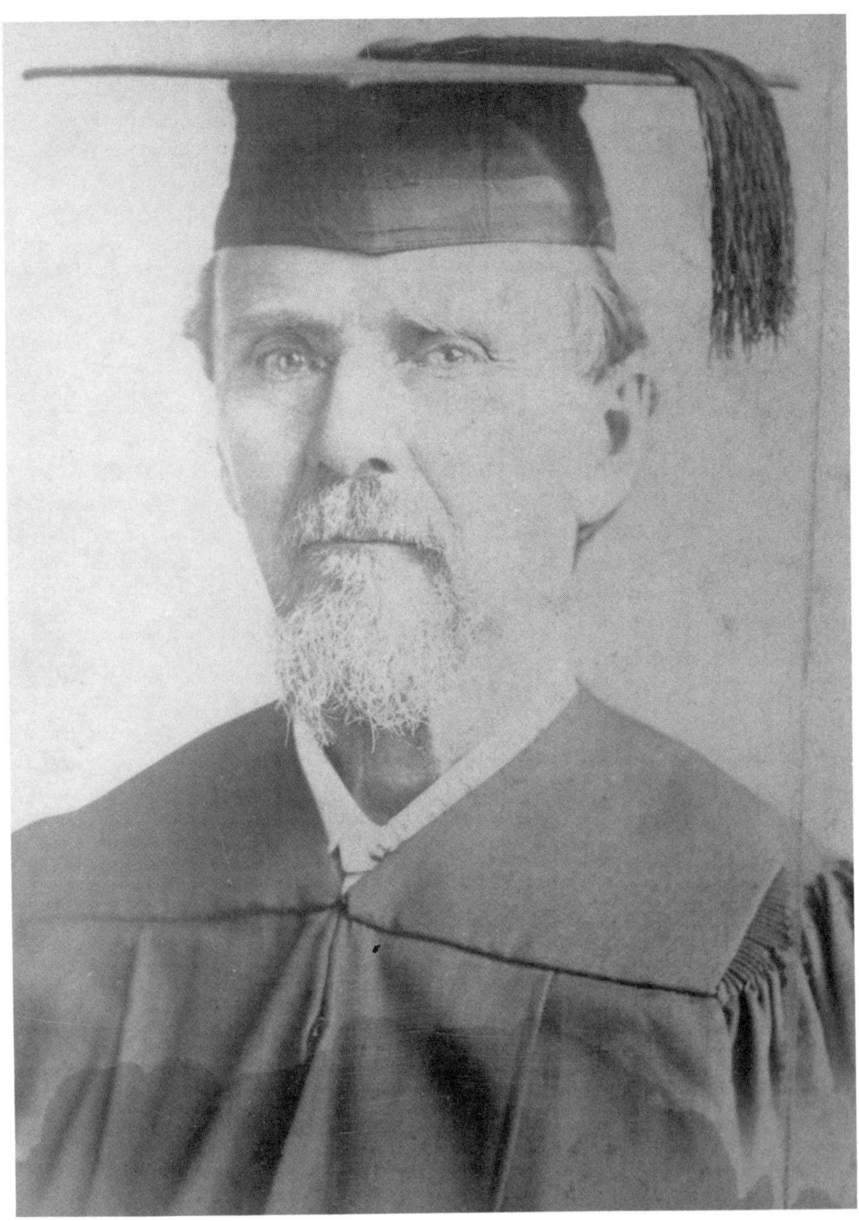

"Official" photograph of A. T. Still to be used by other Osteopathic schools

Then came other questions equally as great, which pertain to conducting the business of a great institution of learning. Many important positions will have to be filled by persons who must have the necessary attainments to do the duty devolving upon that office. Then all must be combined and have one head that is mentally qualified with long experience to select competent persons to fill all places of trust ond honor in the whole institution, with the nerve and judgment to execute.

December, 1896

Definition of Love.

DR. A. T. STILL.

Love is the true odor of life,
When moved by contact of eye,
Oceans of inexpressible acts of strife,
Come from friend, man or wife.

It has not yet been described by man,
It binds man to man, how? unknown,
It comes never to leave again,
It fills our mind's to feast when alone.

It comes and stays,
A loving flame of soul,
And asks no change of ways,
But to find a friend and unfold.

It is the odor for smell, taste and sight,
Comes with self as part of laws,
Comes gentle, and never with might;
Without a word of self or cause.

To embrace, to fondle and draw to
Itself to feed the being unseen,
That law of life only can make or do,
Willing to allow nothing to stay between.

Love begins in self and ends in you,
And asks to roam no farther during life,
Is content when found in friend, child or wife;
And no other ending can even partly do.

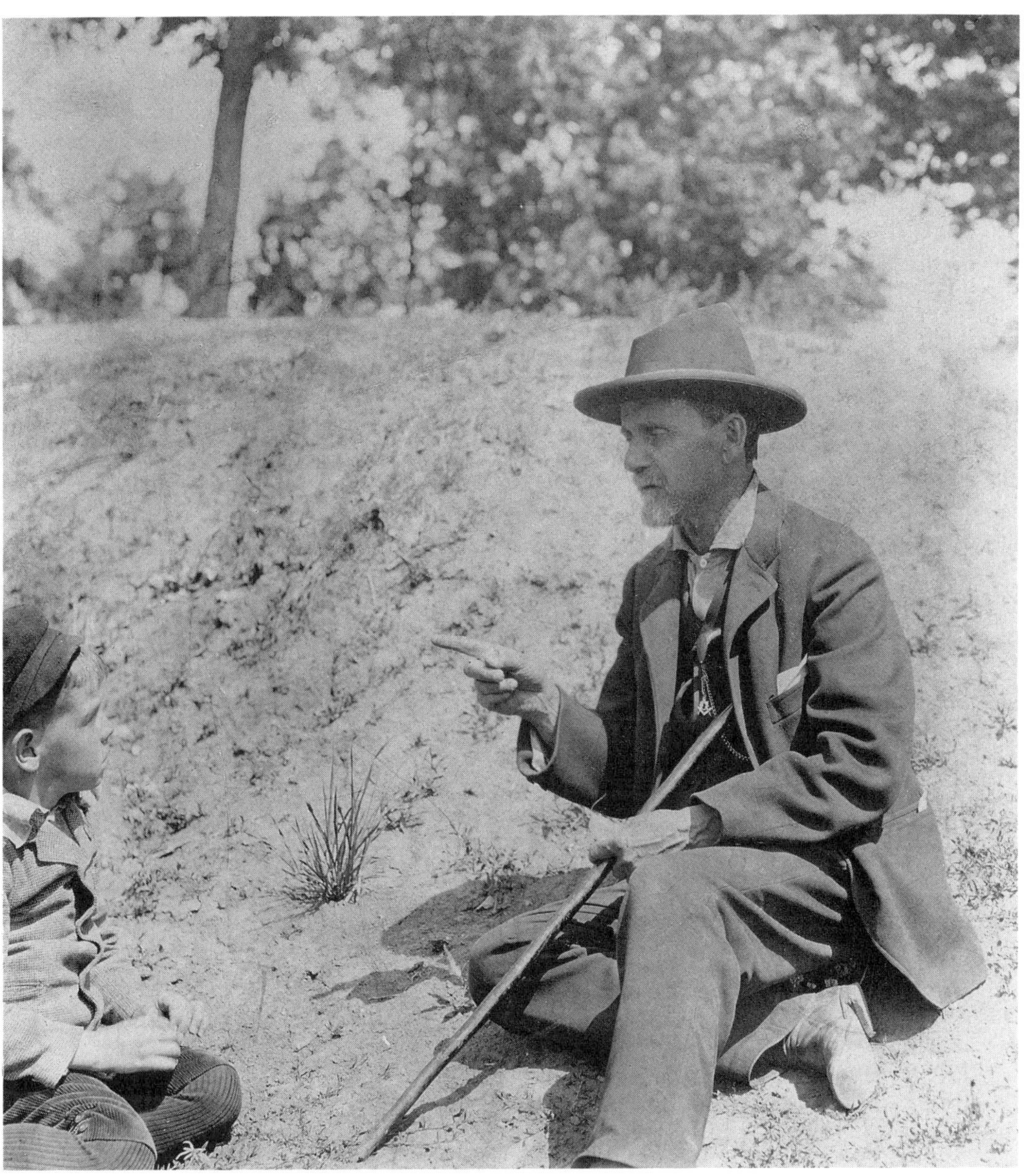

A. T. Still talking with youngster
Date and place perhaps about 1902

December, 1896

HOW TO LIVE LONG AND LOUD.

The time is now at hand for Christmas, New Years, and great big dinners. Big turkeys, big pies, mince, apple, goose and chicken pies, with oysters as big as Cleveland in the stuffing, and cheese with celery, sausage with sage, garlic and onions to kill, nut cakes and soup, ice cream and frozen vinegar, slaw with jersey cream, and walnut cakes with it, and fillibusters and codfish and taters, sweet and irish, and grannie's kind of pies, flavored with pure good old whiskey or brandy, all served in an air tight room, heated to kill by a furnace to 120 f. and not a single vent of pure air.

Now to eat, is the command. Eat means to sit still for two hours and cram your bodies with three to twelve changes or courses of dishes. Then I thought of the fighting preacher who always prayed before he went into a battle among shot and shell. He said: "Oh, Lord, I ask thee to save my body if possible from those vultures of lead and iron; if not able to save my body, oh, please save my soul." Now the battle is open. I see the gunners and aids all in line. The rockets are high in the air, which say the first course is so close you can see their eyes, and the command from the general is to charge along the whole line and show no quarters. Eat up the enemy if you can. The first line is a regiment of bread black and white, ham, butter, celery, cheese, turkey, coffee, tea, slaw and cream, lots more. We downed the first line. I felt good and brave to know I had helped to down the first great line of the enemy. I wanted to go home and tell our wonderful victory, and asked the commanding general for a furlough. He said no, and handed me his field glass and said "look at the second regiment; you may fall at the feet of that regiment and be tramped and left there for the beasts of the field, or sent to Dr. Smith's room for an autopsy." I took in the sight, saw the arms of the second great and extended division, that we must charge and slay at once, or be forever branded cowards by drum head court martial. Oh, my! can I stand another such engagement as the last? I dread their arms. They are the essence of danger. Sausage by the yard at the enemy's side.

I fell and was trampled to unconsciousness, as our general said I might be. All was dead within me but my dreaming powers, and they kept up a perpetual panorama of the lives and customs of the fouls and beasts; how they ate and how they lived; the iion, panther, eagle, vulture, elephant, and many other long lived animals. All the animals from the ape to the eagle, told me big dinners composed of a hundred kinds of eat and drink would ruin the stomach of all but the buzzard, that never was known to be foundered.

All long lived birds and animals that live on but few kinds of food should be a lesson for man, not to eat and drink 'till the body is so full that no blood vessel can pass in any part of the chest or abdomen. Our great dinners are only slaughter pens of show and stupidity. Some would say, "it is such a nice place to talk and visit. Does an owl hoot and eat at the same time? Let me eat quick and trot and I will have health and strength.

PHILOSOPHY.

How to Learn to be a Great Thinker.

Now I will make a philosopher of you, if you will obey and follow the rules I will give you, if you have the germs of reason with average culture.

Rule first—Is the machinery of the object, then the duty each part is to perform. Now I will take as an example to explore or know what this machine is designed for, a hog for our subject of exploration. For conclusion as to the design nature had in its construction. Now the first order I give, you must obey or fail: Look at the hog's snout. I mean snout and nothing else. Now let the tail alone. I said snout; not foot, but snout. You have nothing to do with the hog's foot; I told you to look at the snout. What do you see about the snout? Look and get its form, and let its uses alone. I want you to know a snout first; its form is all I want you to look for. Now you see the snout do you? You must not think of anything about which end of the hog the snout is on or its use or attachments. You cannot succeed as an investigator if you leave that snout before you get the form in your mind. Now you are master of the form of the snout, you can look how it is attached to the end of something by this time. You see a plow to turn over the ground, now go from your discovered plow to attachment to head which is fast to neck, neck to the body 'til hog is complete.

Moral: When you wish to learn anything, take some part to study and stick to it until you master a part at a time, 'til you know all parts. Then put them together in their places and your work is done. Nature does the rest as is indicated by all forms of animal life. Learn the parts and places and they will show their uses, if not, you have failed to use your reason and are lost, time spent and you none the wiser. Study the snout or you will forever fail.

SURPRISE FOR '97.

Dr. Still is out, and we go to press. His last move is a chair just visable to his oldest operators. It was under lock and key until the mail started with papers for the patent office. By it an expert can do more and better work than six of his best and most experienced workmen who have ever been in the school or treating rooms. All work is done by the hand of the operator and not the chair in the least. The work is what tells. More of it in February.

TO DR. STILL.

Little words in kindness spoken,
  A motive or a tear,
Oftimes heals a heart that's broken
  And makes a friend sincere.

A little touch of the healer's art
  Gives joy where pain was known,
Osteopathy plays a part
  With muscle, nerve and bone.

Sympathy silent and grand
  Goes out to rich and poor
Charity lies in open hand,
  When poverty knocks at the door.

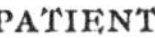
PATIENT.

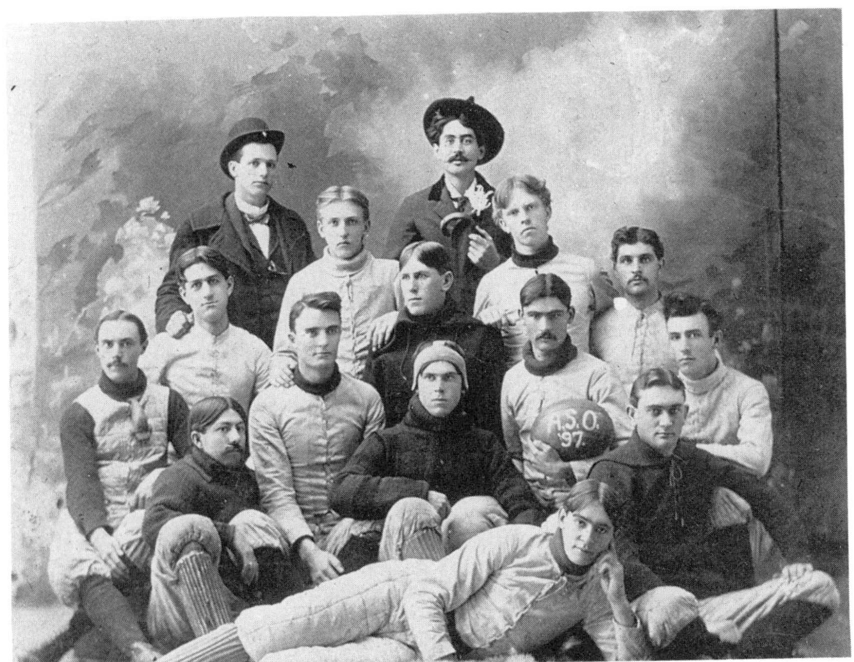

First A.S.O. football team, 1897

December, 1896

DR. STILL'S LECTURE.

The following lecture was delivered by Dr. A. T. Still in Memorial hall on the evening of Dec. 21st. The hall was filled with students, patients and visitors. The doctor said:.

Ladies and gentlemen, patients, students, Americans and foreigners:—I am glad to see you here to-night. You have come to hear something of the science of Osteopathy. The word "Osteopathy" is not expressive enough. A person who examines a lexicon to find the meaning of it is not satisfied. Os signifies bone—pathology is the science of disease. So we concluded here in the back-woods that we would just name the baby "Osteopathy," bone pathology. The reason we used the word bone is because it is like the handle of a hoe, it is the principle by which the motion is given to the instrument. We find all the fibers attached to bones, except the nerves. The nerves are somewhat independent of the bones, still, they penetrate all of them, surround them, it is not known to what extent the nerves do penetrate the bones. The bone is supplied with blood, which would indicate that there are nerves of action there and nerves of nutrition; when you cut into a bone you find nerves of sensation.

Nearly a quarter of a century ago a question came into my mind as to why it was God, not accident, had placed man on the face of the earth and that in sickness he should be in such a crippled, helpless condition. We called for help. We resorted to remedies. The patient died and another patient got well. We didn't know whether we had cured one or whether he had killed the medicine and then the disease and got well anyhow. These are facts. I began to think "What is man?" I might have started with the question "Who made man?" but I concluded I would let that job alone. "What is man?" I find one lying on the road stretched out full length, another one doubled up, another one erect, one in motion, one still, inactive. I began to look at this machine, not as an engineer, because as an engineer I was just as ignorant of the human body as the mule I rode. I called her Bets, and that is all she knew about it. The engineer of the human system ought to be as able to control the engine of life as the common locomotive engineer is to control the locomotive—run her fast, we expect that—run her slow, we expect that—stop, we expect that. There are the three principles that that man has to work on. Then, his machinery may not work at all. What do you expect of that man? Do you expect him to give a lecture on the financial issue? Do you expect him to stand on his head? There is your train stopped and your journey only half done, and the children crying at home, one of them had a broken arm when you left. What do you expect of that engineer when the machine stops? You expect in the first place, that he will use as much good, practical sense then as he ever did in his life. If he has good sense what do you see? You see him jump off the cab. He goes along the side of the train to see what is the matter. You see him stoop down. "What have you found?" "O, I have found that wheel locked here, got hot, and it is locked." "Can you get it out of that condition?" "Yes, I cool it off and put a little oil on it and it will go along." You come to another place. He says "Whoa," when he gets to the depot, and the engine goes right by. What do you expect of that engineer when his machine will not stop at your station and he cannot make it stop by the ordinary methods? You expect that engineer then to run along by the engine while it is in motion, let the air out of the brakes, and you expect that engine will obey the word "stop" and it does stop. If there are no air brakes he applies the chain and that clamps the engine and every wheel of the whole outfit, and she stops.

In every pursuit of life, it matters not what it is, you expect the leader to show and exercise reason, just as you did with that engineer. He examines the boiler, the drive wheels, the long and the short shafts and the brakes. If he don't do that he is a failure. How can he do this? In the first place, before he can be an engineer of something, he must know what that something is, and must know where the power is generated. He must know how to apply it. He must know how to move it. If it is an electric engine he will examine the connections and see that they are all right. If it is a steam engine, he will see that the steam valves, the steam chest, the steam pipes, and the supply pipes that keep the water coming into the boiler, are all right. If the engine threshes along, steam up, all the valves open, you will expect that man to give a reason why. You know he will do it if he is an engineer, and no hesitation about it, He will examine the mud valve; possibly the water is all out and he is running her on an empty boiler, Another time it stops, and what is the matter? You look at the water guage and it is clear to the top, the whole boiler is full of water. Do you expect that engine in that congested condition to run? The most limited knowledge of an engine would suggest, let out a part of that water, so you can generate some steam and fill the steam chests and meet the heads. Suppose then, after all these conditions are met, that the train will not start. What is his conclusion? Here we stand. We have an engineer that does not know much about it; he does not know enough to see that the steam heads are on a center and it wont turn. If he don't know enough to start that with a crow bar you will all stay there till you freeze. You have to change it from its center. He must know that or he is a failure. If he should report to the chief mechanic that he could not get his engine off of the center, they would undoubtedly take him off the engine into the machine shop and would teach him a few lessons as to what is meant by stopping on the center.

I want to tell you ladies and gentlemen that every well conducted business has a head. It has its branches, its executioners—from the courts of the United States down to the county court, each has its head. He works all the branches connected with it. If he does not he gets nothing done. Your government has a head, it has a president; and his word is the electric battery for the whole nation. Each officer who is under the government must obey at the word "go." If not there is stagnation in the government. When you go into the military department, what do you expect there? System. You expect to find a head, or general of the army. It has branches and subordinates down to the private. Without that there is failure. You claim to be in a Christian land; not where they rob and kill as they do down there in Cuba, or some other places. You claim to be here in a good land, where people are good. Good people ought to think pretty well, they ought to think kindly of the Mechanic who made all the mechanics and everything connected with them, I want to make this assertion: That for the last twenty-five years my object has been to find one single defeat in all nature, to find one single mistake of God. But I have made a total failure in this respect.

When I reason I must have something to reason from and something to reason with. I make to myself, and I have as much privilege to do that as the savage has to make him a wooden God, I make to myself a God of Intelligence. And then and there I begin to ask questions, and as most of our made gods are dummys, I ask the question and I answer it. By reason I propound a question and wait, and by reason I am led to a conclusion.

One of my breasts is sore, a lump in it, and I don't know what is putting it there, and the doctor don't know either. He says he will cut it out. Will that stop it? I don't know and the doctor don't know and you don't know either. You bleed and you groan, and maybe another one appears somewhere else, or you may die. The engineer, or the man who reasons as an engineer, would go over your breast and see if one of the shafts, that we call a rib, wasn't thrown across another shaft or running up a little too close. The blood must get through some place to make my breast and to make yours. When it has done its work it must have the privilege to take the remainder off. When we commence to reason and look around what do we find? We find a body with over two hundred pieces of timber in it. We call them ribs and shanks and femurs and spines, and all those things. Here is a brace, here is a joist, miter, etc. We need in this frame of man crooked shafts and rafters—we find almost none at all straight. The fact is, not a straight bone can be found in the body. We begin to look at the machine, and if a man will use his reason he will find that there is a constructed house and inside of that house is a principle that we commonly call life, and in that life a principle called mind or reason. We find motion that requires power; we find that the temperature is not very high, therefore it is not steam power. We find it not above a hundred. Steam must be higher than that. What have we? It must be electricity, as that needs only common temperature. Where is this electricity generated? Go on with your investigation, saddle up your horse and take a ride, your mental horse, and take a ride up between your eyes; you will find yourself passing between two hills and going over a little bridge; on the right is a heap of brain and on the left is another, and in the center is what we call a septum. We find a great big lump of matter that we call the big brain; we run over that hill and we find a little hill, the small brain or cerebellum. Below that we have what looks like a dutchman's maul with the spinal cord for a handle. We go down the spinal cord till we come to the cauda equina or horse's tail, with thousands of electric wires branching off. If you clip one of these everything below it is inactive, just as that light would be if we clipped the wire. Osteopathy is based upon the wisdom of God, and when a man has passed a grade of from 90 to 100 in anatomy under our rigid examinations he will know where to find the right electric button. I wish I knew what button to turn when a man is drunk on whiskey. Tell me the difference between what you pronounce insanity and a drunken man and I will get you a yellow coat—and then you will be a gold bug. What makes one crazy when he drinks whiskey? It strikes the terminations of the solar plexus, the great nerve that spreads around the stomach, and affects the heart causing it to pump the blood faster through the arteries, paralyzing the brain, and the blood does not return; therefore you are drunk. The question that Osteopathy has before it now is to know why alcoholic stimulants makes a man drunk, and why you call a man or woman crazy who is perfectly sane all day and suddenly goes into a spell of insanity, as you term it, and remains so until he becomes exhausted, and when this exhaustion is gone they are just as rational as the man who got drunk last night. That is a proposition that is taking my time day and night. I want to take your husband out of that asylum and sit him at your side. For hundreds of years the world has trifled with the thought of insanity. It generally results in housing the insane up, hampering them, chaining them, and forcing doses of caster oil and jalap down their throats. I have never yet pictured out a good old Methodist hell to be half as bad as an asylum. I would rather see my daughter shot and buried than taken to one.

Osteopathy is a science; not what we know of it, but the subject we are studying, is as deep as eternity. We know but little of it. I have worked and worried here in Kirksville for twenty-two long years, and I intend to study for twenty-three thousand years yet.

There is another subject I am going to tell you about. The fat man gets fat because he cannot help it. We have some very scrawny ones that wont do to fry at all. My investigation so far is a great step toward solving the problem why one woman is fat and her sister is not. I believe that before twelve months passes around I can jerk the fat off of you. Why so? So far in the last two months that I have been investigating this, I find that lean women, or a great many of them, have had abscesses in the side of the neck near the glands in and about the jaw, near the 5th pair of nerves. I believe we are on the verge of finding how to get rid of that annoyance, too much fat. Nature's God intended every particle of that fat to be utilized in support of muscles and other tissues. You will find that the arms of those persons are as hard as bologna sausage. That shows that the overplus has been thrown overboard. I am after that fat, I am after the insane person, who is to be pitied as the inebriate is to be pitied, and it is the duty and determination of this School of Osteopathy to solve just such questions. I could almost put my finger on a person who was decided insane and sent to the asylum, but who only had asthma. I could place my hands almost on another one who was placed there because he had the headache. He had his neck set here and was alright until he was injured again, when his head commenced aching. And rather than let him come to these contemptible Osteopaths a committee of doctors decided that he was insane and there was great danger that he would kill his family. They took him to the asylum, and in order to get himself out he told them he was better when disease was preying on him almost to the very center.

We expect to come back about the 4th of January and begin another year's work, and we expect to keep at it until we can walk by the side of sane men and women who have once been in the asylum. I am invited by a United States Senator to visit the insane asylums of the great state of Ohio. I am not sure but what I will go, but I don't know enough yet to take hold of it. Some men that know more than I do tell me what effect a drink of whiskey has on the blood. I will go to the head and take out the insanity. A very dangerous man came here a while ago. His father and brother stayed with him all the time. He is now enjoying soundness of mind and good health. He told me that he knew there was something wrong but he couldn't tell what it was. He wanted to hit something, to destroy something, and it would be a pleasure if he could do some heinous crime. I have no doubt but that it is a delight to an insane man to shoot the brains out of his wife; he anticipates it with as much pleasure as you do what you will get in your stocking tommorrow night. I have talked with them and asked them about this, and they say that at the time they knew everything, but the idea of destruction of life or doing some great crime was pleasing to them.

I want to make you all welcome here tonight. We have not had an opportunity for four months to talk to anyone while the building was being erected. I am going to shave and get some sand-paper and sand-paper my neck and then I will talk to you. If I undertake to do anything you need not ask me any questions, I will execute it regardless of consequences. Had I not done that in regard to Osteopathy, just as I have done with this house, you would never have had any trouble with it. Osteopathy was a single fight. It was a fight for truth. It never struck a wave that made it tremble. When people would call me a crank I didn't get mad at that, I didn't get cross at all. Says I, if you had as much sense on this subject as the sheep I would feel hard towards you, but you are perfectly excusable. I would ask the very fellows who laughed at me how many bones they had in their foot, and 75 per cent of them could not tell. Each of those bones in the foot has a place to supply, muscles are attached to them, arteries and nerves pass around and between them.

Here in the throat you have a button that has a good many colors in it, that button has the color of diphtheria, croup, scarlet fever, measles, whooping cough, tonsilitis, sore breast for the mother, and spots on your face You better get acquainted with that button and quit putting powder on your face. Now, when you go home don't think you will find buttons sticking out all over your skin.

What is the coldest part of your body, men, women or children? And how do you prove it? When you open your dry eye there isn't a bit of water on it, and before even thc lachrymal glands can act. as soon as the air strikes it it converts the moisture in the air into water, the oxygen and hydrogen unite, the eye being colder than the atmosphere. It is the mystery of God himself how that water is spilled in the eye, when there was no water on it. It is a mystery that we ought to think of. You get acquainted with the machinery of man, and if you will do nothing else but master that, you will find something always new. One says; if I just knew how to make a few moves I could stop flux etc. Then he would go and tell the people, why I just came from Kirksville, I understand all about it. This fool with a little $3 book says he is an Osteopath. If he understands Osteopathy, I do not, and I am the discoverer of the science. The greatest wonder is that after Osteopathy ha sproduced its cures it can make more pretenders and counterfeiters in a town of 1000 inhabitants than any thing I ever knew of. You take one of them, and they cannot describe a single muscle, cannot give the origin and insertiou of any three muscles in the body, and let them choose the muscles. Do you want such a man as that for a doctor? If you do, it is all right. There are plenty to wait on you. They will treat you for so much. They know just as much as the old docter because they hitched up his team three times.

I want you all to come out here some time in January. I want you to feel at home If I were to talk to each of you in detail it would talk my head off in less than a week. A patient that has been to all of the physicians in Europe and America, can ask a string of questions that would almost go around Cleveland, and they are just as hard as the glittering diamonds of Africa.

I want to tell you that this science will handle all fevers—typhus, malaria, typhoid, scarlet fever, croup, pneumonia, and right along down the list. It will handle any fever that it reaches in time without ipecac, quinine, digitalis, belladonna or aconite. It will do it just as surely as when you turn one of these electric buttons the light goes out. I have proven that nature has provided the body with all that is necessary for our comfort and health. Take the lungs they are made so they will act as well in New Orleans as in Alaska. Why is it? When you go down south they widen out; it takes a little more room when you get there. The same lungs will do you on any part of the earth. You do not need to wait for a shoemaker to make you a new set of lungs to go north or south with. The lungs will suit themselves to the change. And when you begin to take calomel, quinine, nux vomica, belladonna, use the hypodermic syringe, etc. you are proving that God does not know his own business. The very instant that you take any drug that is not a nourishment to the body you have proven God to be a failure in just that much. I work by the intelligence of God and live by it. Good Night.

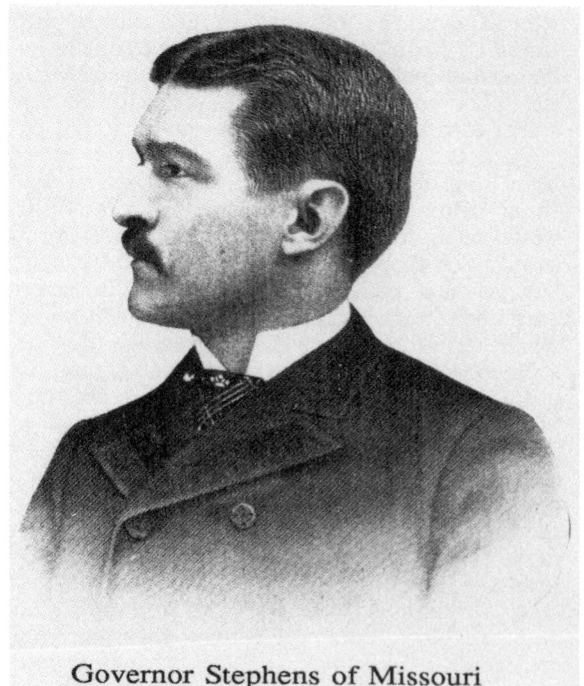

Governor Stephens of Missouri

March, 1897

LEGISLATIVE.

The bill legalizing the practice of Osteopathy in Missouri was passed by the House February 25 by a vote of 101 to 16. March 3 the bill passed the Senate by a vote of 26 to 3. On March 4 Governor Stephens signed the bill, and it is now a law.

The law requires a personal attendance of four full terms of five months each in a regularly chartered school of Osteopathy, and provides penalties for its violation.

Ratification at the Infirmary Saturday, March 6 at 2 p. m. All are invited.

***

The practice of Osteopathy is now legalized by special act of legislature in Missouri, Vermont and North Dakota.

In North Carolina the bill has passed the senate, and has pretty good prospects of becoming a law.

In Colorado a bill is now before the senate. The senate committee to whom it was referred gave the friends of Osteopathy a public hearing, and, as the Denver papers say, were very favorably impressed by the showing made.

In South Dakota a bill has been introduced and friends are doing all in their power to secure its passage.

In Michigan it has been recently decided that Osteopaths can register under the present law, but an effort is being made to secure the passage of a special act.

March, 1897

THE NEW JOSHUA.

Since October, 1874, my pen has been silent as to reports of how the child, Osteopathy, has been treated. When I opened the cage in which I kept the boy that I believed, in time, would be the greatest fighter that ever appeared on the world's stage of reason, many stayed long enough to see that the child was a boy, red headed, had a Roman nose, a good sized neck, an eagle's eye, talons and wings of great length, which they said meant to fly very high if necessary, and the eye meant to select the choicest gems at will, and the claws said in the best of language that to penetrate deeply is the rule of reason and wholly indispensible, and after a careful investigation said, that child has the build of a gritty and sensible fighter. Others said, what do you want to fight for in time of peace? I told the multitude that in days of peace was the time to prepare for war. I began to train my boy for the olympic games of all future days. For years I kept him in close training to be a skilled fencer for I knew much hard fighting would have to be done as soon as the boy kicked old theories that had no merit but age and tradition to boast of, and I knew my Joshua would soon command such suns and moons to stand and make them obey to the letter. Some would say, but in a low whisper that young one was an illegitimate child, its father could not be found and it would at all times be known as a bastard; farther than that, no illegitimate could be allowed to run at large in Missouri. But it soon grew to manhood and sued its accusers for slander and the suit was put off from term to term for over twenty years. A great and good man by the name of Lon V. Stephens arose in the highest court of Missouri and said, "I am its father and will give it Missouri for its inheritance;" and he executed his will and put the great seal of the State of Missouri with his signature of authority, on March 4th; 1897, and named the boy "Joshua."

A. T. S.

March, 1897

OUR SCHOOL NOT A DIPLOMA MILL.

It will cost you five hundred dollars to be an Osteopath and not a cent less. We have now been in the teaching business five years and made some cheap Osteopaths. Made some in six months, some in seven, some in eight and nine. They get wise and want to start Osteopathic schools and write books. We have made some in two, three and four years; none of the latter have become teachers, presidents of Colleges of Osteopathy nor written books, and promised to make men and women of great knowledge in six weeks or six months for $25., or $250, and say anything that is untrue to get your money. I have tested all lengths of time to know just how long it takes to be qualified to go out into the world as a good and safe person, one that I can recommend, to take charge of your lives and ready to meet all kinds of disease. If my word, with six years trying to impart a good knowledge of this science, is worth anything to you, I will say, less than two full years of ten months each, cannot make and endow any man or woman with any more knowledge than hit and miss, and I cannot truthfully tell you differently after my long experience in teaching. Any person who tells you different, knows but little of Osteopathy; its second year's teaching is the soul of the science. Fortunately but few if any are out for cheap schools, short time and shoddy methods of teaching. I will keep my school up to the highest standard or not teach at all. I cannot afford to deceive you for your money's sake, and will not. My school has a good character at home and abroad and has legal honors bestowed upon it in a number of states. I am here to keep and maintain a school that all Americans will be proud to speak of when in any part of the world, and its diplomos never taken at a discount for any cause, by the most learned of all nations. Next year we hope to be able to go deeper in the mysteries and beauties of the laws of life as found in the books of the Infinite. A. T. S.

March, 1897

"DIVORCED."

BY DR. A. T STILL.

Revolution after revolution have originated in America—political, religious and scientific. Governments have changed with the velocity of demand. These revolutions run from the congregated assemblies of our law makers, military, religious and scientific professions, and the navigation of the seas down to each individual why has granted to him the right to secede or differ from any of the above named systems. He or she has the right to ask and obtain a divorce from husband or wife when proof in sufficient quantity is produced; and letters to that effect are granted by our highest courts by common consent of the people. As I was wedded to Alopathy early in my life, I lived with it, put up with it, suffered under it, until it made my life miserable by continuing the association, and I asked a divorce. I asked, and put in my petition on June 22, 1874, for a divorce. I based my charges upon the foundation of murder, ignorance, bigotry and intolerance. The fight in the court through which I had applied for a divorce was very hot and determined. A decision was refused from 1874 until October 30, 1894, previous to which time the judge of the circuit court carefully examined my claims and referred my case to the secretary of state, who, after causing a careful examination, granted me letters patent from the state of Missouri, with her great seal, and said, "You are hereby set free from further obligations to Mrs. Alopathy."

"CASTING OUT DEVILS."

In bible times disease was looked upon as a special visitation of providence, or the forcible possession of the body by agents of the devil. If of the latter classification, many were the ingenious methods employed to drive these devils out of the unfortunate victim. An insane patient, for instance, was thought to be possessed of a peculiar kind of devil that could by a certain "hokus pokus" be driven from the victim's body and made to take up its abode in the lower animals. There are no well authenticated clinical observations recorded upon this subject, but there are several interesting cases told in both sacred and profane history.

-++++-

The pervading idea among these superstitious ancients was that disease was an entity to be attacked and driven out of the body. And, incredible though it may seem, that idea has been the guiding star of all healing methods from time immemorial to the founding of Osteopathy. True, a few of the advanced thinkers of the medical profession have declared that disease is a condition, and schools have gone through the form of accepting theories of this character; but despite their declarations they continue to treat disease as entity. The great mass of the profession have been totally unable to get out of the entity rut, and medicine with its boasted research of more than two thousand years, still clings to the old superstition that disease is a mysterious, tangible something, which gets inside the human organism and must be beset by another something which has a natural antipathy for the supposed cause of the disease, and which, when introduced into the body of the patient, will search out and exterminate the troublesome little enemy to health. Wedded to this superstition, our medical friends have searched every nook and corner of the earth for specifics that, liberated in the human body, would destroy the cause of certain diseases.

-++++-

Nowhere do we find this old superstition more thoroughly at the helm of medical research than in the present day germ theory of disease. The "devil" to be cast out is no longer a plain devil, but a scientific "Microbe," which goes about in search of fashionable victims, and which would probably scorn the idea of taking up its abode with a herd of swine. Its name and occupation are made known by the number and shape of its horns. These little devils differ from the devils of the ancients only in size, and had the poor ancient had the advantage of a microscope with which to tone down his imagination the difference between old devils and those of the microbe persuasion would probably be but slight.

-++++-

In their desperation to prove the supposed correctness of this old superstition, modern medical writers have piled up volumes on the chemistry of disease and its specifics, and experimenters have analyzed almost every atom of the known universe, and studied the minutia of the effects of bodily disorder, to the total neglect of the broader and more important phenomena of animal life. In their long and fruitless search of the outside world for specific poisons that would drive their "devils of disease" from the human body they have totally ignored that great engine of life itself, and have failed to recognize the presence of native forces which the Creator placed within the mechanism for its own government.

Here is where Osteopathy took up the fight and where it won its victory. The founder of Osteopathy looked upon disease as an abnormal condition, and reasoned that the means of restoring the normal should be in the human engine itself—not in some remote corner of the universe or hidden miles under the sea. While the medical profession has searched all the world outside of man, the founder of Osteopathy searched man himself for the means of controlling disease, and he has been rewarded for his trouble by discovering that the great Machinist placed within the human body everything necessary to run it smoothly without drugs.

March, 1897

DR. STILL TO STUDENTS.

Some advise us to teach our classes in Osteopathy as to gain the approval of the legislatures, and thereby gain recognition. I care nothing for pleasing legislatures by taking to them large bundles of useless, blind rubbish. I want the students and diplomates of Osteopathy to go from this school with a better knowledge of anatomy, physiology, and the laws of nature and their ability to ward off disease than is taught by any other system of curing on earth. Let them do the work, meet sickness and come to camp with live children and live adults, and not with the wailing sounds of funerals. Let them do that, make qualified men and women, learn them what man is and what disease is and how to cure it, and you can no more keep the mother away from an Osteopath than you can keep the houseflies off a darkey's head. Cure her baby and she will do your legal fighting. Save her girl, and pap will roll up his sleeves and help her. So keep out as much trash as possible. We are safe if we do the work. You can learn how if you attend to your business. Osteopathy is the very essence of symptomatology, diagnosis and cure. Learn it, be it, and you will have filled the law. This school is to teach you. It will be the judge when you are ready to go, and will send you as soon as possible. We want you in the field at work and wish you to pay strict attention. We will get you off as soon as you are ready to go. We want you to know anatomy and physiology by books and dissection, and Osteopathy from the rooms of the clinics and when you do you must go, for the world wants you and needs you badly. There is but one way for an Osteopath to show his competence, and that is by results.

March, 1897

QUICK RESULTS ARE NOT THE RULE.

The common error made by people who apply to an Osteopath for treatment is in believing quick results can be obtained in every case. It is by no means uncommon for a sufferer whose physical mechanism has been creaking and wheezing along badly out of line for a dozen years or more, to come to an Osteopath expecting to be cured in a few treatments. Perhaps a score of quack physicians have taken turns at filling the poor fellow's system full of poisons which nature will require years to throw off. Yet the patient has heard of people who were cured by a single Osteopathic treatment, and expects a like result in his own case. While cases of many years standing have been cured in a single treatment, and others have been restored to health in so short a time as to seem remarkable, a majority of cases require more time. Many of the most truly wonderful cures have been those in which results came only after a long course of treatment. In some cases the obstruction which is the cause of the trouble, can be removed directly by the Osteopathic operation. In others, where the trouble is more complicated or deeply seated, the operator must give such assistance as will enable nature to remove the obstruction herself, and nature, like the mills of God, grinds slow but exceedingly well. The dislocations, contractions and contortions, rendered almost permanent by years of neglect, and aggravated by improper treatment, cannot always be corrected quickly. One case may be cured at a single treatment, while another, the outward appearances of which are the same, may require many weeks, perhaps months.

April, 1897

DR. STILL.

Dr. A. T. Still, the revered founder of Osteopathy then arose. The applause lasted several minutes. When quiet was restored, the "old doctor" said:

Mr. Chairman, ladies and gentlemen, students and faculty: We have voluntarily assembled ourselves here today, March 6, to begin the celebration of a very important event, express our joy and thanks to the house, senate and governor of the state of Missouri—to thank them for granting to the American School of Osteopathy a statute law by which the school is granted the privilege to teach and issue diplomas to its pupils, qualifying by said act who shall be licensed to practice this science in the state of Missouri. Much deliberation and thought was given by the committee to whom this bill was entrusted. It consisted of eleven of the best lawyers of the state of Missouri, which was the committee on criminal jurisprudence; and imbued with the spirit of progress, they as judges of law, formulated the bill to regulate the practice of Osteopathy in the State of Missouri.

After due deliberation they did recommend its passage, and it was passed by an overwhelming majority by the lower house, duly prepared in form and sent to the senate, and by that body referred to the eleeomosynary committee, which also recommended that it do pass and become a law. The bill then passed the senate by a vote of 26 to 3. As soon as the necessary form of law could be complied with, the broad-minded and sensible governor, Lon. V. Stevens, did affix his signature, and the bill became a law of the state of Missouri.

At this period in my remarks I will give you an interesting coincidence, at least it is so to me. In the troublesome days of Kansas, when slavery and freedom wrestled for the supremacy, one J. B. Abbott and myself were lieutenants of the same company and regiment, and fighting for freedom in that territory—freedom of thought, press and person, without regard to race or color. In the year 1855 the pro-slavery element, being in the ascendency and backed by a pro-slavery government, did order one Sam Jones, who was United States marshal of the district in which we lived, to arrest Lieutenants J. B. Abbott and A. T. Still, under a pretext that we were violators of the territory law, and take us to Lecompton, the then capital of Kansas, for trial, sentence and service. As we thought the chances for justice were all against us, we withdrew from public gaze to a hiding place which we knew of in the timber and brush, on the banks of the Kaw river. While hiding out and away from the sight and probability of being found we felt secure. J. B. Abbott was an eastern man, and full of knowledge and customs of the eastern states, being a goldsmith and generally skilled mechanic. I had great respect for his opinion, and we conversed freely. I felt it a great privilege to listen to his suggestions on many subjects besides the freedom of Kansas. Among the most lasting impressions he made on my mind while in hiding, was that the practice of medicine was not a science and was far in the rear of general progress of the day. He told me that if he was not mistaken, I would not have to live many years to see something come forward that would take the place of Alopathy, Eclecticism and Homeopathy. Being in love with Alopathy and its methods of practice, I could but look on the man in astonishment to hear him talk so wildly as I then thought. I have lived to see his prophecy fulfilled to the letter. I have lived to love and respect the man instead of dread and fear of his teachings. I have lived to see the substitute come, and on the same day that his remains went into the earth, with thousands left behind to mourn his loss. While thousands mourn his loss, tens of thousands are made to rejoice all over North America, for on that day Governor Stevens affixed his signature to an instrument of writing and gave to the child Osteopathy, which was the outgrowth of those brush hidings and conversations, the state of Missouri as its inheritance Now allow me to tell you that my feelings are far from making any noisy demonstrations about my great victory over the enemy. Suppose at this time I should have heralded by publication and other ways that I had gained a great victory, would I not make a very great mistake? Would it not be a wiser expression and a better use of language to say "I have passed one more mile post that leads us to a higher chamber, a place where all mental gems that shine are cut from the stone out of whose rent flow rivers of life to be drunken by all who thirst for knowledge?" Would it not be better to say "I will trim my vessel for longer voyages into seas that have never seen a navigator, even of a dugout in all time past?"

You see at a glance that the bill Gov. S tevens signed asks no superior privilege for any school of Osteopathy, but states by positive statute who may practice said science in Missouri. The bill requires four full terms of five months each, with personal attendance in such legally chartered school previous to obtaining a diploma, which shall give the holder the right to practice, or treat as an Osteopath. I think it is a good law that exacts of every person who treats the sick or claims to practice as Osteopath, Homeopath, Allopath or any other school, to be able to prove that he is what he claims to be. I say hurrah for Stevens and the law makers of Missouri, Vermont, North Dakota and any state that punishes all who try to pass counterfeits of any kind. Osteopathy has a good character over all the world as far as known, and without law to define who shall treat as an Osteopath, the world would soon be over run with all kinds of deceivers. Law is made to prevent thieves and liars from obtaining money by false pretenses from the afflicted or the well. Let us have more such law.

Now that we are legally on equality with all schools of the healing arts, we will answer a few questions of the many and a few blind statements of the ignorant and uninformed of the extent of the claims of the American School of Osteopathy. It teaches the very frequent use of soap and water, combs, toothpicks and stomach pumps for the drunk and poisoned. We use the saw and knife but very little if at all. We use forceps but once at birth when alopathy, homeopathy, would and do use them one hundred times. Right at this point I will say Osteopathy knows of and has a high respect for surgery, general surgery in its fullest meaning. Osteopathy is a complete system and science, fills the bill in general diseases, midwifery and surgery at any time and place. When a person tells you that Osteopathy is not a complete system of itself and cannot do all that comes before it just as well and better without the aid of any other system he tells you what is not true; and he who says or teaches differently is either excusably ignorant or has an ax to grind in which he is interested. We do cut, saw or chop off a leg, arm or any part of the body when we find that such limb or part cannot be kept without danger to the life of patient. Two years well spent will take you into the higher chamber of our philosophy and prepare you to know that you have been in a school that rounds up a student and puts on a finish that will shine before him all his life.

I believe there is a time for all things, and will close by saying, we are all happy, bells, dogs, anvils and fire-crackers, and will use much of this day and night in music and greeting, thanking all who have taken a part with our joys by word, deed, or even a smile to remember one year from to-day, you are all invited to meet with us again.

***

April, 1897

PUBLICITY.

My opinion and rule of action has been firmly fixed for twenty-five years in this belief, that he who seeks publicity will find seclusion as his reward, and he who seeks seclusion will obtain publicity as his reward if there be any merit in his purposes; therefore I do not ask any person, or persons, male or female, to become students of my school, nor do I ask the afflicted to come to me for treatment. I never have, I never will. If you ask for intelligence of this science I will freely impart; if you ask us to relieve you of disease and pain, we will kindly do for you the very best we can. This institution in all its branches, literature, and remedies, must build its own character or fall, all without the aid of advertisements, either through the JOURNAL, any other papers or traveling agents. We will answer all communications, and leave the choice with you, whether to enter the school as a student or the Infirmary as a patient.

A. T. STILL, President.

MORE CRUTCHES FOR SALE.

Mr. E. B. English, of Quincy, came over for treatment the latter part of December. He had been a sufferer for some time from a spinal affection which deprived him of the use of the right leg, and also effected his right arm and other parts of his body. Owing to the peculiar nature of the case it was an impossibility to begin a vigorous treatment at first. However it was not long until Osteopathy began to take hold of the case, and during the past week Mr. English is to be seen on the streets without crutch or cane. Asked if he believed in miracles Mr. English replied: "Not often, but I am a firm believer in Osteopathy."

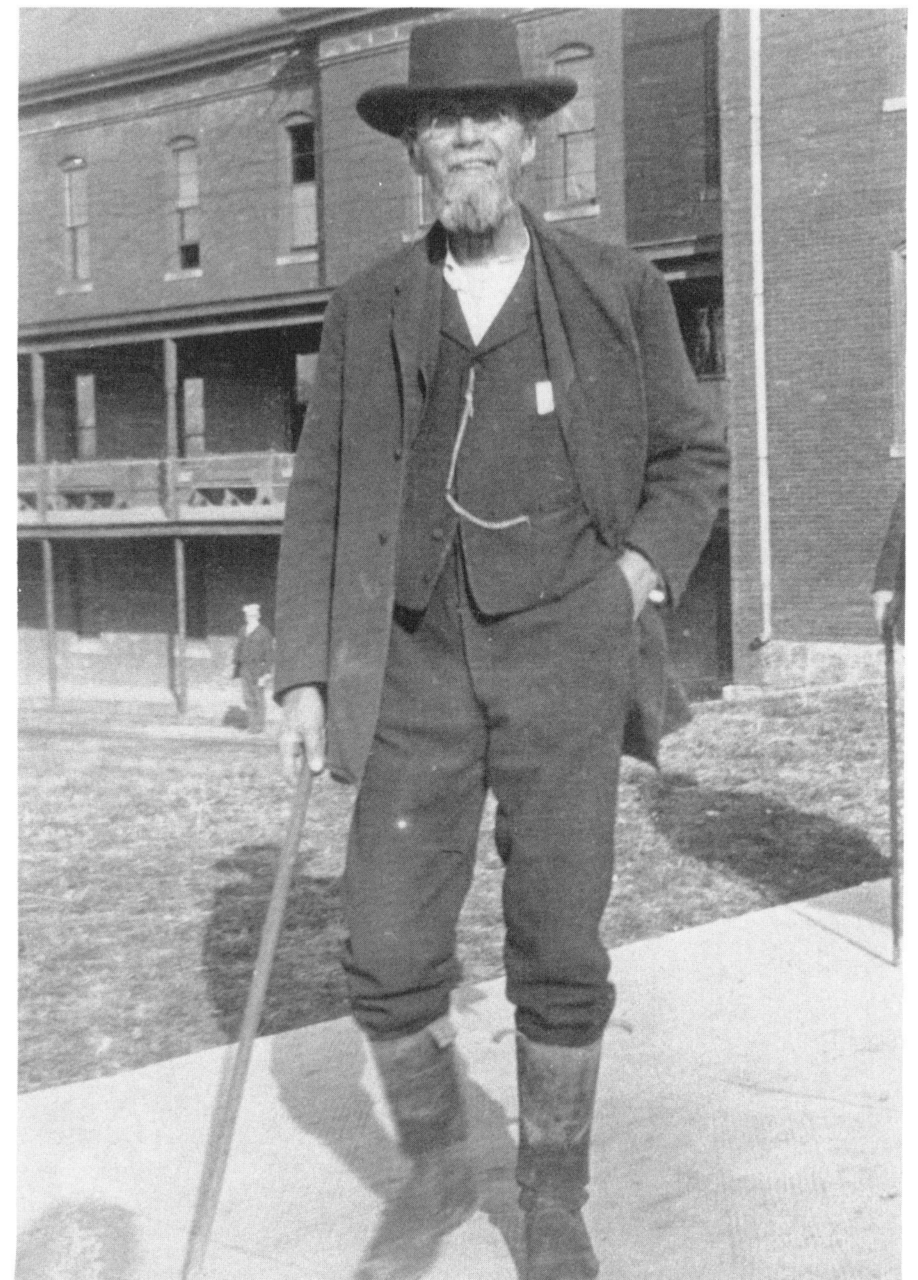

Then if that philosophy has passed from theory to the degree of proven truths by experience then the gate is open and practica land marks are before us in open view and lead us to view smallpox as ~~an~~ a foreign body ~~the~~ of poison that found its way into the body and should be met by antidot of greater energy, by insersion or absorption or any method that would bring the two poisons together and turn their attention from injury to the body to that of antagonising each other.

Thus the hope that cantharides would enter and destroy small pox in fetal life, by its superior energy, which we know to be the case, because we can blister a man to death ~~befor~~ with cantharidine long befor varioly would reach the degree of Eruption irritation

To those who have been
out and meeting the wise the
fools the truthfull and the lyers
confidence men and women
~~those~~ the sick and the well
I will say you have great
reason to be proud of your
short stay in Kirksville
you have found men and women
who are wise and far above
Earths wisest men they get wisd
from Zeno yallow moon and
all the great men of the skys
These mediums don't claim to be
wise themselves but get wise
from the dead phylosophers

A. T. Still's handwritten notes

How to Get to Kirksville, Mo.

Quincy, Omaha and Kansas City Railroad Co. is the Kirksville Line.

4 DAYLIGHT PASSENGER TRAINS EQUIPPED WITH CHAIR CARS **4**

CONNECTIONS

CHICAGO, QUINCY, ST. LOUIS,	From North, East and South.	OMAHA ST. JOE KANSAS CITY	From West, North and South.

See that your tickets read via QUINCY, OMAHA AND KANSAS CITY R. R. into Kirksville, and arrive in daytime and in comfort.

W. G. BRIMSON, General Manager.

A. J. BANDY, General Passenger Agent, Kansas City, Mo.

J. W. QUAIL, AGENT, Kirksville, Mo.

AMERICAN
School of Osteopathy,
INCORPORATED MAY 14TH 1892.
C. E. STILL, Secretary.

KIRKSVILLE, MISSOURI, ...189

E — D.
You can say for me A. T. Still
That I am 65 Years old aug 6 1893
My father was an M.D. of the first
Medical School that was in the State
of Ohio. I was rased- by a drug Dr.
he was called a good Dr of his day.
he was. and did just the M.D.s do now.
Blister physic puke purg sweat. give whisky
Opium Calomel Quinine Digitallis
Arsenic Tartemetic bleed keep grub and water
away and let none live who did not have
animal power greater than the disease and
drugs. deat was the rule. recovery was the exception
for 34 years I wated and read all that was
written for one single abiding truth from
any school of drugs. My hunt was a total
failure. My verdict was the whole thing was
"Cut and Try" from begining to to end
and like the great M.D. Prof. Gregory of the
Edinburg Med. College said to his medical class,
Gentlemen, ninety-nine out of every 100 medical facts
are medical lies.

A. T. Still's note from 1893

As O.P. is now over 20 yrs old
And known to be truth
upheld by many millions
of the of the people of

America & Europe -
we will dilate only enough
to say that It it has
done singly and alone
that which all other
systems have totally
failed to do, Ensland
cure Asthma measles
flu and diseases of
all seasons climate
or locality It is the
engineer of life with
a full knowledge of
the laws and working
of the machinery of life
that nature can do
its work -

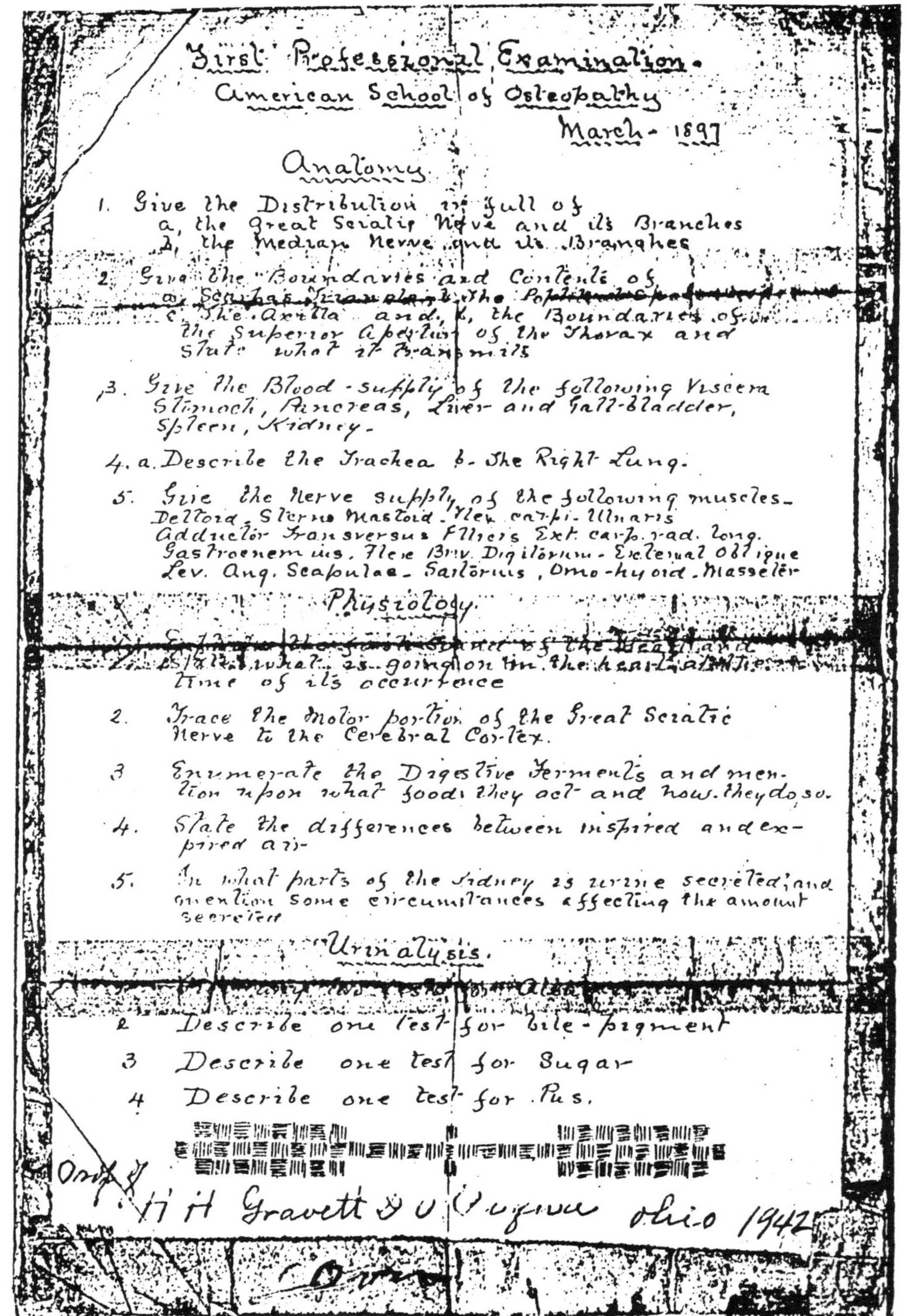

First Professional Examination.
American School of Osteopathy
March - 1897

Anatomy.

1. Give the Distribution in full of
a, the Great Sciatic Nerve and its Branches
b, the Median Nerve and its Branches

2. Give the Boundaries and Contents of
a, Scarpa's Triangle, b, the Popliteal Space [illegible]
c, The Axilla and, d, the Boundaries of the Superior Aperture of the Thorax and State what it transmits

3. Give the Blood-supply of the following Viscera Stomach, Pancreas, Liver and Gall-bladder, Spleen, Kidney.

4. a. Describe the Trachea b. The Right Lung.

5. Give the nerve supply of the following muscles - Deltoid - Sterno Mastoid - Flex carpi - Ulnaris Adductor Transversus Flexors Ext. carp. rad. long. Gastrocnemius. Flex Brev. Digitorum - External Oblique Lev. Ang. Scapulae - Sartorius, Omo-hyoid - Masseter

Physiology.

1. [illegible] of the Heart and State what is going on in the heart at the time of its occurrence

2. Trace the Motor portion of the Great Sciatic Nerve to the Cerebral Cortex.

3. Enumerate the Digestive Ferments and mention upon what foods they act and how they do so.

4. State the differences between inspired and expired air

5. In what parts of the kidney is urine secreted; and mention some circumstances affecting the amount secreted

Urinalysis.

1. [illegible]

2. Describe one test for bile-pigment

3. Describe one test for Sugar

4. Describe one test for Pus.

Orig. [illegible]
H H Gravett D O [illegible] Ohio 1942

First Professional Exam at the A.S.O. 1897

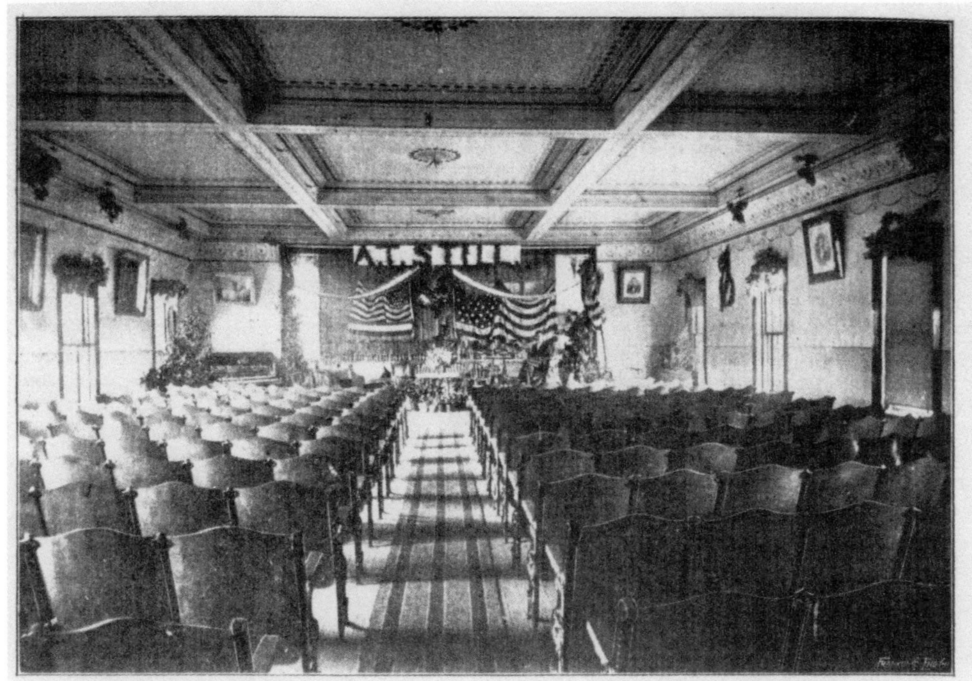

MEMORIAL HALL, AMERICAN SCHOOL OF OSTEOPATHY.

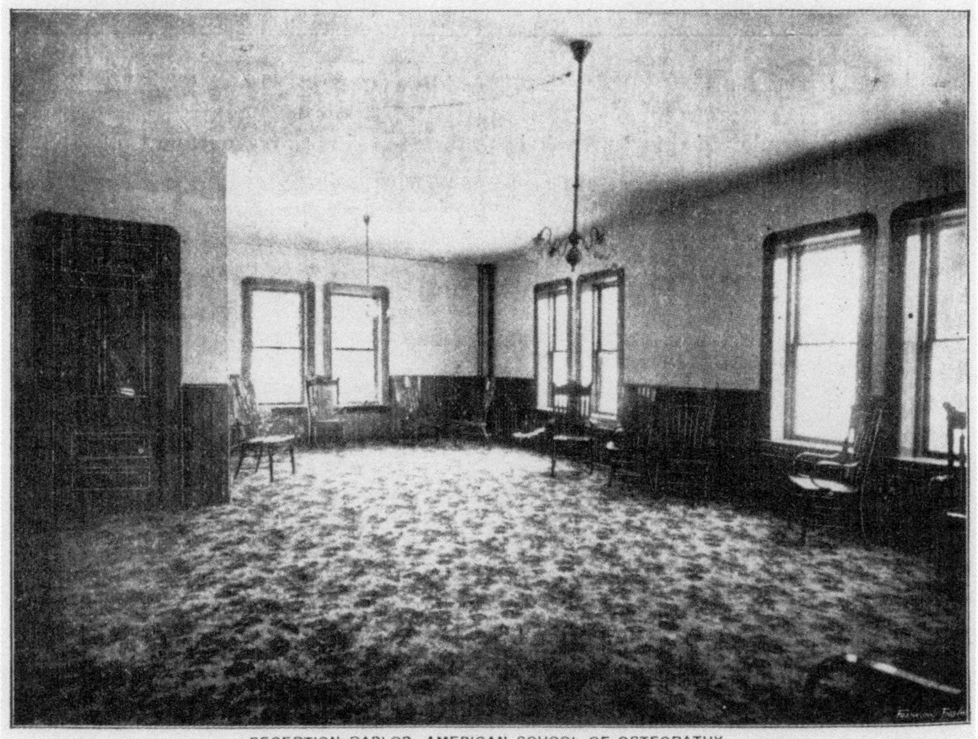

RECEPTION PARLOR, AMERICAN SCHOOL OF OSTEOPATHY.

June, 1897

DR. STILL'S VISION.

A. T. Still.

FROM early youth I have been a great seer of the visions of the night, one of which I will proceed to tell you as best I can. My descriptive powers may be too short; my ability to explain by words may be too limited to communicate to your understanding graphically what I have seen night after night. It is the most attractive vision that has disturbed my dreams from birth till now. The house in which this panorama seems to dwell is as wide as thought; as long as all the ages of the past. Its seats in numbers were as the sands of the sea. Its roads were paved to the uttermost parts of the earth, all centering to the one place. I seemed to be only a silent spectator. I saw legions of the finest carriages, coaches, cabs, bicycles, horsemen, footmen and rolling chairs with their waiters. And all these vehicles or methods of travel were loaded to fullness with men of all ages of the remembered and great forgotten past. With glistening knives of all forms, tweezers, tenaculums, blow-pipes and microscopes of the greatest known powers. They all alighted from their different modes of travel. They rested, feasted and slept through the refreshing hours of the night, awoke early the following morning, ate their breakfasts, took their morning exercise, and at the sound of the bugle they all assembled.

The chairman, a very dignified elderly gentleman, arose and stated the object of the meeting, and said: "We have tried to formulate a scientific method that should live with coming ages, by which we could successfully antagonize the diseases of the earth, which prey upon and destroy too great a per cent of the human race prematurely. And I have to say from a conclusion based upon sworn statements of all sages of the different medical schools, that their foundation is wholly unscientific and unsatisfactory, from conclusions based upon results. All victories belong to that champion that has no knowledge of defeat, whose name is the 'czar of death.' We have brought into requisition brigades, divisions and nations, and met the enemy in open fields, only to lose our flags and mourn over the loss of our beloved dead."

A new idea came over the congregated legions that the victories lost should be attributed to the abortive use of drugs as prescribed and used by all schools, and a resolve passed over the whole congregation to meet the enemy with the knives of surgery—the knives of standard surgery.

The battle raged and the wailing over the dead increased. Lamentations seemed to prevail and hearts sunk. An armistice was called. Another general arose with the appearance of greatness, armed himself to the fullness of all he could desire with instruments made for the purpose, and said:

"I believe I can meet and conquer disease."

And the chairman rapped aloud his gavel and said, "We must have truth, and demand that truth itself must have facts for its voucher, or it can have no place in the finale of the reports of this assembly. We are sore and tired of the words, 'war, defeat, surrender and lamentations,' and said record has found no victory to chronicle for drugs, and a very limited supply for surgery. If this body of thinkers wishes to be kind and liberal to all, with but little hope of abating the relentless hand of disease, the chair will say, 'Proceed, doctor, and give us the facts you now think you possess.' Remember, no more experimenting at the probable cost of life will be received by this committee of the world. They say, in the rules adopted to govern this meeting, that all theories must and shall be proven to be true or false by the propounder being forced to submit to and be treated by the tenets of the system which he claims to be truth, before he can be placed on the special role of this council. And I give you all notice that this council never will adjourn until a system of cures be adopted that stand based on the law that is without beginning and eternally the same. All speakers who represent any brotherhood of cures will be patiently listened to by this meeting and given all the time that is necessary to give history by notes and observations as to diseased persons he has met and known to be cured, killed or permanently injured by his methods. We want the good and bad of all systems; how their remedies affect the body and mind. We are told by one of a later date, who champions the system of 'Orificial Surgery,' that the brain can be acted upon by stimulating the nerve terminals; and his theory must be vindicated or fall, after being fully tested as given by the by-laws of these men, who put all assertions to the most crucial test, known as the 'fruit of the tree test.'"

The judge cried aloud and said, "This meeting will now adjourn for rest and refreshments, and before you leave I will say I want the committee on 'Allopathy' to rest four days and on the fifth assemble. Each man must arm himself with a fine mental sieve that nothing can penetrate but known facts. I am sworn by the people who sent me to this council of inquiry to bring on my return the truths, and not assertions; and know by careful analysis that the truth when rendered to them on our return be chemically pure and in exact conformity to the known laws of nature, which can only come from the mind of the infinite. Nothing less will be received. On our report depends the length of our days, for we are dealing with a jealous and enraged people, and must be able to report to them in such manner that there be no doubt left in their minds as to the methods of relief. I tell you the cup of forbearance is about drained and a furious explosion is bound to come. This council can do much to ward it off. We must wake up and act or suffer. I tell you, men and brethren, I have had a spy in the camp and on the track of Osteopathy for five years, and it is most wonderfully true."

❧❧❧❧❧

June, 1897

SINCE Osteopathy has been made by law equal to any other school of the healing arts, it will be as bold in the future as in the past, to give the reasons why it asked ldgal equality. First, we wanted the epaulets of law on our shoulders, so we could meet the enemy in open fields and measure sabres, and from now on we are in line and will try shot and shell, and meet the champions of drug in open field, to charge in any engagement for the belt.—*A. T. Still.*

June, 1897

FROM now on the JOURNAL will be devoted to the history, science and defence of Osteopathy. It never will ask you what it shall write any more than a man will ask you what God he will serve, or what form of service he will render. When it has a truth to publish it will be given. It will be devoted to the education of its pupils and the world of progress. It will be bold to assert its claims, teach you what is meant by Osteopathy, and not leave that to persons not qualified to give you the truth by their ignorance of the science. It will give you the facts as to diseases treated by this process. It will come to you full of truth for you to read and sleep on. It has entered the contest and will never be satisfied until its teachings are found in every house of reading over the whole earth. We will not bring as tropies anything less than the medical flag of a state. We have two or three now and they are gems in the constellation that clusters around Osteopathy.—A. T. STILL.

❧

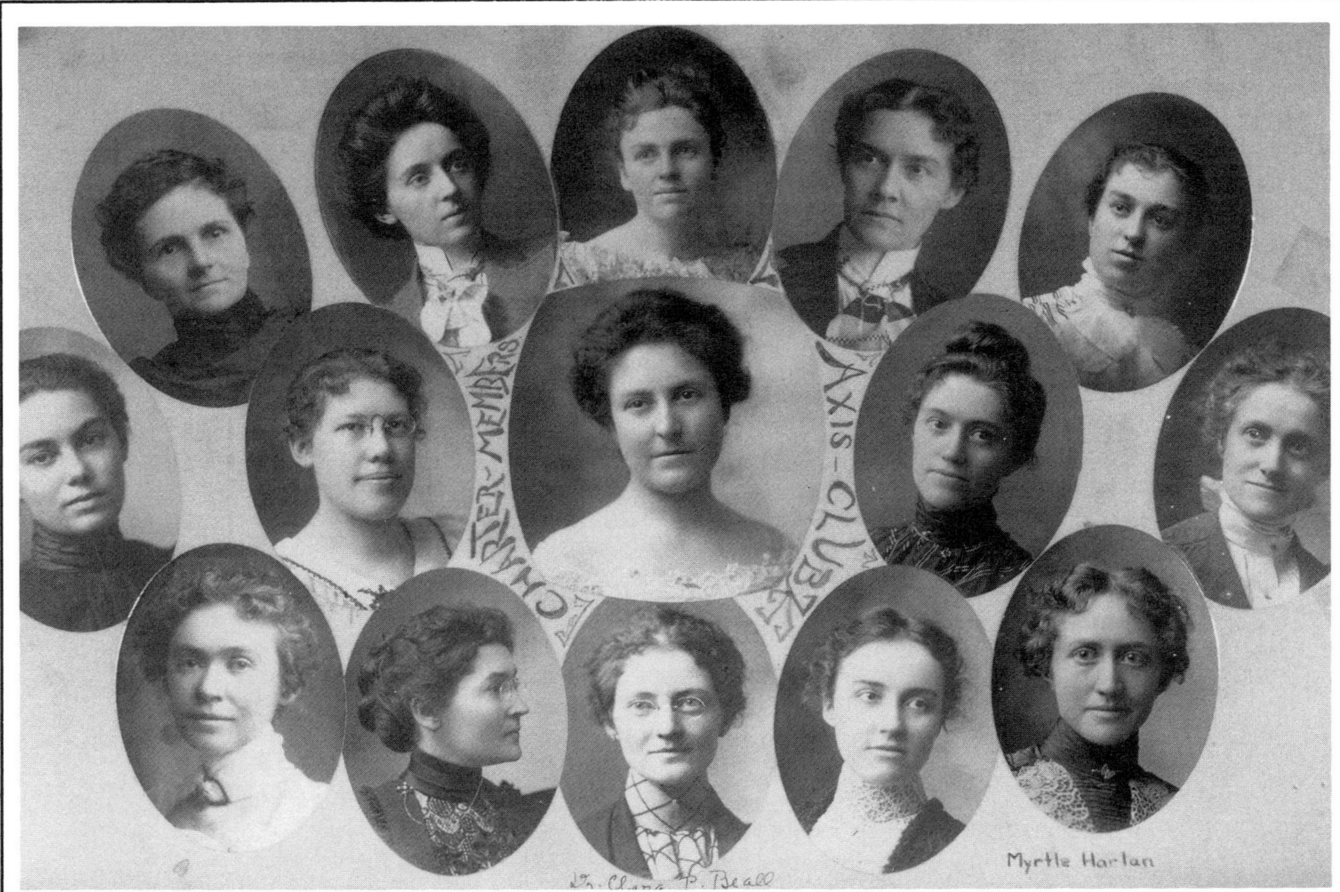

Charter members of the Axis Club

August, 1897

PREPARATORY STUDIES ESSENTIAL.

BY A. T. STILL.

WHAT books and studies are necessary to a complete education in the science of Osteopathy? is a question to which I have given much thought, and after a quarter of a century in this work I have reached the conclusion that every successful operator should fully understand Anatomy, Physiology and Chemistry. Your knowledge of these three books and the principles which they teach must be thorough. When I say Anatomy, Physiology and Chemistry, I mean if you fully understand these branches you are a star of the greatest magnitude.

I want to ask you if you have ever taken the time since you entered the classes to think of the length, breadth and depth of the meaning of these words? Do they not imply a perfect house, builded by a competent builder—a Being who knew what was needed to make a house fully equipped with the machinery for all demands of the spirit that was to dwell therein?

What would you say of a brag architect, who had the name of being a wise and faultless builder, who would say, "Your house is completed," and hand over the keys; but when you tried to fire up the furnace you should find he had left it without a smoke-stack? Would you think he knew anything about excretions? You would not, or you are ignorant of that part of Anatomy that treats of renovations. Did he put in a water-closet, with tubes running to it from all parts of the house? If you do not know, look at your Anatomy; start at the bladder, and follow all openings that run to it, from the brain to the soles of the feet, by that renal law of drainage which you find in the porous system of man and beast.

Before you receive a house you should go into all the rooms, try the doors, windows, closets, lights and ventilations, from foundation to roof. That is your duty before you receive the building.

You must be well versed in Anatomy, or you cannot judge the plumbing. You must understand it, or you cannot truthfully say that the house is well braced. Without it you cannot tell what foundation the house of life is builded on. You must know the shape, place and use of every piece that belongs to the whole superstructure.

By the bones you learn the frame-work. By the ligaments you find how carefully and exact the bones are fastened, each to all others. By the study of the blood vessels you learn the channels of supply and renovation. By a knowledge of the origin and insertion of muscles and tendons you understand their uses in manipulations as a machine of motor and locomotive power. By study of the fascia and synovial membranes you see why one muscle can glide over, under or around others and not irritate the harmony by friction. You get to the skin, which is the roof and weather-boarding of the whole house, with millions of pores to ventilate and purify by excreting impurities. Open your book and behold the brain, which runs all the machinery of force, to carry on all the duties required to make and keep the man normal in all parts and principles. The brain is his power of wisdom and strength, which runs analytical chemistry, preparing and blending all kinds of matter to be applied in the building, with the wisdom found in the Biology of the association of the living with the dead matter, which takes on itself life for hours and days, as wisdom commands.

You see, if you can see at all, that life comes to a man as a skilled chemist, fully endowed with force to do, and wisdom to select and shape, atoms suited to construct nerve and blood channels to supply strength and material to build man or beast—wisdom which is present and in working order at all times in all beings. It plans and forms each part to suit all other parts of the being it constructs. It takes the material of crude nature in its arms, and that is all we know of it until we see bone and muscle, clothed with life and form to suit the place for which it is intended.

This is the chemistry of man, made for him; and all other systems of chemistry have but little claim on him as a market for their products. The Osteopath who goes into the world with the idea of Chemistry attached to him as useful to help the Divine chemist that is in your brain, blood and battery of life, is only a boy who ties rags to rags to make his whip long and does not know it will wind around his little head when he wants to "pop." He needs the rasp of intelligence to rub his scaly eyes until he sees in man a fully equipped being from the mind of God, supplied with chemical, biological and all other machinery that man or beast needs, or all he could ask for if he had the mind and skill of God himself.

Does God know how to make and equip man? If he does, all you are required to know is how to keep the engine lined, fired and oiled; it will run its miles without any of your dopes or suggestions. Study the normal, and keep man in that chair, and you have run the length of your mental rope.

In all time past man has felt and acted as though the Creator had provided all things for him that he could ask or desire but one, and that was what to do or take when sick. We have lived under the tradition that man is made sick as a punishment for a few apples that Grandma Eve took, and has never been well since. I wish she had let them alone, if that was all she knew about the chemical and biological effect of stealing apples.

One says: "Do you object to the study of elementary chemistry?" Not at all, if you have not studied it previous to entering our school. I think it will help you very much to begin to think of the wonderful chemical laboratory that is eternally at work in man. This chemistry is less understood than any branch of Nature, and its workings for life and health are more to be admired than all other blessings bequeathed to man. An atom cannot have a welcome place in man if it has not had its fitness and purity passed upon at the school of life and truth, of which God is chief chemist.

Chemistry is a branch of our scientific literature that is unlimited in its variety and benefits to man. It begins and shows us the affinities and antagonisms of all known elements.

It is a guide to all our fine arts. Beginning with earth, through all its products, man is the crowning work of the skill and wisdom of all Nature, and halts to see the beautiful workings of that unequaled laboratory of life as it operates in him. No equal stands on record to date. He is not only refined to the least atom of his form, but his atoms of body are more refined and better adjusted to a higher plan and plane than all other forms of animal life. It had to be made and kept so, as the duties he had to perform were to control the world and all its elements by reason. Therefore all the machinery must be higher in form and quality to suit the coming demands. Thus we are warranted to reason that the department of chemistry in man is greater and more effective; that from crude material to the throne of reason, with power to select and purify previous to construction, by all rules of reason, he must be of a higher order of matter, skill and knowledge.

You should study and acquaint yourself with chemistry, as you are now preparing to go into the world as adjusters of the machinery of the chemical and physiological laboratories of life as a profession. You should understand the chemistry of the fine arts, that you may be more able to know by comparison the uses and what to expect in the economy of man and beast.

All nature lives by chemical action, and you should arm yourself with a useful knowledge of all that pertains to man by analysis, comparison or otherwise.

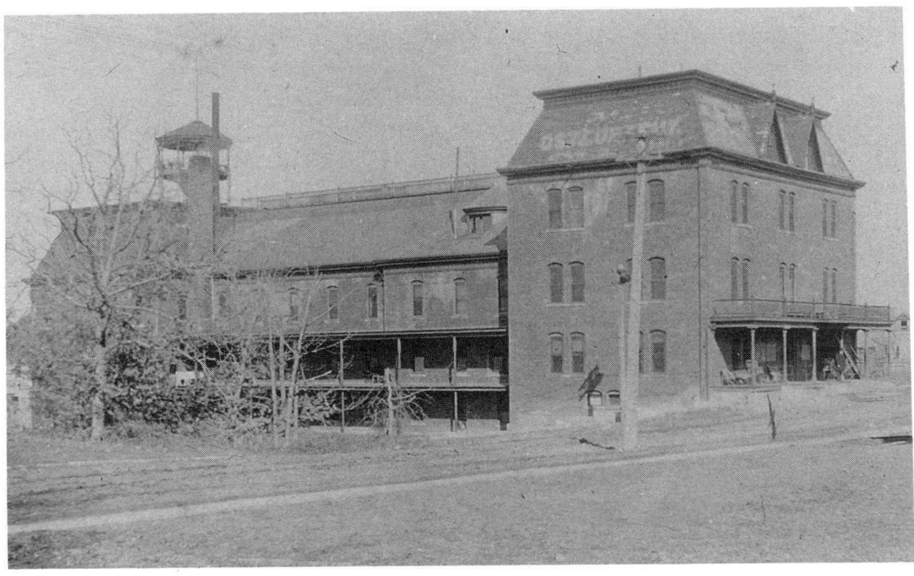

A.S.O. building looking toward the northeast

November, 1897

WHAT CAN OSTEOPATHY GIVE?

By A. T. Still.

WHAT can Osteopathy give us in place of drugs? is a great question which the doctor of medicine asks in thunder tones. Tell him to be seated and listen to a few truths and questions. "What can you give us in place of drugs?"

We have nothing to give in place of Calomel, because Osteopathy does not ruin the teeth nor destroy the stomach, liver, or any organ or substance in the system. We cannot give you anything in place of the deadly Night-shade, whose poison reaches and ruins the eyes, both in sight and shape, and makes tumors great and small. We have nothing to give in place of Aloes, which purges a few times and leaves you with unbearable piles for life. We have nothing to give in place of Morphine, Chloral, Digitalis, Varatrum, Pulsatilla, and all the deadly sedatives of medical schools. We know they will kill, and that is all we know about them. We do not know that they ever cured a single case of sickness, but we do believe they have slain thousands. We cannot give anything that will take their places. Their place is to ruin for life; and Osteopathy considers life too precious to place its chances in jeopardy by any means or methods.

In answer to the inquiry, "What can you give us in place of drugs?" I will say, we cannot add or give anything from the material world that would be beneficial to the workings of a perfect machine—a machine that was made and put in running order according to God's judgment—perfect in the construction of all its parts, designed to add to its own form and power day by day, and to carry out all exhausted substances that have been made so by wear and motion.

If this machine is self-propelling, self-sustaining, having all the machinery of strength, all the thrones of reason established, and working to perfection, is it not reasonable to suppose from the amount of wisdom thus far shown in the complete forms and workings of its chemical department, its motor department, the nutritive, the sensory, and the compounding of elements, that the Master Mechanic has provided the avenues and power to deliver these compounds to any part of the body, and to make by the newly compounded fluids any change in the chemical quality that is necessary for renovation and restoration to health?

When we see the readiness of the brain to supply sensation and motion, and are notified of an unnecessary accumulation at any point of the body by sensation or misery, we want removed that over-accumulation which is making in-roads on life through the sensory ganglia, to all its centers. We know when fully possessed by diseased fluids the fort of life must yield to the mandates of death from climatic or diseases of the seasons as they come and go.

If life yields to the poisonous fluids that are generated during detention and chemical changes, why not conclude at once that the motor power is insufficient to keep in action the machinery of renovation through the excretory system? Reason proceeds at once to reach the oppressed points. Through the vasomotor being irritated the venus circulation becomes so feeble as to allow diseased fluids to accumulate, locally or generally, through the system to such a length of time that they become deadly in their nature from the power of separation being overcome and lost.

Osteopathy reasons that the special or general power of all nerves must be free to travel through all parts of the body without any obstruction which may be caused by a dislocated bone, a contracted, shrunken or enlarged muscle, nerve, vein or artery. When enlarged or diminished they are abnormal in form and action.

If you have a thorough and practical acquaintance through Anatomy and Physiology, with the forms and workings of the machinery of life and health, and treat it as a skilled physiological engineer, then you are prepared to say to the doctors of medicine, "We have found no place in the whole human body where you can substitute anything but death in place of life." Remove all obstructions. All means ALL, intelligently done to completion, and nature will kindly do the rest.

Let me in conclusion ask the drug doctor if he has been able at any time to compound substances that can be introduced into a vein that leads to the heart, and not produce death? Do you not throw all substances into the stomach with the expectation that the divine chemical laboratory will throw out that which is incompatible to life? Are not all your hopes placed upon this one foundation, that we make the horse of life trot slower for fever, and walk faster in the cold stage? In short, Doctor, is not your whole theory based upon guess-work?

Nature's God has been thoughtful enough to place in man all the elements and principles that the word "Remedy" means.

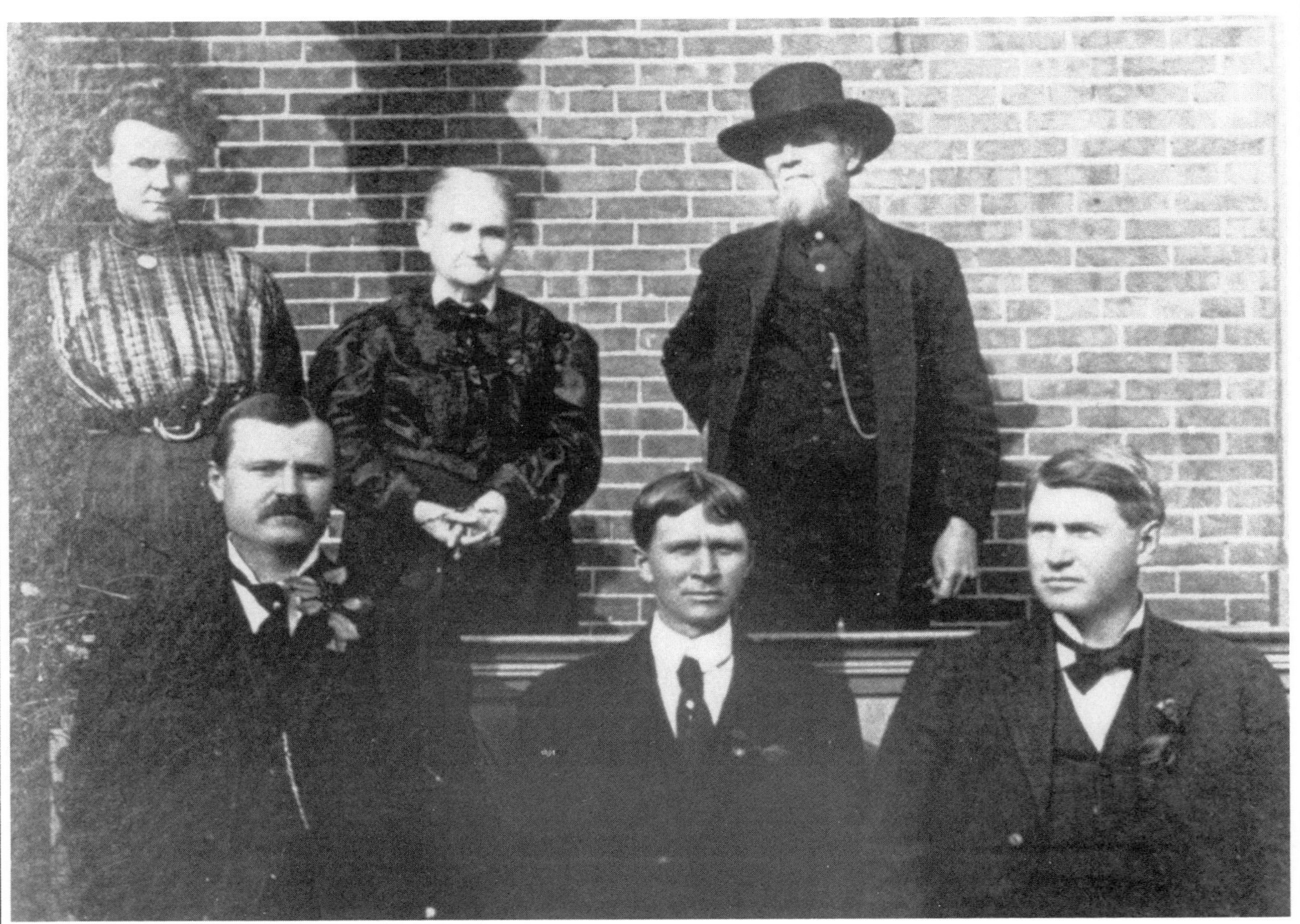

The A. T. Still family about 1913. Top: left to right, Blanche, Mary Elvira, Andrew Taylor. Bottom: left to right, Harry Mix, Herman Taylor, Charles Edward

November, 1897

DR. A. T. STILL'S DEPARTMENT.

THE JOURNAL was called for long before a line was written for its pages. Multitudes of patients who had been cured by Osteopathy insisted that a paper be published by me, that the people might know something of this science. I felt timid to begin the duties that naturally belong to a person who would embark as a writer of truths and principles that were so little known to the world. I felt I could not do justice to the pen nor the subject. First, because my life had never been that of a writer, therefore I felt my productions would meet with ridicule by the formal reader. But when in mind I set at naught that hinderance, I saw a greater trouble: that was, to describe the engine of animal life graphically, which would require a person of great anatomical knowledge. I knew but little of how they could work, and could learn nothing by council. I stood before anxious men and women who wanted me to write the hows and truths of life. I felt I was badly alone with no one to tell my troubles to. I went to those whom I thought should be of assistance, but their minds had received no ray of light that was able to penetrate, to any degree of depth, the subject of human life, as is seen in the union of mind and matter. I saw at once that the laws which govern this being were hidden at the very centre of the great mountains of mystery. To obtain a knowledge of the contents of that inner mountain, the pick and shovel, and the explosive power of the dynamite of reason had to be freely used, and the contents analyzed and separated by a qualitative and quantitative analysis. Those metals that were to stand the crucial tests of all acids should and must be obtained, labeled and set aside as suitable material with which to construct the foundation of human life.

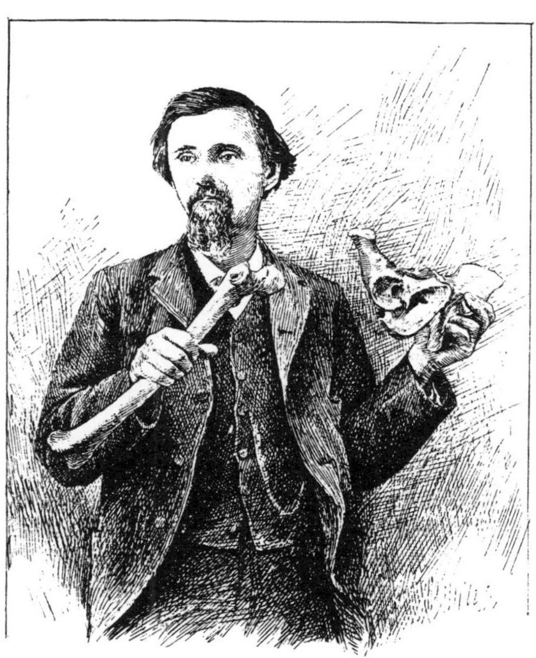

By this time I learned in my investigations that I could not pass before the public as a worthy journalist and supply my readers with clippings and immemorial quotations. The human mind had arrived to this, the eminence on which truth, with the fact, would be demanded. Without further apology I will say to the readers of The JOURNAL, such as I have, freely give I unto you; and that which appears to meet with your reason as truth, make such use of as you think best.

⁂

FROM the day of Moses until the present time, by habit and education, we have been taught to believe and depend upon drugs as the only known method of obtaining relief from pain, sickness and death. By habit and use of drugs in sickness through so many generations, we as a people think there is no remedy outside of them, and as the mind has been so unalterably fixed on that thought for so many years during all ages of the past, people have felt it a duty if not a necessity to be governed by established customs.

We feel when our friends are sick, we must do something to relieve them. If household remedies fail we then call in the doctor and turn the case over to him and he will call counsel when he feels he cannot manage the disease, then if the patient dies, the family and friends are satisfied that all had been done for the sufferer that was possible. Every known remedy and skill had been exhausted and we must be content with the results. Though death has prevailed, we feel that we have done our duty.

I wish to say to the graduates who are about to go out in the world, when I entered this contest I took as my foundation to build upon, that the whole uuiverse with its worlds, men, women, fishes, fowls and beasts, with all their forms and principles of life, were formulated by the mind of an unerring Deity, and that He placed all the principles of motion and life, with all remedies to be used in sickness inside of the human body. He had placed them somewhere in the structure if he knew how, or he had left his machinery of life at the very point where skill should execute its most important work.

Now I have given you some reasons why I believed I was warranted and it was my duty to proceed cautiously to test nature's skill as a doctor. The how to do was the all-absorbing question of my mind. I finally concluded that I would do like unto a carpenter when he knows he has the elements to contend with, and desires to cover an old house with new shingles. He knows if he takes the shingles all off at once, he exposes all that is in the house to rain, hail or what may be in the elements. A wise carpenter would take off a few at a time, and cover with new shingles what he had exposed before he would proceed farther. I knew it would not do to take the shingles of hope (drugs) off of the afflicted all at once. I felt it would be a calamitous move to so act, with my limited knowledge of cause and effect. I was called to treat a case of flux and being a physician, and familiar with the remedies for such disease, questions like this arose, "What is nature's remedy?" "Has it a drug store?" "Does it use sedatives for flux?" "Does it use sweating powders such as Dovers, etc.?" "Does it use astringents?" "Does it require alcohol in any form in prostration?" and if it does, "what does it use it for, and why does one die with flux, and another get well, after having used the same remedies?" "Would our dead patient have lived had we kept our drugs out of him?" "Did the convalescent patient have the power to resist both disease and drugs?" You may answer these questions, I cannot. One is dead, the other alive, and that is all I know about it; and my brother councilman expresses the same feeling, and says, "I do not know."

When all remedies seemed to fail in my first case of flux, I felt I had done my duty and no censure would follow in case of death. Myself and council had agreed that this case was bound to die. Without any instructions or text book to be governed by, I concluded to take one shingle off from the spinal cord, and see if I could not put a new one on that would do better. To my great surprise I found the flux stopped at once. That shingle contained all the opium, whisky, and quinine that nature required to cure flux. That shingle took the pain out, the fever off and stopped the bloody discharge from the bowels, and my confidence in drugs was badly shaken. I soon had opportunities to treat many more cases of flux, all of whom recovered without the use of drugs as recommended by our standard authorities, which has convinced me that nature's laws are trustworthy when thoroughly understood. By investigation I was led to a better understanding of the cause of flux. That flux was an effect, which could be traced to a cause in the spinal cord or other nerves, and the remedy should be addressed to cause and not to effect. I felt proud to be able to say to the people when I threw all the known remedies for flux out of the window, "I can now give you a reliable and demonstrative substitute that I found on a prescription which was written by the hand of the Infinite."

I kept up this method of removing old, and putting on new shingles until the house was entirely covered. I have written this bit of history for the express purpose of warning you, students of Osteopathy, against the danger of breaking down when you have difficult cases, and calling in the supposed aid of drugs, because you do not know what set of nerves are disturbed, and you are made to assert that what you have said about the power of nature to cure is false, or, you do not understand your business. If you will allow yourself to think for a few minutes, who of the Osteopaths out in the field are trying to treat Osteopathically, and yet have a drug doctor running around with them, you will find such persons to be feeble in Osteopathic power, with less than one year in school previous to the time of offering their services to the people. You are very apt to find on their card "such and such M. D's. in our office," with a great long apology for ignorance and say they do thus and so to please the people. Every drug that is tolerated by an Osteopath in disease will shake the confidence of your most intelligent patients, and cause them to always take

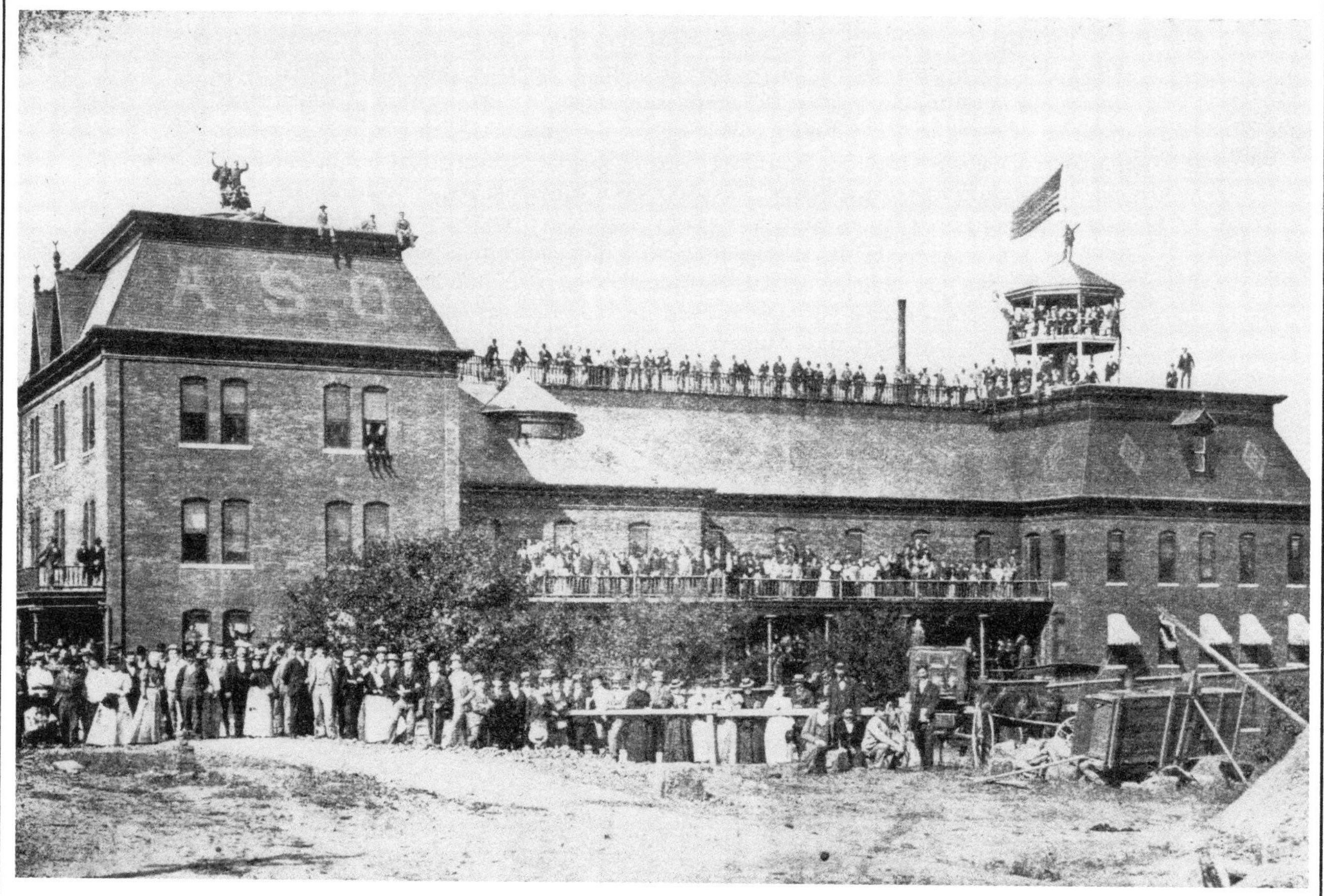

The A.S.O. school looking to the northwest

your word, skill, and ability at a great discount. I would advise you to bathe your heads long and often in the rivers of divine confidence, and pray God to take care of you with other weak minded people who pretend to know that which they have not studied.

Much more could be written on this line, but I think I have said enough to warn you against being a kite-tail to any system of drugs which is your most deadly enemy. A doctor will use you for what money he can get out of you only. Osteopathy is now legalized in four states, and you do not have to compromise your profession or dignity by associating with anything. Your opportunities from the American School of Osteopathy to master the science have been good, your foundation is solid, and I want you to come back with heads up, and on your return, I want you to say, "I have transacted my business as the institution teaches, without the aid or assistance of drugs, and I have proven that the laws of the Infinite are all sufficient when properly administered.

***

THE exact time when man's foot appeared upon the face of the earth no record shows. A knowledge of his advent might be profitable. The unwritten history of the human races with the genius or lack of genius might be to us the open book of knowledge, as it is not supposable that the mind of man has just become observingly active in the last few centuries; while absolute evidence of a purer and deeper reason than we have been able to control, stands recorded on the faces of many valuable "lost arts" which we have never been able to equal. It is but reasonable to suppose that the mind that constructed man was fully competent to undertake and complete the being to suit the purpose for which he was designed, giving him physical perfection in every limb, organ, or part of his body; and at the same time gave him all the mental powers needed for all purposes during the life of his race. And with that perfection in the physical, it is supposable he approached very nearly to intellectual perfection. Now a question arises: When did man begin to degenerate physically and mentally? Let us reason on this line. The stock raiser carefully preserves the best developed and most healthy of his herds for breeding purposes, that their offspring may suit the purpose for which he wishes them, and as a result he raises stock from the poultry house up, with marked improvement in form, strength and usefulness. Should he be foolish enough to kill off all healthy and well developed males as they appeared in his herds of cattle, horses and other stock for one or two centuries and keep the crippled, deformed and maimed for breeding purposes, would anyone with average intelligence say or think for a moment that such stock improved his herds? On this line we will look at the procedure of all nations. Has it not been to select the strong and healthy men, drive them out on the field of battle, destroy a million or more of the strongest, as the records of the war of the sixties show today? Since that war closed the fathers of our children had to be the crippled, worn-out and degenerated physical wrecks. Such men are the fathers of all children born during the last thirty years. Every healthy young lady who has married and become the mother of one or more children since sixty-five, had to, and did select her husband from a war or hereditary wreck. From that degenerated stock of human beings our reform schools and asylums are filled. And the beams of the gallows are pulled down by these mental dwarfs. Run this train of reasoning back for a few thousand years, this degenerating force bearing upon the offspring, is it any wonder we have the lame, blind and foolish all over the country?

Now if we have been mentally degenerating, killing our best men back for a thousand years and still have a few who are fairly good reasoners, what was mental power then compared with now? They could think from native ability, we only through acquired ability by our methods of education. Should an original thinker appear occasionally from the crippled and maimed, he will have much to contend with that is not pleasant, unless he is generous

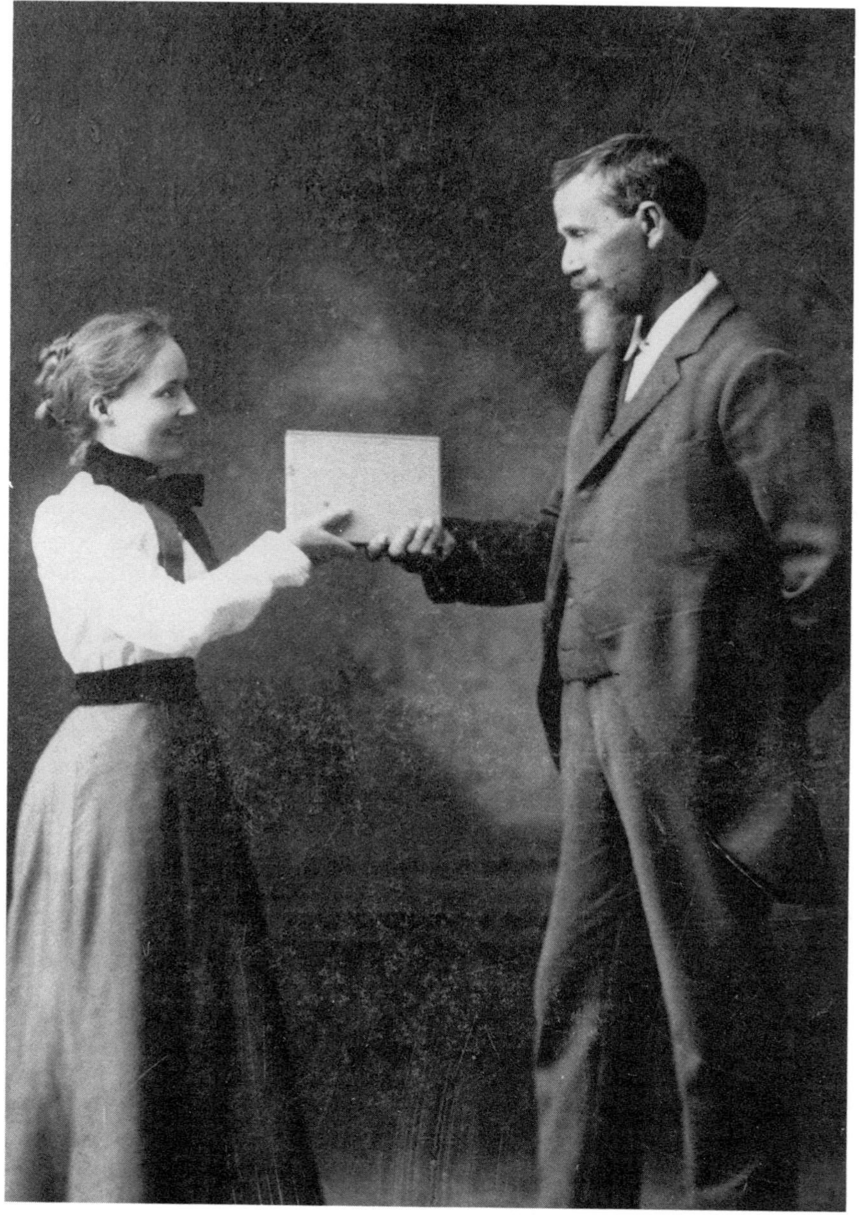

A. T. Still presenting a copy of his autobiography to Jennie Lorene Moore, 1897

enough to credit the cause to an effect produced by the lack of mental and physical forces in the sires just described.

Men and women who are able to reason, cannot afford to wear out their forces by spending time in tiresome discussions with the blank masses, who are very fortunate to have intelligence enough only to make a living under the methods that require the least mental action.

It would not be gentlemanly nor ladylike to allow a feeling of combativeness to arise, and spend your forces with such persons. Pre-natal causes have dropped them where they are, and a philosopher knows he must submit to the conditions, and is sorrowful in place of vengeful and vindictive. And all that is left for him to do is to trim his lamps and let the lights defend themselves.

On this line we have much to think of. Anciently they did think: great minds existed then, as evidenced by the architecture displayed in constructing temples and pyramids. As in philosophy, chemistry and mathematics—they stand today as living facts of their intelligence. In some ways we equal and even surpass them. Before the establishment of religious and political governments, national and tribal creeds, to sustain which the powerful minds and bodies by thousands and millions have been slain, and their wise councils prohibited by death. Reason says, under the circumstances, we must kindly make and do the best we can in our day and time.

No doubt their religion was far superior to ours before they began to fight over their Gods and governments.

Some evidence crops out now and then that their methods of healing were natural and wisely applied, and crowned with good results. As far as history speaks of the ancient healing arts, they were logical, philosophical, good in results and harmless. It is true enough that we have great systems of chemistry that are useful in the mechanical arts, but very limited in their uses in the

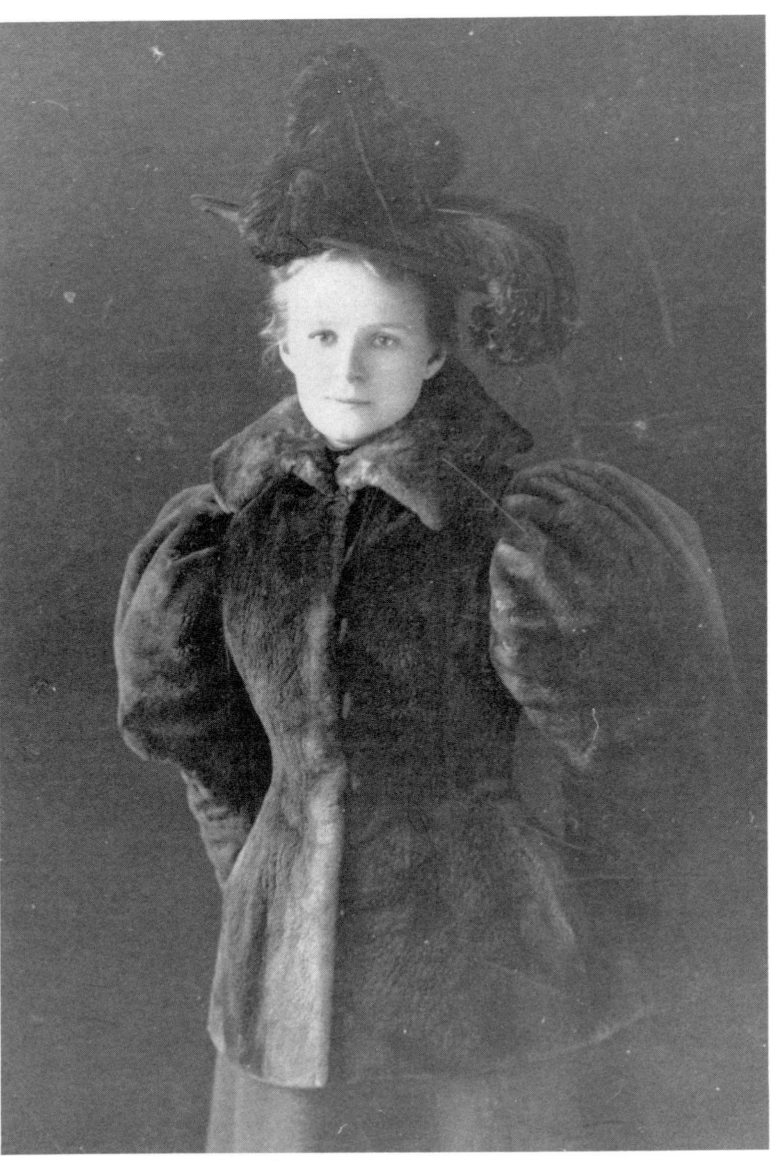

Blanche Still

healing arts. In fact a very great per cent. of the gray haired philosophers of all medical schools unhesitatingly assert that the world would be much better off without them. These conclusions are sent forth by competent and honest investigators who have tested all methods and medicines, and observed carefully the results from a quarter to a half century, and say, let us call it a "trade," as the use of drugs is not a science.

The author will now say, the health hunter, in the majority of cases when he administers his drugs, gives one dose for health and nine for the shining dollar.

As it becomes necessary to throw off oppressive governments, it becomes just as essential to do away with useless customs, without which no substitute has ever been received.

Allopathy, a school of medicine known and fostered by all nations, drove on with its exploring teams, gave up the search, went into camp and builded temples to that God who purged, puked, perspired, opiated, drank whisky and other stimulants, destroyed its thousands, ruined nations, established whisky saloons, opium dens, insane asylums, naked mothers and hungry babies. He still cries aloud and says: "Come unto me and I will give you rest—I have opium, morphine and whisky by the barrel. I am the God of all healing knowledge, and want to be so recognized by all legislative bodies." "I do not wish to be annoyed by Eclecticism, Homeopathy, Christian science, Massage, Swedish movements, nor Osteopathy." "I hate Osteopathy more than all the rest combined, it scratches me and all my disciples; I cannot destroy it. It uses neither opium, morphine, nor whisky, and it is impossible to catch it asleep. It has scratched our power out of four states during the last twelve months, and no telling where it will put its paws next time. We must prepare for more war; I have heard from my scouts that on its flag the inscription reads thus: 'No quarters for Allopathy in particular, and none at all for any school of medicine farther than surgery, and war to the hilt on three-fourths of that as practiced in the present day. The use of the knife in everything and for everything must be stopped, not by statute law, but through a higher education of the masses, which will give them more confidence in nature's ability to heal.' "

ANDREW T. STILL.

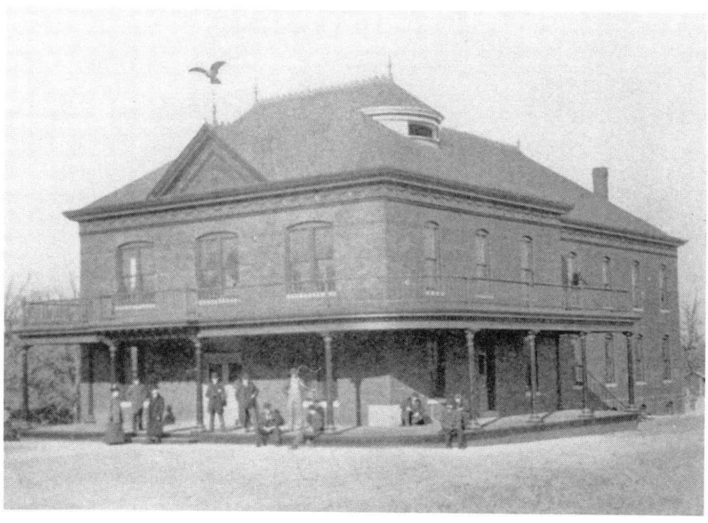

The Infirmary shortly after it was completed

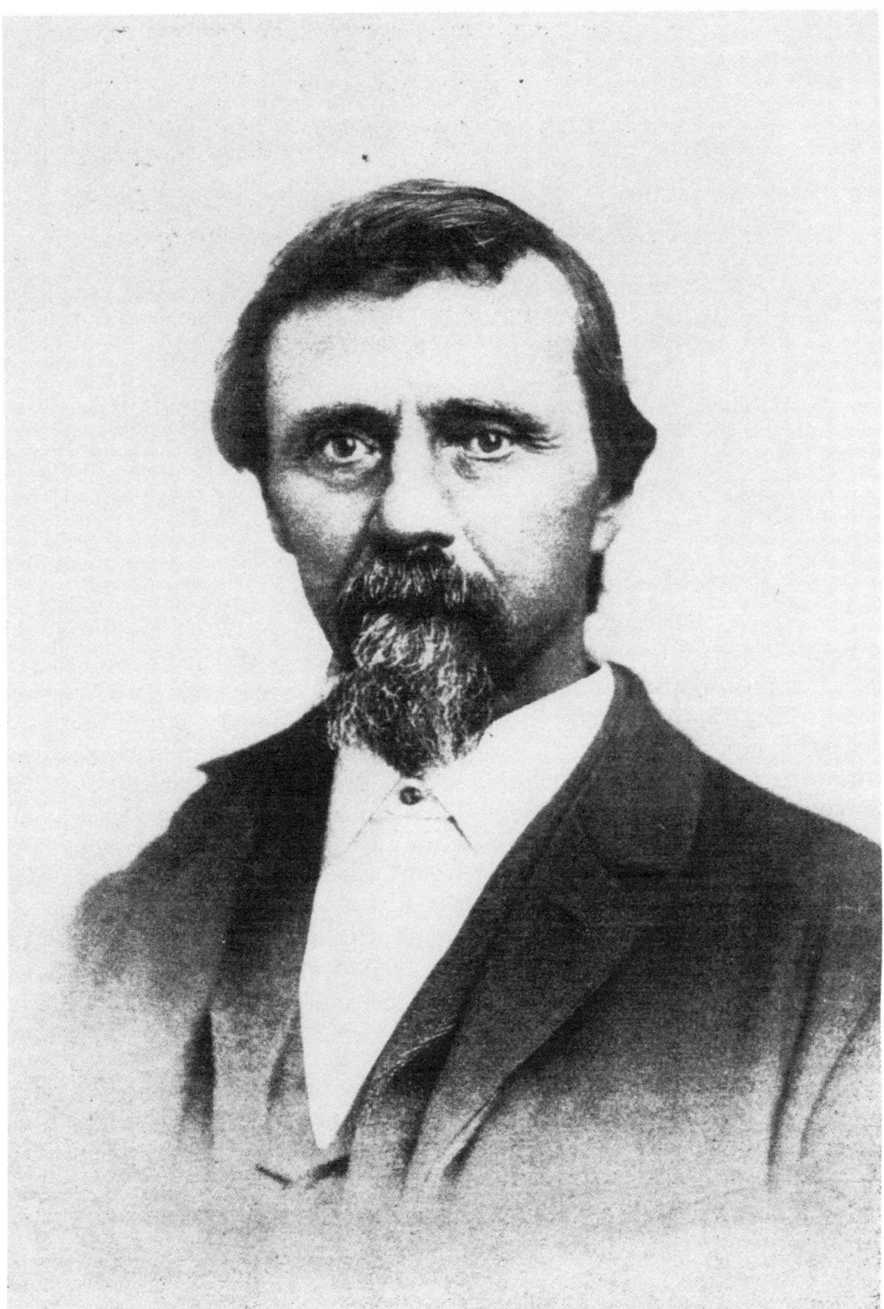

DR. A. T. STILL'S DEPARTMENT.

CONVULSIONS are an effect, and to know the cause has been the anxious study, not only of the doctors of medicine, but of every household in all ages. Convulsions have no partiality—they are just as apt to take hold of a czar as a peasant—a general in the heat of battle as a man in the ranks—a minister or priest who is reverently thanking God for life and health, as a layman—the mother as she nurses her babe from her loving breast, as the babe. All are equally liable at any moment in life to be attacked by spasms, rigid in nature, which deal their blows on the nerves to unconsciousness, and often do not relax until death closes the doors of life. "Spasms" are the unsolved problem of all the philosophers of past time. The question of their solution is open today, with the prayers of four billions of people for the success of the philosopher who can solve the mystery of catalepsy, epilepsy, apoplexy. The doctors of all schools of research join in the hope that someone may catch and tame that demon who is the terror of the whole earth from the cradle to the grave. I feel it would not be manly for Osteopathy to omit to say something on such a momentous question as spasms. I feel there is no harm in giving a history of a few observations and results of experiments with that dreaded disease for twenty years with drugs and another twenty years by Osteopathy.

When I used drugs, some patients got well, but the greater number continued to have spasms right along, though mild and strong medicines were faithfully and hopefully used. Many lost their minds entirely; others became feeble minded and idiotic. Questions like this arose: "Have I failed to cure the spasms and ruined all the powers of reason by administering such powerful remedies as popular authorities on convulsions have recommended?" The truth is, spasms are the unsolved mystery of the time, without reference to methods or doctors.

To an observer a spasm presents a general rigidity of the muscles of the whole body, beginning with the ligaments which attach bones to bones, and all the ligaments of the whole system. With this condition presented to our observation, questions arise and a great many of them. We see and know that here is a case of spasms, in which we see all voluntary nerves and muscles under subjection and entirely inactive. The person struggles until exhausted; the spasm abates but the unconsciousness continues for a longer or shorter period. Finally consciousness returns, with motion of the whole body apparently in normal condition. On examination we find nothing on which to predicate an opinion as to cause. We frankly say we do not know the source of this trouble. We think and talk about "maybe-so" causes. In our ignorance of the facts, we are just as apt to say "tapeworm, or other intestinal worms," or something that has been eaten, or drank, that has produced an irritation of the general nervous system by the presence of foreign bodies in the bowels. We use purgatives for the purpose of removing such irritants, and we use them freely and often. In a few days or weeks another spasm appears, as powerful or worse than the first. We feel the trouble is not from the irritable bodies in the bowels, after they have been thoroughly cleansed by the most powerful and searching purgatives known to the profession. Another council is necessary in order to find, if possible, some other cause than the one just stated and rendered doubtful by use of drugs recommended for purgative and cleansing purposes. The second spasm is far more powerful than the first; consciousness and motion are much later in making their appearance, leaving the patient more exhausted. At this time we change our reasoning from the bowels to the general nervous system. We place our patient on such remedies as will break down the periodical rigidity of the system. We choose and administer such medicines as the wisest counsel suggests in treatment of nerve diseases. We prosecute the treatment more heroically than in the previous attack. We push those remedies day and night, week in and week out, hoping to destroy the cause, but in due time another spasm appears, more violent from the start, than the previous ones. It keeps up its fury until the patient becomes exhausted, the spasm relax for a moment then take hold with renewed energy, and keep up this process for a day, two days, a month or six months, with from thirty to seventy-five spasms a day, notwithstanding drugs are used by the mouth, inserted under the skin by the hypodermic syringe, and by medicated injections in the bowels. The attending physician is constrained to say there is no efficacy in drugs. At this time of trial and affliction, the patient dies in the spasm and leaves the doctor confirmed in the opinion that medicines are of no avail in convulsions. The doctor dreads spasms, because he has had the evidence that he has been at sea without a compass time and again.

After long years experience with spasms and trying to do something to relieve the sufferer, I gave up the subject as hopeless. For a number of years I had nothing to do with spasms. Finally I was impressed that the cause might be pressure of some section of the vertebra on the spinal cord, by dislocation of some joint of the neck or spine. On examination I found the bones of the neck or spine to be in an abnormal condition. I decided that the bones were partially dislocated, and held so by ligaments and muscles, which might press upon some system of nerves that should supply nutriment to other nerves, which failure would leave the motor nerves without nutrition; and they had no other method of telling us that their store of nourishment was exhausted than by contracting all motor nerves, and holding the system in that condition until the nutrient nerves could supply the demands, set the machinery of nutrition in motion and feed the motor nerves.

My opinion is firmly fixed if we suspend the supply of nutrition from the motor nerves we have spasms, which will last until they are supplied. The demand is absolute.

Since acting upon this philosophy, results have been satisfactory. I have treated many cases of periodical spasms successfully. I have confined my explorations for cause to the spinal column only. In every case I have found it to be abnormal both in bone and ligament. I am proud to be able to report that the majority of cases have recovered entirely. My investigations have not been under the most favorable circumstances because of attention to other subjects.

My sons and opera tors in the Infirmary are handling and disposing of a very great majority of such cases. With report of success already obtained we intend to prosecute investigation with the expectancy of finding more of the causes of spasms, also much of the so-called insanity, located in the spinal cord. We have had encouraging success in hundreds of cases which came previous to partial loss of mind either with spasms or so-called insanity. I believe relief can be obtained in the majority of such cases. This opinion is based upon the observation and results obtained by Osteopathy.

***

THE man who lives an honest life has influence from merit only. God himself has put merit only in all things. Policy is the soft soap of liars and hypocrites, which a man never borrows nor buys unless he doubts his own merits. A just and wise man needs no such help. Influence is asked for by men and women who have not enough merit to sustain them when they make a business move in life.

If a man desires an office he should never hunt for men or papers to loan him influence, unless on reviewing his past life he finds on the scales, that he has been found wanting, and is not the object of the admiration in his county, state or nation that is needed for a successful race. But if he wants an office or position for the money he hopes to get, and his only object is to obtain and occupy the position, that man is a stranger to merit.

When such a person goes to men of character for assistance, he knows his own word will be taken at a discount by those who know him best. He makes many promises which he does not expect to fulfill. He wants influence to hide his faults. A question: What influence does gold need beyond native merit?

None; neither does it need recommendation written nor spoken beyond its native usefulness; no amount of influence would be of the least benefit to it.

I speak at this time as I feel, from long observation of men who depend upon merit with its triumph in all engagements in the battles of life. He who lives an honest and upright life should fear no man, rich nor poor, of any political, religious nor scientific position.

Why should we coolly pass the man of toil for two years, and then kiss him and his household with our lying lips, when we know that all we want is his vote cast into the ballot box for the election of a policy man, who is like a cow-herder who raises cattle for sale, just as some men will sell their friends, when they get good prices.

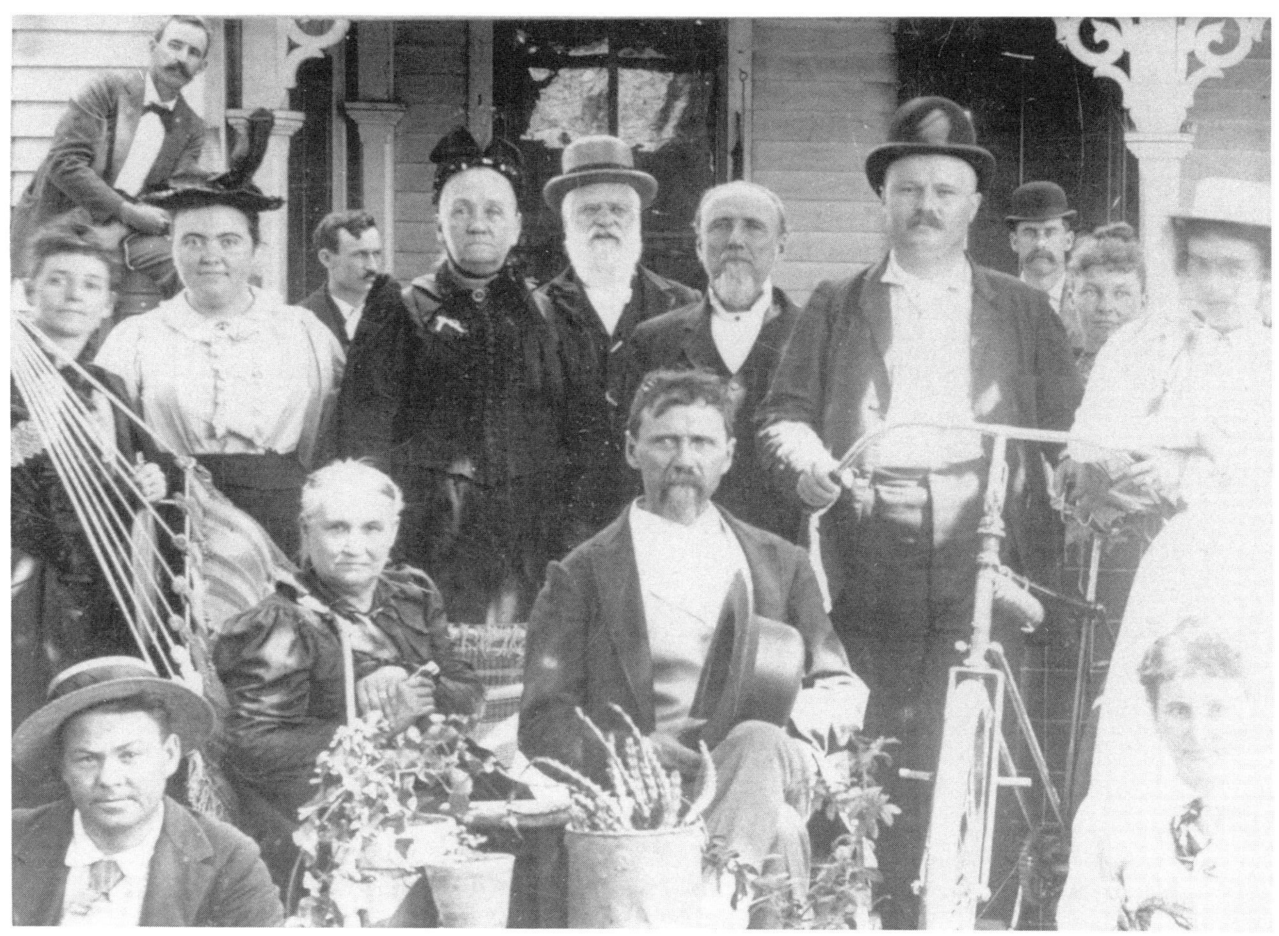

A. T. Still and Mary at a picnic about 1897

Why should an honest man ask for influence when his neighbors know all about him both good and bad? Why should a nominee for president, congress or the legislature, stump the county or state in which he was born farther than say, "I will obey your orders?" His character and caliber have stumped for him each day of his life, and he will get all the votes he merits, and that is all he should have; in fact a policy head is just like a dehorned cow's head, big at the neck only.

A policy hunter always has "friends for sale" written on the black bulletin of his heart. Instance: Judas of old; or any policy man. Who can trust such a cowardly pup? You have only to go to the church and other gatherings to see him bow and smile; he puts in but little money, prays loud and long, and asks God to care for the widow and orphan, but reserves the right to be called "Holy Willey." He loves the Lord for the wool that he can get from the flock. He would not go to heaven if it was not for the "influence" of "Old Nick."

A policy man will soon show you when he gets you in his grasp that you are his slave, and your liberties are lost. He has you and your babes under his political, religious and business whip, and will never smile again at you as a "wonderful blessing to all earth," but command your knee to bend in reverence to his powers, wash his fine carriage, hitch his team to it and hand him the whip, which he will apply to you and the horses which he has taken from you by a liar's policy, blinding men by cloaks woven by the most threadbare policy looms.

His tongue is that of a liar, his heart that of an assassin, his hand knoweth naught but to steal, he commands obedience with this injunction: Do as I tell you or I will organize mine host and crush you and all your friends and efforts for all time to come."

Let us pray! Oh Lord let me go to heaven when I die, but if there are any policy people within its walls I prefer oblivion to doubtful felicity. Thou canst punish me by any reasonable method, but I do think it would be too bad to have me spend an eternity where policy men and women dwell. Thou knowest I dread their tongues above all hells or half-way places. Give me merit, O Lord, for I feel that the very pillars of the throne of God stand upon merit.

***

I AM OFTEN asked this and similar questions: "Dr. Still, what caused you to study out the great truths of curing the afflicted without drug remedies?" As you have asked me that question, I will give you this as a partial answer. First, I tried the virtue of drugs, as taught and administered by Allopathy, then noticed closely the effect from the schools of Eclecticism and Homeopathy. I concluded all were a conglomerate mess of conjectures and experiments on the ignorant sick man, from the crown to the hod. I learned that a king was just as ignorant of the nature of disease as his coachman and the coachman no wiser than his dog. I had passed through measles, whooping cough, and the full list of contagious, climatics, and diseases of the seasons. I was raised by a graduate of medicine, who trained me to observe the start, progress and the two endings of disease. The one to get well despite drugs and disease; the other to die amidst pills, prayers and all human efforts. I was familiar with the word "God" from a child up. My father was a good man (or tried to be.) He gave me castor oil, rhubarb, gamboge, aloes, calomel, lobelia, quinine and soap pills, then he would ask God to bless the means being used for my recovery. When I grew older I followed in his footsteps all but asking God to bless the means and poisonous filth I was using in my ignorance of cause and effect. I thought the filth I had given would kill or cure if it was its nature to do so, and in time nature's scraper would scrape out the system and the patient would get well.

I began to look for a God of truth who did not guess all things. I learned to believe that there was a respectable God at the head of all things—one who did not use morning bitters to tone him up for the coming day's work. I began to learn that all his work when done was placed above criticism or even a suggestion. I concluded I would prove him and see if he was as smart as I thought he was. I put his work on the race track of reason and experiment. It got the purse of victory every time and all the time.

I got ready to attend the fall races. I got up in the judges' stand where they ring the bell to "go." Nature's little pony came out on the track. He was not much bigger than a goat. He sided up by the fine steeds of drugs, and at the word "go," he lit out at full speed. I was afraid the fiery steeds would run over him. The race grew more interesting each quarter-post he passed, and he won the prize in fall diseases, because he depended upon Nature's law. The horses of much ribbon and big saddles tried their very best; they broke gait, ran and plunged in wild confusion, determined to pass Joshua, but he got the purse, blue ribbon and all, in the fall races.

They found that Joshua had nothing to do with jockey racing. He went on into winter and spring diseases; he commanded them to stand and they did stand.

When the races were through and the fiery steeds found there was no use to measure speed with "Joshua" they made many suggestions. That, as Osteopathy was a great truth discovered and demonstrated by Joshua, it could be made a great money scheme; that millions could be made out of it; that its literature should be placed upon all newsstands because of the anxiety of the people to know something of the pedigree of this little horse of so many victories on all race tracks, where the speed and efficacy of remedies should have a fair trial and the ribbon be awarded to the successful contestant; that the notoriety thus obtained will give in favor of Joshua the lever by which we can make countless millions, if we use it.

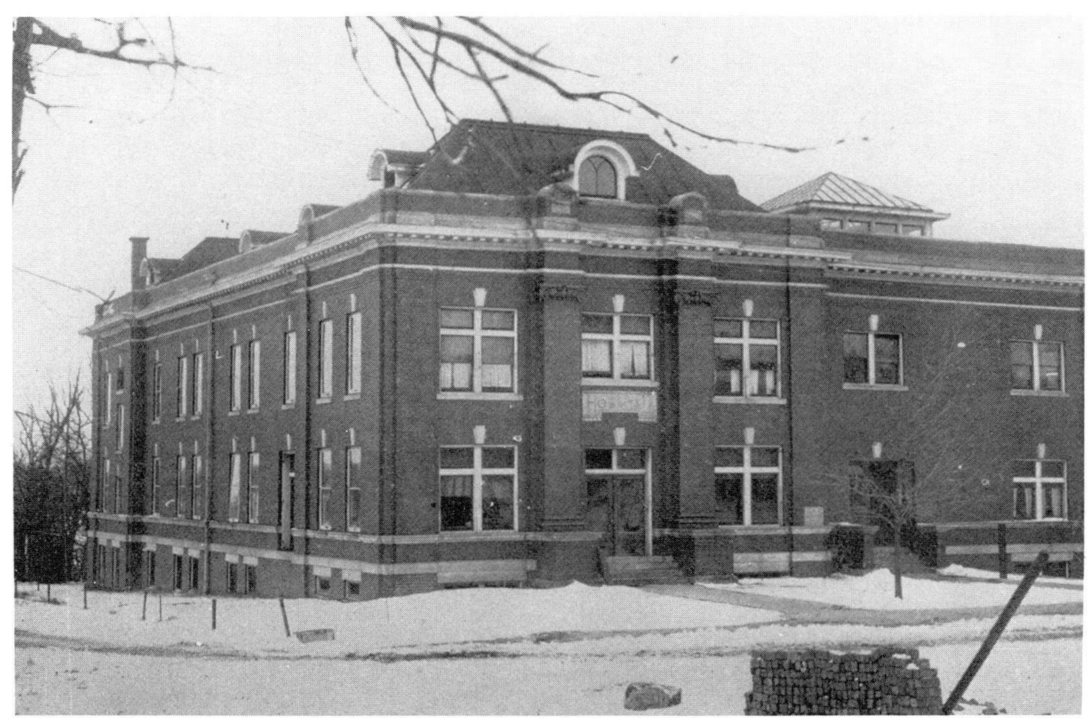

A.S.O. Hospital

Joshua stopped and looked at the sun and moon which he had commanded to stand, which order had been obeyed at once, and while looking at those wonderful planets he said: "I will go into no jockey races, combines, or organizations by which one dollar or cent can be taken unjustly from suffering humanity. Fame and money are not what I want, unless it be given me at the tracks where the ribbon of merit is awarded to the successful horse, without jockeying or collusion whatever."

Osteopathy is not the outgrowth of printer's ink; but of what it has been able to do for the afflicted when all other methods had failed to give relief. The mouths of the once afflicted and now well are the oracles through whom the growth of the work of this science has been made great and world-wide famous. It is the cures, not paper stories.

It is not my intention to write nice pieces for the orator to quote from, but to suit myself only. If a journal can be made self sustaining I will be fully satisfied. It cannot be conducted as other magazines because it is in a sea of furious waves and will load to suit its comfort all the time. Some say the Journal will be criticised; the lack of criticism is what I fear.

***

IS MILK while in the breast or udder a living substance? If a living substance while in the breast what of its vitality after it gets cold? Is it not reasonable to conclude that the child should drink the milk directly from the breast of the mother, in order to graft the living material into its being while in a living condition? If milk takes on itself animal life while in the process of production would it not die like other animal substances as it cools from blood heat to a lower temperature? Is it not reasonable to think, in the passage from the teat to the pail, that it gets mixed with the deadly gasses of the common air? Do they not naturally unite as elements of change? If so, what is milk when life is extinct? Does it not have to enter a new process of being reatomized, and take on life anew before its atoms can enter the blood system and be applied for use as muscle and bone? Much evidence favors the position that cold milk is far below the nutrient power of warm milk, that passes from the mother's breast to the young stomach warm and alive. All other milk is surely dead, and must be made over and used while in the greatest vital condition to get the best results. Nature would seem to say by its work that the machinery of the mother ought to prepare food for the child after birth to suit the strength of the young stomach, for a period long enough to allow the stomach to harden to suit the demand for crude substances. The process from crude material to living flesh is surely a grand process. No dead atoms can be received in an artery as a part of a muscle. Nature uses no unsound principles nor substances in plans and buildings. Wisdom can be seen plainly written on all works of life. Form must be perfect in all parts of the machinery of digestion, which begins with rough food and ends with blood, which is proof of the choicest skill and greatest wisdom.

Before each atom of blood leaves the heart a separate covering is placed on all corpuscles of blood except the white, whose duties are not definitely known. They possibly mend up broken veins, construct fascia and other white parts of the system.

Physiology leaves us to conjecture much of the hows and whys of nutrition, before it appears as blood in the arteries. But reason takes us to the wonderful fact that all that nature does is through living substances which it produces as it uses them. Thus no great supply is kept on hand before it is used, neither could there be and live long. We know blood and milk corrode and harden soon after cooling. Evidently they are dead, and these changes are for dissolution, as milk surely dies as soon as the animal heat leaves it. Thus the process of converting it into gasseous fluids, with other substances taken in to suit the laws and processes of dissolution, previous to completing its total destruction as milk.

Similar processes follow all dead substances that enter the body and blcod. Nature is careful to bury all her dead in the air and earth. Milk and blood do live and die, and the mother should remember that her breast makes better food for her babe, and it will flourish and grow better on it, than on the finest slops of all baby killing substitutes on earth. Let us sing:

"Praise mother's milk and fonntain, too:
No substitute equals what she can do."

CORRECTION.

IN DR. STILL'S article on Milk, page 316, first paragraph, commencing with sentence on tenth line read: "Does it not have to enter anew the process of being atomized and take on life before its atoms can enterer the blood" etc.

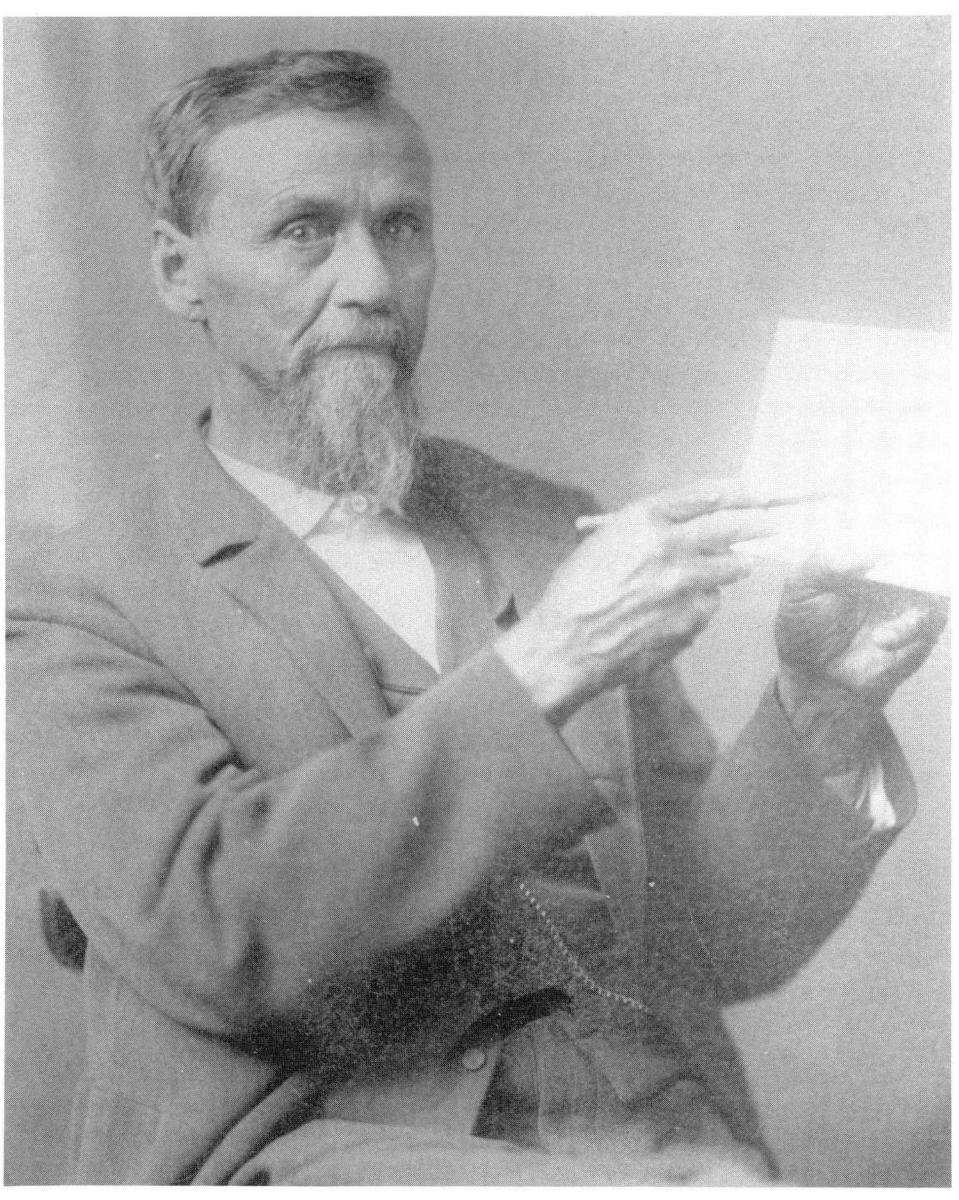

A. T. Still, 1898

January, 1898

DR. A. T. STILL'S DEPARTMENT.

Will We Ever Meet?

A MAN'S days dribble along, drop by drop, but all come at last. Some are reasonably good, but all fail to do or bring the thing most wanted, joy. Joy is the ripe apple of the tree of man's aspirations. But it is stung in so many places by the bugs of prey, that malcontent keeps an open grimace on its face filled with sorrow.

Time gives us joy only from the vessel that roams the seas, which comes into port now and then and gives us a taste, then turns her bow seaward for another voyage. She may never return to fill our cup again; she navigates the seas of time only. Joy may be on that vessel which meets all storms and brings to us a cargo of comfort. But, alas! there is none on this boat for us. We wail with broken hearts, and our sweetest music is the echo of our moans.

Hope often turns our hearts to drink of the unseen rivers of joy, and says, "it is for all; come drink freely and quench all thirst."

But the cup we have to use is of the kind that changes all drinks to bitter. It has the power to change all fluids before they reach the lips of man—even obliterates the sense of taste for all things except the most bitter solutions.

Why should man ask the sun to repeat its daily rising, while time holds the cup of gall to his mouth, to drink that heart pressing compound of acrid poisons which enters only to add torment to his empty chambers? If one day is like all others, why ask for more? Does he not know that hope is a lost star and he is left forever in the dark? Has he not learned that joy is not found in eat and drink, but is in the heart and brain of a man who can and does love? It comes and dwells with him and her, who has it for sale or to give away. He and she are happy when they can say and feel that man's love, joys and hopes are all born of minds that never do eat at a selfish man's or woman's table who does not try to have it loaded with kindness, with a welcome for all, without regard to race, color, creed or condition. He cannot hope to purchase joy with gold; he must plant the seeds of love in the richest soil of his heart, and cultivate it by the best methods known, and try to improve on all systems.

Man is surely what he makes of himself. If he wishes to be miserable he can be so by his unpleasant ways to others, who are just as good as he is in every respect, save perhaps less wealthy. But by your abundance of kindness you should reach far beyond all points of fame, to that manhood and intelligence that eclipses all those brilliant stars, who have on their banners nothing that shines but gold, with its joyless lustre, which can be changed by the hand of adversity, in a day. Let us learn to love and make all happy, and spend our days in the sunlight of peace.

When we call back from the graves of time, a few of the sunny days and by the longing of our souls, we love as we weep, love the day, and even fail to feel for a moment, that time has feasted and swallowed those hours long since, we see that it is simply a vision we behold on the mirror of memory, and our hearts quiver with the thought that those days have long since gone under the dark clouds of time.

The eye fills to overflow, and despair veils itself with the dews of eternal night, and all we can do is to weep, love and moan, as hope is forever lost. We feel that oblivion has come with its mantle to veil our joys beyond vision, and leave us to know that the happy days of our childhood and youth are all now with the hopeless past.

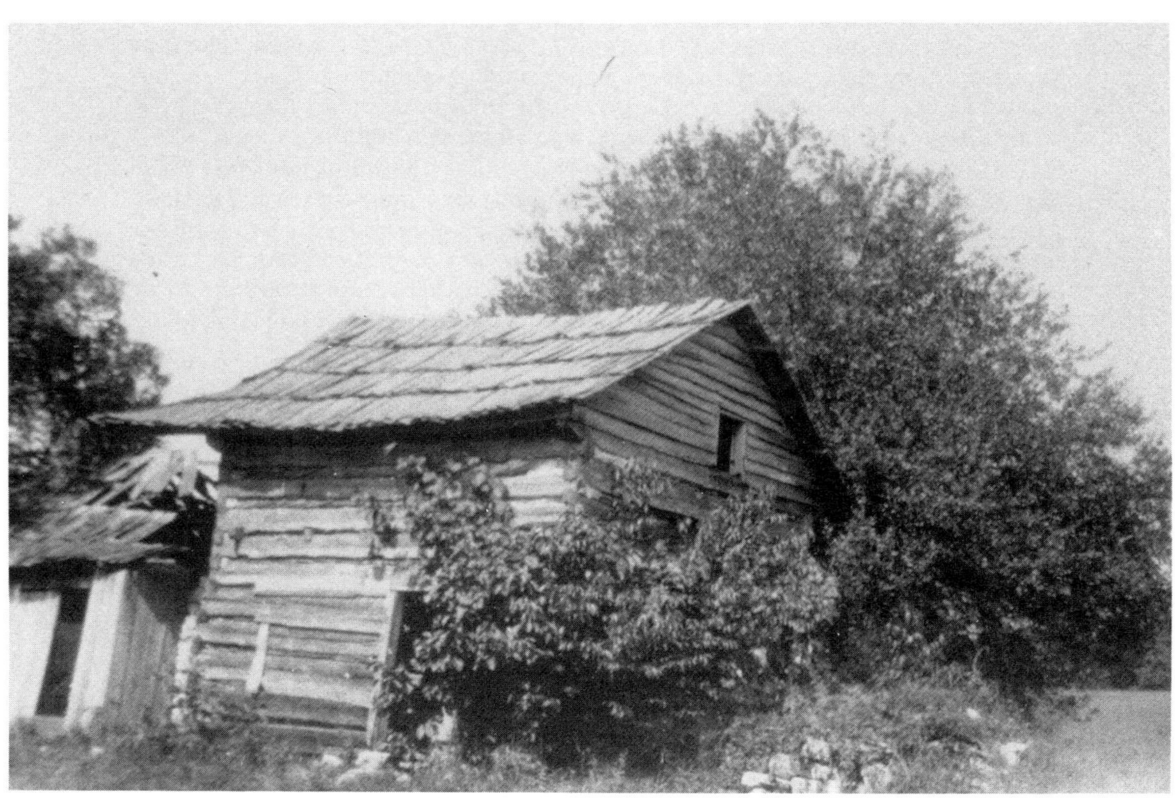

Abram Still cabin in original location 1927

Silently we slumber, or be awake all night, till morning's sun wakes bird and beast, to eat and drink of the joys of another day.

All move and speak, but father, mother, and friends, who do not arise from their night's slumber to join the host that seems so happy. Could their sleep let them loose only to smile once more, rivers of joy would burst forth from our hearts, and empty the oceans of the briny contents of our longing souls. But their voices sleep with their lovable dust.

As we long to hear even a whisper of love from her who toiled all day, in and out, for our joy, and all we have of her is the wet pillow of a child's love for its mother.

One would say to us think of the day when we will meet father and mother with other departed friends, and taste "joys immortal." Does that only come at the end of this life? If they can speak to us then, why not now, and turn this bitter cup of day and night into rivers of honey? Then love would be the sweet fruit of the promised tree of life. Give us one word from their silent lips, and take all earthly joys.

I suppose I am as other mortals, eat, drink, labor and sleep, but my days are all as a vision. I see and drive my horse, he goes on knowing not to where or for what. I am behind him, which is all he knows. I, too, am driven by the whip of time, I go day after day, why and where I know not; millions do as I do, live as I live, and end as I do, journeying to a pit that holds a corpse, which is all we really know.

Why should I dress as the "polished gay?" My heart rises and falls then as now. Let me dwell and die in the forest with beasts of prey. If they feel as I do they will not molest me. Let me be my own audience—talk and sing myself to sleep. It surely is good to dwell alone, talk alone and drink of the river of time, until my lungs hush and my hand closes forever the window blinds of time, and mine eyes for all future days. It is peace I want, and a day of joy that never ends, though that day is spent in my tomb with all who forever rest only in their graves.

PREVIOUS to building a ship the architect who draws the plan and specification must have the skill of a master mechanic. He must so construct the hull as to give the greatest known strength. He must select and locate beams, braces and all that is useful to give the greatest power of resistance to furious winds and lashing waves. When completed and the ship ready for the inspector, if done properly he will find engines located in their places with powerful bolts, every shaft, pipe, furnace, water, oil, coal, and all that pertains to the engines carefully provided for.

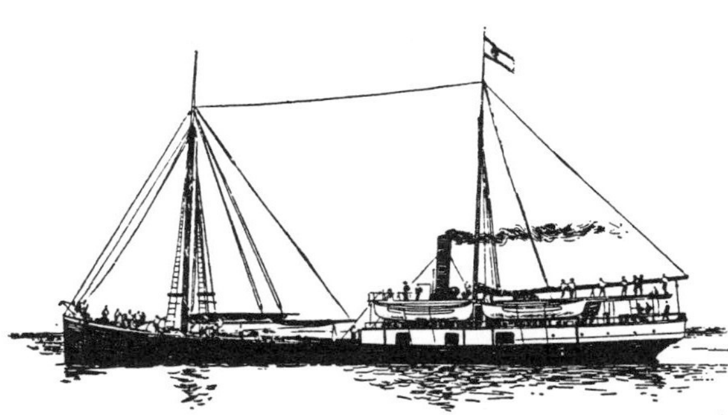

He inspects from hull to highest point on the vessel, from bow to stern, from starboard to larboard, with rigging all complete. Then he marks the vessel "sea-worthy."

The captain orders the engineer to fire up, and at the sound of the bell turn his vessel seaward for a long voyage. He steams on and on day and night, week in and out, completes that voyage with many others successfully. She starts on an another voyage full of passengers and valuable lading, she has so far met and conquered many severe storms, and on inspection nothing had given way. This vessel was considered almost master of the elements.

But at this time she enters the beginning of a more powerful storm, which doubles and quadruples, the angry forces hitherto brought to bear upon this vessel. This storm with its increasing fury lasts for days and nights, and the only salvation for this ship-load of human souls hangs upon the power of hull, faithfulness of the engine, and the skill of the engineer. He must steer to the wind and hold it there all the time. To do so he must increase his speed on account of the fury of the storm, as all lives depended on this one thing. Notwithstanding the pressure is very high, he orders his fireman to roll into the furnace rosin, tar, bacon, or any substance that will generate heat, which order is obeyed to the letter. He succeeds in keeping his ship headed to the wind. And when the fuel is fast deserting him the storm ceases within a few knots of the ship's destination. But just before entering port, the vessel begins to go round and round, and on examination the engineer finds that the steam-pipe that supplies one cylinder which has stood many storms has at last given way, and he has a case of "hemiplegia." One side of the vessel is wholly powerless.

The captain fires the gun of "distress." The officer of the lighthouse hears the signal and sends the lifeboat to his rescue. On landing, the inspector finds this once powerful vessel, that had triumphed over many storms for years, disabled and sends her into dock for repairs. Every bolt, brace, pipe, and all parts of the engine, hull and rigging had received more or less injury, by the great labor and strain in passing through the storm just described.

High heat and great pressure of steam, with the fury of the storm have produced irreparable strains and the vessel will be seen on the high seas no more. Prudence would say, she should ever retire from heavy labor both of hull and engine.

We give the student this illustration with the view that he may expect the most powerful vessels to mark a collapse. Equally so with man when out on the ocean of life. He may stand many storms but will meet one that will send him into port for repairs, which on inspection will be condemned, and the boat silenced by the fiat of force.

Long voyages of mental and physical labor have weakened his engine. His store of vitality has been greatly exhausted from the many struggles he has had; and he must give up all labor that will strain either mind or body for a time, as their continuence will only hasten the finale, which is death.

The master mechanic may do much by way of repairing very great injuries and enable the vessel to bear light burdens and take short voyages. Experience says, keep near the shore and live as long as you can.

Man is dual in nature, physical in form first, mental in action, powerful in union. But all his powers are limited to suit the being, man. He must economize his mental and physical forces in order to live long and happy.

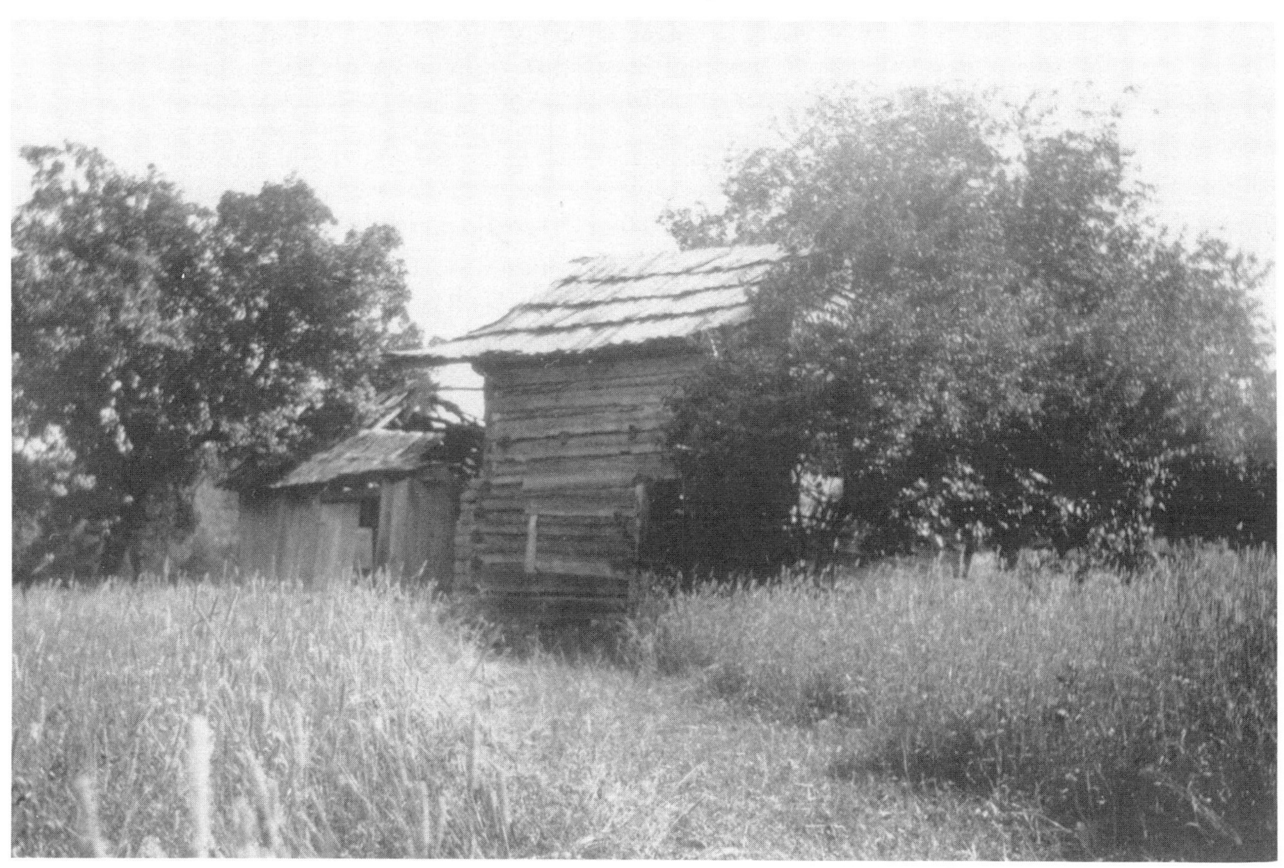

Virginia cabin in which A. T. Still was born

LECTURE TO THE CLASSES IN THE CLINICS OF OSTEOPATHY.

WHEN you have learned all that can be taught in a systematical way, then you have an opportunity to go for a higher knowledge of anatomy than any school has ever been able to teach. Your first term is in Gray's anatomy, in which you have to pass above 80 on a scale of 100 as an accepted grade.

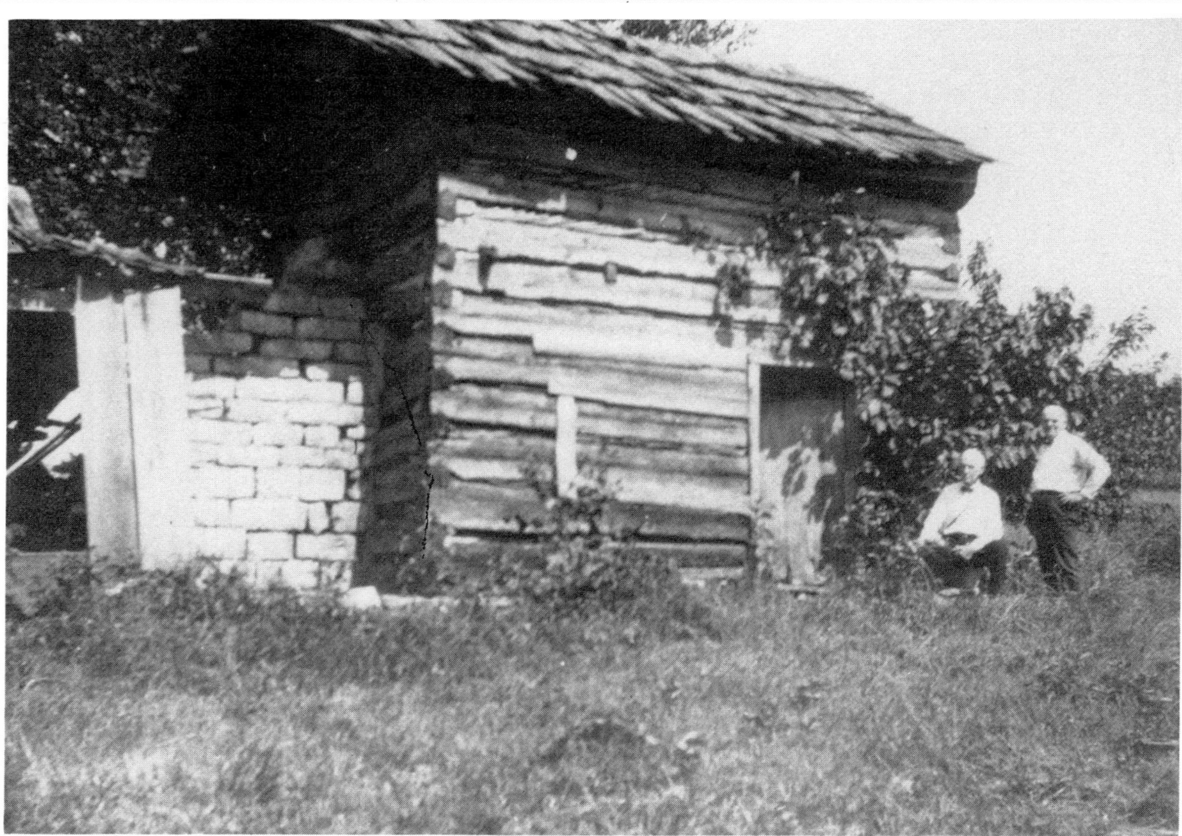

Dr. Harry H. Bill & Dr. Harry Lyndan Chiles view cabin before its removal to Kirksville

Then you are prepared to enter the higher class of anatomy under the rigid training of Dr. William Smith, who is possibly the best anatomist now living. I have never met his equal. His papers show that he graduated as M. D. after five years' rigid drill in the University of Edinburgh, Scotland, one of the greatest schools of medicine in the world, then devoted two years more to the subject of dissecting, of which he surely is master. For the past three years he has been dissecting, and demonstrating anatomy, in this school.

After entering the rooms of the clinics you are required to use the knowledge of the branches which you have studied, for then you are required to think and act as an engineer, who is supposed to begin to apply his knowledge in a practical manner as an operative engineer.

Thus those sour and tiresome days begin to reward you with light, which you now begin to receive while operating under the instructions from those whom you have felt even angry at for holding you from the rooms of the clinics until you could be well prepared to enter this, the most responsible place in which the operator meets and realizes the importance of knowledge.

Here I will inform you of a very serious truth: the danger of allowing a person to come into operating rooms who is ignorant of anatomy and physiology. He would prove a failure as an operator, lose confidence in Osteopathy, go off disgusted, enter some medical college, and like the old sow, go back to the wallow of drugs and drunkenness. He gets his medical diploma—and if he knows no more about medicine, than he learned of Osteopathy, he is only a pitiable failure all round—then wants to establish a great

Infirmary of Osteopathy, using the word Osteopathy to delude the ignorant, and the title M. D. to screen him from the rigors of the medical law.

As your grades from the preceding rooms and branches therein taught show your proficiency to be high, we now welcome you to the rooms of the clinics, and if you give your attention as faithfully here for the coming few months as you have in the past, you will receive your diplomas from an incorporated school of Osteopathy, which is the only one now on the face of the earth (so far as I know) that has all the facilities, with the most competent teachers that money and experience can obtain.

You have paid your money honestly to this institution, and you shall have value received if within the power of the corporation to give it.

In order that you may be well qualified to enter the world of responsibilities, we teach you all the branches taught in any medical university. For fear you do not understand what I mean, I will detail by saying, we teach anatomy, physiology, histology, urinalysis, chemistry, symptomatology, diagnosis, prognosis and treatment, with the knowledge of drugs and their uses, poisons and antidotes, midwifery and surgery as taught by them and from the same books.

Why should you feel timid when you meet the medical doctor, when you are his equal if not his superior, in all branches in which he has been taught;

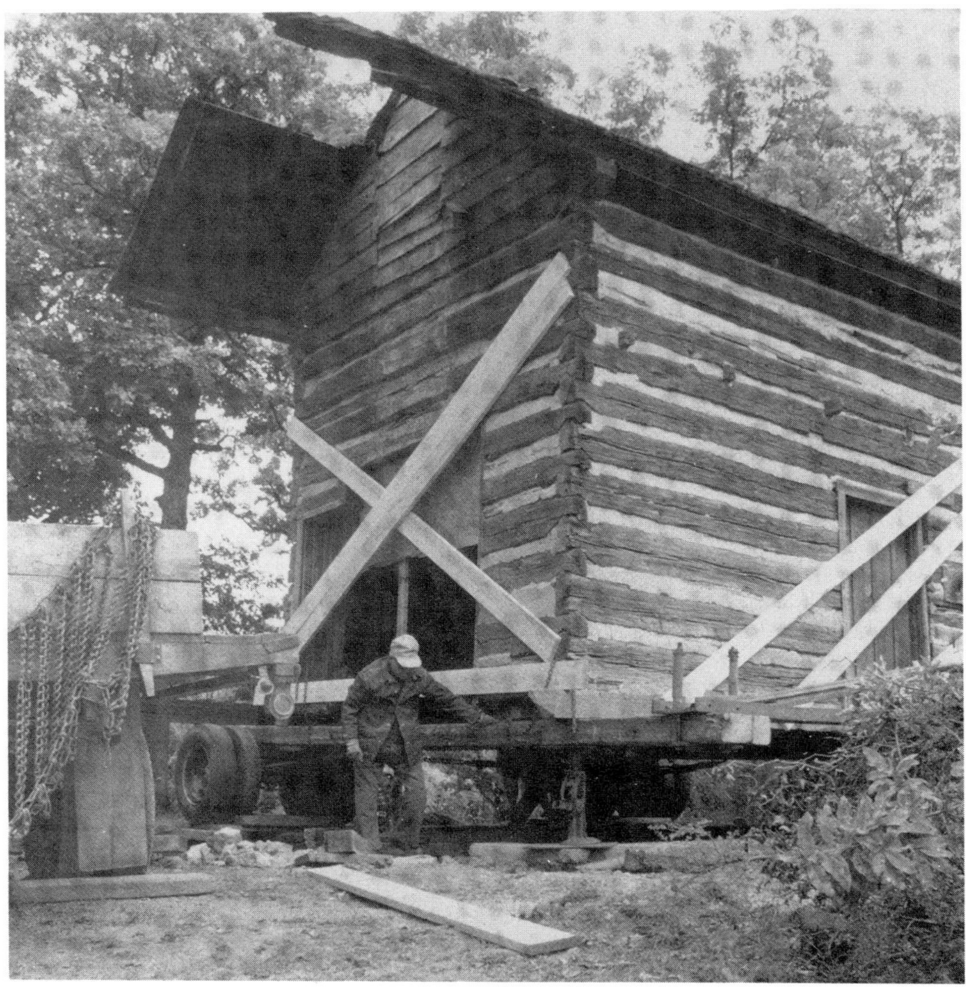

Resetting the cabin

also master of the philosophy and principles of Osteopathy, which has proven by its merits to be the highest of the healing arts. You have filled all requirements of the law, and have taken the degree of Diplomate in Osteopathy. This document is an honorable recommendation to the crowned heads of the globe. And you receive it bearing the signatures of men whose last and least thought is to obtain money by any hocus pocus method, bragging or publication.

By your request I have built and equipped this institution, which is open to the scrutiny and criticism of the literati of the world, and is pronounced good, and even "very good," as the Lord said when he had created man.

In constructing this building I was careful to build it myself, and by my own means, every brick and brace from foundation to dome is free from the odium "joint stock company." It was not built to boom and sell town lots, nor was it built to obtain money, but to teach the principles of Osteopathy, of which I claim to be the discoverer. Not one principle or truth has been evolved since the year 1874. Neither was it known and practiced previous to that time.

I am the discoverer of the science, and the first man to put its principles on record and in practical use, demonstrate to the world that asthma and all other diseases are effects only; cause was abnormal nerve and blood supply. Also birth was natural and should not be the hell of mortal life, the dread of which suffering has caused millions of unborn children to be slain in the womb

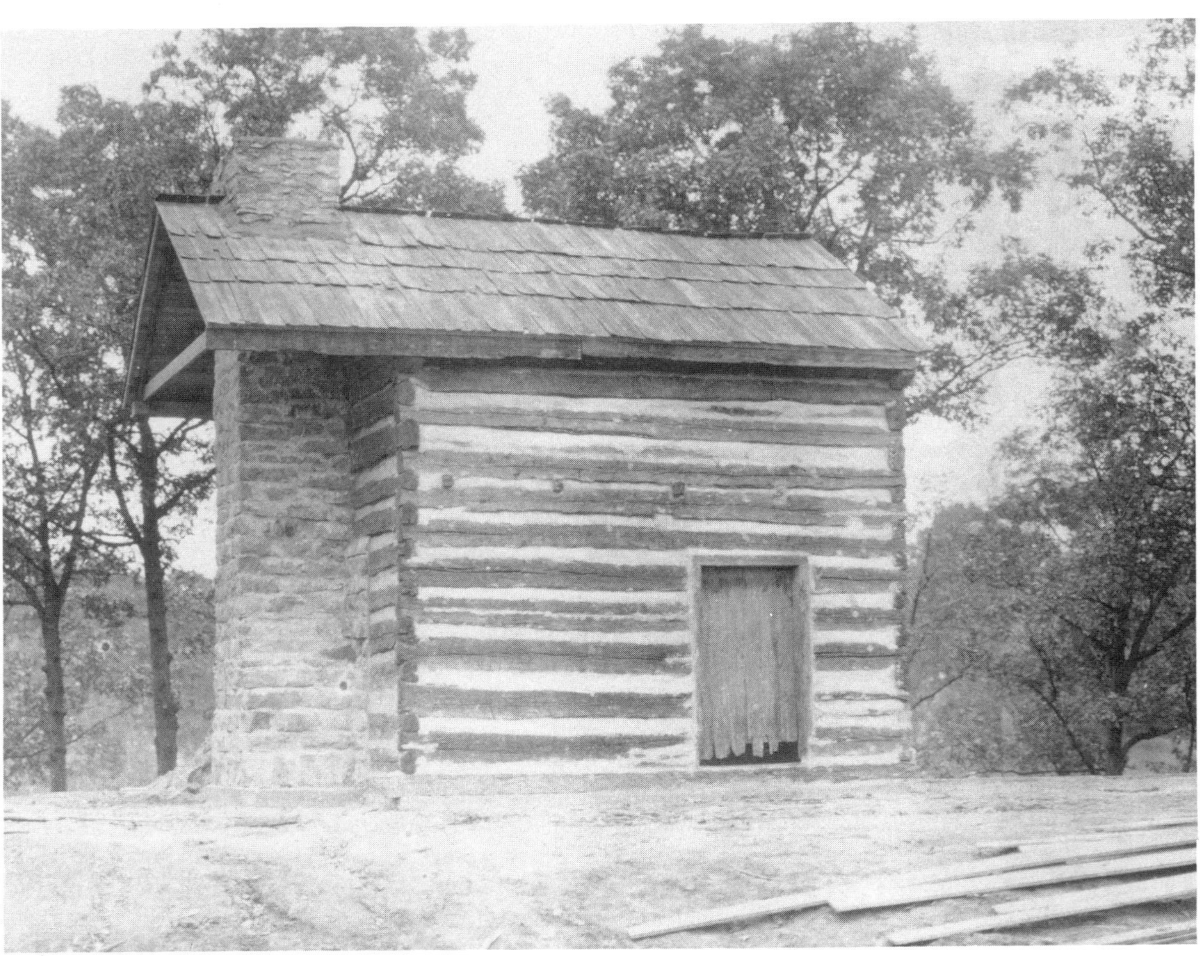

Cabin located on north edge of A.S.O. property

of the mother. Farther, that all normally formed women were entitled to reasonably easy delivery, and without the use of forceps, at the end of two to four hours duration, when in the hands of a skilled operator.

TO
ANDREW TAYLOR STILL
FOUNDER OF OSTEOPATHY
THIS TABLET IS ERECTED
BY THE
AMERICAN
OSTEOPATHIC ASSOCIATION
ON THE CENTENNIAL OF HIS BIRTH
AUGUST 6TH 1928

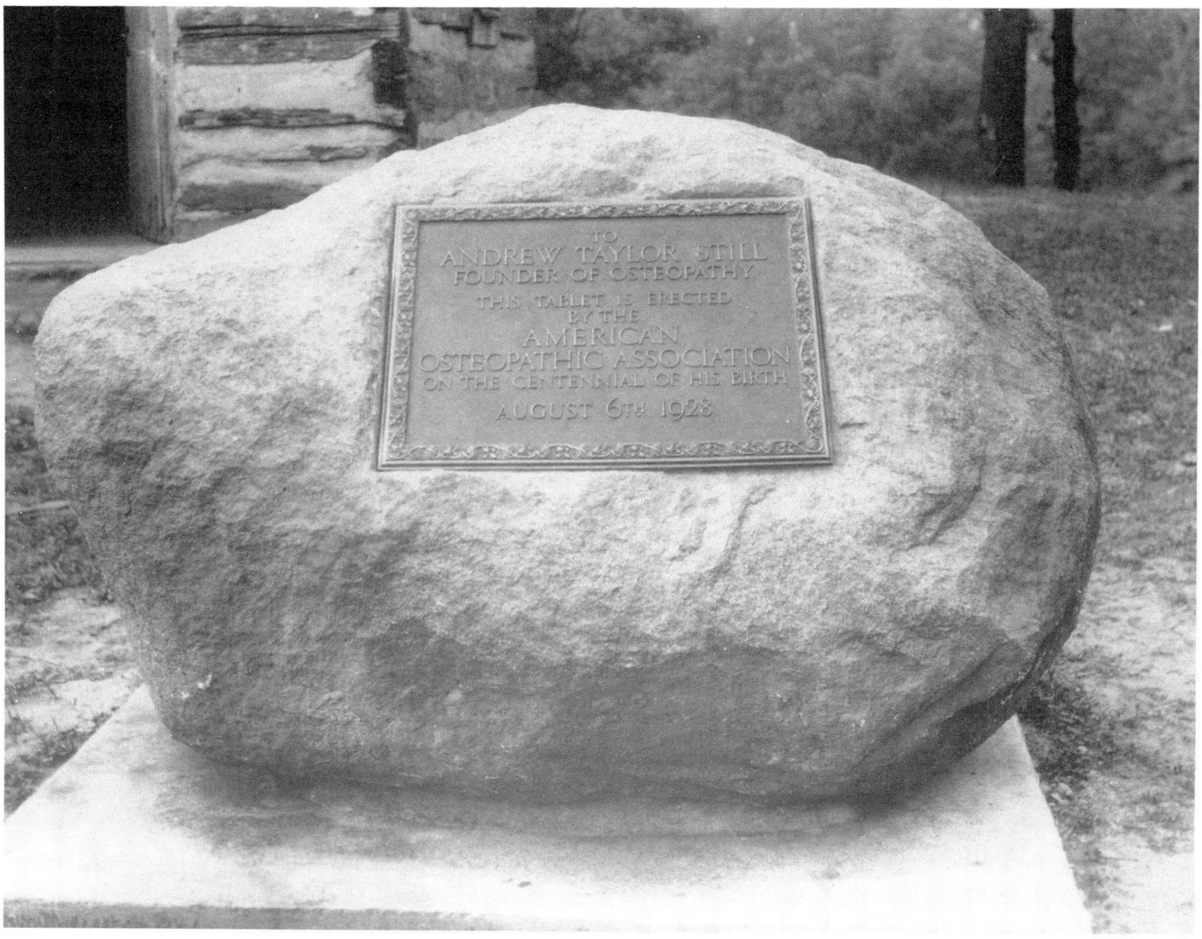

I wish to emphasize this one fact to refute such assertions as this, that Osteopathy has been known and practiced for many thousand years as I teach and practice it. Talk is talk, and I think and pronounce any such assertions without truth or foundation in history. Ignorant men and women may swallow such trash, but I think you will live and die with the knowledge that I am the discoverer of Osteopathy with all its blessings.

I have never seen the man who could suggest or present one principle great or small that could add to the knowledge of Osteopathy I already possessed. I have learned more from the dumb brutes than I have ever been able to obtain from man, as the beast comes nearer to nature's laws, on which the principles of Osteopathy stand.

With many men their first suggestion is that we can make a "mint of money." Such persons I always part from without shedding a tear. And say to them, "if that is your only object you must git."

I have caused to be taught in this school all the branches that are taught in the most learned medical institutions of the world, for the reason, that I want you to go out of this building well posted and able to enter all engagements, prepared to do your duty and to know your business as Osteopaths; and if you do not succeed all is lost. For the brains of the medical world say that the systems of medicines are bungling failures. I will further say, you will often meet men of limited mental powers who will tell you in their ignorance of the powers of adjustable nature to heal, that they have found out that drugs must be used in many cases. I would advise you to look at their wise heads and international step, and sing that good old song:

Show pity, Lord, O Lord forgive,
Let a repenting rebel live,
Are not thy mercies large and free?
May not a sinner trust in thee?

My crimes are great, but don't surpass
The power and glory of thy grace;
Great God, thy nature hath no bound,
So let thy pardoning love be found.

O wash my soul from every sin,
And make my guilty conscience clean;
Here on my heart the burden lies,
And past offenses pain my eyes.

My lips, with shame, my sins confess,
Against thy law, against thy grace;
Lord, should thy judgments grow severe,
I am condemned, but thou art clear.

Yet save a trembling sinner, Lord,
Whose hopes, still hovering round thy word,
Would light on some sweet promise there,
Some sure support against despair.

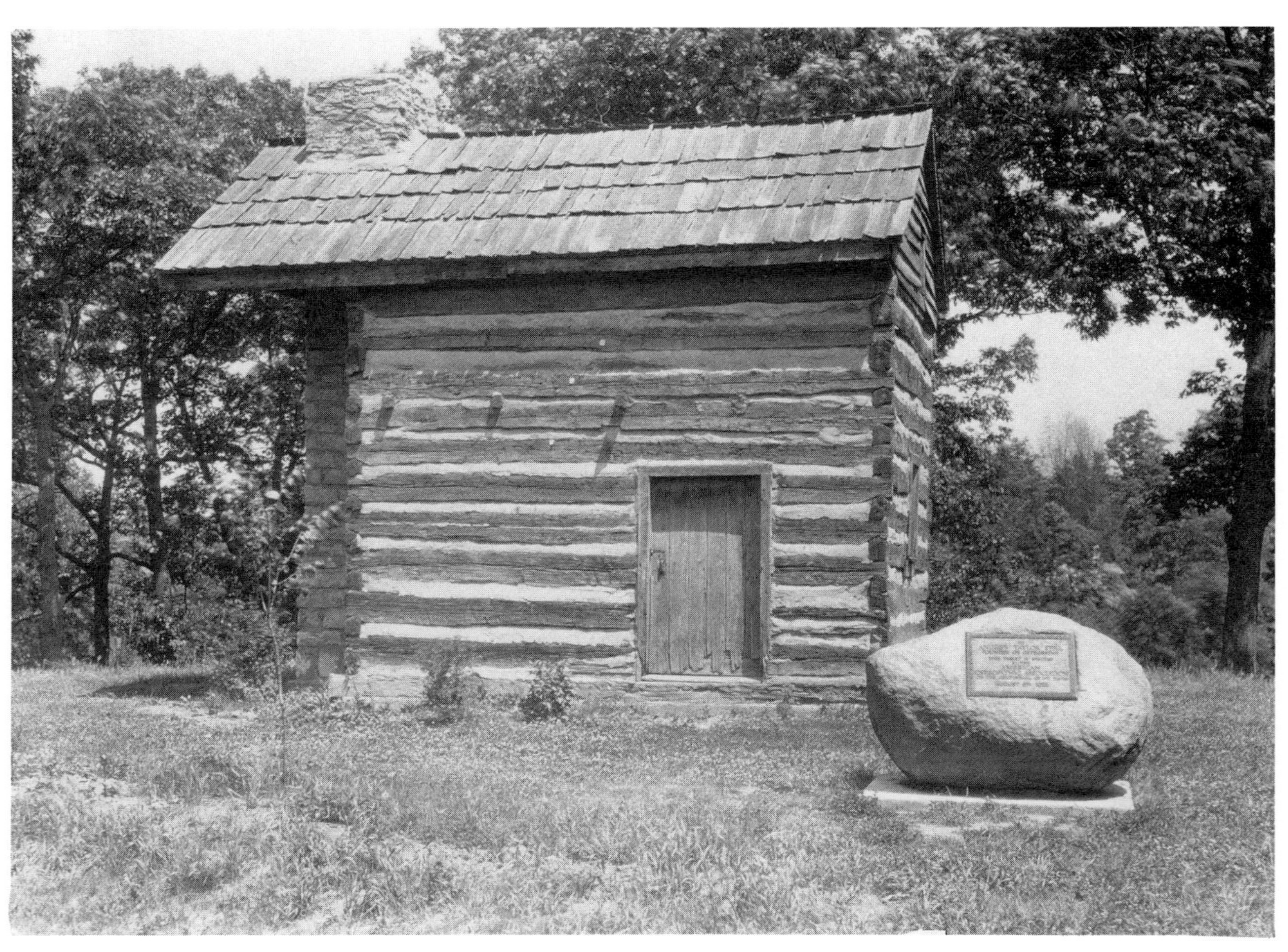

February, 1898

DR. A. T. STILL'S DEPARTMENT.

WHAT IS LIFE?

THE philosopher who first asked that question no one knows. But all intelligent persons are interested in the solution of this problem, at least to know some tangible reason why it is called life. Whether life is personal, or so arranged that it might be called an individualized principle of nature.

I wish to think for a time on this line, because we should make a wise handling of the machinery of the body.

If life in man has been formed to suit the size and duties of the being, if life has a living and separate personage, then we should be governed by such reasons as would give it the greatest chance to go on with its labors in the bodies of man and beast.

We know by experience that a spark of fire will start the principles of powder into motion, which, were it not stimulated by the positive principle of father nature, which finds this ovum lying quietly in the womb of space; would be silently inactive for all ages, without being able to move or help itself, save for the motor principle of life given by the father of all motion.

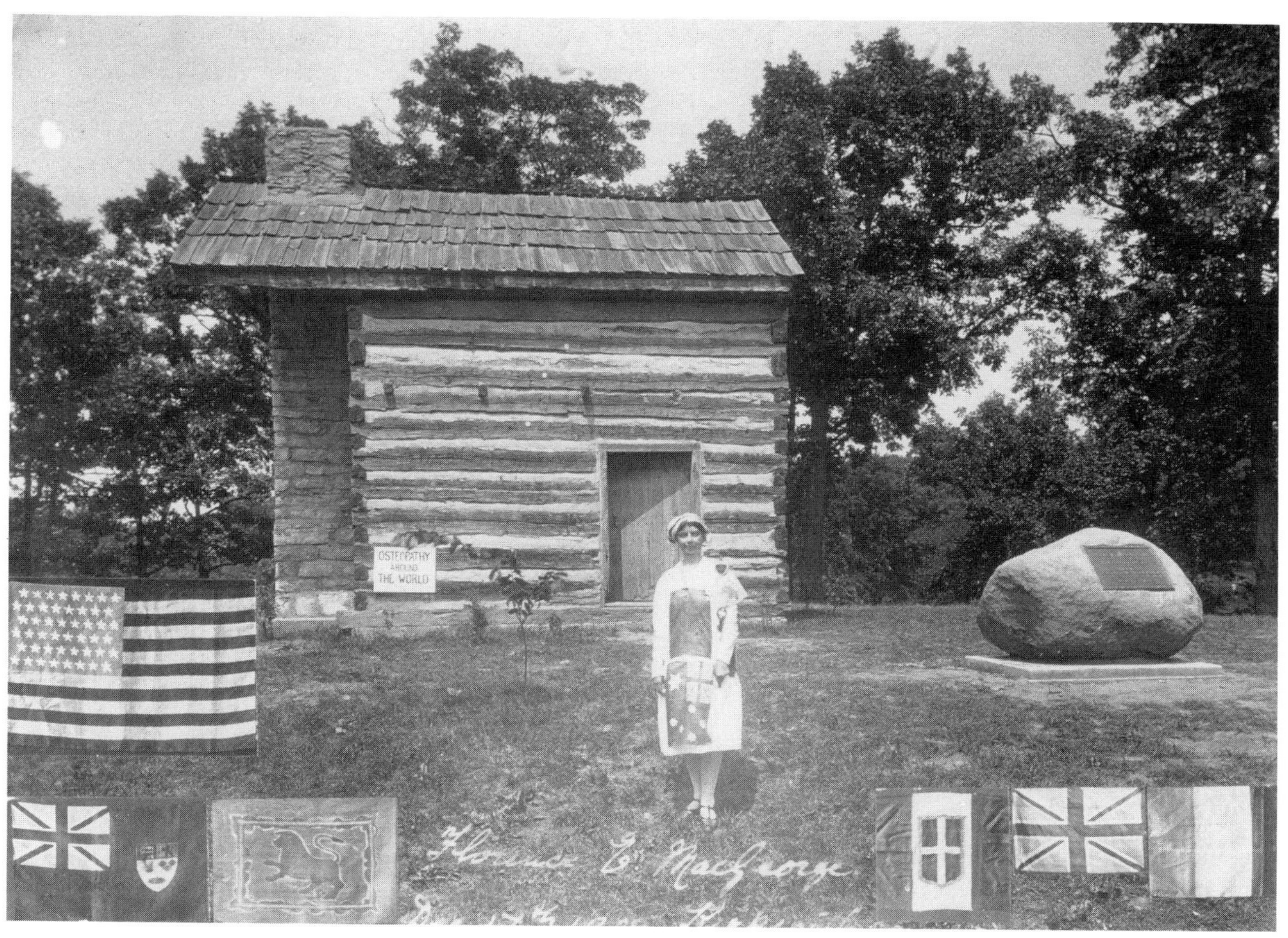

1929 celebration before the "Still" cabin

Right here we could and should ask the question: Is this action produced by electricity put in motion, or is it the active principle that comes as a spiritual man? If so, it is useless to try, or hope to know what life is in the minutia. But we do know that life can only display its natural forces by action of the forms it produces.

If we inspect man as a machine, we find a complete building, a machine that courts inspection and criticism. It demands a full exploration of all its parts with their uses. Then the mind is asked to see or find the connection between the physical and the life laws. By nature you can reason on the roads that the powers of life have arranged to suit its system of motion.

If life is an individualized personage, as we might express that mysterious something, it must have definite arrangements by which it can be united and act with matter.

Then we are admonished to acquaint ourselves with the arrangements of those natural connections, the one or many, as they are connected to all parts of the completed being.

As motion is the first and only evidence of life, by this thought we are conducted to the machinery through which it works to accomplish these results.

If the brain be that division in which force is generated, you must at all hazards acquaint yourself with that structure of this machine; trace the connection from brain to heart, from heart to lungs, and all organs that can be acted upon by the brain, whose duty it may be to construct the fleshy and bony parts of the body. Trace from the brain to the chemical laboratories, and notice their action as they chemically unite and prepare blood and other fluids, that must be used in the economy of this vitalized, self-constructing and self-moving wonder commonly known as man, wherein life and matter have united, and express their friendly relation, one with the other. While this relation exists we have the living man only, which does express and prove the friendly relation that can exist between life and matter, from the lowest living atom, to the greatest worlds. They can only express form and action by this law. Harmony only dwells where obstructions do not exist.

The Osteopath finds here the field in which he will dwell forever. His duties as a philosopher do admonish him, that life and matter can be united; that union cannot continue with any hindrance to free and absolute motion. Therefore, his duty is to keep away from the track all that will hinder the complete passage of the forces of the nervous system, that by that power the blood may be delivered and adjusted, to keep the system in normal condition. This is your duty, do it well, if you wish to succeed.

***

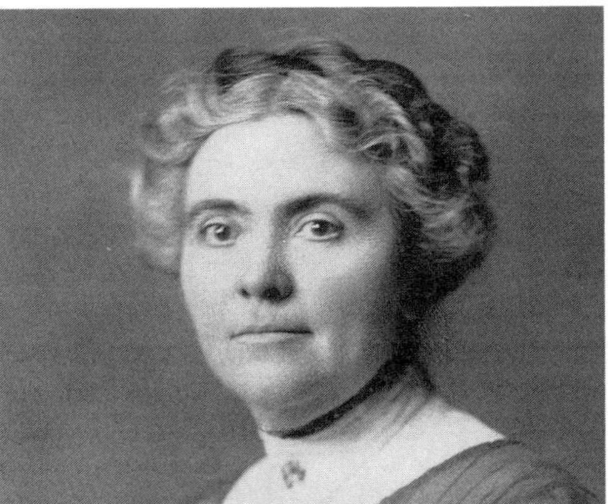

Dr. Jeanette "Nettie" Bolles,
first woman graduate of the ASO

February, 1898

PROVERBS.

WE OFTEN say we love our friends and neighbors as ourselves, and better too. Let us see if we do: We say such "an person" is so good, so kind, so lovably lovable that we want to embrace them, and give them the kiss of brotherly love and charity. We never see them but we feel to sing from our souls, "I want to be an angel." I think all day of the good things he did for me. Never a Christmas passes by but he sends granny and me a nice turkey and dram. "It was so good in him—turkey fat, and whisky just as old as ma. Oh my he is so good."

But as the moon changes often, so does man's love; he says, "I do not feel as I once did, I feel somehow or another that I don't like him quite as well as I did. I try to, but he did not send me the turkey, nor dram neither this year. Oh my, I don't see why he treats us so 'mean,' but I'll get even with him yet. That $300, I borrowed of him to pay the mortgage off our house and team, I didn't give him my note for it, and I will not pay it. He cannot prove he let me have it, so he can't. He called me up in the stable loft and counted it out, and said he didn't want anyone to know he let me have any money at all. You bet no one will know it neither. I won't pay one cent of it, and he knows he cannot make it by law, because my wife has everything in her name.

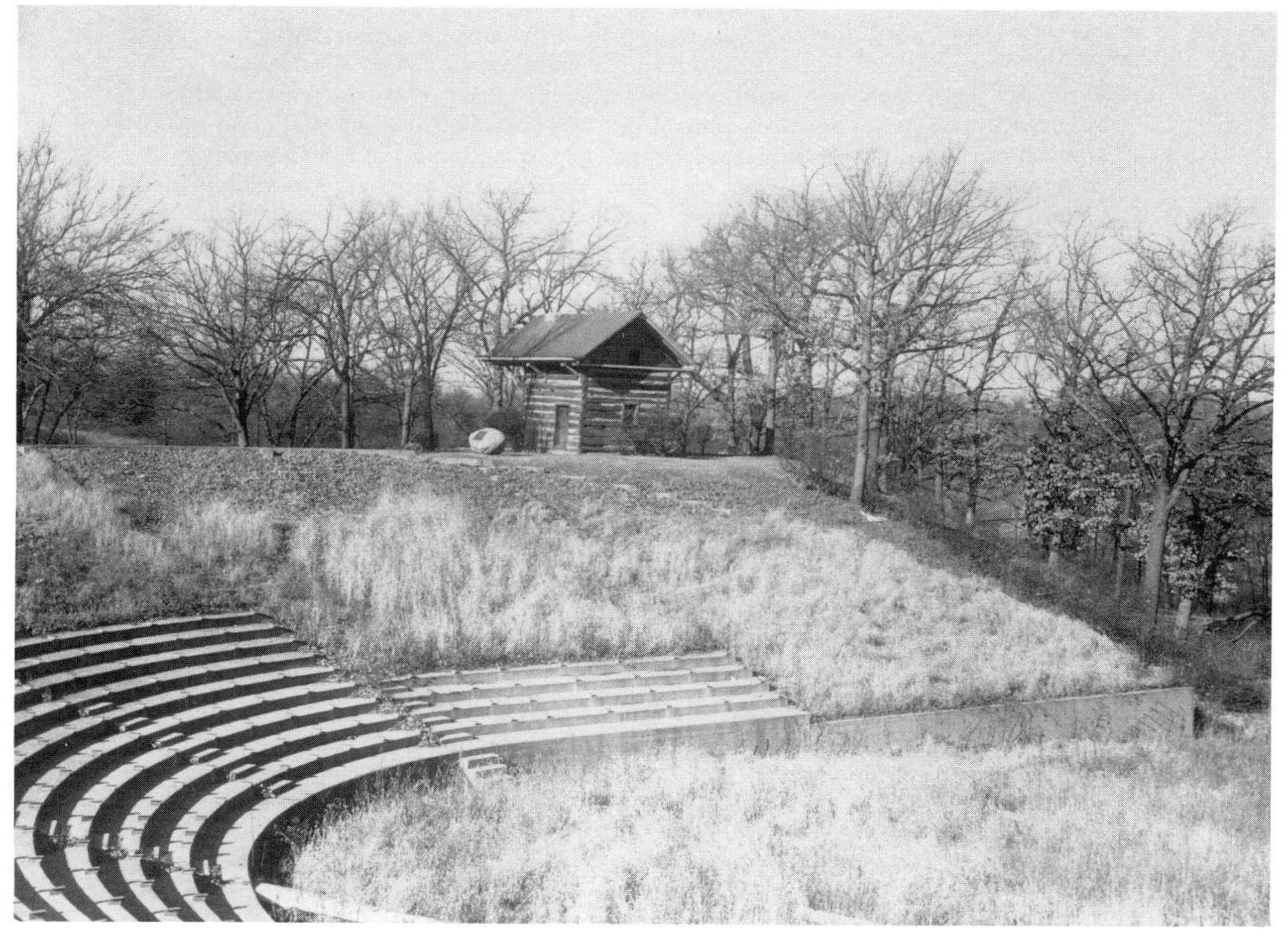

Cabin cited above Laughlin Bowl

"I told you the moon changed often, so do I. I will change love to hatred any time to save $300. I don't care if he did save my house from the sheriff. What if the people do talk, I don't care, I wish I had got $3,000 instead of $300. I don't like him now and I don't care who knows it. He can keep his old turkey and whisky too. I'm going to join the church anyhow, as soon as there is rain enough to fill up the ponds.

"I believe every fellow for himself, is better than all your love your neighbors as thyself's. A man's love is like a rotten egg , it is liable to pop, and will pop, when you pull your sucking bottle out of his mouth. He is a good calf as long as the milk lasts, but Oh my! how he rears and scrapes when the milk is shut off, and he is turned loose in the pastures to hunt grass for himself."

I do not say that all men are deceivers, but I do believe there are enough such lovesick hypocrites in America to whip Spain in two hours, and leave 16,000,000 to go to Klondike.

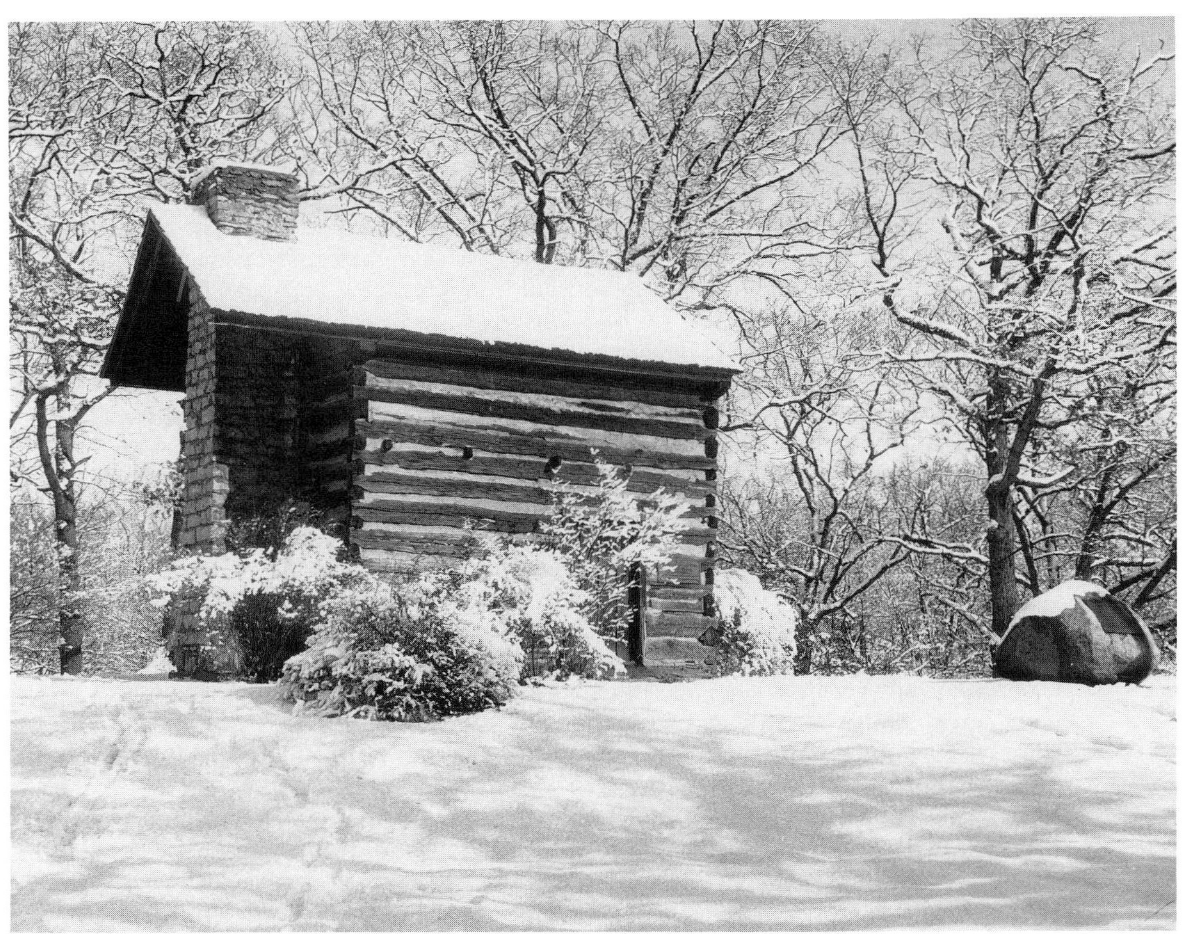

1964 winter scene of cabin behind hospital

Man Was Man.

HOW or when man came on earth no man seems to know. One says he grew to the condition of man by a process of swiftness of head and foot; that on the race ground he beat all monkeys, apes, jack-rabbits, toads, geese and cattle, and won the belt of beauty and wisdom, and that all beasts had the same chance that he had.

Another story is, that he was made of dust; that may be so, but if true he had a dirty start, and perhaps that is why he is doing dirty tricks.

Another class of reasoners say proof is quite plenty, that his form has not changed in the least in four to ten thousand years, and they think he was the same then as now in form, force and reason, and he was so wisely made and supplied with mentality and all other qualities, by a wise mechanic, and when he was turned loose as a finished job, he could not grow out of his first shape, neither could other beings such as birds and beasts, change forms nor minds. That the germ of life was the plan and specification to begin and finish man, birds, fishes, and beasts, by the powers and wisdom given in the germ, that the original or "first" man was a germ of life from his father who was prior to him ad infinitum. His God is credited with perfection in all the skilled arts, before he, it, or nature began to make man, beasts, or worlds. Perfection was known by that law to mean, that nothing was to be omitted in the work, and when finished it was above criticism from start to finish, in all parts; for a completed being could be found in that body, and all could and would be as designed by that power that makes all his machinery work without jar or friction.

Who or what made man is a question of but little difference to us. But we have a question that has a useful place in all minds, which is this: When he is sick, how and what to do to his machinery to make it do the work of grinding out ease and health? To know what part has failed to do its work, and is the cause of this weakening of force, supply, and renovation, and allowed deposits to accumulate and strain or destroy the effective workings of parts or the whole person. What we want to know is something that is useful to us. Whether we sprang from monkeys or buzzards does not help us as much as to know how to quit getting drunk every time we take cold; how to get sober doctors into our families who know enough of man's form and disease, to stop fever and pain without drunken poisons, or anything in the shape of drugs.

Man will continue to load his stomach with such trash when he is sick until the doctor gets such trash out of his head. We must remember that men who labor for body and soul, do not have the time to study his form, and its power to drive blood in search of impurities, which accumulate previous to the beginning of disease. How many families have a boy or girl who can tell the names of the bones in the lower limbs? How many bones in the foot? How many more bones in the right foot than are in the left? And which side of Eve the rib was taken from to make Adam? Whether his liver looks like a bucksaw or an owl? And which leg the liver is in? and so on and so forth.

If your heads were as sharp as the toes of your shoes, I would not talk so loud, but we have to yell at deaf people.

⁂

Wonders.

WONDERS are daily callers, and seem to be greatly on the increase during the nineteenth century. As we read history we learn that no one hundred years of the past has produced wonders in such number and variety, as this the nineteenth. Stupid systems of government have given place to better. Voyages on the ocean have had months by sail reduced to days by steam. Journeys overland that would require six months by horse and ox, are now accomplished in six days by steam and rail. Our law, medical and other schools of five and seven years, are now but two or three, and the graduates of such schools are far superior in useful knowledge to those of the five and seven. And no wonder at that, for the facilities for giving the pupil knowledge are so far improved that the knowledge sought can be obtained in less time. Our schools are not intended to use the greatest number of days that are allotted to man. But at this day, schooling and learning mean, to obtain knowledge in the quickest way that a thoroughness can be obtained.

If there is any method by which Ray's third part arithmetic can be taught so as to master it in thirty days instead of thirty months, let us have it. We want knowledge. We are willing to pay for it. We want all we pay for, and we want our heads kept out of the sausage mill of time-wasting.

A great question now stands before us. What are the possibilities of mind to improve our methods of gaining knowledge, shorten time, and getting greater and better results? I am free to say the question is too momentous to form an answer, as each day brings to us a new wonder, from some man or woman who reasons on cause and gives demonstrations of effect.

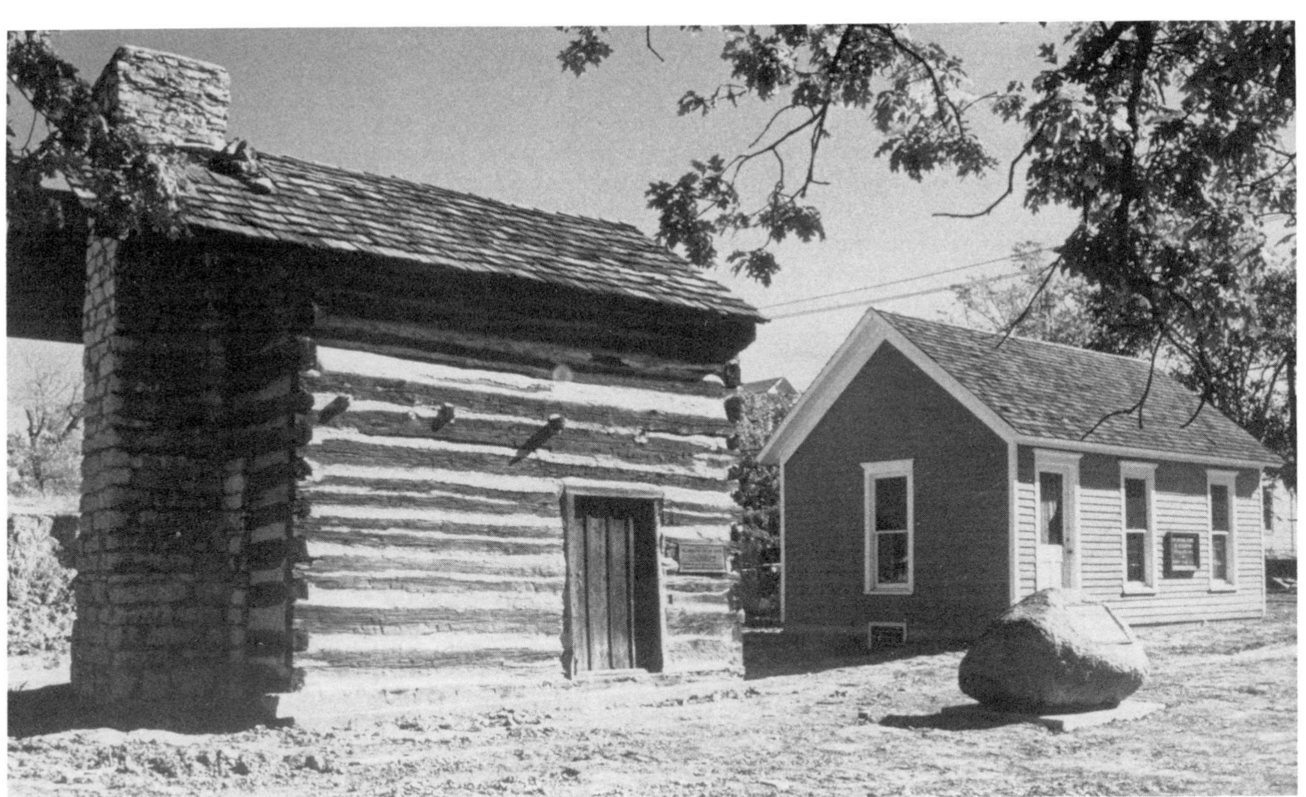

Cabin and First School in current location

Ladies as Students and Graduates.

I HAVE always advocated that a woman had as much sense as a man, or she would not have been called his help-meet and companion. A question: What man wants to spend his days with a woman fool? I think she is in as much danger of spending her days with a fool as he is.

I opened wide the doors of my first school for ladies. Another and a much greater reason I will offer and emphasize. Why not elevate our sister's mentality, qualify her to fill all places of trust and honor, place her hand and head with the skilled arts? I know no reason why she should not study anatomy, physiology, chemistry and all the machinery and laws of life.

I believed at that time she could, and at the end of five years trial I know she can; for she has proven herself to be equal to man in all places of mental skill.

Another reason, she has wisdom to offer her sex, in place of the gossip of the day. A mental revolution is wanted, a better race is needed. A scandal-vending mother gives birth to a son who will be the blackguard. A child is surely what it is made by pre-natal causes. Get something in the mother's head besides idle gossip, then when the child's brain is forming from her blood you may hope for a bright child, youth and man.

I will say by way of encouragement that all ladies who have graduated from this school and gone out in the world, have done well financially, and are made the guests of the best society of the land. They are received and honored as ladies, and well paid for their skill. Places are open and ready for all that have a diploma from this school. And for the first time I will say, come on and qualify yourselves to take your places of usefulness. Do your part well, and a feast awaits you.

***

The Mind a Gem.

WHY should a man not be proud, when he knows his head contains that of which he is not worthy? Shall we call it a gem, whose brilliancy cannot be covered by the darkest veil ever woven by the genius of adversity? Does he not know that his mind is far above all the beautiful gems worn and displayed upon the hands, breast, belt or any apparel of kings, queens and the honored of all nations? Does he not feel and know, that he is the possessor of a gem, the genius of reason, cut by the lapidarist of thought and adjusted to suit his person, by the skilled hands of the knowing artist who knows how and what to cut? Does he not know that the possession of this great gem when worn, is the insignia of nobility?

One exploring thought is bound to make the discovery, and bring home to the mind the glad tidings, that you and I do possess a treasure, whose beauties no poet can describe. In its display of colors the red-light of hope, joy and prosperity, are hanging upon every limb of the tree of life, whose foliage reaches to the very paradise of God.

Have you not great reason to rejoice that by this mental gift you may fathom the mystery of this, and other lives.

Think of that ever productive tree of thought, loaded down with the cocoanuts of joy; whose milk feeds to fulness the stomach that energizes, and gladdens our hearts with the twilight of the rising sun of prosperity, which illuminates and sweetens our days.

Mothers, what is that which makes your hearts rejoice? Is it not a ray of light coming from the brilliant blazes of thought that prompts your soul to leap with joy, when your children stand around you, whose minds are the choicest gems, receiving and transposing light, with all its beauties tinted with the seven colors of reason, whose variations and cautious blendings make to our eyes all that is beautiful? It is those beauties seen in and on your children that cause the inexpressible heavings of your heart to burst forth from a mother's soul, while she sees the beautiful lights of the action of mind and intelligence. Haven't you reason to be proud beyond the power of language to express? To feel and know that the mind above all other gems is to be the most admired.

February, 1898

DR. A. T. STILL ANSWERS QUESTIONS.

A WORD from me to men and women who wish to have a profession by which they can make an honorable living for themselves and those dependent upon them : I will say, if Osteopathy is your choice, I think you will become, as all those who have taken diplomas from this school, proud of the day when they entered the mother institution of Osteopathy. No money could cause them to lay down their diplomas which are from headquarters, and will be honored wherever they go, whether far or near. I can further say that all Diplomates who have bidden adieu to their alma mater—both ladies and gentlemen—report universal satisfaction. Many are far away in different parts of the world. All write that they have never lost a victory ; that they are kindly received wherever they go. They are proud of a diploma from headquarters which they earned by hard study. To them it is a token of approved merit. I would say : Keep your sons and daughters at home if they have to be coaxed. We have never put a solicitor in the field. Our school must stand or fall by its merits, is our motto. You can make money, and make it reasonably fast, by sober industry, because when people find that you are much better posted in anatomy, physiology, and diseases, than are the ordinary doctors, and cure many diseases that they cannot, or even relieve, you will generally get a large practice, which will pay you well, because you can give the relief they want. They will pay you thankfully, and send you more patients. A list of over fifty ladies are now in the classes, and they would be a credit to any school.

Another word to young ladies of mind and ambition, who wish to make a living and be independent. Many thousand young women annually go to great expense to get a musical education. When completed they try to do something in that line. They find the world is overstocked with music teachers and give up disappointed and disgusted. I will say no such trouble has ever met a lady Diplomate of the American School of Osteopathy. Everyone has sent love and thanks, that I had advised them to study Osteopathy; that a diploma from this school will hold soul and body of any lady who possessed it, above want or trouble, and make her free and independent.

CHANCES TO GET WORK.

The world is now ready for Osteopathy. Ten thousand good places are now demanding something to take the place of the deadly drug, that gives no proof of its ability to cure the sick. Their prayers are earnest. They want Osteopathy badly. If you should choose Osteopathy I have no doubt you will be pleased with your choice. We can teach it with all that belongs to it, because we are fully qualified by the very best talent and facilities the world can afford.

I would advise all persons to come and spend a few days; visit all the classes, talk with the students and professors, patients and graduates, and judge for yourselves, then enter the classes if you are fully satisfied that this is the place of your choice.

March, 1898

DR. A. T. STILL'S DEPARTMENT.

AN ADDRESS BY THE PRESIDENT TO THE GRADUATING CLASS OF THE AMERICAN SCHOOL OF OSTEOPATHY FEB. 1st 1898.

BEFORE handing to you your diplomas, which you have earned by faithful and hard study, having passed satisfactory examinations in all branches:—It has been ordered by the trustees of the A. S. O. who have been constituted and legally authorized by the state of Missouri to issue certificates of qualification to all who shall have passed such examination. Such certificates are usually called diplomas. That you may the better understand what is meant by diploma I will give the definition of the word as given by the revised Encyclopedia dictionary by Hunter and Morris, English and American:

"Diploma: A writing or document conferring some power, authority, privilege, or honor, usually under seal and signed by a duly authorized official. Diplomas are given to graduates of a university on their taking their degrees; to clergymen who are licensed to officiate; to physicians, civil engineers, etc., authorizing them to practice their profession."

All diplomas have local and significant values. Local because they cannot extend beyond the jurisdiction of the grantor. Instance: A diploma granted in the state of Missouri has no power to go beyond the boundary of said state. But by courtesy and the rules of reciprocity a diploma issued in the state of Missouri may be respected in the State of Illinois and other states of this Union. A commission or diploma issued by the U. S. government is only good within its jurisdiction.

As each state has its individual statutes by which it is governed and you are receiving a diploma from the state of Missouri, after conforming to the laws of other states you will be permitted to practice, in such states that do not have prohibitory laws. A number of states do not have any statute law that would bar the practice of Osteopathy; also four states by legislative act have legalized Osteopathy within their limits, Missouri from whom you receive this document being among the number. I have the honor at this time to hand to you your diplomas, on whose face appear the names of the Professors of the American School of Osteopathy.

By many who are ignorant and jealous of this system you will be advised that you should attend some medical college for the purpose of learning the use of drugs. When such advice is given, remember you have passed a rigid examination in all branches taught in medical colleges, as is shown on the face of your diplomas. No doubt your qualifications have made you competent to teach 75 per cent of all such persons for twelve months. I would advise you to examine them and if you find them professional blanks close the conversation and pass on.

Osteopathy has no use for drugs as remedies, but a great use for chemistry when dealing with poisons and antidotes. It recognizes and has a useful place for surgery in both of which you have been well informed.

I will now draw your attention to the significant value of the diploma. If you have any power of reason you must know, and I will say you do know, that only by comparison can we arrive at an absolute knowledge of the difference in value of all things.

In speaking of the significant value and the comparative difference and moral force existing between two diplomas, one from a long and well established institution of learning that has the wealth to furnish all things necessary to a finished education, which school has been very careful in selecting experienced persons to fill the chairs in all departments, and the graduates who have completed their full course in all the branches necessary to that profession, be it law, medicine, sculpture, or any of the skilled arts, and whose graduates have gone forth into the world and proven by their work that such school or schools had the ability to give the necessary and useful information. Now in order to compare we will take a diploma from a school whose character has not been established, would you not arrive at the conclusion by comparison that there was a difference in the significant value between the two documents.

With due respect for all others we will take one from the world renowned medical university of Edinburgh Scotland, whose thoroughness in all branches, is today established beyond doubt or inquiry. Would'nt your judgment say, give me my diploma from an old established institution.

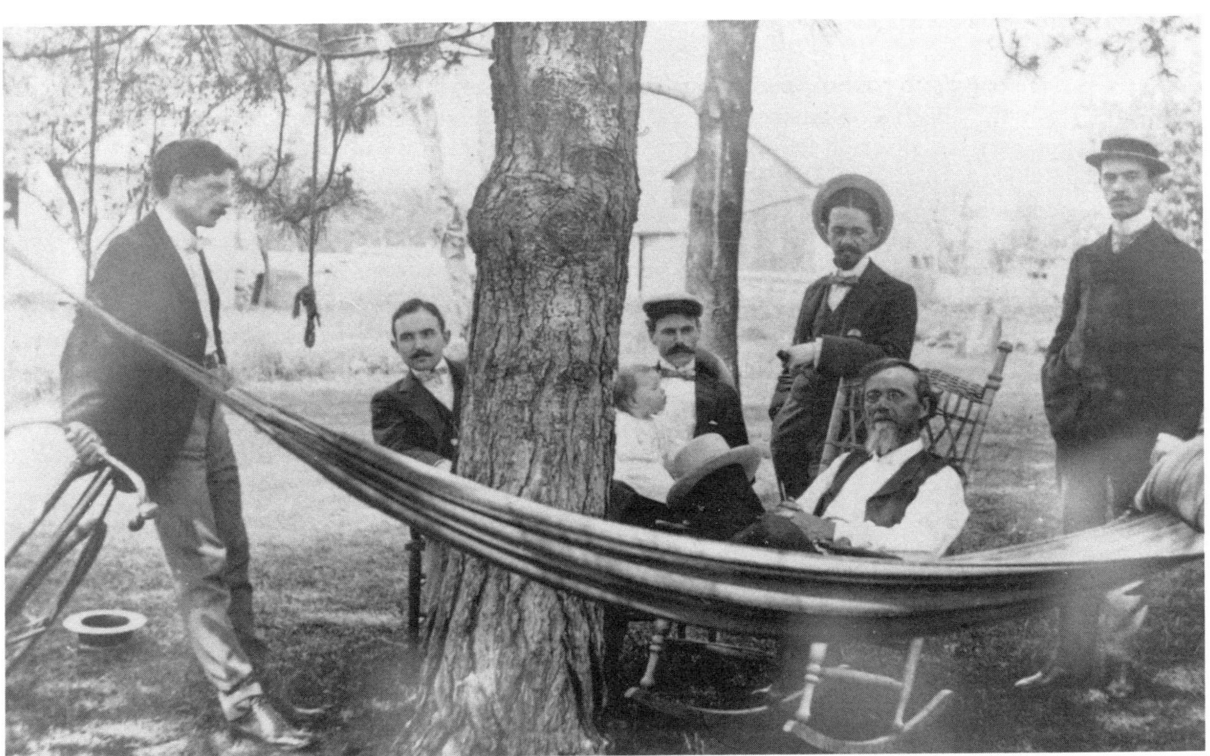

A. T. Still relaxing with students 1897

This comparison has been between old and established medical institutions for the purpose of bringing before your minds a foundation upon which you can decide whether you want established merit or prospective merit. As the American School of Osteopathy is the oldest and best prepared to teach the principles of Osteopathy, I believe that your diplomas will best sustain you in any part of the world. Because it has been as carefully guarded as any mother has ever guarded and cared for her children, morally, intellectually and justly, for one purpose only, which was to unfold the principles whereby life and health could be sustained by natural law, which requires no assistance but rest and nourishment, when all parts of the human system are in their natural positions.

On this foundation Osteopathy has stood for twenty years, and successfully combatted diseases of all kinds, without the aid of drugs. To the intellectually strong: the principles of Osteopathy will crown you with success, provided you adhere to them, while the wavering man will fall by the way-side.

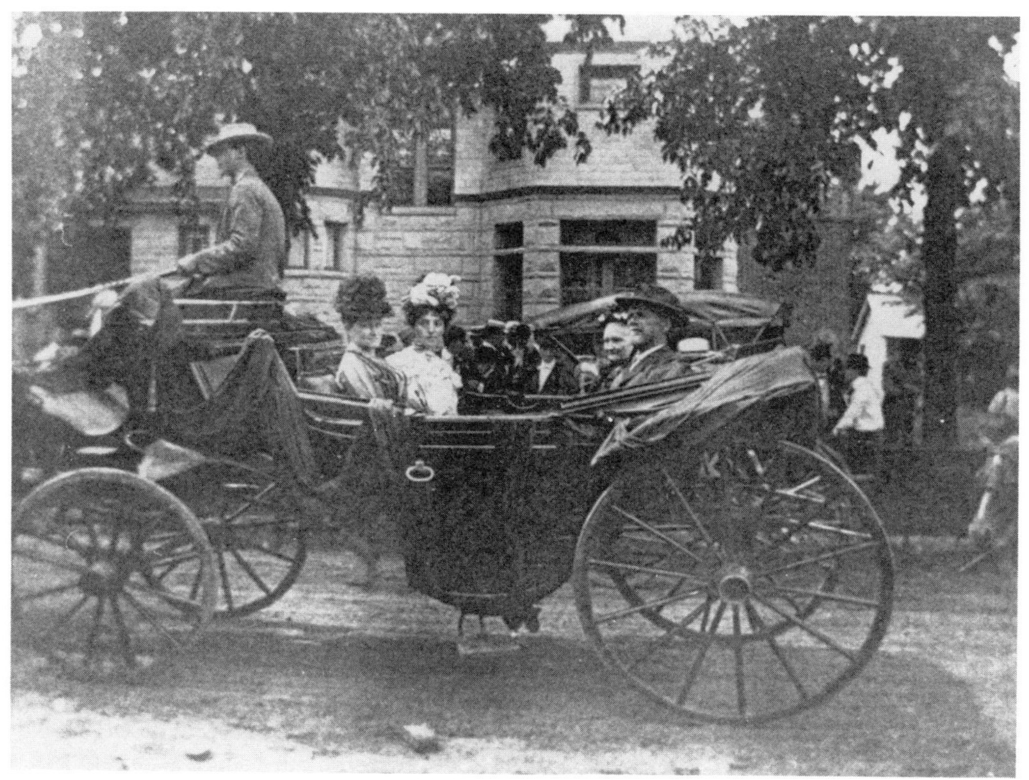

A. T. Still and Mary pass before the Baird house, c. 1890.

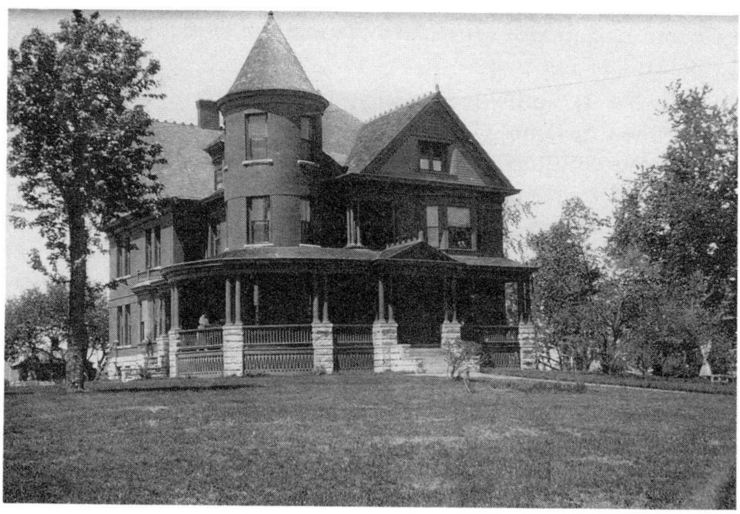

The Still home at the turn of the century

OUT ON THE OCEAN.

I SUPPOSE all who have passed, by hard study, to the degree of Diplomate of Osteopathy, feel they have learned all "pap" knows and more too. But as I am "old and childish" I can talk and tell the children funny stories for their amusement. I wont lie if I do talk. I will say I was very poor when I stepped on the iron clad battle ship for a voyage on the seas of stern realities. My wealth was ten dollars which was the full measure of all my financial credit. I could borrow no more. I was poorly clad and had but one friend who would stand by me, and that was my mother's grit that was in my blood which considered to back down was a shame and disgrace. I used the tactics of experience, economy, truth and industry. I studied all cases that came to be treated, I broke the bones so I could get the marrow to eat. I needed mental strength. No diet ever helped me but the marrow of mental perserverance. Many bones were hard to break, but I found good fat marrow every time. As I ate I grew stronger in my mental powers.

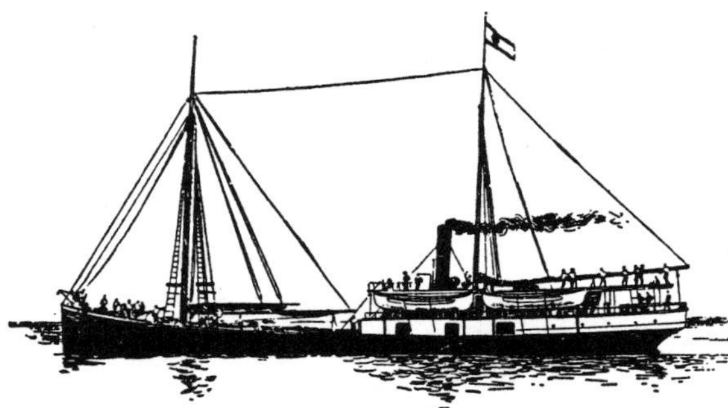

Now my little girls and boys, I never saw the sun shine twenty-four hours at a time. I have seen it rise nice and clear, and long before night of the same day, I have seen cyclones of wind, fire, hail and rain, ruin crops of great promise, and the wealthy man who ate his dinner in joy and hope, also ate his supper in poverty and despair.

Of course you never will be ruined by hailstones nor human leeches, because you know what button to touch to make storms burst far away from you and kill the rascals before they confidence your pocket and head. You never will be toyed around by business men who never did any business, but run business schemes and rob honest men of their earnings.

Haven't we learned in two years that "Pap" is a business fool? Why he could be rich, but he has no business git to him. Just give us an open field to plan and fight business battles and you will see what muscle can do. He says drones hover around honey and eat but do not make any. I did'nt know what he meant by drones, I supposed it was to walk home if we failed. I'll never do that; I will take my bicycle with me. I'm no drone if that is what he meant.

I asked Pap what he meant by drones, leeches and such words. He said it was your neighbor's calf sucking my cow. Why I have'nt got a cow to suck: it can't be that. Go again and tell him to make it plain so we can understand what he means. Well, this is jist what he said, go off and 'larn' as I did.

Good-bye, little boys.

PAP.

March, 1898

My Observations In Lung Diseases.

AS VOLUMES have been written during all the centuries of the great past on lung diseases each pen has generally been directed to irritation, coughs and waste of lungs. We learn from these writers very little if anything at all. Little is said of cause, but much of effect. They tell us all about symptoms, and substances coughed from the lungs; tell when and how it started; tell us that ulcers and abscesses go with consumption; tell us there are tubercles in the lungs, and others will form, and in time bleeding will often accompany or follow a hard spell of coughing; that pus is often found in the urine, lymphatics and blood.

By the microscope we compare and see a great difference in the appearance of the consumpted lung, and the healthy one. We see effect, talk of effect, treat effect, and our researches stop when we conclude in council, that the child is as its father or mother was before death, who had a cough and died as their parents had before them. Thus we decide we have a case of hereditary consumption. This is their opinion and assertion. But they have failed to prove by any fact that consumption is hereditary, that a child was ever born with consumption or the seeds of tuberculosis in its blood or body.

With all this array of assumed wisdom we learn nothing of cause. And the writers have never seen nor said anything except on effect, if we are to judge by their writings. The thought of hunting for cause had never entered their minds, neither has the gravity of the subject. If we judge them by their actions, they felt that to go beyond effect would be criminal, and their searchlight of farther investigation ceases to shine.

Thus all hope is removed from thesufferer when he is told by the symptomatologist that he has heriditary consumption.

I think it is a very serious matter to read the death sentence to a human being from the bench of stale habit, and by the judge who rises with dignity and says to the person, guilty or not guilty you must die. Such judges are stationed in every city, town and village all over the world.

I know this to be true. You also know this to be a correct statement. Having spent the entire one-fourth of a century to acquaint myself with the human system, and the lungs in particular, by anatomical, physiological, experimental and practical knowledge, in working with the human body in its wisely constructed machinery, with its battery of force, its engine of supply, its chemical laboratory, its nutrient provision, its power of renovation and purification, a machine of such high perfection, that the spirit of life can joyfully dwell therein, I began to reason thus: that as so much wisdom had been displayed in the construction of man with all parts and principles blending in harmony, surely the power and quality must exist to dissolve and expel all tardy and improper accumulations from all parts, and keep and maintain it in such condition during natural life.

With this thought in view I began the search for a better knowledge of the exact reasons why one should begin with a cold and cough himself to death, which cough in many cases had lasted for a great number of years.

I believed that God was right, and had made the machine in the highest order of perfection. In this view I examined the greater and lesser nerves of nutrition, motion and sensation. I separated the nerves by division. I blended by association all nerves of the whole body to ascertain if by union there was not strength, which could be concentrated on any part of the system for the relief of the brain, heart, liver, stomach, bowels, or any branch or division of the body.

I found that nature had provided all things necessary to sustain animal life, modify temperature and remove disease. I found but one trouble and that was to know the cause and treat the case accordingly. To me the cause of the disease known as consumption was absolutely plain, and easily comprehended. I have been experimenting with good results. No bad effects have followed.

I expect to keep up the investigation for an indefinite time. The whys and hows I get those results I shall not publish nor communicate until a later date. I want to extend my experimenting through the four seasons of one more year, in order to make as scientific and truthful a report as possible, as a successful experimenter, with that dread disease consumption, which I believe has very little right to take and keep possession of the lungs, the cause of which I think is plainly indicated.

I believe the time is short, and very short, when consumption will cease to be the most dreaded disease of the human family. As I have solved the question and removed the dread of measles, mumps, whooping cough, scarlet fever, diptheria, flux and many other diseases I feel assured that the road is open, the journey easy, and the victory mine by the tenets of Osteopathy.

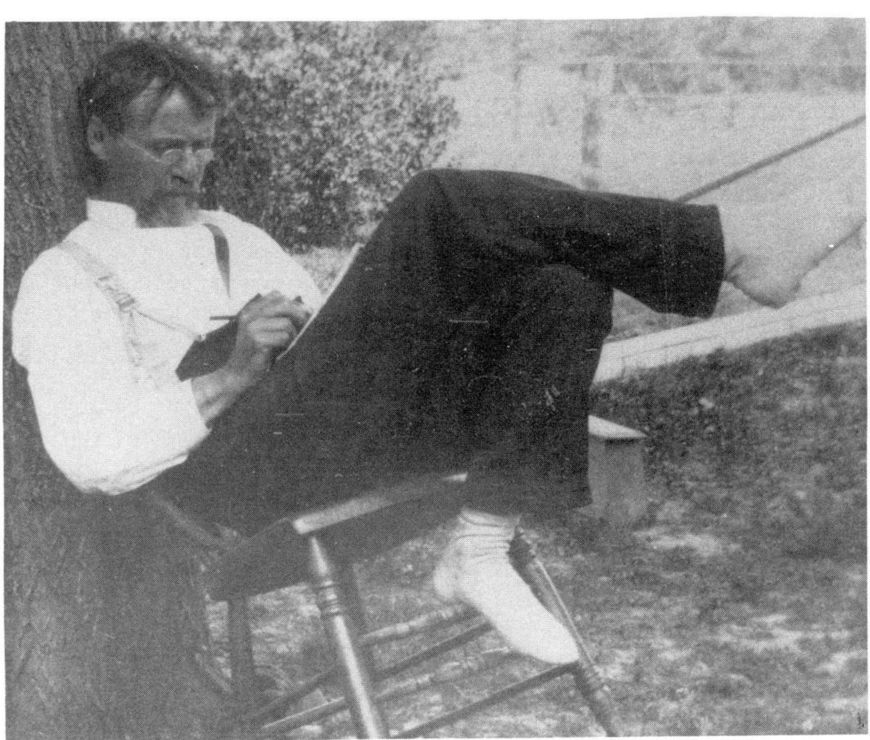

A. T. Still writing his autobiography at the Sol Morris farm in Millard

April, 1898

TEXT BOOKS.

WHAT is a text book? For an Osteopath, or any person engaged in the study of the art of healing the afflicted. I have but one answer. To heal the human body of any affliction, one must have a complete knowledge of the body. Gray's Descriptive Anatomy, as well as all other similar works by eminent and competent authors on the subject, are in my opinion the greatest text books that any student or operator can have with him, as a safe guide to produce the results desired when combatting diseases. It guides him first to the frame work, by its teachings of the bony structure, its attachments of bone to bone, with ligaments described and illustrated;—muscles, blood supply, where from and where to—nerve supply, with its connections to the brain, and each and all auxilliary systems necessary to circulation. It gives their forms and uses for the student and operator to reason from, and conduct his thought by physiology, histology, and chemistry, that he may see and comprehend all of the parts and principles in the great machinery and labratory of nature, when all this is fully understood he is ready to enter the rooms of the clinics, and receive instruction on the principles and philosophy of Osteopathy. When he has completed his education in this manner, he is ready to say by knowledge that anatomy, physiology and chemistry are all the text books he wants and needs. I consider the above the most perfect text books that can be given to man, and the Osteopath who spends two years in the American School of Osteopathy, and has not made this discovery has not, in my judgment, improved his opportunity. Remember that these utterances are facts.

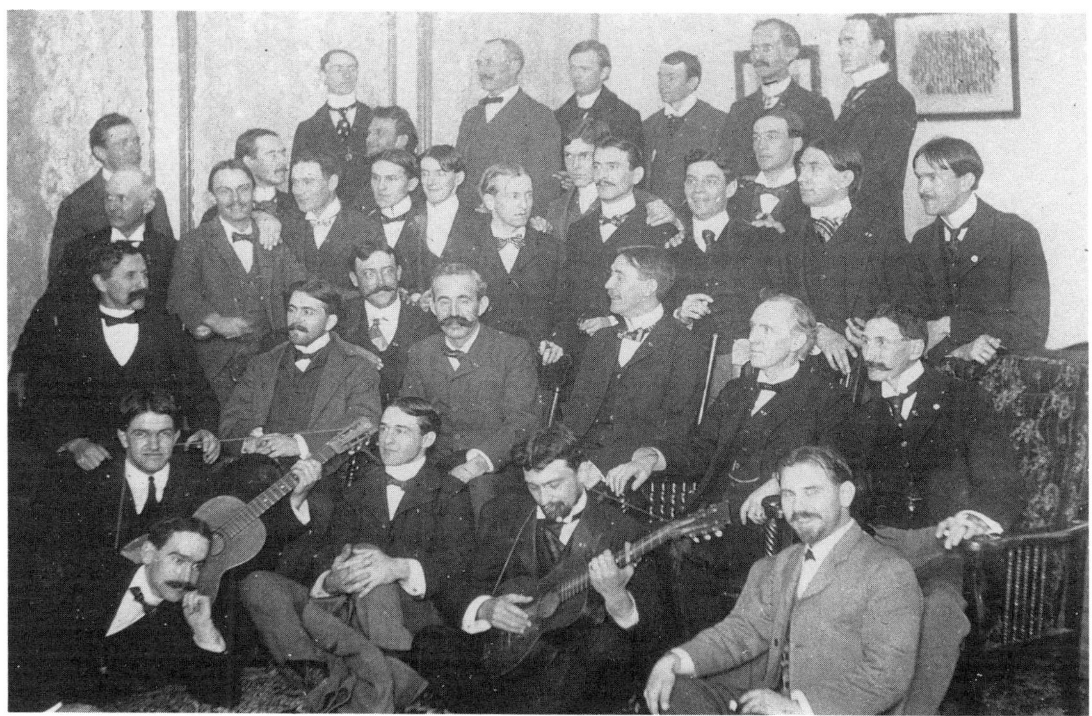

First Osteopathic Fraternity, The Atlas Club established 1898, photo from 1899.

DR. A. T. STILL'S DEPARTMENT.

Chew, Swallow and Digest.

But few persons ever give a thought to the laws of nutrition. We chew, swallow and digest. Some substances are so hard to separate that it takes all the powers of the great muscles of the under jaw to push the teeth through them. Then the labor begins in earnest on that chunk of beef or half cooked old turkey gobler's breast, that has been embalmed with spice, sage and pepper sufficiently to keep a thousand years. After long chewing, twisting and failures, we often have to take the bite in our fingers and pull it to pieces to get it small enough to swallow, for we know we risk our lives if we try to swallow it as it is. Thousands have choked to death in this way, and to avoid that danger we put the muscles of the jaw to a great strain.

I want to set you to thinking just a little, for it is your bodies I wish to save from an untimely, or the imprudent man's early grave.

I will speak first of the labors of chewing and swallowing. Each process differs from the other. Chewing first, swallowing next, and digestion last. Digestion never starts its work until the other two have finished the work of mastication and swallowing. Three sets of nerves have to take active part before nutrition has reached the climax of physical perfection.

In reducing substances to fluids, qualified when passed through the thoracic duct to the lungs by qualification to a higher process or otherwise; to be forwarded from there into the heart, which will send the blood by its force to the brain and other departments of the body, to receive such elements by addition as would qualify the blood for its various uses through all divisions of the body.

If the reader will stop and reason for a few moments can he not see that chewing, swallowing and digestion are separate and active principles, which cannot all act at once. Therefore when the nerves of mastication are in motion the process of digestion must be suspended. Right here we are forced to conclude, that when digestion becomes active chewing and swalloiwng must be inactive during that process, and the sooner their duty is completed, reason would teach us digestion would commence its work at an earlier date. Knowing this to be a natural truth that no two of the three forces above described can work at the same time; would it not be the best philosophy in this day of electric speed to hurry the process of mastication and swallowing through their labors, that they may stop in order that the chemical process of digestion should have an undisturbed opportunity, to accomplish that great and most wonderful feat of nature, which is to change dead substances to living matter?

Persons who have not studied the physical laws of life, innocently or ignorantly crucify the chances for physical and mental comfort, which can be seen, felt and comprehended only by an intelligent man or woman, when by accident or otherwise they are invited to partake of, and go through the military drill of the six o'clock dinners, which are considered very limited in display when the changes are less than seven, very moderate at ten, and fairly filled at thirteen. This process of animal torture with suspended digestion, ligate pressure of abdominal aorta, vena cava, renal, pelvic and all nerve centers of sacrum suspended by pressure of the loading of the foolish and indigestible compounds, that have been forced into the stomach by the most idiotic stupidity of the present age.

An intelligent observer, and not much intelligence is required, provided he understands some of the laws of anatomy and physiology to see and know that the cause of so much apoplexy, paralysis of one or both sides, gout, heart disease, Bright's disease, appendicitis, piles, shaking palsy, bald heads, and insanity both periodic and continued, all have their origin in some big dinner.

One would say it is such a pleasant place to talk, but with all these facts before us I would say, less talk, more sense and better health.

At this time allow me to ask a few pointed questions. What do you suppose a Kentuckian would do with his servant if he should treat his fox hounds as you have treated your stomach? He would give him a raw-hiding, then have him hitch up a four horse team, send him to Tennessee with a draft and order for a wagon load of dogs. When the darkey returns with the dogs his master gives him another whipping and says, the next time you feed my dogs to death I will hang you.

"Massa will you please tell me, can a pusson feed a dog to death?"

Much is said about the pleasures at the table, I will admit there is much pleasure at the table while eating, but more can be found in the parlor, for this reason; the circulation if the blood is pressed and stopped extensively by the pressure of an overloaded stomach; every nerve, vein and artery is being pressed to misery. Why not get up and take the weight off the abdominal aorta, vena cava and all the systems that must have room to act to let digestion get to work before the food rots in you? You have forced the blood to the brain by taking up all space to go to other places. Is it not reasonable to think a blood vessel will burst in the brain and pour in its contents until you have a case of apoplexy etc.?

★

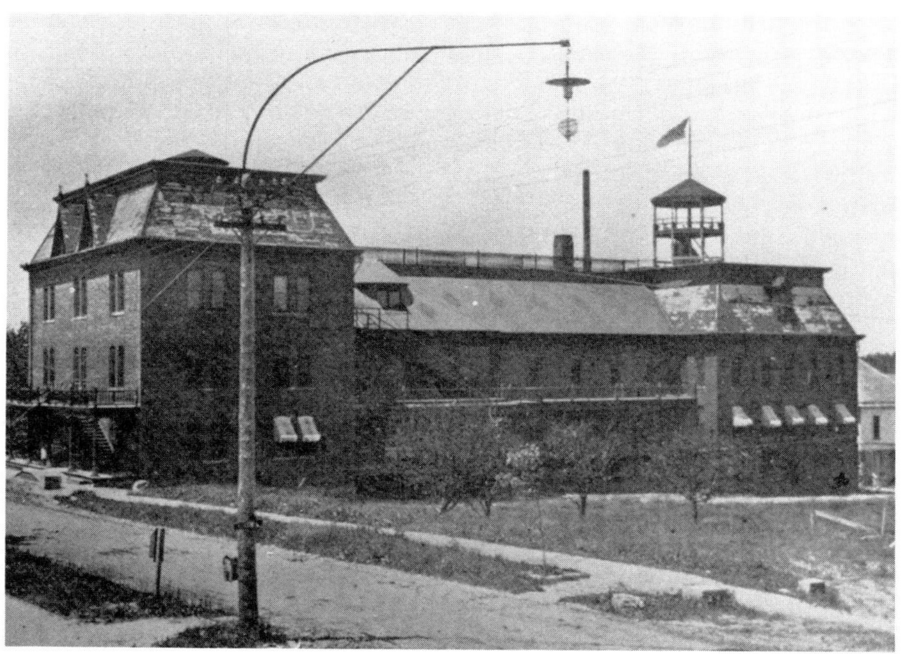

The Search Lights Of Success.

NO truth ever took place among men and was adopted for its value that did not exist in nature. Self created, self living and comes with the gray hairs and whiskers of lo ng ages. It has ever stood in the open fields, and with the label on its breast written in all languages, "I am for you," and has even broken ranks to catch the eye of man. "I at first spread in full view the full broadside of my vessel, that tipped all shores with bow and stern; but man did not, would not, take his eye off the boats of empty tradition long enough to read the labels of this great vessel, whose length reached from shore to shore." One said I wish I was on that long boat, I believe a person could get a long sleep on it. A person may stand in the best of places and listen to the arguments of truth and not move a muscle of mind or body for years, and will not because he fears it will not be popular. He is a liar and a hypocrite of the first and of all kinds of water. He is a coward and a sneaking paltroon, and lives by short weights and hypocrisy. He is much more to be dreaded than the man of much sleep. He wears the yellow rose of jealousy, and is ever ready to say when the hard fight for truth is over and the enemy is dead, I too want to be a pall-bearer at that funeral, and makes an ass of himself. He knows he never spoke one word to encourage the growth of that now wonderful truth, that he is splitting his throat to tell the people about.

Does he travel in the front line of progress with a search-light of an honest explorer? No, he is naught but the mill-stone of untruth around the neck of honest investigation. He takes hold of this unfolded truth with the tongue of a liar and hand of a thief, and says "I am the Edison of all discoveries, the commander of the sun and moon. I am far in advance of all thinkers as the size of my hat shows. I have gotten all the knowledge that mortals can give."

*

The Head Of The Family.

MAN is the head of the family, so declared by sacred writ. Has he not great reason to be proud of this appointment? For is he not also master of the beasts of the field, the fishes of the sea and the fowls of the air. All of these facts being indisputable, is it not reasonable that he should lead in all things?

The woman is the weaker vessel, and generally very weak; would it not be expected that this divinely endowed gentleman should lead in all things? If so, let him rise in the morning, make fires, have the room warm and comfortable to receive the weaker vessel. Is his arm not stronger than hers? If so, let him cut the meat, grind the coffee, churn and dress the butter, wash the dishes, make up the beds, put on and fill the wash boiler, do the washing and ironing, box and spank the children, in order to save her strength. She has many duties which the head of the family can assign to her, which are lighter and more pleasant. Such as playing the piano, riding the bicycle, curling her hair, light gossip, entertaining company, receiving the news of the day such as deaths, marriages and the latest scandal. He is admonished not to be weary in well doing for in due season he shall reap if he faint not. He must ever remember that these light afflictions have some glory at the end of them.

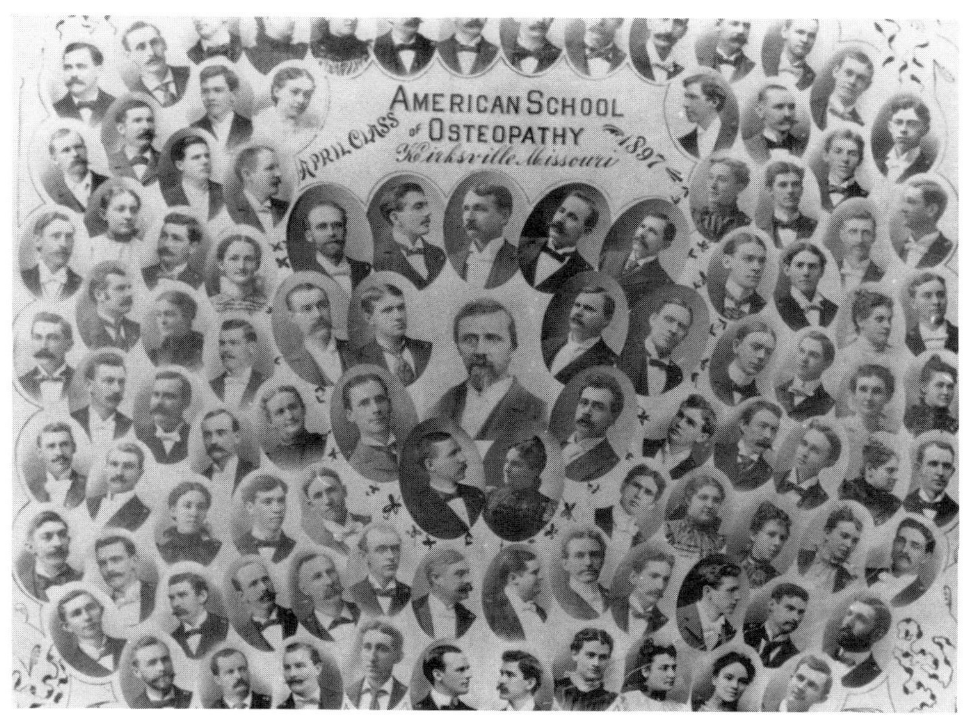

June, 1898

DR. A. T. STILL'S DEPARTMENT.

To Think.

HISTORY should be an association of facts, so as to become desirable food for the mind. Thinkers by birth form one class, and thinkers by note another. One thinks and talks for display, the other talks and thinks to improve his day. To think easily you must stand solidly. To stand solidly you must guard well the construction of your foundation. Level the upper surface, and square all sides and plumb accordingly. A foundation should never tip to any point of the compass after being leveled, if it should it is an evidence that something is wrong with the under pinning. The amount the foundation tips to any point marks the amount of neglect that is shown and by a lack of careful preparation of the strong pillar on which you wish to stand.

A writer cannot do justice to that he does not comprehend, no amount of words, quotations or plagarisms can disguise his ignorance.

If you should undertake to describe a muscle, you only do it by an intimate knowledge of all, material, mechanical and otherwise. How could a person speak the Chinese language by using English adjectives? What has his effort proven short of his ignorance? You can tell what you know and no more. Now this means when you describe a muscle or any principle in the human body, throw down every other consideration and consider with your own mind, and see if you are in possession of such truths and facts as can stand the most crucial examination, short of that of Deity himself.

Four is four, and two, one half of four. take no truth that cannot be divided into four parts, and when all added together are equal to the original only, then your stories will not need to be disguised to hide their lack of brilliancy.

*

June, 1898

To The Inquirer

SUCH questions as the following arise: Why not use time honored remedies? On what does Osteopathy depend? Where does it find remedies? What is the basic principle on which it depends or hopes to restore the normal condition in disease? A wholesale answer would be about this, a belief that God is competent to begin and finish a being, know all its needs and furnish to fullness.

First anatomical shapes, bones as frame, muscle and ligaments in shape, size and number to suit vessels and conductors, batteries, engines and a living being. To conduct the whole and supply with qualified substances and principles, there are evidences all along the process of life.

Of what use is Chemistry, Anatomy, Physiology, Histology, and Urinalysis? Why not use the old systems? Why not mix Osteopathy with drugs?

There is danger of drifting clear away from nature before its merits can be or are proven to be all sufficient in sickness.

Before you experiment with any dangerous poison, of cut, try and hope, you find just as great mysteries in the effect of any single drug as in the whole human body. Thus in our ignorance of one law of life as a machine, we increase perplexity when we add a new or foreign element to the competition.

Until man has proven God's ignorance or failure in providing for all his needs, Osteopathy feels a delicacy in offering to do for the afflicted anything that is not to be obtained by the wisely provided machinery of man. Has God failed! Keep silent until we prove such to be the case; prove that the drug in the body cannot restore us to health.

★

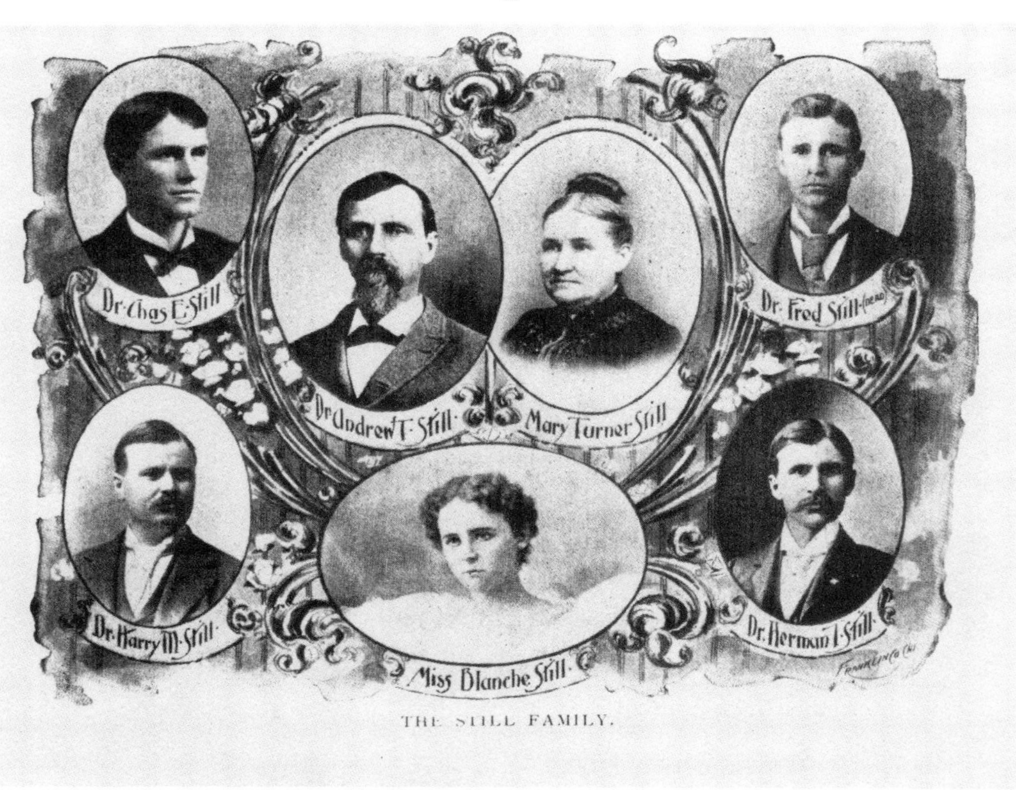

THE STILL FAMILY.

June, 1898

Completeness of Life.

WHEN we use the word complete we wish to direct the attention of the reader to the embryo of animal life, though microscopic in size. No evidence is recorded in proof that to that germ of life is received a single additional principle. All we know or have been able to learn of that atom of life is, that it is a being with plans and specifications, with powcr to build a man, woman, beast, bird, or fish. Not only that, but as it unfolds it makes its own laboratory, qualifies and fits each atom to suit the part for which is made. It goes on and with its work, builds machinery to fill and meet all coming demands for our comfort and kind. The power of self defense in bird, beast, man and fish, prove conclusively that a germ of life tho' small is the work of wisdom, with power to live, act, form and defend its kind. Thus we have the laws of hunger, eat, drink, grow, move, sleep and defend self and offspring.

One defends by its teeth, others by horns, others by poisoned teeth and deadly odors, which the enemies to its life cannot endure and live. All are furnished in that microscopic germ. Power to form the deadly poisons by its own peculiar processes of generating such defences as that being required for its personal protection.

If it is to swim in or under the water that germ of mind thought out and formed a fin or float to suit. Then to the birds of flight, the wing and feather comes as true, as found in specification of its form and all its requirements. Nothing is omitted, no additions can be suggested or find a place. Thus we are admonished to stop and say, life to each specimen of being is the trustworthy principle of all forms.

When we think of life we have to dwell in seas of mysteries from start to finish. We see what it can do, we do not know how big it is, we do not know that the life of an elephant is larger than a humming-bird. We do not know how it acts, we know there is motion, farther than that we knew nothing. We see no more wisdom in a horse than in a bee. If we know what life is then we could go farther with the feast. But we must be satisfied to know what it can do, and what it cannot do.

The life of a cow can make hair, hide, horns, legs, eyes, ears, tail, liver, heart, lungs, an udder and four teats, so made to fit the mouth of the calf or the hand of man who may desire that fluid as a nourishment. She may be lovable or deadly in her nature. She seeks her own food and drinks, masticates her food a second time. Goes to the shade when necessary to shield her from the summer heat. Makes her bed in such places as the wind strikes her with the least possible fury during the cold season. She is the result of the great power of the germ of her existence. With all her powers she cannot make a feather, neither can she make an egg, yet she has all she would ask, or that would be any benefit to her species.

A germ of another kind when it passes through the process of development, would make the furious lion the king of beasts.

From morn till night we are confronted with the great question: What is life which begins its work a germ, and concludes with a mammoth of many tons, and he too with all the powers of his life cannot make one rattle for a snake, nor the wing of a grasshopper? There is no evidence that the beginning germ of the mammoth was any larger than the egg of the mosquito.

At this point we will leave the fowls of the air, the beast of the field, the living terrors of the forest and take up man. He too has life and mind, both of which have always been before his eyes, the unsolved mystery of life. As much so to-day as he was when he first set his foot upon the face of the earth. He is endowed with all the attributes common to the animal, also a more extended power of reason than they, yet he has not been able to solve the problem of life with all his knowledge.

Motion is all he knows of life. Results are all he knows of mind. And he who observes the most of the workings of natures' law is surely the shining star of intelligence among men.

He who would change natural law is an assassin to his best friend.

Ruts have men and notions in them who sleep with a good relish for generations, not knowing they have eyes to see and minds to reason.

Let us swallow a seed of knowledge and let it grow by metal cultivation to a tree of ripe fruit. By it we drink from the ocean of reason. All roads take us to such fruit as truth has in store for us. Reason is the oil of joy. Joy is the wise man's God. When reason fills our whole body the hand goes with the mind and does all that mind would demonstrate as proof of the ability of nature to vindicate its merits.

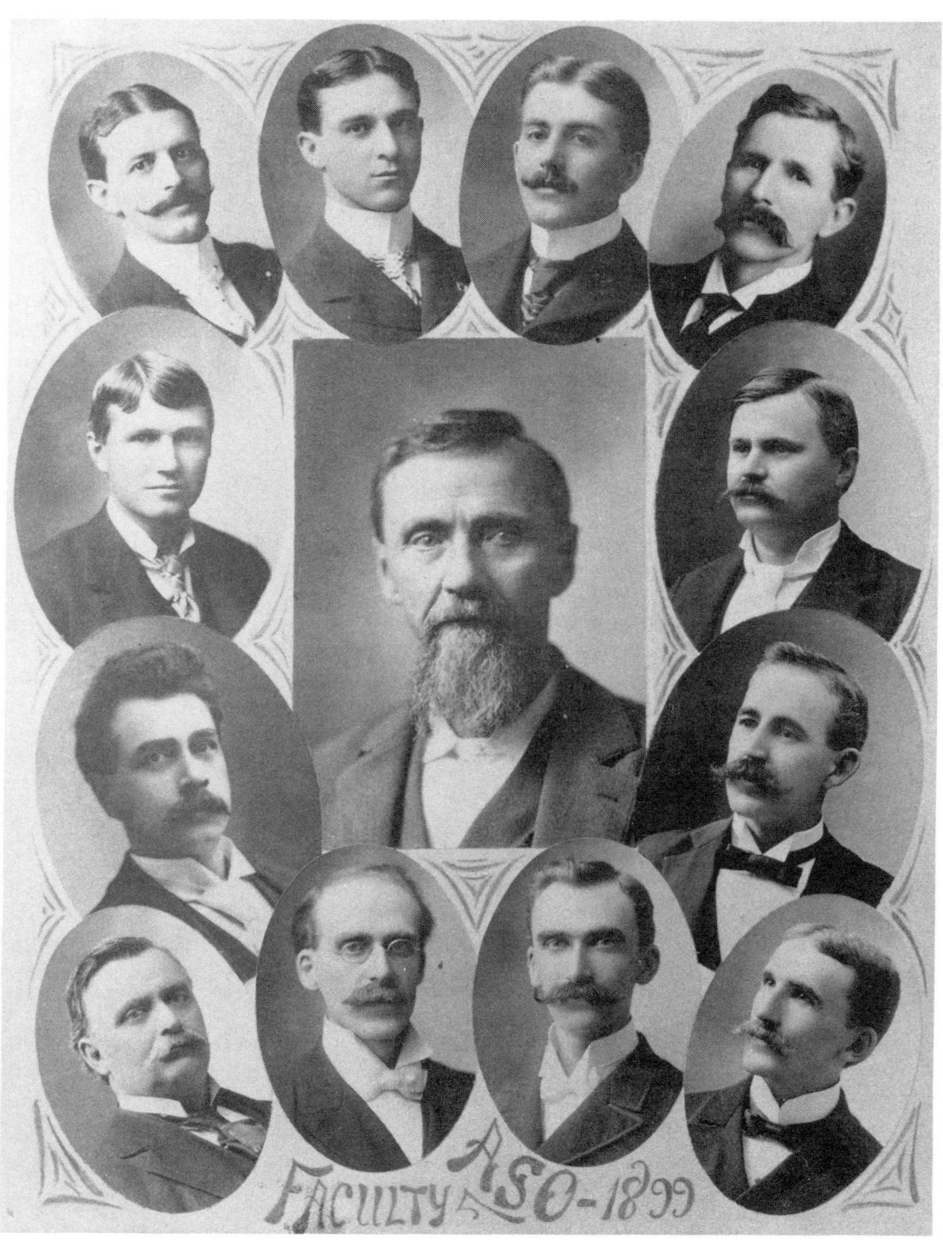

June, 1898

I heartily endorse the work of the Research and Review Club and the men composing it. The splendid work of the Research and Review Club has awakened all to the need of such auxiliary organizations in the American School of Osteopathy, to such an extent that I feel like encouraging the formation of such clubs for study while in school. And I also recommend the gentlemen named in this club as competent Osteopaths.

A. T. STILL.

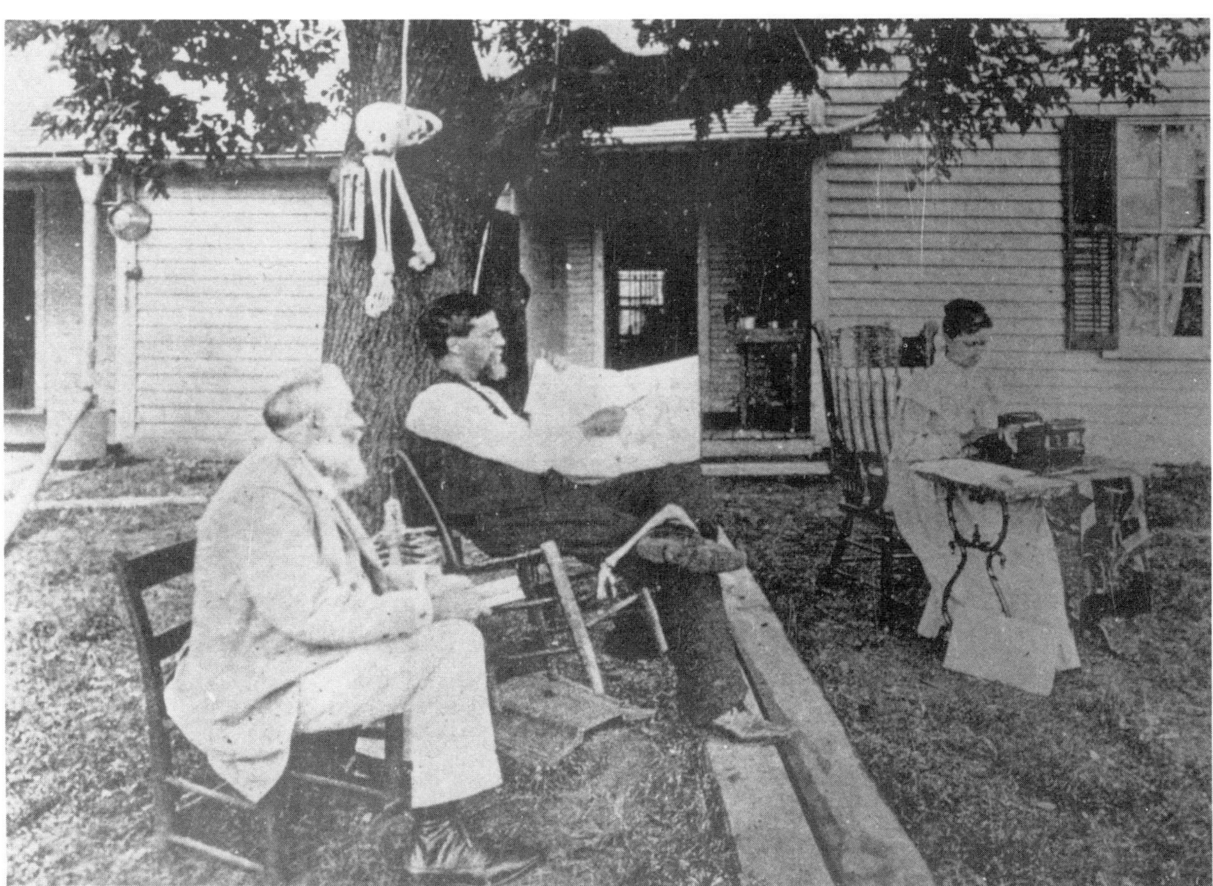

A. T. Still, *center*, describing his theory of osteopathy

July, 1898

THE BELOVED DEAD.

OUR beloved dead should ever be honored and never forgotten. But to quote them as authority for wisdom and learning that would be equal or superior to the minds of today, would be very unwise in many cases. Take the work of the mechanic of today, who prepares ships to battle with force. See him enter the sea with his vessel and plow the furious storms on the ocean; he goes just as he pleases, he knows the time he will be in port—say London—or any other place desired. He knows the number of miles between points, he knows his vessel will not be tossed to and fro just for the amusement of the laughing waves of the sea, but that he will split all billows and leave them far behind him, and come into port on date, as wired, in from one to six months less time, than the greatest ships of our beloved dead could do, with the best sailing rig of their day. Would it be wisdom in us to read their books of art and apply their thoughts to our day? I think not. What do you think? I do not wish to spend my days with Chinese deadly stupidity. See what that sleepy life of 6000 years has done for that great empire of wealth, with its hundreds of millions of population. Their freedom is now gone and the vultures of the world laugh at their ignorance, while they tear the vitals of that once great empire. This is the wisdom and result of their pig tail reverence for their walls of defence, that have ceased to defend for long ages, Still they stick to the ever failing customs of their beloved dead; and like some of the M. D's of today do not know that the chariots of time are loaded with progress and wisdom. Suppose America had been unwise enough to trust the cannons and war ships of Washington and Napoleon, what would be our condition today? Our boasted liberty would flee like a feather before the wind, and we would be the servants of the bloody kings and emperors of the world, as a reward for our stupidity, and for not knowing that to quote, live and do, as our fathers did in their day, would be death to all that is sacred to us now. Should we stop at this point without making the application, many would have a blank, an empty feast.

The object of the above is to reach the mind of the student of Osteopathy with the facts above quoted, a knowledge of which has been the compass that has guided the minds of the skilled artists of this and all other progressive ages, not the masses, the average mind, nor the wealthy—but for him whose skill of thought was able to comprehend and foreshadow coming events, and ward off calamities by his forethought and skill. I wish to call the attention of the reader to the fact that independent philosophers are few and far between, they who are able to manage wisely and keep a healthy political condition for the inhabitants. It would seem that great statesmen are not made, but born for the purpose. The military man who should guard and defend the peace and happiness of a nation is only born once in a while during a nation's life. Instance: Washington, Lincoln, Grant, of America; Bismark of Germany; Gladstone and Salisbery of England, and so on through the list of great and good men of all nations. A successful statesman or a military man formulates and executes his own plans. It is almost impossible to call around him as council, men endowed with mental skill that would be of any benefit to him. Thus each champion of success must raise his own star, and stand by his own convictions, and abide by results.

★

YOUR Osteopathic knowledge has surely taught you, that with an intimate acquaintance with the nerve and blood supply, you can arrive at a knowledge of the hidden cause of disease, and conduct your treatment to a successful termination. This is not by your knowledge of chemistry, but by the absolute knowledge of what is in man: what is normal and what is abnormal; what is effect, and how to find the cause. Do you ever suspect renal or bladder trouble without first receiving knowledge from your patient, that there is soreness and tenderness in the region of the kidneys along the spine? By this knowledge you are invited to explore the spine for the purpose of ascertaining whether it is normal or not. If by your intimate acquaintance and observance of a normal spine you should detect an abnormal form, although it be small, you are then admonished to look out for disease of kidneys, bladder or both, from the discovered cause for disturbance of the renal nerves by such displacement, or some slight variation from the normal in the articulation of the spine. If this is not worthy of your attention, your mind is surely too crude to observe those fine beginnings that lead to death. Your skill would be of little use in incipient cases of Bright's disease of the kidneys or any disease of the whole system, climate or season, or contagion. Has not your acquaintance with the human body opened the mind's eye, to observe that in the labratory of the human body, the most wonderful chemical results are being accomplished every day, hour and minute of your life? Could the labratory be running in good order and tolerate the formiug of a gall or bladder stone? Does not the body generate acids, alkalies, substances and fluids necessary to wash out all impurities? If you think an unerring God has made all necessary preparations, why not so assert, and stand upon that stone? You cannot do otherwise and not betray your ignorance to the thinking world. If in the human body you can find the most wonderful chemical labratory mind can conceive of, why not give more of your time to that subject, that you may obtain a better understanding of its workings? Can you afford to treat your patients without such qualifications? Is it not ignorance of the workings of this Divine law that has given birth to the foundationless nightmare that now prevails to such an alarming extent all over civilization, that a deadly drug will prove its efficacy in warding off disease in a better way than has been prescribed by the intelligent God, who has formulated and combined life, mind and matter, in such a manner that it becomes the connecting link between God and a world of mind, and that element known as matter? Can a deep philosopher do otherwise than conclude that nature has placed in man all the qualities for his comfort and longevity? Or will he drink that which is deadly and cast his vote for the crucifixion of knowledge.

★

HAVE we not a feast of mind, a world of hope, as we survey the whole human body, in irs wisely formulated parts, each and all bound together by cords of love, with the deepest soul stirring harmony in all action as seen in man. Each organ and all other parts laboring together, seeming to know that they are parts of a stupendous whole, and must assist like a watch of many wheels, in which all must move, all the time, and with infinite exactness, in order to truthfully report the time. Should any part of any wheel or spring fail to do its duty, the whole machine fails and shows that the watch is diseased and cannot give a healthy report of the time sought by the owner. The same is the law of animal life, from brain to the least nerve fiber, as I hope to show you further on. Before we lay aside the watch let us run by comparison a moment longer. We find by comparison, it is our greatest lever to obtain truth. In man we learn that his BRAIN is the source of power from which all parts are made to act. Just so we find in the watch the mainspring to be the power of all motion seen and used, by wheels, levers and pulleys. As this watch has many duties to perform it becomes necessary to prepare it with separate parts for each duty; when we muster them into one company, and when all parts labor in unsion (if under proper spring power and the parts are in form and place) you get the hour indicated correctly. How is it with man? Can he mark perfect health with a small nerve of an eye-lid hurt by an irritant? Go on to a strained finger, toe, leg or arm, or even a rib. Would you think that person's health would be just as good as though such variations from the normal did not exist? You cannot afford to say yes, when reason would condemn you. Then by reason we conclude that to be perfectly healthy, we must have a normal body in all parts, or disease will mark the degree of abnormal positions of some or many of the wheels found in animal forms. If this philosophy be true there is but one assertion that is true, and that is, *all parts must be in place without the variation of the one thousandth part of an inch.*

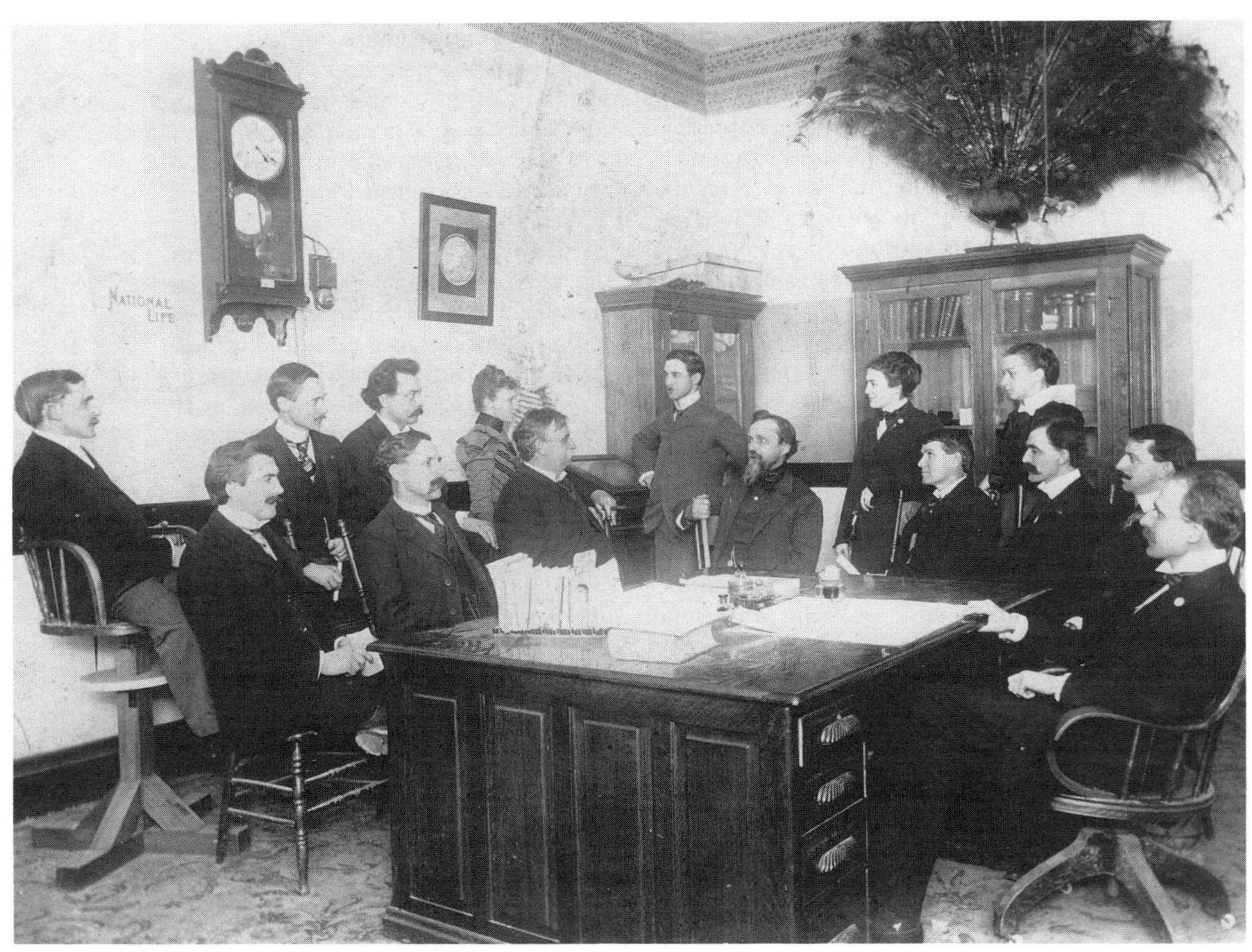

ASO faculty, c. 1898

July, 1898

HISTORICAL ADVICE TO THE PRESENT, PAST AND FUTURE GRADAUTING CLASSES.

Dr. A. T. Still, President, A. S. O.

As the time for my annual report will soon be here, I will begin by reviewing all the days, hours and ways I have done from the beginning six years ago to this date. Twenty-four years ago I saw enough of nature's power to adopt it as the best way to cure the sick and afflicted. I studied how, and made many successful applications on diseases of seasons, climate and contagions, which proof gave me, after twelve years experimenting, a very heavy practice and some money.

At that time many came and asked me to teach them how to cure the sick. I hesitated, as teaching had not been the business of my life, but as I had four children whom I wanted taught the principles and philosophy which I had proven to be master of disease in so many places, I concluded to hire Dr. Wm. Smith, of Edinburgh, Scotland, to give them training in anatomy and physiology, which was the foundation on which I had succeeded in all the diseases I had cured by the new method "Osteopathy," and without a drug.

After I had arranged with Dr. Smith to teach my sons there were others asked to be admitted to the class, which was done and we had a class of about twenty. School began in November, 1892, and ran through the winter. In March 1893, Dr. Smith left me, and went into practice as physician and surgeon in Kansas City. The following winter, I employed Mrs. Nettie Boles to fill the place vacated by Dr. Smith. I gave her Gray's Anatomy and the Quiz Compend, and told her to do the best she could and she did well. By this time our class had doubled. Mrs. Boles conducted the next school of over thirty.

As she had arranged to go to Denver, Colorado, and could not lead my next class of over fifty, I looked around for one to fill her place and concluded to try a nephew of mine who had been four months under Mrs. Boles, and see if he could teach Gray's Anatomy with the aid of a "Quiz" and my own help. I was a little afraid of his ability, and sent him and three of my children to Chicago for eight weeks drill in dissection, under the renowned anatomist, Prof. Eckly, so that they could tell a head from a liver. In the mean time I wrote to Dr. Smith to visit me. He came and while here I asked him to take a position in the school as demonstrator of anatomy, which he kindly accepted. There is no need to speak here of his ability as a teacher, his work speaks for itself. He commenced with a class of about 130, which has increased until to-day it numbers near 550.

By this time you see the growth in numbers, with about a doubling ratio annually.

I have no difficulty at any time in keeping my business well officered for any purpose that the growth and requirements of the school may demand. Nor do I anticipate any difficulty in the future. Many that have served as teachers and clerks have gone out in the world to make their fortunes, some by teaching, others by the practice of Osteopathy. Thus at every vacancy made, just as good men and women stand ready and fully competent to take the pen or broom.

During the past three years I have built at an expense of $150,000 a convenient and commodious house, with about eighty rooms for teaching the branches necessary to an Osteopathic education, and in which to treat the sick, in order to demonstrate to the student the reliability of nature's law, to cure the curable and relieve the dying.

Now by way of encouragement to you who are about to receive your diplomas with my signature and those of the professors of this school, I will say, for twenty-four long years I have never met a discouraging reverse. Every day has only marked another step in progress. Right here I will say that sometimes I have been greatly annoyed with a lot of old business bungling failures, they have been very loud mouthed in offering to furnish me business brains, cheap. As far as I have ever trusted one of them I have been "burnt" and deceived. They have, do, and will, hang around the graduating classes like buzzards over a dying hog, telling them that they can make mints of money, and that their business ability will help you to make a success in starting Osteopathic schools and Infirmaries. My advice to you would be to have but one walking stick at a time and use that yourself. Manage your own business. Use your own brains. Handle your own money, and keep out of corporations. You are still my children and have asked a father's advice. Read the above before you leave my roof, after which I shall use no parental authority—only pray for your success.

July, 1898

I AM JUST A MAN.

(A soliloquy and a vision of the night with a lesson.)

I AM just a man, so are you. You have plenty, I have nothing. You and I entered school on the same day, both graduated at the same time. Our grades were recorded just the same. We were both married about the same time to women with apparently the same intellect and physically the same. My children are feeble in form and restless, yours are quiet and well developed. Mine cry for bread, while yours slumber with fullness. Yours go to school, learn quickly and are brilliant stars for their ages. Mine are not. Your children have lucrative positions, mine are servants. Your mother lives with you, in peace and plenty, while mine is in the almshouse, without the comforts of either bed or table. Your father's body rests in a beautiful cemetery. My father's bones are playthings for the students of anatomy. I love my father and mother next to my God. The scalpel of the student tore from my father's bones all his flesh, and from his breast dug out piece at a time, every fiber that contained love My conditions are such that my mother's sacred flesh, with all her vitals, are bound to be torn from their moorings to her loving breast, because I have not the means to save her from that bloody scalpel, which tore all parts asunder and away from my father's bones, which were the pillars that bore up his love. Alas, the edict of poverty has said my loving mother shall be the open gaze for the dissecting table, and her heartstrings of love shall be cut in twain. I have not the means to feed her, neither have I a competency to purchase her a coffin of the cheapest grade. I own no foot of earth in whose bosom I can deposit her loved form. As I weep, rivers of love pour from my soul, and I feel that anxiety that I have felt for years. I pray until my physical body is as weak as a child.

At this period of my grief I can hold out no longer. I must slumber. Oh my! Oh my! I am now in the midst of a vision of the night. A history of the panorama of the past is passing before me. I see when a child,

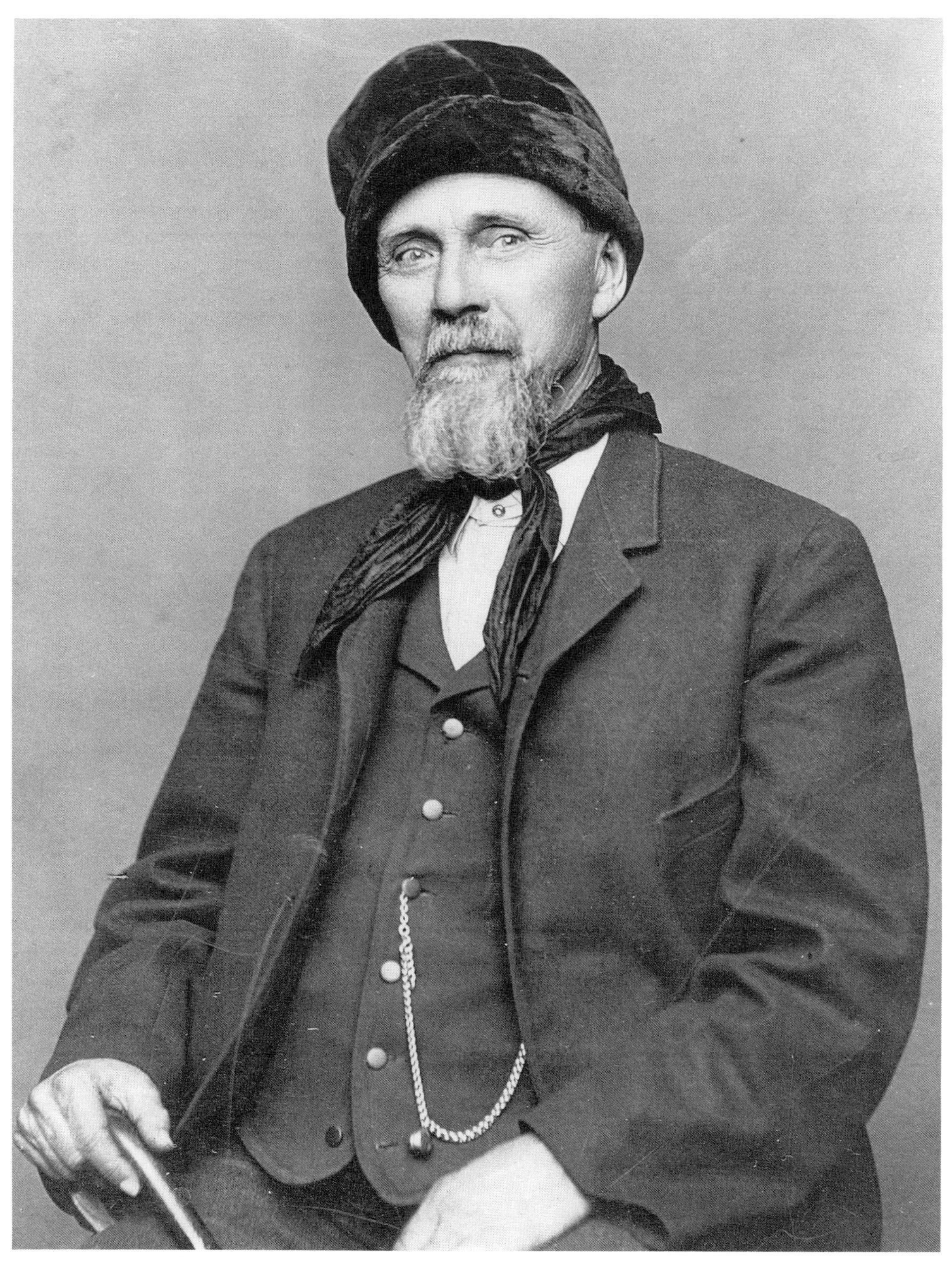

A. T. Still

I was healthy and robust, I knew nothing of sickness and pain. When at labor I could execute all work entrusted to me with equal and at many times superior speed as those that worked with me. In my school days I had plenty, kept up with my classes in all grades. In short, my youthful days were a paradise. When I married and went into business for myself all the doors of prosperity were open and encouraging. I went into business with a fair amount of money ; for a few years I seemed to prosper wonderfully, but like a good many young men, was not willing to let "well enough alone." My deposits in the bank were fairly good, luck and prosperity above the average. At this time of my vision, I see a wide-mouthed dragon of destruction, he smiles and caresses me, and says get on my back and ride and I will carry you to success and widening prosperity. Unthoughtedly like an ignorant child I found myself astride his back. I journeyed on and on with him, and he said unto me I am the champion of success. With what money you have and my ability to manage business I can lead you to success after success, until with your bountiful supply, you will want no more. As he was old at business, and I young, I handed over to him all my means, and rode along on his promises. We came to the side of a dark river, he straightened up on his all fours and smiled as he pitched me over his head, down, down into that river of financial despair, whose length was great, and its banks were high, and I have rolled and agonized within its black billows ever since the day I mounted the back and listened to the advice of that old deceiver, who is always ready to lead the young political or business aspirant to success. He has all my money, all of my hopes, and has left me the bitter cup of despair to drink from, all the rest of my days. And my vision passed off with these words, the world is full of just such beasts of prey.

A. T. STILL.

June, 1898

HIRED HELP.

IT takes two persons to make a contract in North America. If a man needs help he can get it, if he has the "spot cash" and plenty of it, to pay as much or more than others pay for the same kinds of work. So you see there is no "thank you business" about it.

When a man hires as a clerk, boot black, or for any other purpose, he will get all he can for his labor; and when he is paid as agreed by contract, you are free, and don't even owe him a "much obliged" to you. It was a job for cash money from start to finish. This has been my experience and observation in regard to business matters generally. I have nearly always been well pleased with my hired help, and hope they were also satisfied with their reward.

PROVERBS BY PAP.

***

June, 1898

TWO KINDS OF DIPLOMAS.

DEWEY sank eleven Spanish ships, a whole fleet of one of the oldest, and once most powerful kingdoms of the earth. Dewey's diploma was earned by hard study and close attention to the rules and methods of the American War School. His name is known and feared and honored by the whole civilized world. Dewey kills for glory and duty, but the commissions sent out from the American School of Osteopathy, are not given to kill and to cause people to tremble with fear of death, but to fight all diseases to the death, and to let the children of God live and know His law is all-sufficient to conquer all diseases without drugs or drinks. A diploma from the American School of Osteopathy, carries more honor than all other diplomas in the world. While the Spanish fear Dewey, the old school M. D's fear Osteopathy more. Dewey's fame is great but Osteopathy has come to conquer the world by its teachings.

PAP.

***

June, 1898

A STATEMENT.

IN regard to Horton Fay Underwood, of New York, who has been practicing Osteopathy in that city for some months past, I desire to say this, that he was a faithful student, while in attendance at the American School of Osteopathy, and that he graduated with high honors. After receiving his diploma, Dr. Uuderwood worked in my service as an operator with great skill and credit to the Infirmary and to himself. I further for the information of those who employ him, say that he is worthy of their confidence. He was second to no operator. His foot is always found in the front rank. This has been my observation. For some unknown reason this notice has already been too long omitted. In the future personal mention of anyone going out from this institution need not be looked for, as a diploma signed by its officers will be sufficient endorsement, and the list of worthy graduates and skilled operators is becoming so large that space cannot be spared in this JOURNAL. A. T. STILL.

What is harmony but health.—A. T. Still.

★

God's pay for labor and time is truth, and truth only.—A. T. Still.

★

When I look upon the work of nature, it doesn't work for a dollar and a half a day; it works for results only-—A. T. Still.

★

Father and mother by nature are really our dearest friends. Next to them sensible economy is our special, daily and hourly friend. It is the tape-line that measures our business sense. He who wastes anything is a business fool. He who saves all he can for the day of need has a well balanced head. She who spends and wastes money when young will shed bitter tears in old age. A. T. STILL.

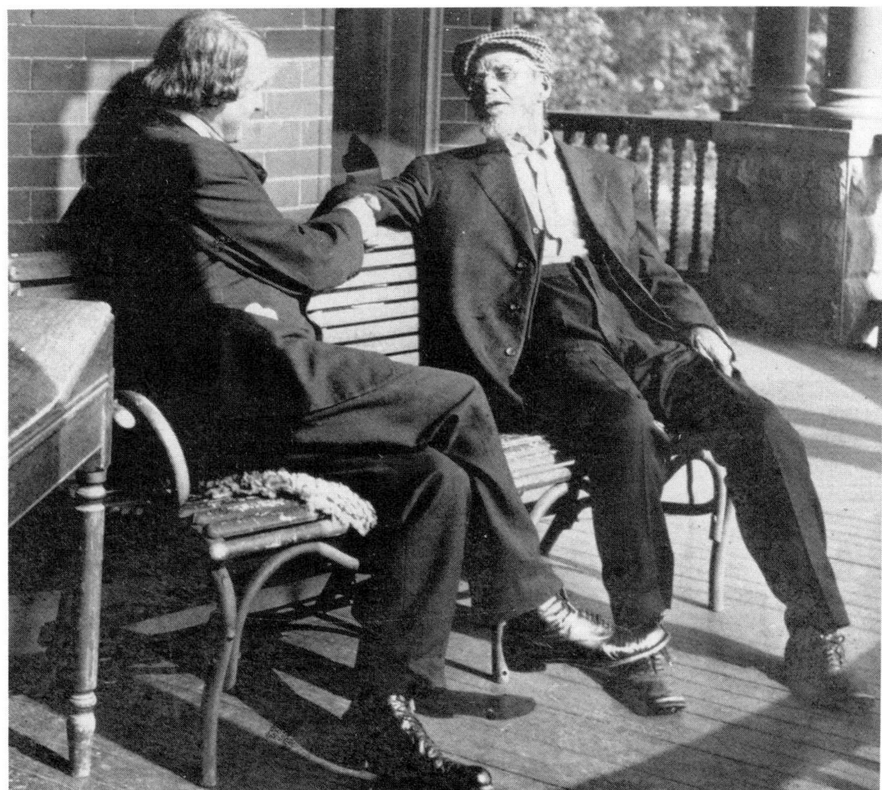

"Pap" talks on his front porch to a visiting D. O., c. 1914

August, 1898

DR. A. T. STILL'S DEPARTMENT.

*

DIGESTION.

ARE the tracks and truths of God in plain view? I use the word God in preference to Nature, Almighty or the Supreme Being, because I believe it conveys the thought of absolute intelligence more forcibly to the mind of our deepest thinkers, as well as the half-way and superficial. Whether "God" be an individualized person or not I will leave that for the reader to decide. But when we take up any one subject for investigation on which mind and experience may dwell for knowledge we see those truths, those mighty principles, always going in one direction which is for the accomplishment of some great and wonderful result. We can halt as explorers at any point, place or position, for the purpose of taking observation, and we reap a great reward, a feast of intelligence in all forms of life that it presents, in every principle that is discovered or unfolded to us by reason.

For a long time I have tried to stand upon this stone of observation. Questions like these arise to my mind: does God or Nature chew, swallow, digest, produce blood, muscle, bone, skin and hair? What is digestion? Where does it begin to manipulate matter for the purpose of making blood, which is simply matter prepared for the purpose of transposing substances from one form to another and for different uses? To what degree of condition of finenesss would satisfy the exacting demands of nature in preparing acceptable matter for producing a muscle? Our popular Physiologists have traveled part of the journey and gone into camp, satisfied that they have acquainted themselves with the law of digestion, with every step from mastication to living blood. Are you satisfied to pitch your tent and go into camp at this point of the journey, as an investigator, believing you have obtained all knowledge pertaining to the subject? If you are I am not, for the reason, that in the stomach of nature, the lungs of space, I see the law of atomizing is only partly fulfilled, prior to the gaseous condition, when the great thoracic duct of animals receives the fluid, commonly called chyle, which I am satisfied is in a lifeless and very crude condition when it arrives at the lungs.

We are told that the lungs take on oxygen, throw off carbon and other elements, and at this time we have "living blood." But as we look farther into nature's great gas generator of space, we find previous to forming worlds that they are first converted into purified gas. Then the association of prepared matter begins by building the frame work of a globe from the hardest substances which we commonly call stone. In the animal body we would say bone. This generator of worlds keeps up the process of producing gas which may and does contain all known elements, these great vital forces conducted by nature to a completed world. Are we not at this point admonished to halt and observe the action in the lungs? which is possibly the greatest and most wisely constructed gas generator that mind of man has ever been able to contemplate. Does not every breath taken into the lungs teach you by the highest school of reason, that the exacting and refining laws of nature do demand, proceed to execute and reduce all substances to the gaseous condition previous to forming it into blood.

At this point of our investigation we will give place to the literary definition of digestion as found in Webster's International Dictionary:

"DIGESTION:—The conversion of food, in the stomach and intestines, into soluble and diffusible products, capable of being absorbed by the blood."

When a philosopher has traced digestion from mastication to the stomach and bowels where it receives various liquids supposed to be solvents and transfers the compound which is called chyme into the thoracic duct, to be conveyed to and into the heart, where it is transfered to the great common gas generator, commonly called the lungs, where one gas is exchanged for another he seems to be pleased to say it is useless to go farther. He sits down under this beautiful tree of "light" and never sees nor speaks of the wonderful works of nature as she converts this crude chyme into gas, which contains all the elements known to the chemist previous to reducing them to solids and semi-solids as the body of man may require in its construction.

Has the philosopher ever conceived the idea that the human body is a complete gasometer, which holds and reduces the gases in the lungs, which are condensed and reduced back to the consistency of bone and muscle, and placing this liquid back into proper channels for distribution? Does not reason teach him that all material forms have been by nature reduced to gas before they can be constructed into bodies of any kind, animal, vegetable or mineral?

Is it not reasonable to conclude that digestion is incomplete in all conditions short of the gaseous state? If worlds are the result of association of condensed gas, what is a bone or muscle but condensed gas?

At this point of reasoning we are frank to say our belief is that every part and particle of flesh and bone that is in the human body has passed through the gaseous condition previous to its appearance as blood and bone. Thus we have a better understanding of what is called digestion, which we believe has received its greater work while in the lungs.

One would say this is a new story about digestion. The story may be new but the law is as old as "God." See the spring, summer and fall, as the part of the year that vegetation grows. How does it grow? A proper answer to the question would be, by eating food suited to its growth. Is that food visible to the aided eye before it enters the vegetable body? If not then it must be in the gaseous condition. If nature can feed vegetation by gas only and goes to that trouble to fill the stomach of vegetation from gas, why not expect the same law in animal life? Reason says it must be, and that the gaseous change is given the blood in the lungs, as we can find no other reasonable place to change chyle to gas before blood is completed.

We think and speak of death but never think of a defect in the gas generating machinery; that it has failed to produce pure gas while in the lungs, which I think may be the cause of asthma, consumption, dropsy, all diseases and death. A good definition of death would be asphyxia by foul gas. If that be true then life must be sustained by pure gas. Then we are bound to stand on the conclusion that pure gas is the law of life, and impure is death. At twelve breaths per minute we generate in the lungs about seventy-two gallons of per hour, and about 1728 gallons each twenty-four hours, that is the air taken in the lungs as the basis of gas, when united with dead and vital substances met in the lungs while forming gas. Then we have about 3455 gallons of gas as a result of such union during twenty-four hours.

★

When Digestion is Completed.

AFTER digestion is completed and the flesh material is condensed after the application and appropriation, what can we think of this process but that it is the finale of physiological action, with the completed construction of the parts and ready to be used for all purposes by the spiritual man. Please say the principle of life or life itself, which is ready at all times to construct in proper form to suit its uses as the end and object of this body during its existence. This principle of being has knowledge, it has strength, with all the active qualities common to man or beast, the fishes of the sea, the fowls of the air, with all the intelligence as given by the Supreme ruler. Without the fine workings of the lungs in refining matter to that degree by which life and matter can exist in the associated form, all efforts to bring into existence a world, a muscle, or the whole being, without doubt, would be a failure. Thus we see the workings of the lungs by every method of reason that we can bring to bear upon the subject are nearer to God or mind itself than all else of the human body. We have great reason to believe and facts to know that the lungs do more work in preparing the nourishment of animal beings, than all else combined. Let us establish an observatory right here and make intellectual beings of diseases, for convenience of argument and ask mental questions to be answered by them. We will address them by the title of Mr. and Mrs. We will begin with Mr. Measles and ask that mighty champion in what part of the body he intends to deposit the seed of death? His answer seems to be given about thus and so: "by the action of the lungs and the elements of air I ride in the air into the lungs and deposit an egg, believing that a living principle commonly known as biogen, welcomes and assists me in the development of measles; here I reach the nerve terminals as one would say, and by secretion am conveyed to the universal fascia, in which I am nourished and watered into perfect manhood, matured measles. Then as I have possession I assert my authority and run the machinery of life until my whole desires are satisfied although death be the result in many cases. When I take possession of the lungs my first thought is to close the secretions by filling them with dead substances as they pass out of the skin. My first strategetic move is to close the mucous secretions of the lungs. Should they continue normal with the ability to combine oxygen and hydrogen, I would be washed out by the water renovation, therefore I close both excretion and secretion until my work is done, and my goods exhibited upon the surface as my ability to work, which child has been universally called a rash."

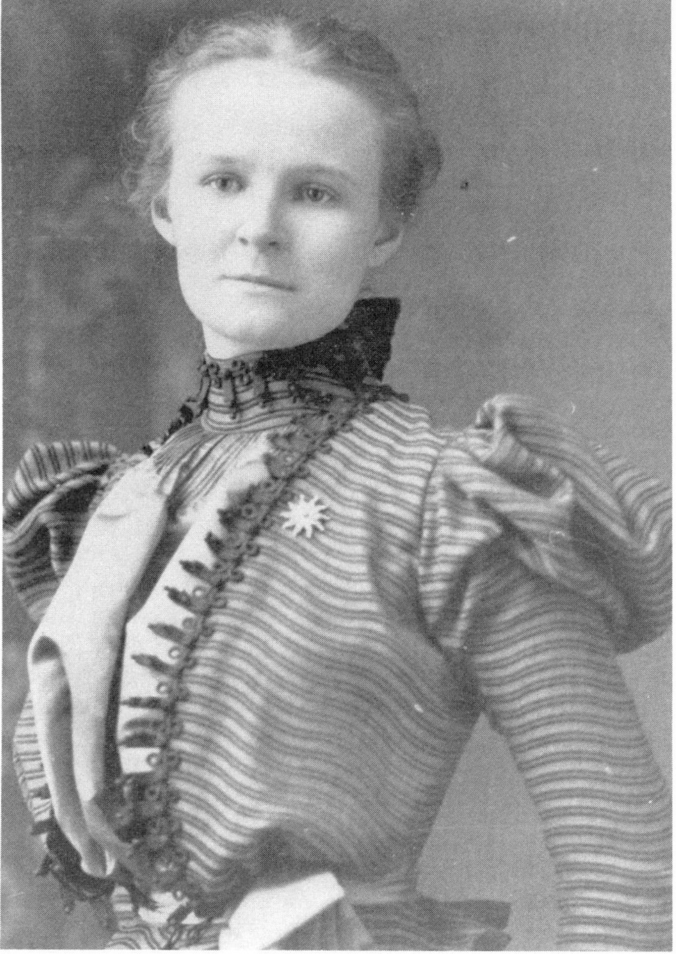

Blanche Still

Another mighty dragon's head appears whose name is "Asiatic Cholera" and says, "I have some work to do," and succeeds in opening secretions and excretions, which process lowers the temperature of the lungs and body to the degree of condensing gases to water in the lungs, secreting and excreting. "In order to make my work successful, I stop all principles of thirst or desire for water, then I proceed to use the lungs as a generator of water, I throw all the powers of secretion into motion until the water fluid becomes an irritant, by the power to fill and strain the excretory vessels throughout the whole body; then I turn the faucets of excretions loose upon the stomach, bowels and skin, and as there are thousands and millions of excretory channels I drown the man or woman, and they die of asphyxia by the water thus generated in the lungs." The champions of other diseases and death all come and put up at one common hotel, deposit their baggage with the clerk, wind up and put the machinery of death in motion, and spread out their goods for inspection. One is small-pox, one summer complaint, one malaria, one brain disease, one throat disease, one of arm, one of chest, one of heart, lungs, bowels, liver, kidney, bladder, rectum, and the lower limbs, and say emphatically that all the tunes of death play their pieces first in the lungs, and so places the sound-board that the dying groans can be heard in all parts of the physical organization.

By further observation we have evidences that the lungs do generate water for all animals and birds. Some birds, the eagle, hawk and buzzard, have never been known to take a drink of water. Many animals have been reported to spend long periods without having access to either food or drink. A lady and gentleman of undoubted veracity related an instance to me where on the night of Nov. 25th, a skunk made its appearance in an outhouse. In the same house was a half barrel which was used as a pounding barrel (a washing machine in those days.) Fearing the scent would spoil the barrel she ran in picked up a cover that just fitted the top of the barrel, and as the skunk could not be found, gave up the chase. As it was nearing winter the barrel was not molested until the following April, when the woman took the cover off the barrel she noticed something moving very slowly. Being somewhat alarmed, she called her husband, when on close inspection he found it to be the skunk that had been scented on the night of which I have just spoken. The barrel was worn smooth and shone as though it had been polished. The man turned the barrel down and the animal had barely strength to crawl. Without taking a second thought he killed it, but says he has been sorry ever since for the rash act, as he thinks it paid dearly for its life, being shut up in a barrel without food or water for four long months.

★

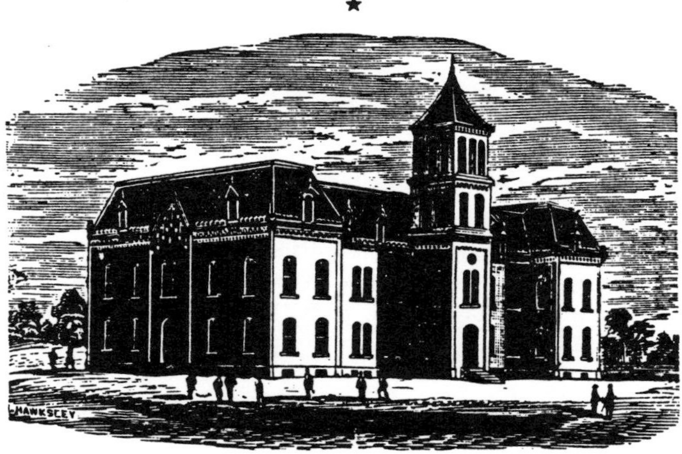

STATE NORMAL SCHOOL, KIRKSVILLE, MO.

WHEN I think of the melodies of the sky and remember that it came from the swan of the long ago as he sailed aloft with angel-white plumage as his robe; I listened to them, I enjoyed their sweetness, they were charming from their perfect harmony in musical tones, so much so that I sought the body to dissect that I might see the construction of that great and natural music box, the bagpipe that was carried and played upon by this beautiful bird. I laid the skin bare on the front side of his neck, which is about two feet long. I dissected away the flesh until I reached the breast bone. There I found the wind pipe descended under the bone in a circuitous route, made a turn until it penetrated the body, then turned until it reached the breast bone again, thence back and turned over the body for a distance of ten inches, then it forked and entered into two sack like tubes, one of which extended to each lung. Those sacks seemed to be the musical part of the bagpipe of the swan. When I took the windpipe out of the lungs with the musical bags I had a trachea five feet long. Why this wonderfully long pipe ran backward and forward doubling itself so often until it got into the mouth of the bird I cannot tell, I can only say this, that the softest and most melodious sound I ever heard came from that bird. That beautiful bird whose music so often comforted me when a child, today is numbered among the extinct birds of this country; the hand of man has destroyed him with all his associates. He is dead, his music is gone, his form is seen no more in the sky, but his memory to me is yet as vivid and as sweet as ever. I often wish I could hear one single note from that beautiful bird in whose construction the God of skill seemed to have displayed one of his greatest efforts. The rustle of the wing of the wild

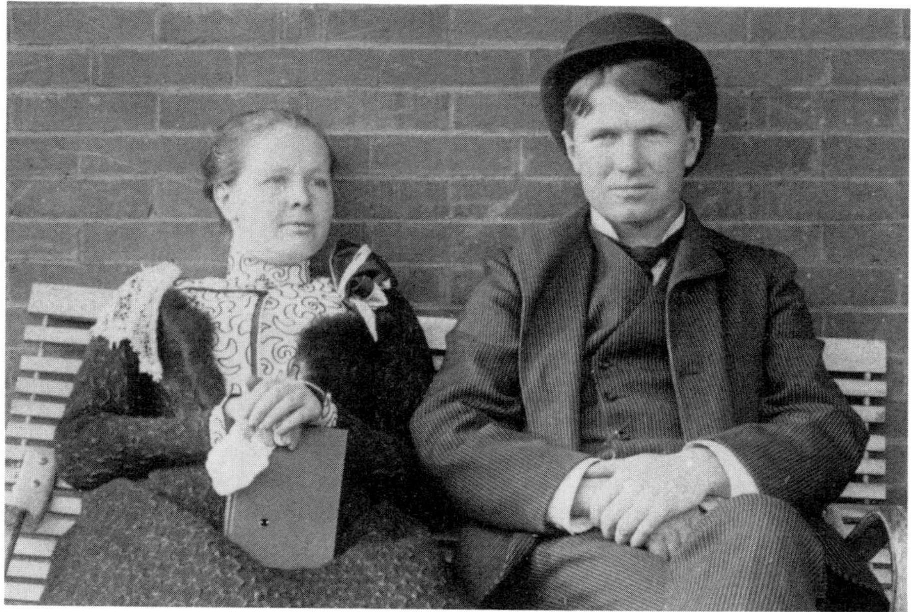

Charles E. Still and his wife, Anna Florence, c. 1900

pigeon which was given by millions upon millions has long since been booked with the swan. The raven, the paroquet and many other of the musicians of the sky are gone. But I have one friend left to cheer and remind me of the days when the swan did sing for my comfort. He does not sail aloft the starry skies but keeps close to mother earth. It is the common American-toad, and when he sings his plaintive lay my eyes fill to overflowing; it brings before me all the days of my youth, the joys and sorrows that surround me. Were he dead too, I could possibly forget the rest, but when my ear catches his low strain I realize that he is the only one left. He and I too will soon cease to disturb the living with the sound of our voices. Oh! that I could describe the scenes of the past that appear in this panorama when I hear the midnight moans of the toad, the last friend of my childhood days.

★

A Word to the Osteopaths.

WHEN you are summoned to the bedside in cases of sickness of all kinds you must remember that you are there to report as an engineer, for the purpose of inspecting the machinery of the physical body, and your duty as an explorer must be to first find the abnormal conditions, which are the results of derangement of either bone, ligament, muscle, nerve or blood vessel, to such a degree as to distract the natural workings of the laboratory of life when in action to produce normal fluids, for the use of all parts of the body. You are not called there for the purpose of giving written opinions of so-called eminent authors, nine-tenths of which have long since had an undisturbed rest in the waste basket that was prepared before the foundation of the world, to receive and retain the latin adjectives of the superficial writer, which he has borrowed from the grandpaps of all stupidity. You are not supposed to enter the sick room armed and equipped with books on symptomatology that contain no symptoms whatever except the symptoms of guess work and ignorance, which have been dead so long in the hand and mind of the speaker that he has not been able for more than twenty years to shed one tear over their demise. But you are called there to show your good sense as a skilled workman who is proud to know that Osteopathy is a science complete in and of itself. A science that is proud to know that it can lend, but can neither borrow nor buy one assisting thought from any medical school or from their writings.

As this school is young, and has a chair devoted to Osteopathy, we promise you that oral lectures with demonstrations will be given you as fast as possible. We say oral because we do not want compilations from medical authors palmed off on you as Osteopathy, and when such chairs are filled they will be filled by men and women who will know what to say from an intimate acquaintance with the subject on which they talk. You can only receive knowledge from him who has knowledge, and that knowledge must come from his head and mouth which will have an easy delivery, if he knows what he is talking about. The Osteopath that depends upon notes for information is poorly armed for the combats of the sick room.

★

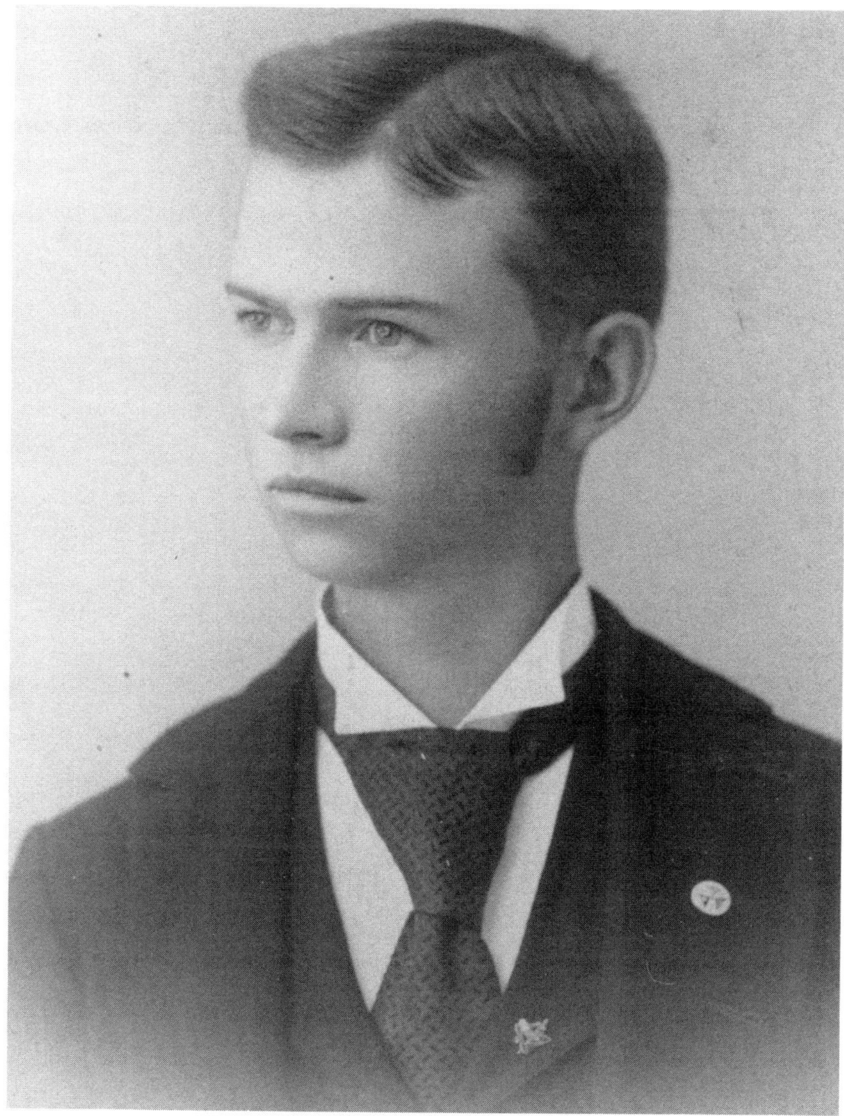

Fred Still

August, 1898

PROVERBS.

I WALKED out into open space in the early night, I turned my back on the full length of the earth, there was nothing between me and my earth support and that world of space. I threw open my eyes and began my nightly gaze. I saw worlds wheel, counter-wheel and march to see other and lesser worlds dressed in infant garb, and lying upon the breast of nature, whose motherly care and fountains loaded with the milk of life was thrown into the life of embryotic worlds. They nestled close to their mother's bosom and drank freely, until those children of the skies developed the pure paternal and maternal orbs and homes, with the countless millions of forms of animated beings, the human races, though all different in appearance, different in language and different in genius. They seemed to be as numerous as the stars and parts of stars found in some great constellation, all vivified by the one common force of light and life and governed by that one unerring principle mind. Many of those children grew at the mother's breast and took complete man and womanhood. Kissing their mother farewell they commenced their journey into space and they carried with them the odor of love and wisdom. They have obtained that love and admiration by the beings that God brought into existence, those worlds and inhabitants living in peace without any knowledge of war, or any of the common wrongs known and practiced by the inhabitants of this earth. There seemed to be great walls around many of them as represented by the rings of Saturn. When I enquired the use of those rings which were placed many thousand miles from those orbs, I was told those walls were to prohibit the approach of any element of man's creation, hatred, wars, grief and confusion from entering or approaching near these harmonious worlds. And the mother of these worlds said, worlds are not created for war, death and disease, but to give birth and growth to man and beast, and so blend their acts and dispositions that they shall give an exhibition of beings covered in the full regalia of love. She said war is not natural nor is it intelligent. It is the act of the poisoned waters of unintelligence that have crept into and spoiled the milk in the breast of that earth-mother, or any other mother world; it is the crazy expression of bad digestion, producing dyspepsia, both of the body and mind. Thus you have the causes of all earthly confusion and unmanly acts.

*

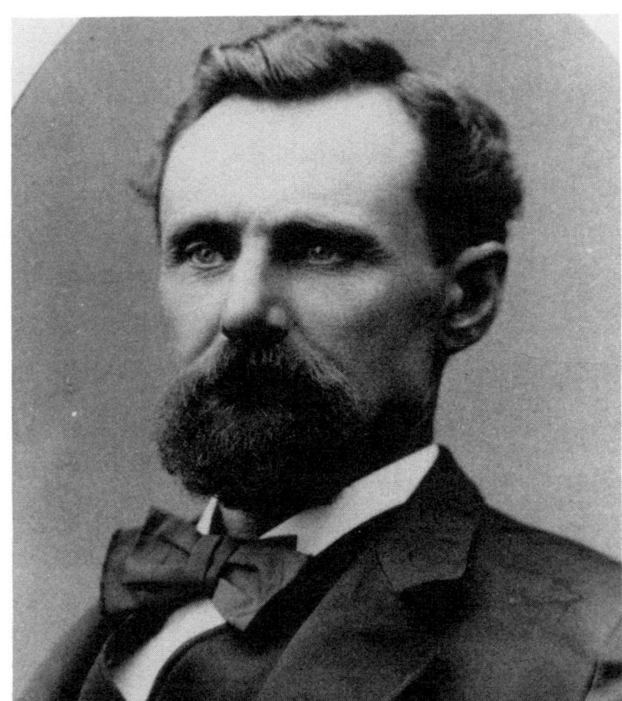

Dr. Thomas C. Still, brother of A. T. Still, 1886

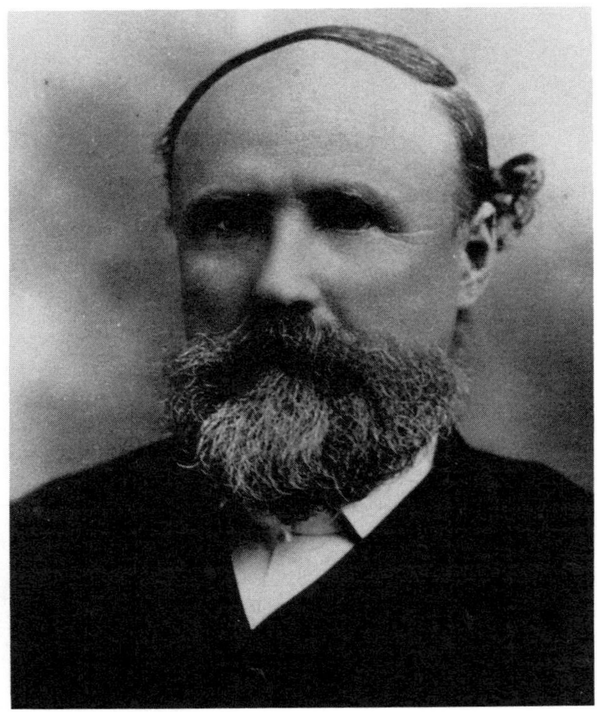

Dr. James Moore Still, brother of A. T. Still, 1889

August, 1898

FOR years seclusion has been my business day star. I have just gone along and attended to my business as I thought best and kept all my plans to myself. I have evaded and avoided notoriety in almanac, and magazine, and newspapers, and circulars in shape of cards and folders. I may be wrong but as I have had a belief that good things would find the front seat by merit, I was quite willing to keep out of the columns of all papers with stories of "my wonderful discovery." Another reason why I have preferred seclusion to publicity, is that so many absolute lies are put off on the sick folks, the voters and even the sinner, that I have gotten tired of people who are so small in merit as to need paper horns to blow their merits. I am often asked why I have not published Osteopathy in all the papers of the world and let the people know of the "wonderful truths of the great discovery." To all such questions I say the persons who have been relieved or made well, must answer such questions. I have never wanted to measure my business by the yard stick of number and dollars, but by merit only.

Our school and business has a JOURNAL in which we publish much of the science and progress of the school, also facts relative to successes of our methods of cures as proven when put to the test of the "beds of affliction." We ask no better method of solid notoriety than the statements of the once "hopelessly afflicted"—now well. If that does not suit the inquirer I know of no better way. We are now well published, but I planted only merit and waited years for the business to do its own growing to the present dimensions of which I am well pleased and hope other schools will do likewise.

Our JOURNAL was not created to be used as a medium for advertising, but to be devoted to Osteopathic literature which will all be new and original as far as possible, as this is the parent of Osteopathy. It will feel free to speak lessons of advice and on subjects of importance pertaining to Osteopathy, feeling that the tree of knowledge is ever ready to let the ripe fruits fall for the use of the JOURNAL of the American School of Osteopathy. Original contributions solicited.

PAP.

★

MY OBSERVATION OF HIP AND SHOULDER DISEASES.

AFTER a hip, shoulder, or any joint, has been out of its natural place for a long time and continues to be sore and congested, it may get well of its soreness, or it may and often does set up a torturous inflammation, by fermentation of blood and other fluids checked in the return to the heart through the veins. Such diseases of the shoulder, spine or hip, are very dangerous from the fact that the high grade of inflammation accompanying those conditions leaves the blood in a thick and ropy condition and forms clots, that accumulate in the veins and is conveyed from there to the heart producing death at once, which would leave the young Osteopath undecided whether the treatment had caused the death of the patient or not. Persons thus afflicted are liable to die without any warning, more than a soreness about the shoulder or hip joint. I will give two cases, one of the shoulder the other of the hip. My sister was thrown from a buggy, her shoulder hit the hard ground bruising the flesh and dislocating the humerus and collar bone. I adjusted her shoulder but the inflammation continued about her neck, scapula, collar bone and under her arm. She had no treatment after the bones were adjusted except the ordinary family bathings with camphor and so forth. She lived three or four years with the lymphatics very large, particularly of the lower neck, region of the clavicle. During all this time there was a swollen condition with soreness commonly called rheumatics. She could use her arm for ordinary purposes, while sewing. Without any warning she simply said, "Oh," and fell dead. That inflammation caused a clot of blood that went to the heart. The other, a sister-in-law, met with an accident which resulted in a dislocated hip which I adjusted some six or eight years afterward, which gave her normal use of the limb and reduction apparently of all swelling, which to her was very satisfactory, and flattering to the operator as a surgical result. It still retained some soreness about the hip-joint which extended up the lumbar region and to her shoulder. The day before she died she seemed to be in ordinary health, but complained of pain in the region of the groin which extended in the inner blood vessels leading to the heart. Some foreign body was pushing itself through the veins. At this time while walking across the floor she placed her hand over her heart and with an, "Oh!" fell dead; no doubt from a heart clot. My observation has caused me to arrive at this conclusion, that when a shoulder, hip, back or any other joint becomes dislocated and is not adjusted before high and general inflammatory condition in the region of joint sets in there is great danger of heart clots being formed from this cause and carried to the heart, producing death. Many from the long continued condition of the venous system could be called cancers. On the other hand I feel justified from my experience in adjusting those conditions. It relieves the sufferer from the unbearable pain about the joint and limb, and with at least nineteen out of twenty a complete recovery.

★

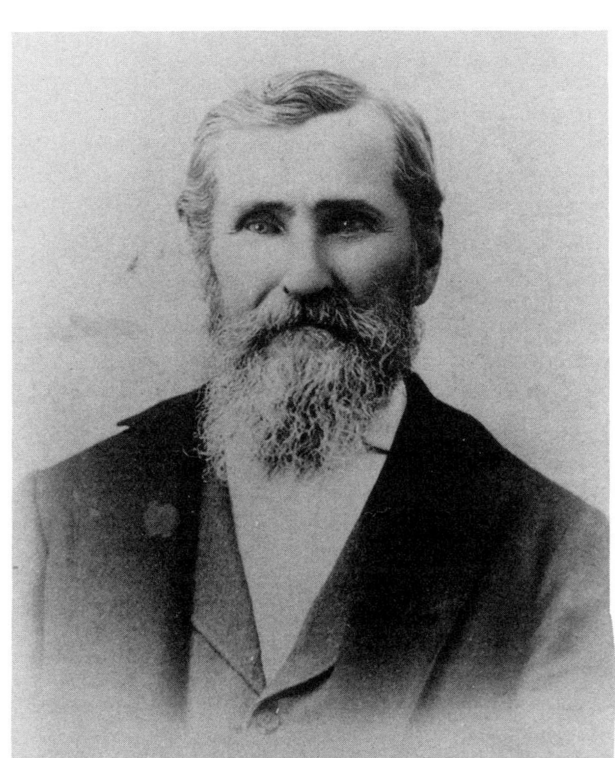

Dr. Edward Cox Still, brother of A. T. Still, 1887

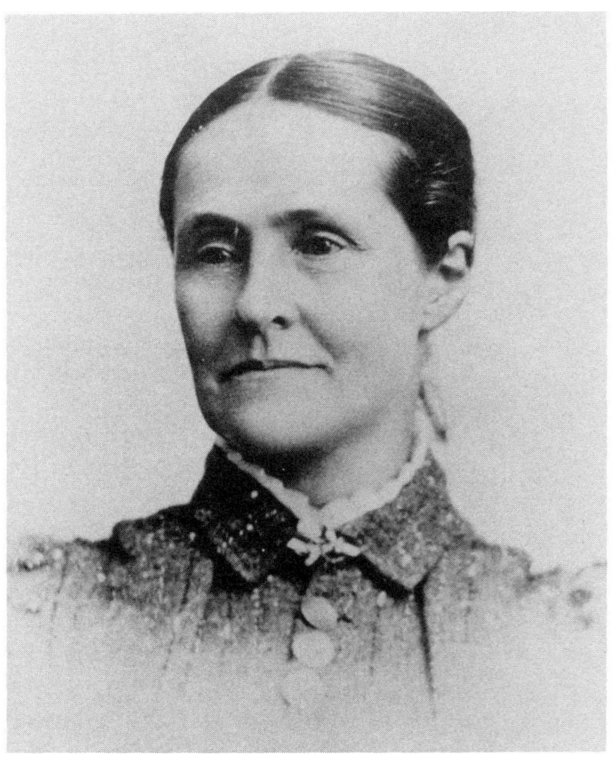

Marovia Clark Still, sister of A. T. Still, 1887

"PAP'S" CORRECTION.

I WISH to state to all students and graduates, that I have never had a "pet student" to whom I gave more attention than others. At an early day I "petted" Mrs. Bolles; later, after she left, I "petted" Mrs. Patterson; and still later, Mrs. Still, by putting them at the head of the Woman's department. I had to be with them much of the time to guard the patients from harm, and help my "pets" to a practical knowledge of Osteopathy, before I could conscientiously put them in charge of the afflicted. In those days I had no choice, as one woman was all I had on hands for the work. Now all have a much better chance to learn, because we have ample arrangements to give all thorough drills in all branches, and they do get it without exception. Such intimations as above alluded to are not true.

A. T. STILL.

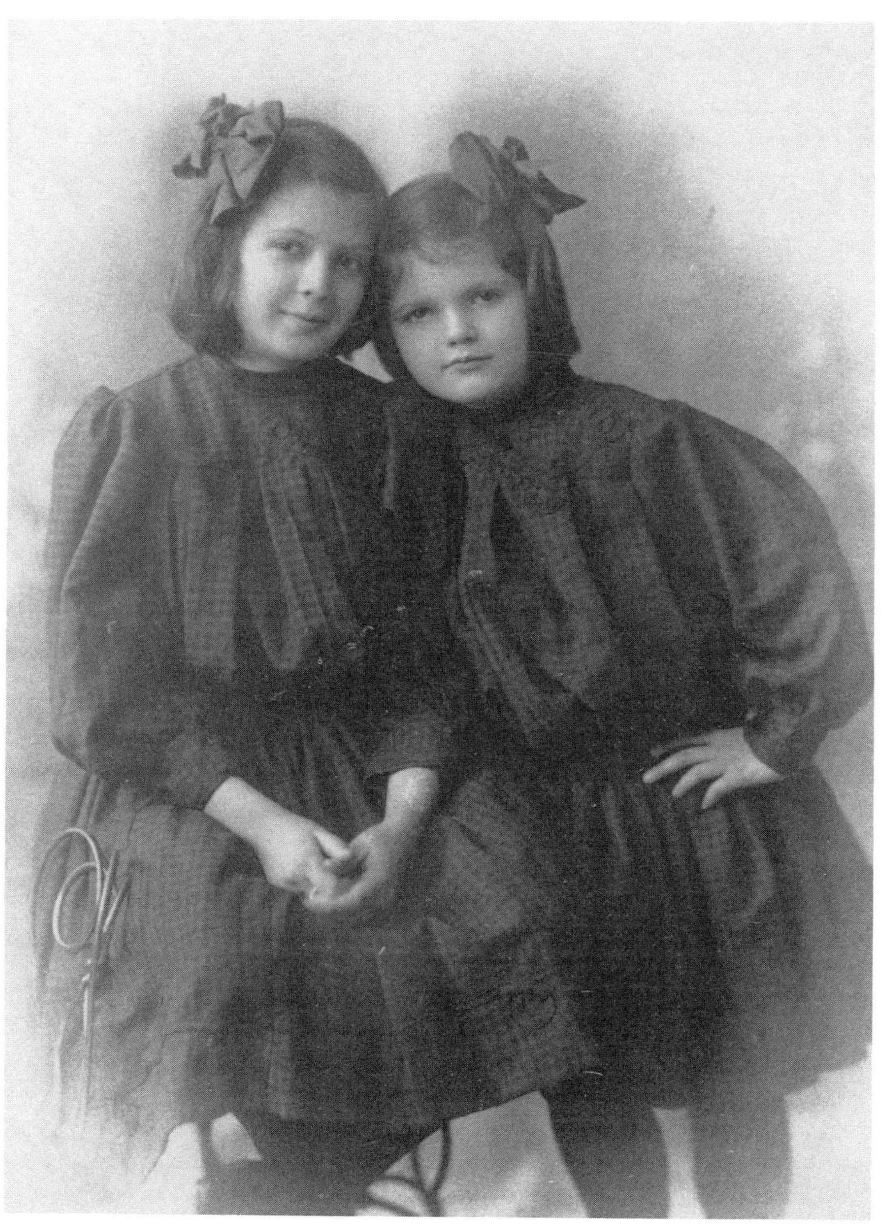

Helen Gladys and Mary Elizabeth Still, daughters of Charles E. Still, c. 1907

Millard MO Feb. 14-1899

H. Bunting K.V. Mo

I am better now.

The Journal is better now. and suits me. I had about concluded to drop it out, to stop needless wast of money. <u>My school</u> was chartered to teach Osteopathy only. Now it must foot its own expenses or go to the waste basket, I am willing to give it a reasonable time to do so. I think that can easily be done if there is any brains in running it, Do the best you can, Kindly A. T. Still

Note of A. T. Still, 1899

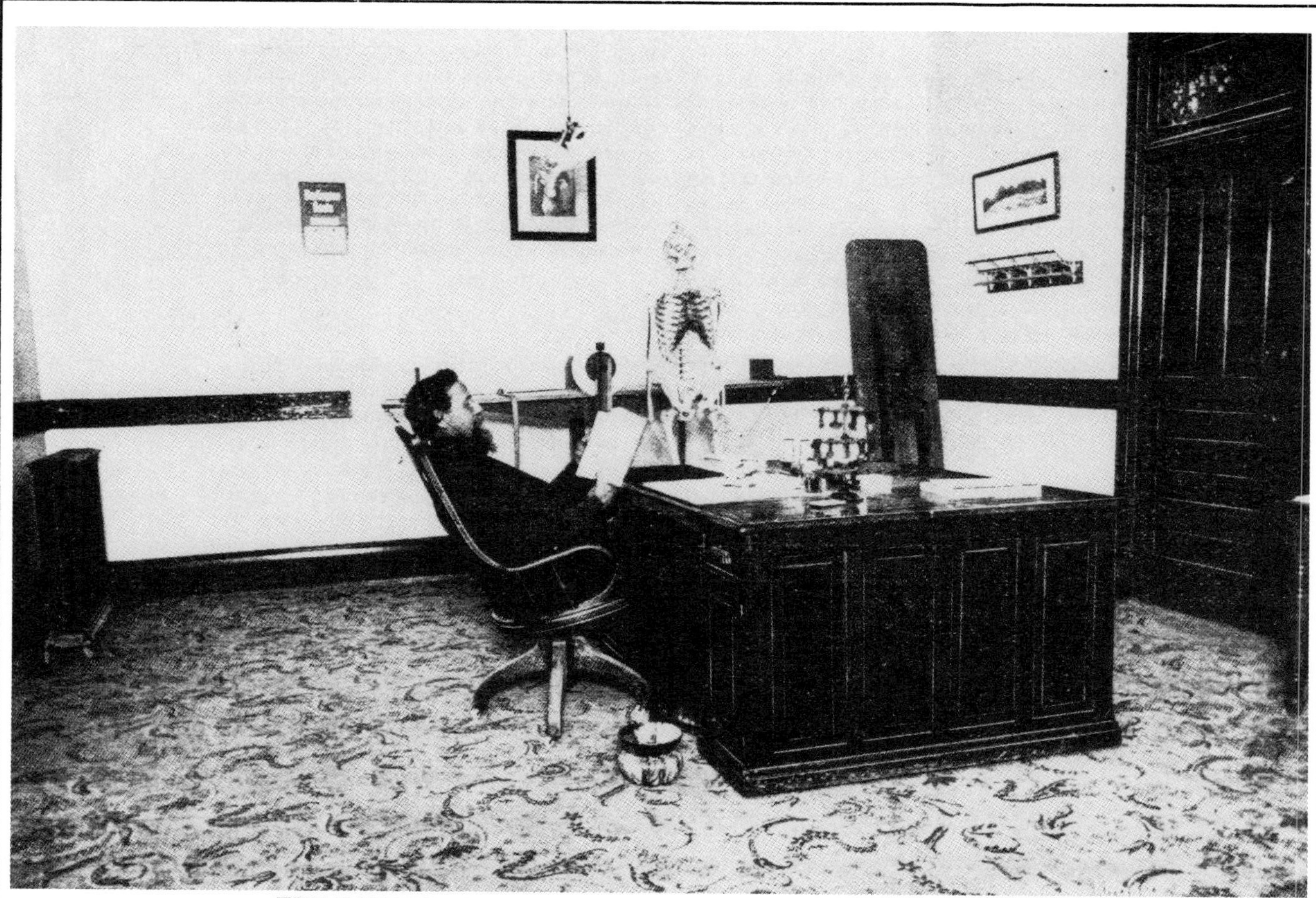

THE FATHER OF OSTEOPATHY IN HIS SEVENTY-FIRST YEAR.

August, 1898

Here is a machine for you to handle, and if you have nothing but words in place of ideas, how are you going about the job?—A. T. Still.

★

Every drug tolerated by an Osteopath in a disease will shake the confidence of your most intelligent patients, and cause them to always take your words, skill and ability at a great discount. I would advise you to bathe your heads long and often in the river of divine confidence, and pray God to take care of you with other weak minded people, who pretend to know that which they have not studied.—A. T. Still.

Let us not be governed today by what we did yesterday, nor tomorrow by what we do today, for day by day we must show progress.—A. T. Still.

★

I do not want to go back to God with less knowledge than when I was born. I want my footprints to make an impress on the field of reason. I have no desire to be a cat and walk so lighlly that it never creates a disturbance. I want my footprints to be plainly seen by all readers. I want to be myself, not "them," not "you" not "Washington," but just myself.—A. T. Still.

August, 1898

★

As an electrician controls electric currents, so the Osteopath controls life currents and revives suspended forces.—A. T. Still.

The great Inventor of the Universe, by the union of mind and matter, has constructed the most wonderful of all machines—man—and Osteopathy demonstrates fully that He is capable of running it without the aid of whiskey, opium, or kindred poisons.—A. T. Still.

If you go out thinking that Osteopathy is a good aid to medicine, you are using the words of incompetency.—A. T. Still.

August, 1898

A WORD TO ALL DIPLOMATES OF THE AMERICAN SCHOOL OF OSTEOPATHY.

WITH the space the JOURNAL has at its disposal, we cannot do any more than to say to one and all, that with the July number we gave notice that "goodbye write ups" would cease, as you all have diplomas that carry on their faces the names of the teachers and officers of the most thoroughly equipped and the oldest school of Osteopathy, and it has long since earned a character at home and abroad as a standard authority, and papers now issned by it are a recommendation to any lady or gentleman holding them. We hope you all will do much good and be well remunerated for your labors. So far the reports received from all are good, with great praise for their alma mater. We could say much more in praise of those who have taken their degrees here, and have then gone out to all parts of the world. So far, nearly every one has been a brilliant success. It is the wish of the JOURNAL to kindly support all diplomates of the American School of Osteopathy. It is your friend and will honestly sustain all the worthy graduates of that school.

A. T. S.

DISEASES OF THE SEASONS.

AS the year is divided into four distinct seasons, it would be wise and proper for the Osteopathic practitioner to adjust his thoughts accordingly. As this is the summer season we will speak about those parts of the body that give away to the effects of heat and cold, as indicated by bowel troubles, liver complaints, and general prostration of the nervous system. Thus you have to contend with, and consider what nerve and blood supply is deranged in flux, cholera morbus, cholera infantum, and summer fevers generally and direct your treatment accordingly.

Later as the season changes we have fall diseases which are traceable to derangement of the spinal chord, from heat, resulting in chills and fever with congestion of the blood vessels of lungs, stomach, bowels and other parts of the system, which are known as periodic diseases.

Still later on we have diseases peculiar to winter; such as pneumonia, pleurisy, and typhoid diseases. Thus your attention is drawn to the sensory and motor nerves of the lungs, plura, etc.

Then come in the diseases of the spring season; such as diphtheria, scarlet fever, measles and various other kinds of rash. If you govern your thoughts as indicated, you will have much less mental confusion to contend with in conbatting disease, being ready for each in turn.

At the close of each season the JOURNAL would be glad to have a short and concise report of your successes and difficulties, together with such observations and conclusions you have arrived at, that there may be a general and systematic consensus of Osteopathic experiences for the benefit of all Osteopaths. Thus local and individual experience is specially valuable to all as diptheria may prevail in one section, yellow fever in another, malaria in another, and so on according to climate and location, and thus each will be able to profit by the experience of all, in the matter of combatting disease in whatever form it may present itself.

A. T. S.

DR. A. T. STILL'S DEPARTMENT.

THE DRAGON OF IGNORANCE.

APPEARED from the muddy waters of that ocean whose surface never sustained a compass by which reason was pointed to any shore. This dragon of tyrannical stupidity closed his eyes and ears to the panorama of the eternal beauties in form, paintings and decorations of color.

This dragon hates and dreads reason, and would sacrifice the child of thought upon the altar of his selfish ambition. He seeks and labors to dwell under the dark clouds of fog. The black smoke and deadly gases are his breath and happy dwelling place. He hates and would kill the child whom he finds sitting in the bright light of the ascending sun of progress. He hates the mother whose body gave that child birth, who unbosoms her breast with milk and love to nourish and encourage that child whose choice is light in preference to darkness. His amusements are the groans, shrieks and moans of that child's loving mother. That dirty old dragon has prostrated nations that were flowered and perfumed with learning, prosperity and progress. He has burned the manuscripts and books of the literati of the world. Like a blood-hound no foot-prints of intelligence can grow too old for his ability to keep on their tracks. He makes hideous gods who are minus of all that is good and lovable; strengthens their arms that they may destroy all that do not love such gods. He was never known to create a god whose love extended beyond the personality of a brute. In his god making he left out every principle of kindness, intelligence and love, except that of his own foolish dogmatism. He would destroy all who sought to acquaint themselves with that God who creates and qualifies all his beings to live and labor for personal and universal comforts. He is always busy traveling from nation to nation. He is very fond of whiskey, beer and wine. He is a successful general; he attends to but one business and that one business all the time. He dynamites, shells and destroys every fort in which he finds liberty and reason. He hates man and all men whose day-star is intelligence, whose eyes observe, minds comprehend and tongues speak the beauties of nature. He hates that God in whom reason dwells. He is never so happy as when he builds and armors a fort and knows it is well officered with well drilled bigotry; he knows such generals will make and keep him happy. He is so jealous of man's happiness and brotherly love that he will destroy the usefulness of the assembled statesmen with his drunken bitters, and is never more happy than when he receives the tidings that his chief executive is on a drunken spree.

September, 1898

Flux, (Bloody Dysentery.)

FLUX is common in all temperate climates. It generally shows its true nature as dysentery, after a few hours of tired feeling, with aching in head, back and bowels. At first nothing is felt or thought of more than a few movements of the bowels than is common for each day. Some pain and griping are felt with increase at each stool, until a chilly feeling is felt all over the body, with violent pains in lower bowels, with pressing desire to go to stool, and during and after passage of stool a feeling that there is still something in the bowels that must pass. In a short time that down pressure partially subsides and on examination of passage a quantity of blood is seen, which shows the case to be "bloody flux," as the disease is called and known in the Southern states of North America, or bloody dysentery in the more Northern states. It generally subsides by the use of family remedies, such as sedatives, astringents and pallative diets. But the severity in other cases increases with time, there is greater pain, discharges have more blood mixed with gelatinous substance even to mucous membrane of bowels, high fever all over except abdomen which is quite cold to the hand. Back, head and limbs suffer much with heat and pain, much nausea is felt at all motions of the bowels. Bowels change from cold to hot even to 104, at which time all symptoms point to inflammation of the bowels, the colon in particular, at which time discharges grow black, frothy and very offensive from decomposition of blood. Soon collapse and death close out the case, notwithstanding the very best skill has been employed to save the life of the patient. He has tried to stop pain by opiates and other sedatives, tried to check bowels by astringents, used tonics and stimulants, but all have failed—the patient is dead.

But a question for the Osteopath: At what point would you work to suppress the sensation of the colon and allow veins to open and let blood return to heart? Does irritation of a sensory nerve cause vein to contract and refuse blood to complete circuit from and to the heart? Does flux begin in the sensory nerves of bowels? If so reduce sensation at all points of bowels, stop all over-pluses, keep veins free and open from cutaneous to deep sensory ganglion of whole spine and abdomen. Remember the fascia is what suffers and dies in all cases of death by bowels and lungs. Thus the nerves of all the fascia of bowels and abdomen must work or you will lose all cases of flux, for in the fascia is all the soothing and vital qualities of nature. Guard it well so it can work and repair all losses, or death may begin in the fascia and pass through the whole system.

Scholarship and Agreement.

This, Agreement, made and entered into by and between the **American School of Osteopathy,** of Kirksville, Missouri, party of the first part, and

Mrs M. Katherine Fitzharris

party of the second part;

Witnesseth, THAT: In consideration of the sum of Three Hundred Dollars as tuition, and other good and sufficient considerations, receipt of which is duly acknowledged by the said first party, the said second party is hereby entitled to attend the said American School of Osteopathy two full years, with all the rights and privileges of a pupil therein.

This scholarship and agreement is not transferable nor assignable; nor will any part of the above tuition be refunded on account of discontinuance in attendance for any cause, except in case of death or disability of second party, when the said first party may, at its option, provide for such adjustment by transfer or refund, as it may deem best.

As a part of the consideration of admission into said school the said second party hereby agrees never to engage in the practice of Osteopathy without first having obtained a DIPLOMA from said School or some other recognized, reputable, legally chartered School of Osteopathy, nor practice Osteopathy in Adair county, Missouri, nor aid any one in so doing; nor never engage in going from place to place in the State of Missouri to remain for a few weeks or months in the practice of Osteopathy; but shall have the privilege of locating in any place permanently, to build up a practice, outside of said Adair county, Missouri.

It is further agreed that any fraud or deceit which may be practiced to gain admission into said school; any wilful breach of propriety or gross immorality; the usage of intoxicants as a beverage; gambling or frequenting gambling places; or persistent refusal to obey the rules and by-laws of said school, shall cause a forfeiture of all money paid, and subject the said second party to suspension from said school.

IN WITNESS WHEREOF, said parties have this, the 27th day of June 1899, subscribed to two copies hereof, one to be retained by each.

THE AMERICAN SCHOOL OF OSTEOPATHY,

By Warren Hamilton Secretary.

M. Catherine Fitzharris

They Never Die.

KIND words like rivers of life are the odors of thought, the dews and muscles of durability, the stay and comfort of the worrying man or woman who tries to reason or travel a road that runs through the forest of darkness, that must be crossed by all who see the lights beyond the brush of the untrodden paths of faith and logical truth.

A kind word lightens the weighted and sinking heart until it can run to the harbor of rest. One kind word is water to the fast wilting tree of hope. There are a few in my heart whose duration has been many years, and are cherished today as rivers of joy, on whose surface float great streams loaded with unspeakable thanks for him, or her, whoever gave me a smile and held even a lamp on shore to guide my boat to the stoneless channels of safe delivery. Those mites from a friend dropped in my cup which I drank as a famishing being, relished, as none other could, but he who had cruised in seas great and small for truth. I think of those smiles and cheering words as the brightest stars and gems of all my days. Our great word "love" fails to express my feelings to those that said, "merit is the choicest jewel of all lives," and will attend all funerals of opposition, because it cannot die, no never! Give me your kind words and keep all else; and when I am dead and my tongue loses its power, I will ask the bones of my tomb to thank you for them.

Old as Time, True as God.

CAUSE and effect as law, are just the same; a thousand years shows no rust. Each day the "man of God" has added to his powers heavier drafts of knowledge, and of the kind that is useful—a kind that will dilate or contract, and eject all unsound and useless words or teachings.

I have said the "man of God" because he cannot be anything else and possess an existence. His existence in form is the effect of life; the cause antedates him by mind and deed. His construction and action in completeness prove conclusively that thought and cause preceeded his coming. He is the effect, and debtor to cause. If he is the result of cause and cause is eternal, and effect also, why not say the race of man is eternal?

With no conclusive evidence that man's existence is as old as cause, his life, or spirit, must be the cause of his form. His form is an effect which was produced by the cause commonly known as life. Cause has no beginning, then by cause and being of cause, he is eternal; and as such is bound to pass all the mile posts of coming eternity, as he has those of the past.

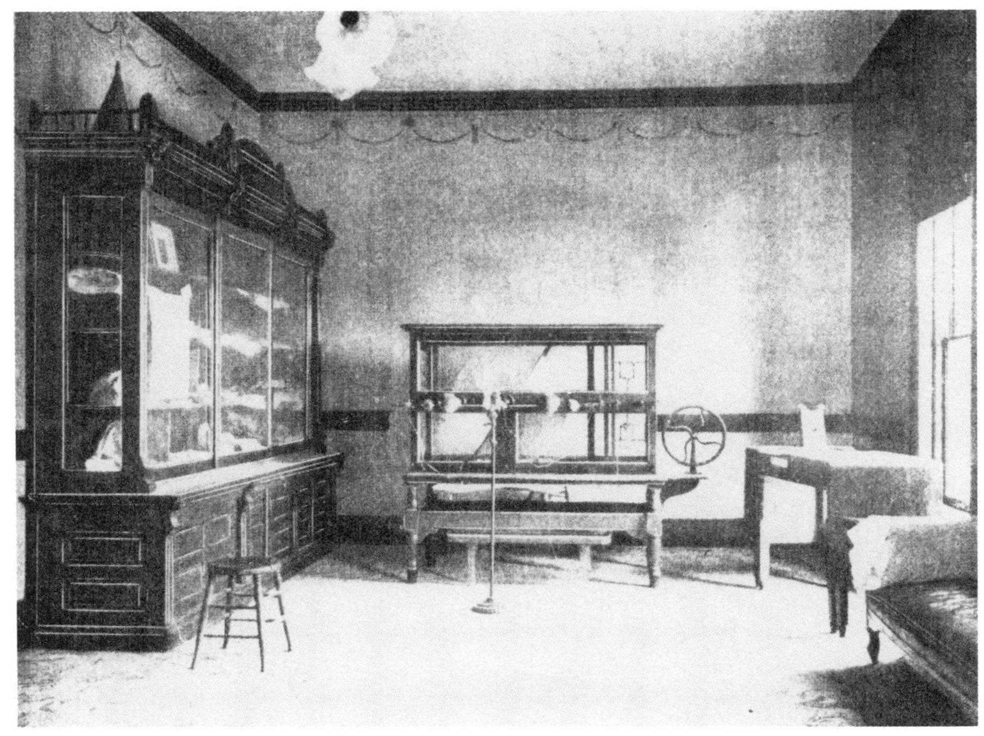

WHERE SOME OF THE MOST ADVANCED X-RADIANCE IN THE WORLD IS DONE.

A CONTEMPORARY conglomerate Medical Journal has said that inside of five years there will not be an Osteopathic school in existence that has not medicine attached to it. We will acknowledge that there is danger of the sow returning to her wallow. With the many that have graduated from the American School of Osteopathy there have been many kinds of heads. Some have brains enough to resist, while others are weak. Some are great thinkers, some are great fools, some have less honor than a hyena, they would crucify all truths, lie to their patients, administer morphine, whiskey, blisters, or any other damnable drug if they could make one dollar or one cent by crucifying every principle of truth. Such animals have been in and gone out from this institution. They brought their drugs and dishonesty with them and will break every injunction of the ten commandments of Holy Writ, and tell a bare-face lie to any old woman, man or child, if they can get one copper more by so doing. They are not now, never have been, and never will be anything but Osteopathic-medical dummies. If Osteopathy ever dies it will be by the encouragement it receives from such unthoughtful, conglomerate concessions who know that God's work is mechanical in form in all things, and the results of the chemical laboratories placed in man and animals are sufficient for sickness or health, or your God is not perfection as commonly taught. You may serve such red-nosed mutton-head gods; I have no use for them or their friends. The God of pure Osteopathy keeps no saloon, practices no deception and tells no lies.

September, 1898

Answers to Questions.

I FEEL to answer through the Journal questions that are asked by thousands of persons annually. And as time adds days and years the number of persons who ask those questions have multiplied to such greatness in numbers that is absolutely impossible to find the time to answer them in detail. And I am not sure that I can answer all of them through the Journal, but will try and so arrange that a few of the most common ones will be answered as best I can.

By my method of reasoning I arrive at the conclusion that man was, after receiving his form, like unto the world on which he dwells, and that in his body could be found all the mineral, vegetable and animal substances that could be found in the beast of the field, the fowls of the air, fishes of the sea both great and small, in short all that was contained in this and all other planets and beings, from the throne of God (himself included), to the lowest form of animated beings; that in the human being all attributes of mental and physical were represented in kind.

With this conclusion I proceeded and did obtain what I have proclaimed and proven to be truths universal in kind and action, submitting to and being governed by one common law. I reasoned that all effects as are shown in disease with the result of the productions of the truths of the one great common law, mind and motion expressing themselves through matter. Motion is an effect of life with its powers. Disease in any form or presentation was another effect. Conception of beings, diseases and worlds, were the biogenic answer of the wombs of nature either large or small, believing while I was in the chambers of sober and intelligent nature where honest reason only can dwell, that it was safe to follow the teachings of that principle that made no mistakes that I could detect.

THE world's systems of cures by drugs are now and always have been based on three principles, namely: opiates, purgatives and stimulants. And the difference there is in the schools of medicine are about all told in the quantities to be given. All give deadly poisons but try to get the same results. Allopathy starts the ball to rolling by big pills, Eclecticism the same, but claims that vegetable medicines are better than mineral preparations. Then the Homeopath closes by pills of less size, and if they fail he drives morphine under the skin and spills it in the fascia, which carries the opium to the brain and produces effects by paralyzing sensation. And on these three principles all depend.

Contented Ignorance.

A PERSON who learns just enough to make money enough to live on and gives no farther attention to mental researches, drifts to a condition of satisfaction with doing today what he did yesterday. He is easy and his mind dreads to study, his body takes command of all his mental energies; he goes no farther and finally stops at the place that he should rush his mind to the greatest activity. But he has tasted ease and enjoys ignorance. He plays chess, drinks wine, sleeps well and comes out on cloudy days to give light by way of giving the sun rest. He feels his dazzling brilliancy and wants all fraternities to join the funeral procession that retires his shining mind from the people who will miss his solar rays and comforts, the satellites of that great head who gave so much light even to fixed stars, and makes the babes say, "Twinkle, twinkle little star." Your life is short but the book of nature is long and full of life and joy.

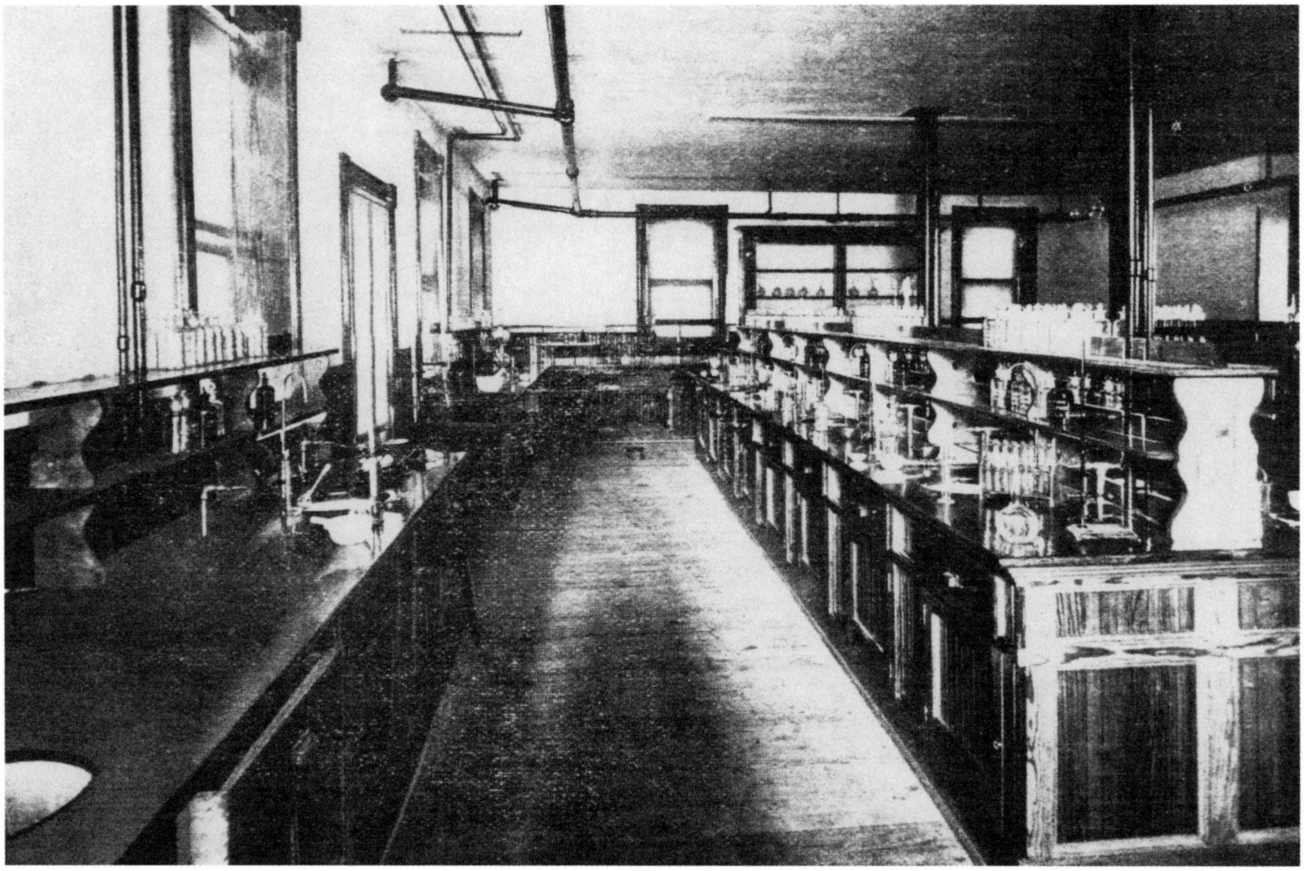

WHERE PHYSIOLOGICAL CHEMISTRY IS MASTERED.

September, 1898

"MEDICAL OSTEOPATHY."

MANY uninformed persons are asking themselves the question, should drugs and Osteopathy go together? Those who ask this question are of the class but ltttle posted in the science of Osteopathy. If drugs are right Osteopathy is all wrong; if Osteopathy is anything in the healing of diseases it is everything and drugs are nothing. This may seem a bold assertion but there is not a true Osteopath living who will not back up the assertion. The man who pretends to be an Osteopath and at the same time uses drugs wants the dollar and is neither an M. D. nor an Osteopath. If he must depend on his drugs at all, why not be honest and depend on them wholly and not attach D. O. to his name in order to draw custom.

Osteopathy and drugs are so opposite that one might as well say white is black as speak of Medical Osteopathy. You can no more mix medicine and Osteopathy than you can oil and water. The man or woman who has this science deeply imbedded in his or her heart and head, who understands its principles, would blush for shame to be called a "Medical Osteopath."

Nevertheless there are certain schools which pretend to teach medicine and Osteopathy. They are said to be the Medical Osteopathic Institutions, which like the bat are neither bird nor beast, and have no classification. They are mongrel institutions, snares, set to capture the unwary and unthinking.

Let us look at the question with calm and unprejudiced minds for a few moments. To acquire a complete Osteopathic education will take two years. Two years is the very shortest time in which the very best trained minds can cover this wonderful subject. What we say is the observation of educated ladies and gentlemen who have gone through the course of study. They admit that two years is short enough.

To acquire a medical education requires four years, as approved by the best medical colleges. There are some which still cling to the three year rule, but all of the best have raised the standard to four years. Now if you intend to be a medical doctor I would advise you to go to the very best medical college, where you will have to study four years before you can get a diploma. Say that you want both medicine and Osteopathy, then in order to be perfect in both you must put in four years in medicine and two in Osteopathy, making six years in college to complete both sciences. If this is true doesn't any sane man or woman know that no school can instruct in both sciences in two years? The man or woman who pays his money into such institutions gets neither medicine nor Osteopathy, but a smattering, enough to make a first class quack.

But some may argue that you might double up on some of the studies; that Anatomy for the Osteopath would do for the M. D. This would onlybe shortening one year, which would make it five years. Then again, suppose you attend one of the cheapest of medical colleges with only three years, and allowing one year for doubling in anatomy, there is no system of deduction known on earth which would place the term shorter than four years, which these people attempt to teach in two years.

I have so often laid down the law that Osteopathy is hostile to the drug theory that it seems almost superfluous to repeat it here. Every man and woman sick and tired of drugs, opiates, stimulants, laxatives and purgatives has turned with longing eyes to this Rainbow of hope. It has been held out as free from whiskey and poisons, and yet these Medical Osteopaths are trying to paint this rainbow with calomel and perfume it with whiskey. It seems strange that divines who make spread eagle speeches on temperance, who claim to love Osteopathy because it is strictly a temperance method of healing, should so far lose their self control as to lead off after the false god of drugs. Are they any better than the man who makes temperance speeches to the public for which he is paid, then takes a drink in private just to stimulate him for another tirade on whiskey? To those pious Osteopaths who mix medicine with Osteopathy, we might quote the following,—Matthew XXIII-14 and 15.

"Woe unto you, scribes and Pharisees, hypocrites! for ye devour widows' houses, and for a *pretence* make long prayers, therefore ye shall receive greater damnation. Woe unto you, scribes and Pharisees, hypocrites! for ye compass sea and land to make one proselyte; and when he is made, ye make him two-fold more the child of hell than yourselves."

What Christ addressed to the Pharisees might be very well spoken of the men who pretend to believe in Osteopathy as a health producing, life saving temperance science, and then wed God's cure with the ignorance of drugs which debases and ruins mankind.

I wish to quote a little of history here, in connection with Osteopathy. About the time I had discovered and perfected the science of Osteopathy, there came to me a man who had suffered with asthma for twelve long years. His case was a serious one, but I cured him in a short course of treatment. This man had been a teacher in a country school, a peddler of lightning rods and a real estate agent. The lightning rod on my house today bears evidence of his skill as a lightning rod manipulator.

He desired to enter on the study of Osteopathy and I took him in as a student, and while under my guidance the ex lightning rod peddler could treat with some success. About the year 1893 or 4, this student left me and set up to practice what he called "Boney-Opathy," under the control and management of "ZENO OF ATHENS," a gentleman who died some 2000 years ago. It was, I think, in 1894 or '95, when he disappeared very suddenly, and next was heard from at a medical school which was expelled from the national association on account of its low standard as a scientific institution.

After two or three years study in the medical college he in 1897 went west to establish an institution to which he proposed at first to give a new name. But after various deliberations and consultations with his managers, they decided on having the word Osteopathy attached to it, because Osteopathy had won considerable reputation. There was money in the name Osteopathy. Was this really honest? Can the institution be an institution of Osteopathy, when it teaches the very evil which Osteopathy cures, viz. drugs? Yet, unfortunately there are many so unwise as to be deceived into the belief that black and white could blend and each preserve its individuality.

There is another institution in a neighboring state pretending to give a course in Osteopathy and medicine in two years. The president of the institution is not an Osteopath, never graduated in any Osteopathic school, but is a masseuse. As a proof that these people teach massage instead of Osteopathy, they recently advocated in a magazine that treatments should be from thirty to fifty minutes; the time required for a masseur but not an Osteopath.

In looking over the faculty one sees surgeons, M. D.'s and practically but one or two Osteopaths. Can such institutions be called Osteopathic colleges? If it takes two years of hard, very hard study to acquire a knowledge of Osteopathy, then why waste half that time in medicine? If it takes three or four years to learn medicine, is any man or woman insane enough to suppose that by adding another science the whole can be learned in two years? Such an idea is too preposterous for discussion. When it comes to the legality of the diploma's issued by such institutions they may be questioned. To be an Osteopath one must be a graduate of a regularly chartered college or school, where they are required to be in actual attendance and study the science in its manifold branches for two terms of ten months each. If you have studied Osteopathy ten months, and medicine ten months, you are neither an Osteopath nor a medical doctor, and who will say you are legally qualified to practice in States that have adopted laws for the regulation and practice of Osteopathy. No true Osteopath can believe in medicine, the very evil it is to regulate. If one wants an Osteopath to treat his ailments he wants a true Osteopath and not one who is a half and half. If one wants a medical doctor he will secure a graduate from a real medical college, not some half and half who is nothing.

If you are going to be an Osteopath don't be a sham, but a genuine Osteopath. Put all your time on the study of the science in some reputable school and when you have graduated have a diploma of which you will not be ashamed, and which the law will recognize and give you its protection.

Take an unfinished course in a mongrel school and will not your conscience always whisper that you are a law breaker.

A. T. STILL.

September, 1898

"THE American School of Osteopathy is a trust," you say! I say it can be trusted to teach, and does teach all that is necessary to make a trusted doctor to go into all combats with diseases. He is taught standard surgery and midwifery and can be trusted to deliver the child in less time and with less misery to the mother than all the old school M. D's on earth combined can do. Our school is a growing trust, that trusts that some time men will see that drugs go down the necks of the ignorant only, and the dopes are given by men who do so for two reason only, first to get money; second because they know too little of Osteopathy, to cure, either with or without drugs.

A. T. S.

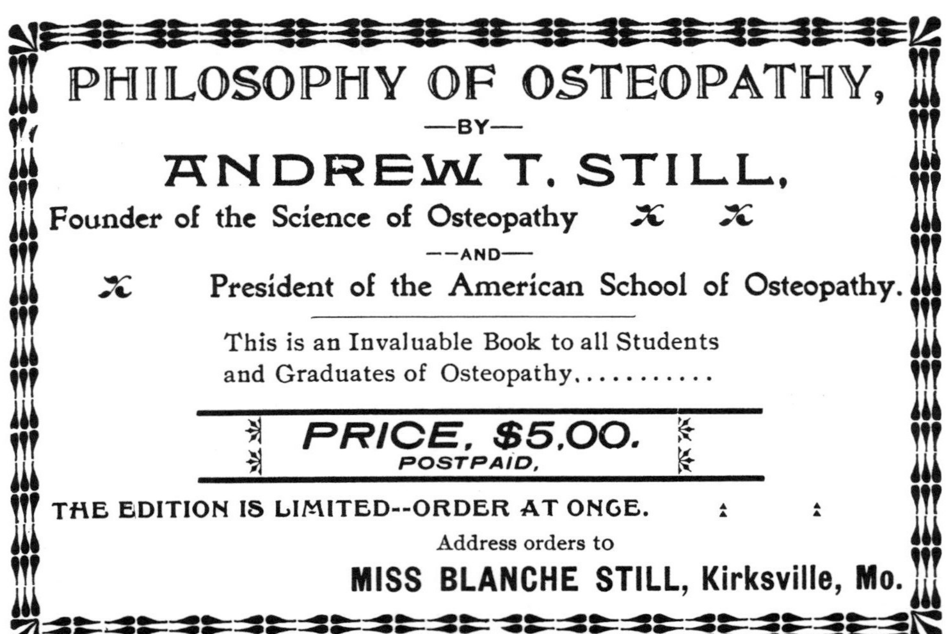

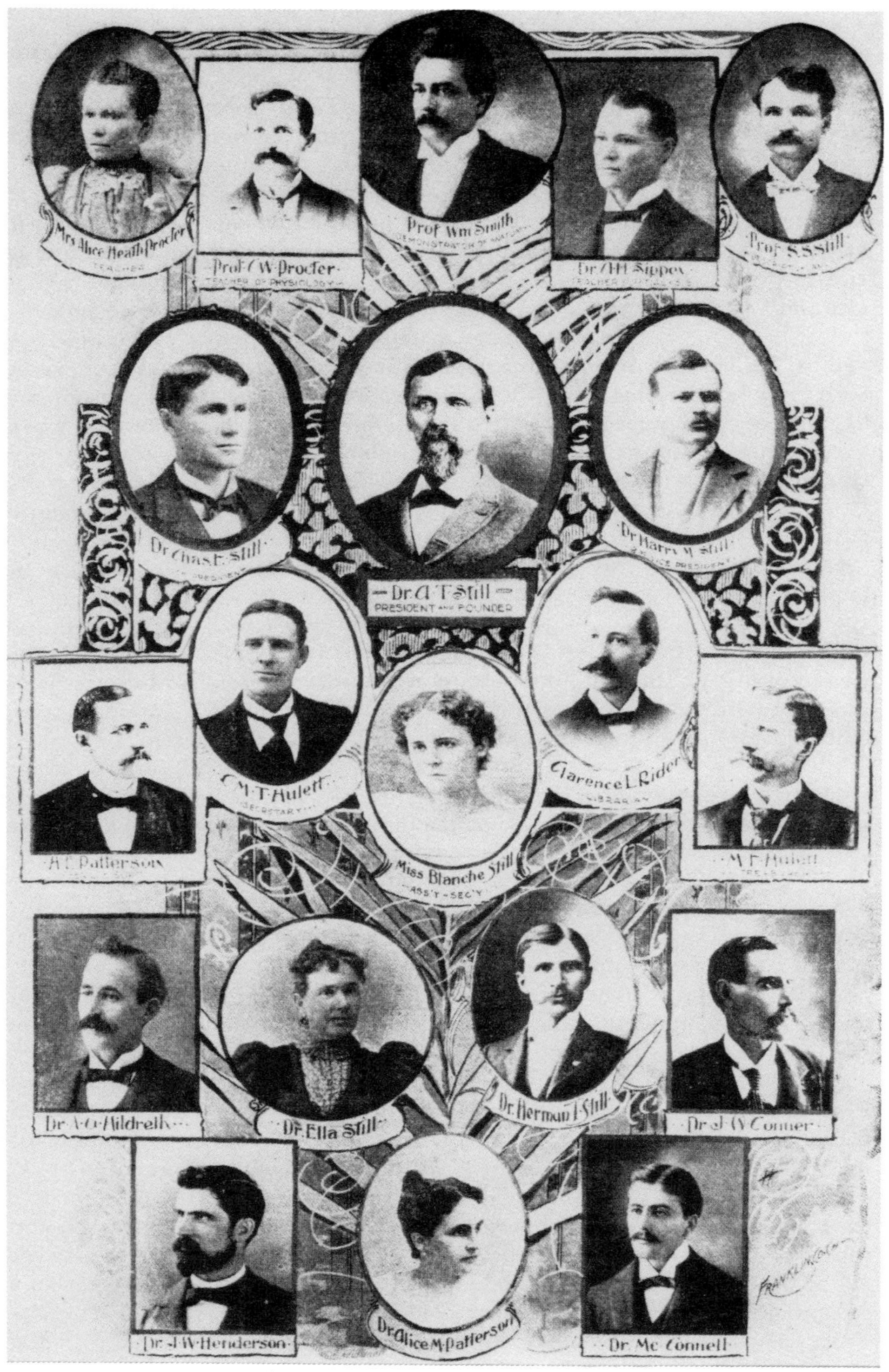

Officers, teachers, and operators, 1897

October, 1898

DR. A. T. STILL'S DEPARTMENT.

Information for Patients.

SOME die and we cannot help it. We would save all if we could, but many come too late; disease has got in its work, and the case is without hope. I would give worlds to be able to cure and send all home well.

One comes in the last stages of consumption, when the whole lung is a mass of ruin, and body dead in all its powers to sustain life. He or she expects to get cured and go to their homes blooming with the red face and powerful sinews of life, just as others have done before disease had done its deadly work.

Another class come with dropsy. They soon yield to treatment, recover and go home rejoicing in health, while another class die and are returned in their coffins. They are dropsical from other causes, which may be the effects of the last stages of cancer.

That the afflicted may know better what to hope for, I write this to inform them that diseases do not all carry the same amount of hope to the sufferer, when they book at my Infirmary for treatment. While about seventy-five per cent. of the cases of asthma are curable in from two to four months, others go longer, because of the low stage of the vitality of the system, to build up wasted lung tissue. There is hope for relief in all cases of asthma and a cure for a great majority.

Many cases supposed to be consumption are not consumption, but asthma in a disguised form. A majority of such cases are curable, and consumption taken before the point of repairing has been passed is curable, I think, in many cases.

Heart diseases are not all alike. The heart and blood vessels often have cancerous growths and derange the flow of blood to prostration, and so found on post mortem examination, others by pressure of ribs on heart or nerves, cause great annoyance, but are generally curable cases of palpitation and other diseases of heart.

Thus you must expect nothing when you come, but to learn just what we think your disease is, and you must patiently give us time for a deliberate decision as to your disease and its cause. We will tell you of the probability of cure and about the length of time required for such.

At this time we will draw your attention to a serious truth, which is this: No two cases are just alike. Nature is infinite in variety. We may have had a thousand cases of brain, heart, lung, liver, stomach,bowels and uterus, previous to your entry, with no two affecting the system in the same way. Yesterday furnishes but little that would be of benefit in deciding to-day what your case is, with its curability or death tendency.

Out of the hundreds of cases of asthma that we have treated there has been a general sameness but no two alike. A case of asthma with paralysis of one side is not like a case with cancer of the breast, neither is it like that of a one legged or one armed man, and the treatment must be different, because of other parts of the body being disabled.

A tortuous pain in the heel may produce convulsions from the heel being bruised, while another heel giving just as much or more pain may have as its cause dislocation of hip, lumbar, or dorsal vertebra, rib or some point of the neck. The same may be the result of miscarriage; it may be followed by spinal meningitis or brain disease itself. You must recollect that one sentence from you has asked a compound question. To be answered correctly we have to review a thousand causes and select the cause of your trouble. True Osteopathy does not feel satisfied to give you an answer in reference to your disease and its cause, in anything like conjectures.

A small wound of a sensory nerve, or a pressure, may produce a raving maniac, convulsions, St. Vitus dance, constipation, leucorrhea, gall stone, bladder stones, eruptions of the skin, consumption and death, because of the center or locality, where this wound is received.

My advice to you previous to coming as a patient of mine would be to be patient mentally, yourself; be reasonable, because on the wisdom of the examination and decision depends our ability to give you a truthful answer.

A severe headache may last for many years. With almost an imperceptible dislocation of some articulation of the neck, which holds a very small nerve tight, which extends to the brain and governs some blood supply this may be the cause of that headache, or if not able of itself to be the cause may partially dislocate the lower or twelfth rib, or unduly tighten some muscle of the illeo lumbar system sufficient to derange the functions of the kidneys; with this addition we have a cause for headache.

Now if you know nothing of the effects caused by such combination it will be well for you to set aside your judgment in favor of knowledge which comes from an intimate acquaintance with the whole human system, which is anatomical in form, physiological in action.

Right here I wish to inform the patient that he must remember that he has not come to my Infirmary as a matter of choice, for many of you according to your own statement, have come here through the persuasion of your friends, and to humor your friends, with no hope whatever of being benefited. Many of you come in a frame of mind and mouth, that makes our first interview with you very unpleasant. Many open the interview with the assertion that they have no confidence in us or anything else, for they have tried everything, and found no relief. At this time the counseling physician has to wade over morphine, whisky and every known drug, with all its crazy effects to get at the mind of the new patient, who has been more injured by the deleterious effects of drugs than the ravages of the disease. Thus you see that we have reason to desire that you end the interview at once. Nothing but humanity would cause us to consent to a continuation of the great annoyance that presents itself at the first interview. The matter of financial profit would bar you at once from treatment, or further interview, for facts and figures show that we spend each year several thousand dollars more for the afflicted than we receive from them. I draw from other sources that you may be benefited. It requires such a large force of costly operators to treat the charity patients, who outnumber greatly those who pay a small pittance, that the one fails to remunerate for the expense of the other. Inasmuch as we have consented to treat you kindly and if possible give you relief, we ask it on your side that you be good to yourself, and us also.

October, 1898

Schools by Comparison.

THE American School of Osteopathy bears no comparison to other schools to date. It is the fountain head of Osteopathy. It is the first school to teach, practice and demonstrate the principles of Osteopathy as taught and practiced by its founder, A. T. Still. His knowledge of Osteopathy and its needs, qualify him ~~to~~ select suitable professors to teach all branches necessary to a thorough knowledge of the science. Next, but not least, the building is suited to the requirements of the school, with all instruments and appliances to impart knowledge to the student, with proper deposits to make all contracts good, from the entry to a completed course, as published in catalogue.

"The American School of Osteopathy is destined to become one of the greatest institutions in the world, because it marks the success of one of the world's greatest discoveries in this century. For more than twenty years has this grand old man, Dr. Andrew Taylor Still, given every moment and thought of his time to the perfecting of this science. And the city of Kirksville, and this American School of Osteopathy, the only one of its kind in the world, should be known as the GRAND CENTER of Osteopathy."

These are the words spoken by A. L. Conger, in Memorial Hall, March 4th, 1897. And as such is this school known at home and abroad.

Pap.

I WANT all persons who may read the Journal to know that I do not now, never have nor ever will allow my name to be used for the promotion of any school other than the American School of Osteopathy until they are at least four years old and their diplomates prove that their alma mater in teaching in all branches is thorough and equal on examination to the American School of Osteopathy.

I will never be a member of any trust, political, religious, commercial or scientific. I want to excel in merit only, and kindly hope it will always win, and hope other schools that may or have opened will enter the race to "beat"—we know nothing equal to individual success.

A. T. Still.

October, 1898

TO DIPLOMATES.

WE are glad to receive letters often from all diplomates of the American School of Osteopathy. We want to know what success you have with yellow fever and other diseases you meet with in different parts of the world; not what patients say in long letters of thanks, but what you know by proof in the rooms of the sick. We will give you credit for what you do. Send reports in your own way and over your own signatures.

A. T. S.

DOCTORS AND JUSTICE TO THEM.

WHEN we opened our Journal it was for the purpose of publishing truths that would be of mental benefit to the reader. I think we should speak the truth of our living and dead doctors they have done the best they could to give the sick relief in all ages. No doubt they have made many blunders or failures but not of choice, but because disease with cause was not understood, but the writer is in honor bound to say that the doctor's untiring perseverance has advanced his knowledge of surgery and all branches of his school; he has given much time and study to the physiology of human life. More dissection is now done in five years than has been done in previous centuries; dissection today does not mean to mangle the human body with saw and knife beyond recognition, but to obtain a better knowledge of form and function of the body.

But little has been known of the physiological work that is going on all the time in the labratory of life that is in all animals. The doctor does the best he can, but unlike other professions, he has to deal with hidden causes, from start to finish. He lives a life of "hide-and-seek." Nature hides the cause of disease in the dense forest of truth, peculiar to its own laws of life and decay. Man never knows just where the seeds of diseases are deposited; he has to deal all the time with effect only, with the cause hidden far off in the clouds of mystery, and there is nothing to govern his actions but to act on such suggestions as symptoms indicate. He knows he in the camp of disease and death, and it is at work dealing pain and misery to his friends, so he tries first to ease the sufferer from pain. He uses such methods as he knows have given ease; he has to risk the deadly effects of overdoses; he prescribes the best he can, consults the books of his school, and works to his utmost ability but death does its work and the patient is dead. We should thank him for the kindly effort; he has been a faithful general, and has done all that his school and a life of long experience could arm him with. In our distress we called for his assistance, like a brother he came and did the best he could. He was with us in our trouble, soul and body and strength, and we should love, honor and respect him for his kind efforts though he failed. He is not to be blamed but honored and respected.

But as time passes its fleeting years on to the pages of history, old customs and methods give place to new and better, we should speak in kindness of the works and ways of our living seniors, and honored dead. We must ever remember that *they* faced the storms and privations of the wilderness and laid the foundation of our great schools of learning; they have more claim than we, for kindly words. I hope to ever be able to drop a tear of love on their sacred memory and view their tombs as a loving child should. Of course, their plows, harness and field machinery, have long since given place to better methods, but that was a step to our day of success in the arts and sciences. They planted the trees of Liberty whose fruits have made us great among the nations; they combated their enemies with muskets and smooth bored canons, and met diseases with such remedies as tradition had handed down to them. Today by the seeds sown by them we stand, if need be, the terror of the seas, by the superior skill we show in war. Our old guns and ships gave way to genius. Just so with our old systems of treating diseases—but even that blessing came as bread cast on water, to be gathered many days hence. Our fathers and mothers did sow, and we gather, and owe all we have to their work.

Much can be said in silly abuse of medical doctors, medical trusts and so on, but he who howls the loudest is generally the least to be trusted; nine out of ten such men are old wolves that sneak around to find a rail off to get into the pen and eat some sheep. I say, let the doctor alone—he is not so bad as he is often called.

A. T. S.

November, 1898

DR. A. T. STILL'S DEPARTMENT.

YES! AND WHY.

THE American School of Osteopathy located in Kirksville, Missouri, is without doubt or debate the best school for the purpose for which it was brought into existence, because it is prepared to teach thoroughly all branches necessary to a complete knowledge of Osteopathy. It has at the head of its management, A. T. Still, the father and founder of Osteopathy, who has devoted every day of a quarter of a century to the study and proof of the efficacy of Osteopathy in combatting diseases, during which time a sufficient amount of money has been accumulated to build, equip and run the institution. To this is added the experience of many years, both in practice and teaching. The selection of the necessary teachers for all branches cannot be done without a thorough knowledge of the basic principles of healing by this method. It is now equipped and in full running order as an institution of learning, created for that purpose. It has gone through all the trials and tests of selecting and retaining the most capable minds to impart knowledge. No position has ever been given to any professor merely by personal preference, but because of his fitness and capability to impart the necessary and most useful knowledge to advance this science. In all cases where unfitness has appeared in the person of anyone to execute with skill and exactness every demand as a teacher or an operator, that place is vacated at once, in favor of talent that is better suited for the duties for such chair, finances not being the question of this institution, but "mental qualification," at all times and in all places, the motto, and has been exacted from beginning to present date; and will so continue to be exacted during the days of the institution.

Another reason why this school is self recommending is that the graduates who leave here and go out to treat diseases, show their skill in controlling disease and they soon go into a lucrative practice, as the teeming bundles of letters which come in with every mail do testify. All, who are diplomates of this school, and are scattered to the four quarters of the earth, assure us that they are happy in their pursuit, proud of their diploma. Because of recommendation and indorsement of this school—their alma mater—the increasing number of students has filled the present building to its fullest extent to accomodate them. Three times during the past four years, the building has been remodeled, and made larger with each addition.

Another reason that this is the best school is that the diplomates of the American School of Osteopathy report that when they go into a new place the first question asked them is—"Where did you obtain your knowledge of Osteopathy?" and when the diplomate answers that he is from the American School of Osteopathy no further questions are asked. The significant value of his diploma, and the character of the institution, places him beyond doubt or cavil. From the first day an Osteopath from this school hangs up his diploma in any office in the United States, he is crowded with patients and business, and is honored and respected, first, because of the known character of his diploma; and secondly, because of the results and satisfaction he gives to the afflicted.

We ask no student to come to this school unless he is confident that the above is true and trustworthy. Keep your money and brains until you know you are right—then go ahead. This institution is satisfied to present the truth and abide the results.

November, 1898

Does Nature Think Before it Acts?

IT IS surely in the line of reason to think so if its work is to be called as a witness. As we view the world of vegetation we see the most wonderful display of wisdom and genius. If we follow vegetation's law to the forest and from there to the vast and extended plain we see astounding wisdom speaking in such thunder tones that the most stupid of our race is made to rejoice, though their minds cannot penetrate farther than the beautiful. The greater mind stands aghast, eyes beaming with wonder and joy. He, too, sees the skill that is bestowed upon vegetation all over tree and shrub. The size of bough, and trunk, powerful in form, strong in fiber, anchored to earth by roots to sustain a body erect of many tons weight, holding its foliage hundreds of feet above earth's surface, with strength of trunk to stand the pressure of thousands of tons of angry winds. Then see the motherly kindness it shows to its children, keeps them in her bosom until ripe as food and seed, and at the proper time severs the tie that binds children to mother, they sail off with the breezes, enter the soil, and plant themselves in the earth and begin the work of building another being to take the place of their waning mother.

When we think of that wonderful engine of life that dwells in the forest and what it does, we feel that wisdom is unbounded in all nature. The searcher passes from forest and field to the briny ocean, only to see trees of greater magnitude, not only as large as the trees of the forest but with power of locomotion and minds to direct, with weapons of offence and defense, whose mind and strength command respect of man and beast of all seas. But as he is used to the old saying that "precious gems are found in small packages" he begins to turn his thoughts to that gem of all gems of the terrestrial plains, hills and dales, MAN. He sees in the study of man, that mind, motion and matter have been united in one, by the mind and hand of the Infinite, and that to study and comprehend man will call to mortal minds the days of an eternity.

Man, that machine, that biological being, calls for greater research than all the trees of the forest and the living of all oceans combined. He is the minature universe, mind, motion and matter made to love and work as one.

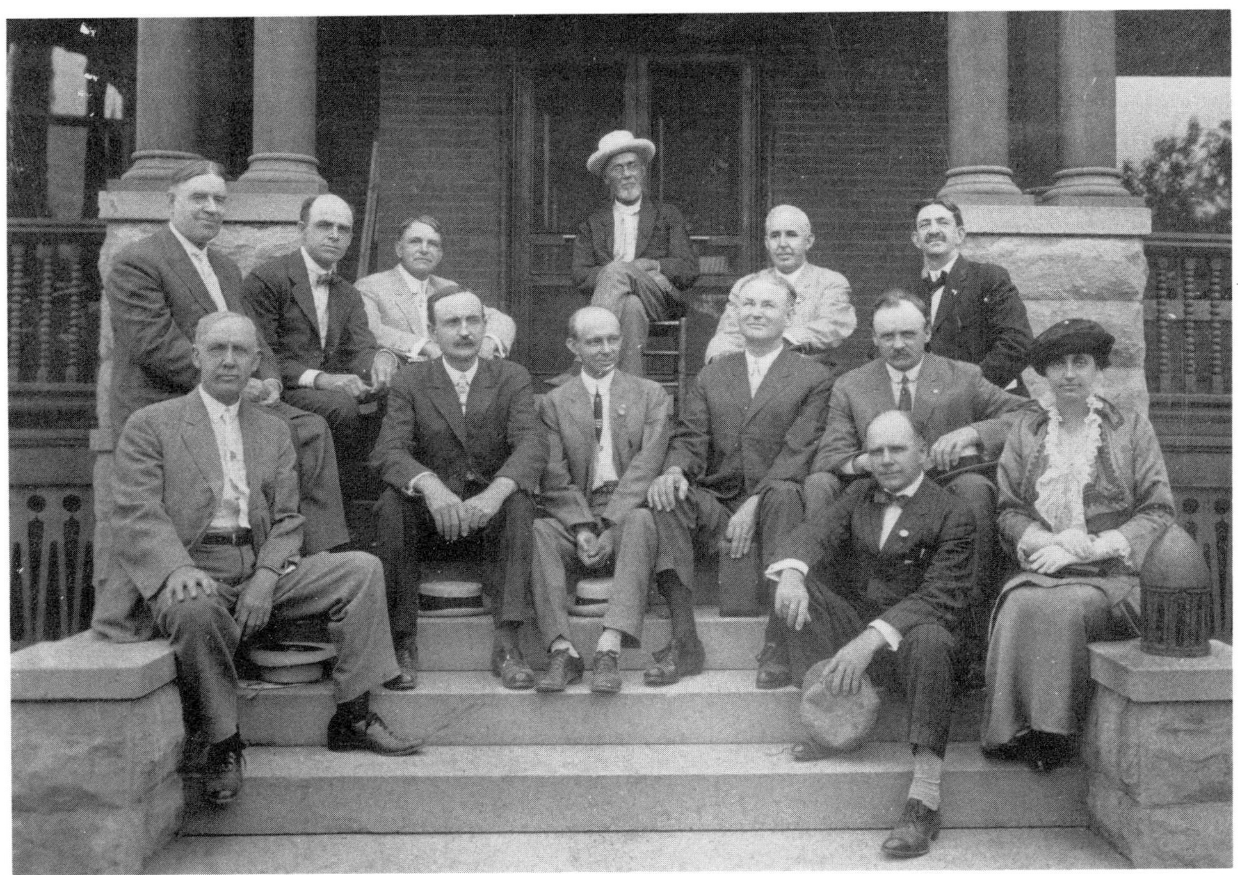

Past Presidents of the A. O. A. on the front steps of Dr. Still's home, 1915

November, 1898

INTUITIVE CONSCIOUSNESS.

BY following a study with practical training, a person becomes acquainted with the principles to such fullness that he can do good work in all parts, and feels no farther effort will be required. He does his work well and feels so, because of his being master of his trade by practical experience and close observation to the study while an apprentice.

Another person of his apprentice class who never lost an hour, cannot do as good work, and lives a life of confused labor, but stands about par in all other branches. The first man has obtained from study something that the second man has not. The first drives through all kinds of difficult problems with ease, while number two is almost a failure in all places. Why the difference? Perhaps number one has worked for and obtained intuitive consciousness, or made all subjects to his mind beings of life, that live under laws made for their being. He who succeeds must study the law of all pursuits or trades. To observe and obey is the only way to succeed; he does succeed by obedience to such laws until mind and body becomes equally sensitive to the fact that man must feel that he is right before he can be successful.

By the law of knowledge and intuition all persons do succeed. Thus we should not be satisfied to know that we are right, but feel so, and act with energy to suit, and our successes will grow with time. We must feel an interest in all we do or we will always eat at the table of disappointment.

It may be possible that we do not think often enough of man's dual nature, and that his body is under his mind, and obeys its orders all the time. By long service under the mind the body becomes saturated so thoroughly with the telegraphy of thought that it feels premonitions of an order to execute some duty before the order is given; perhaps from the fact that the body is full of the essence of mind and its action. I will drop this thought and say, that the above is only an immature suggestion. I believe the greatest blessing we can obtain is to have sensation in union and action with mind and body if we would succeed.

Pap's First Text.

HONOR THYSELF THAT THY DAYS MAY BE LONG ON EARTH: Now, brethren and sisters, the greatest honor a person can enjoy is to know that he has told the truth, every pop all day, every day each week.

Now look at a few idiots who go into various kinds of business. He or she begins the day's talk by saying "this is the coldest day I ever saw," when it is scant zero, and she is an old maid of forty-five winters. He says, "My dog, he's the best dog in the world," when the truth is he's blind and has had fits for ten years. Now, son, don't tell this dog story any more. Just stop right there. If you go into business,—school, mercantile, or any other business,—tell the truth about it. Don't lie and cheat in order to make gain. A man's heart may be full of wine, but one dirty lie will sour all his joy.

Don't say you were a pet student and got a special drill on all branches, and that you were the only object of admiration of all the professors. If you do tell such trash to strangers they will set you down as a fool, and not to be trusted. Your babe is as ugly as mine, and both are as green as a mess of boiled dandelion, so just be easy about your fine qualities. People will weigh you, and give you all the credit for good that you merit.

The way of the righteous is easy, but the road of the untruthful brag is a life of remorse. If I had my choice, I would take a thousand thieves before one liar. What would the universe be if God were a liar? Be honest and God will endorse all you do and say.

"Pap."

As I am often called "Pap" by the students and diplomates of my school, I will try and treat you as a "Pap" should his children. When he or she has received his or her parchment from the American School of Osteopathy and has earned it by faithful and hard study, and passed on all that has been required of them by the school which is of a high grade in all its branches, and when I affixed my hand to your diplomas, I did so because I thought you worthy of them. I felt you had done honor to yourself and the school.

I am proud to say of each and every graduate who has spent the required time in this school, that I feel sure they are well prepared to enter the field of labor and do good work in any climate, season or place, if they keep an eye fixed on the principles taught them by this school; they can at the close of each day be wiser and feel more joyful of the step that put them to study man, the master-piece of the works of God. I want you to feel and know that I have no "pets" I bear the same love to all. Write me often, I will be with you in sunshine or in shadows.

Lovingly yours,

PAP.

December, 1898

DR. A. T. STILL'S DEPARTMENT.

"Women and Girls Gab Too Much."

SHE chatters, giggles, and is perfectly happy when she tells all the gossip and mean stories, minus the good, she has heard about of every woman she knows in the town or ten miles around. She tells all and gets a new list of imaginary "Did you hear its?" and goes off to the next house to ease herself by trying to lower some woman that is as good or better than she is.

What good does it do her? I will answer that question by asking another: what good does it do a man to get drunk and make a disgusting fool of himself? Had he kept himself busy in some useful pursuit and kept away from whiskey, he would have been a useful and respected gentleman, but he got into and staid with such company until he got the habit fixed so strong that his manhood failed him and he went down to a place where fools and vagabonds only dwell. She, too, gave way to tattling and circulating little dirty reports, until she has gotten as crazy to know the last scandal as a drunkard ever was for whiskey. She is a tattler and a nuisance, hated and dreaded by all who know her.

Now, girls, I will tell you what makes a tattler. Woman loves to talk, and if she is not loaded with useful knowledge, she will talk some anyway. A voice says, "we know that what you say is correct as a general rule; and would like to have a few suggestions." I will have to go to my storehouse of experience. At one view through the mental telescope that reaches far back in my life, I begin to review the mental record that I have kept stored away for useful purposes for over half a century. I think I can point out the "whys" that so many meritorious, good designing young ladies lose sight of usefulness. After she has received her education in painting, drawing, music, stenography, type-writing and most of the ordinary accomplishments, she is met with this fact and answer at all places where she offers her services, that the place is ably filled by old occupants; the more she tries to obtain some position by which to make a living, the more she is convinced that all places she is qualified to fill have long since been taken up by others. Thus she is left without a hope to be able to make a living for herself. As I have given this subject much study and have sons and daughters of my own whose welfare has always been uppermost in my mind, and have explored all fields of usefulness for their good, I could not do so without taking the conditions of the whole human race into consideration. I have always felt a determination to hunt until I could find a suitable position which I could recommend to our women. I believe I have made the discovery. I have long sought and have tested its merits. From a child I have known the goodness and wisdom of the mother part of our race; a desire to relieve pain and sickness is certainly as natural as for her to breathe. Now ladies, at this period in my narrative, I will say, I also became interested in the welfare and ease of my race. I have prosecuted the investigation for over a quarter of a century. I have proven to myself the perfection of Nature's work and that man has within him all the qualities for ease and comfort, and when disease makes them uncomfortable, he or she who is familiar with the machinery of life can give them ease and comfort, and restore the person to good health. In the case of the ladies, they have proven their ability to adjust the human body. She gets her pay and she is proud of her diploma, proud of her being, and proud of her position and proud that she is far above a gossiping nuisance.

Ladies, I talk thus plainly to you because of a love of my race. If you desire to know more of the "hows" as to making a comfortable living, visit the American School of Osteopathy, and after due consideration, I think you will find what I have told you to be the truth. All the ladies who have taken my advice thus far send me greetings and words of love from all parts of the civilized world in which they now labor.

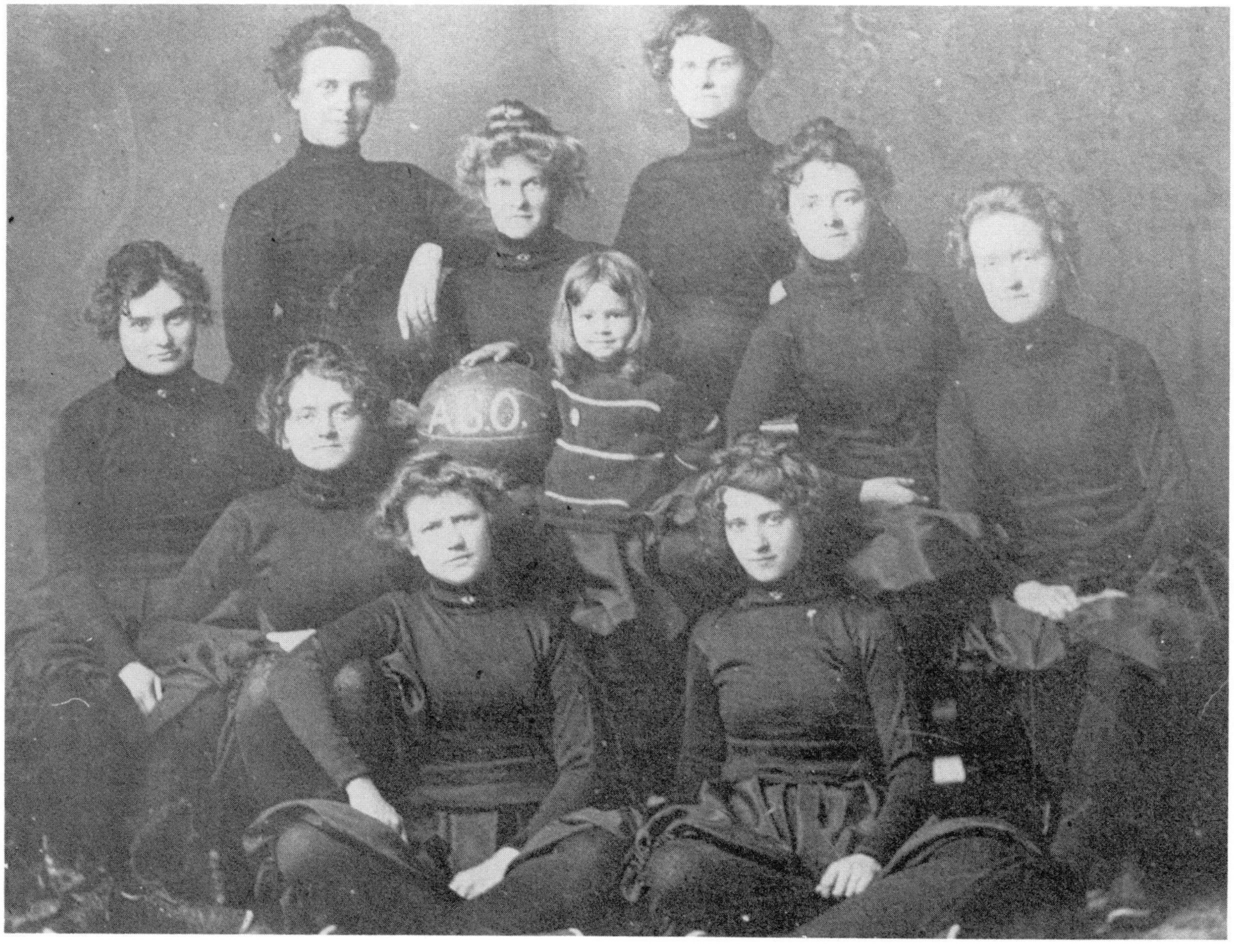

Women's Basketball Team, late 1890s

December, 1898

IT WAS my good fortune or bad fortune to introduce Osteopathy in its swaddling clothes a quarter of a century ago in North America. It was a good sized boy baby, with strong lungs. It has talked to the people of the beauties of the discovery that it had made which are a few of the principles that govern animal life, which, no doubt, are as old as the days of Eternity. After twenty-five years of close investigation, I have made no discovery of any defect whereby I could suggest an amendment. I have used freely the scalpel, the microscope, and the chemical labratory; made a free use of the opinions of all philosophers with whom I could consult; at the end of each season of investigation the conclusion has universely been that the laws bear upon their face absolute evidence of perfection, and are so taken and accepted by the learned people who have time and desire to investigate the truths of Osteopathy.

While I have taken no pains to give this science notoriety by publication, it has been more or less known for ten or fifteen years in the capital of the United States, and today is known, more or less, in every town and village in the states and territories, and is also known in foreign lands.

I will say for those who desire to know more of this science that whenever you see a diploma from the American School of Osteopathy, you will find the possessor qualified to give you the necessary information and to demonstrate the facts of the science by his or her skill and ability which they have obtained during long months spent in obtaining a thorough education in the American School of Osteopathy at Kirksville, Mo.

My signature only goes to those parchments after long acquaintance in the school room with the receiver thereof, and the signature of the trustees and faculty of the school is all that is necessary or that we can do by the way of recommending as to character and qualification. As I know all have had a good opportunity to become well qualified for the duties of a a healer, I will make mention of no particular name or person more than to say that without merit these diplomas would not have been issued to the persons now possessing them, and for me to say who is good or who is bad would be a contradiction of what I have already said—that he or she has our highest recommend on their diploma.

Osteopathy in Congress.

FOR many years the great state of Missouri has been represented by such eminent statesmen as Vest and Cockrill in the Senate, and the worthy and great statesmen, Hatch and Clark in the House, all well known to the world in general.

Hatch, though now dead in body, yet lives in the memory of his friends. He and myself were personal friends; he was great and honorable, and as representative of my district, though a democrat and I a republican, I was a great admirer of him for his honesty and intelligence. He always had a kind word and would inquire often with interest how I was progressing with the new science, while I was practising at Hannibal, Mo., during the early development of Osteopathy.

Our Ex-Congressman Clark, also has been an out-spoken friend of Osteopathy.

While in the south part of the state near the home of Senator Cockrill, I also met him, and found him to be be very kind and encouraging.

Senator Vest always treated me with gentlemanly kindness. Though these gentlemen were not Osteopaths themselves, they have been able to speak of Osteopathy more or less intelligently at the capital of the United States, for lo, these many years. Therefore, I am warranted in saying that Osteopathy has been planted and cultivated to some extent in our national capital for at least fifteen years.

I could speak of Ingalls and many other men who have represented Kansas, and their encouraging expressions of the science of Osteopathy; I could also make mention of Senator Foraker and his wife, of Ohio, who have been treated at the Infirmary, and many others of note.

The people of the Dakotas, of Nebraska, Oregon, California, Minnesota, Michigan and Wisconsin all know of Osteopathy; in fact, there is no state that has not some knowledge of Osteopathy, recognizing that it is a science based upon the visible and intelligent works of Deity, as a remedial science.

Osteopathy is now being ably represented in the capital city by H. E. Patterson and his wife, both are diplomates from the American School of Osteopathy.

Osteopathy in Washington, D. C., and all Other Places.

DR. H. E. PATTERSON and wife, are both diplomates of the American School of Osteopathy. Their diplomas, like all parchments from this school, are the best recommendation we can give.

A. T. Still.

December, 1898

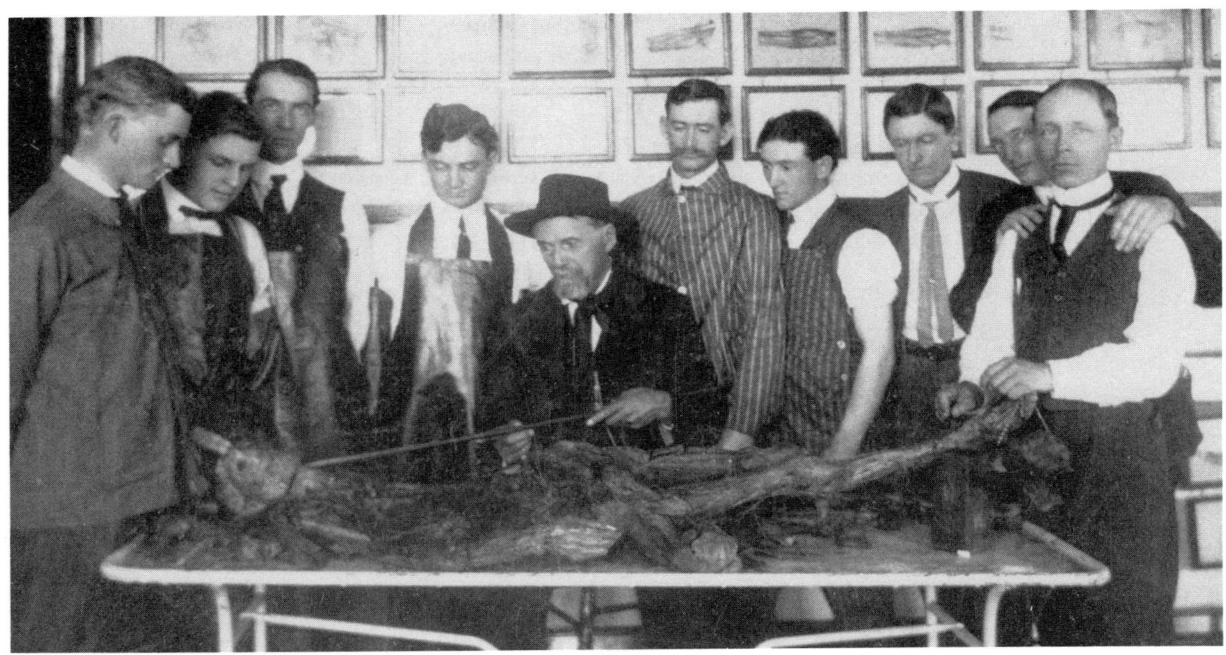

Dissection class about 1903

DR. STILL'S ADDRESS.

LADIES AND GENTLEMEN: "Previous to handing you your diplomas which you have earned by hard study and strict conformity to the rules and regulations of this institution—and as I represent the parent institution of osteopathy, not only of Missouri, but the whole world—I will say that I represent it officially under a legal charter granted by this State for the purpose of teaching the science which I have chosen to name osteopathy, the principles of which no record can show to have had any priority, whatever, among the philosophers of the world. And as to-day closes the last hour of official responsibility with you, I will say when you consulted me in reference to the study of osteopathy, then and there I told you, both ladies and gentlemen, that my experience had taught me that it is one of the finest, if not the finest, science now known. And I did not only recommend, but did insist that you should follow it for the following reasons: First, for the valuable knowledge you could obtain of the human body, with all its parts that work so beautifully in the economy of animal life. Second, the pleasure of the study. Third, as a remunerative, honorable, life-time profession, in which you could do much good and receive the necessary reward. I did believe, then and there, when I advised you to take up the study that the world needed you and wanted your services. And when prepared to meet and treat the afflicted of all kinds of diseases of age and sex, that I would rejoice with you when this day came for you to receive this parchment, the highest token of learning and confidence to which we could subscribe our names. As we are about to take and give the parting hand I will say that my confidence in the usefulness of this science and the good you can do has strengthened in my mind. I believe now as then, that my advice was good for you. I believe in all coming days that you will be proud and happy that you entered this school. I will now recommend you to the highest school known, the University of Experience, in which you will see bright and dark days when you come to deal with promiscuous humanity; and your work will be like unto a visit into a fine fruit orchard ; you will find some very beautiful fruit, ripe with age, delicious to smell and taste, because of the flavor and nourishment it affords to the mind of the hungry explorer; other fruits are dead and rotten, from the stings of the wasps of deception. Though they come to you girdled with golden belts, remember, that the flattering wasp always carries with him the stiletto of death. They are not the philosophers' stone, quietly and firmly pass them by, and try to clinb higher and higher into the fruit tree of knowledge. Be honest. Be just, and a satisfactory reward will come to you, with the same certainty that the rising sun will dispel the darkness I stand by you as President McKinley stood behind Admiral Dewey. I. I have confidence in your skill and ability, and am willing to trust you as commanders of the science taught by the American School of Osteopathy, and am confident that you will enter all 'bays' and come out as he did, victorious."

As Dr. Still did not know in advance whether he would have strength enough to take a personal part in the program he committed this message to paper. With the enthusiasm of the hour, he felt a speech by proxy inadequate and just before the awarding of diplomas stepped to the speaker's rostrum and supplemented his first farewell with an eulogy of Dr. Littlejohn's address and a second God-speed to the graduates. He said:

"After listening to Dr. Littlejohn's masterly address I feel like saying to him and to you all what my old father said to his boys after he set us to plowing and doing other things which we came to do by degrees to his entire satisfaction: 'Boys, you are doing mighty well—I am not sure but you are beating me at it—yes, I think you are.' "

Then followed the presentation of diplomas by President Still during which he addressed some word to each one as the parchment was bestowed. The Glee Club closed the exercises.

Class day exercises were held January 31st at 2 p. m. A crowded house greeted the class representatives and good-natured chaffing and good humor characterized the exercises. The program was rendered:

Music............Orchestra
Invocation............Rev. W. L. Darby
Class History............A. L. Evans
Music............Orchestra
Class Poem............Dr. C. M. Case
Class Representative............M. C. Hardin
Music............Orchestra.

Every train out of Kirksville for several days after graduation day bore newly fledged Diplomates of Osteopathy to the four points of the compass for their fields of labor.

February, 1899

THE PEN OF AN OSTEOPATHIC WRITER.

ANDREW TAYLOR STILL, M. D.

AN Osteopath after dipping his pen into the ink of research with the expectation of informing the world on this science should be very careful to place his pen square on the line that contains nothing but the opinion of the writer. He who has given intelligent study to the science to make him a writer of authority, will find no trouble in finding a subject on which to write a long or short piece, because without doubt the science of Osteopathy covers enough ground to enable him to write something of his own. In his descriptive writings he must confine himself to the principles of Osteopathy which will give him an abundance to write if he will confine himself to any one division of the workings of the machinery of life from the top of man's head to the sole of his foot. Osteopathy has its uses for anatomy, thus the writer has a prolific field in which to write. So it has a great place and use for physiology and the chemistry of man. All these subjects are starting places, and are able to suggest all he can record, and the world is ready to hear from him. Like the historian who wishes to record the real condition of a nation, he must confine his thoughts and pen to that nation ; the geographical description of the country, the people, with their religion, politics and schools, number of inhabitants, with their skill, industry and so on, and so long as he confines his pen to the description of that nation, he is doing some useful writing. But when he takes up his pen to write the high truths of Osteopathy he must write what he knows about it, and not bore his reader with a long list of quotations from Allopathy, Homeopathy, Eclectism, Christian science and so on through the whole list and methods. The subject of Osteopathy is too prolific for a finished Osteopath to have to borrow lines from any other writer, and if he is too lazy and stupid to think and give the people something good to read he had better be too lazy to write and not bore the people with anything but pure and unadulterated Osteopathy. I would advise each diplomate from the American School of Osteopathy when he goes out in the field of practice to purchase a blank book and write down for his own use his observations of diseases of each season, and at the end of the year review his successes and failures. Then, with a new book, commence the second year, and study Osteopathy with all his might and make a record of his observations that will be much better for him than anyone else that will read those notes. By the time he has written his third year's observations he will have taken many hearty laughs over his first year's bosh.

Suppose an incompetent writer, or one who has just finished the course and received his diploma, should take his pen and begin to dilate on Osteopathy, how much farther can his pen reach than what he has learned to say by rote as questions and answers? He has never lead as a teacher of the principles of any branch ; all he knows is what has been told to him by books and professors, which leaves him wisely prepared to drill himself in the school of experience, which is the place to reduce theory to knowledge, in which place he must learn all he will ever know of Osteopathy ; as not blind faith in what we have, but what he proves and knows is what is demanded of him.

March, 1899

A LESSON LEARNED IN SUMMER AND FALL DISEASES.

ANDREW TAYLOR STILL, M. D.

OSTEOPATHY has made rapid progress in showing its efficacy as a successful system of curing the diseases coming to North America and has been largely recognized in nearly one-fourth of the states of this great nation and Europe also; still out of the 80,000,000 people less than one-fourth of them have heard that there is such a science as is taught and practiced with such satisfactory results as by the American School of Osteopathy, and since the reader is kindly disposed to give all discovery an attentive hearing before giving judgment, we think it is due the inquirer to give all the information we can through the JOURNAL OF OSTEOPATHY.

In the summer and fall, we have fevers and bowel complaints. Our summer complaints generally begin late in the hot weather with running off of bowels, which looseness keeps up from a day or two to a week with pain in the bowels before stool, and with head-ache and back-ache in the lumbar regions; there is generally an aching and soreness of the muscles of the body, and limbs and some fever with chilly feelings; great thirst and loss of appetite; the tongue is generally dry with a crust, as the frequency of the stool increases, pain in the head, spine, limbs and body also increases with an increased temperature to 100 and upwards, which becomes continous day and night. Now is the time that the patient wants: 'no cut and try'' work, but that the Doctor is worthy and qualified to conduct the management of his cases wisely.

Just at this time the father begins to goad himself keenly to act wisely and leave no chance for rue in case of the death of child, wife or whoever it is—that the best had not been done. If he calls in an Osteopathic Doctor and he should fail, the parent reflects, "how can I go for the old family Doctor? What if he won't come?" and all the "ifs" and "buts," troop in to worry him; lastly he will say to himself—"how can he cure fevers without giving some medicine to cool fever and ease pains?"

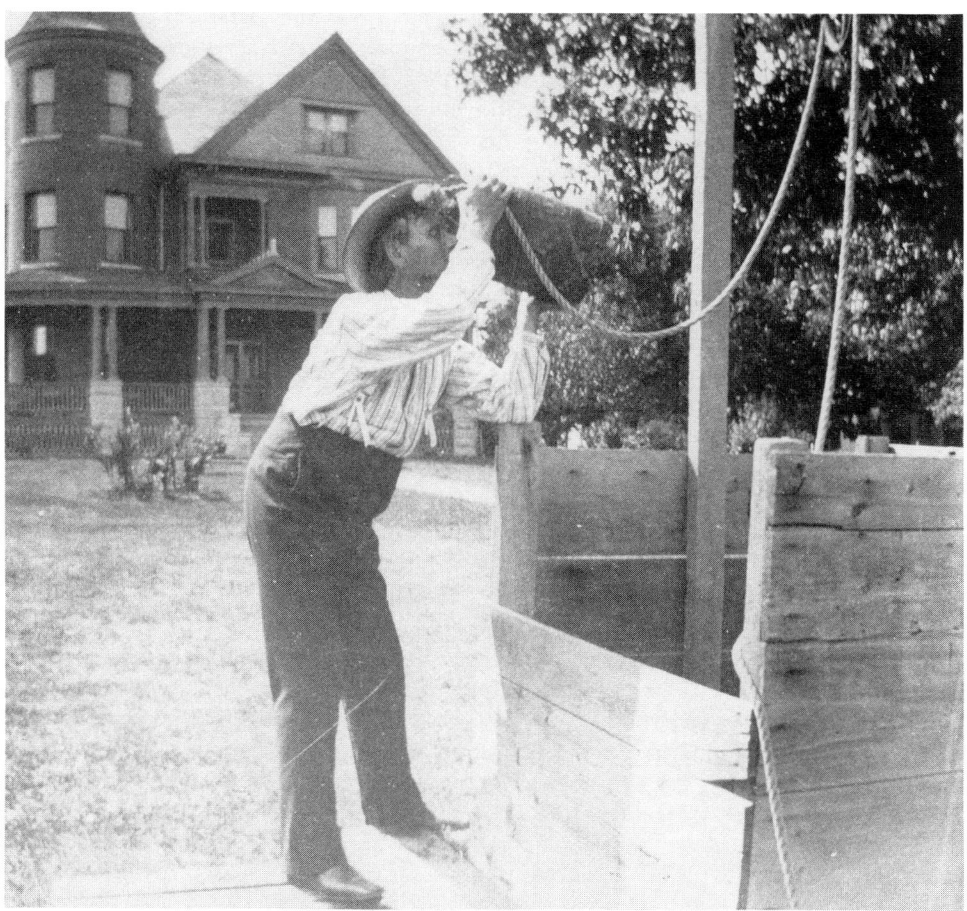

A. T. Still at the well in the front of his home c.1900

These things an Osteopath must meet. He is now among people of good general intelligence on all subjects, except Osteopathy, having fevers and other diseases. This parent will say to him "Osteopathy may be true and can do all and more than is claimed for it, or it may be a total failure and only worth to be set down as a dangerous humbug, but I cannot afford to run any risks in this child's case, as it is a very dangerous and doubtful case;" the sick one dies but fortunately it did not die in the hands of an Osteopath;the parent is free, he has done all that he thinks is his duty and he has no ground for remorse nor sore reflection for the child did have the best of care and all the medicine that Dr. Clarke had ever used before for the flux and many new medicines that the Doctor found in his new book; but they all failed to save the child's life.

The father still feels kindly to the Osteopath and opens out with interested curiosity and wants to know if the Osteopath honestly believes that Osteopathy can do anything with bloody flux? At this time the way is open to reach the bereaved father's reason; then the practitioner tells him what flux is and why it kills both old and young; in the afternoon of this day's reasoning with the father another son of five summers takes with vomiting and purging mixed with blood; the Osteopath is now asked to go to his house with him and give an opinion in the case; the Osteopath walks over and finds a bad case of acute bloody flux of a violent and very dangerous type and so reports to the parents; they ask the Osteopath if he will try to relieve the child of his misery and suffering; he tells them he will try and will do the best he can; he takes the little boy in his lap and gives the little fellow a treatment first to stop the fever, and the headache; then he treats to relieve the bowels of fever, pain and running off; he comes back next day and finds a well boy, but weak; no drugs were used and there is a house full of friends made happy converts to Osteopathy by results only.

At this time all are so happy and hopeful not only to have heard of the wonder but to have seen its claims proven by curing a child of flux in the worst form in a family that has jnst lost a boy while under the best medical skill of this day and age. The Osteopathic doctor now enters a new field of troubles since he has proven to an anxious people that diseases can be cured without drugs. He finds he has placed himself in a position where he must talk to the people and tell them some things of how an Osteopath can cause the human body to become warm when cold, and how to take fever down and how to stop pain and soreness without medicine, either noxious or pleasant. He can easily say "man is a living engine and is driven by brain force; and the lymphatics pour water on a fevered body and put out the fire; and the blood builds up the waste tissue and wasted energy; and the excretions carry off the poisons from the body" and all of that kind of talk. He finds that an Osteopath flourishes better with the wise than with the ignorant for he must tell them how and why he cures all kinds of fevers, diphtheria, croup, pneumonia, and all diseases as he meets them, and gives birth without forceps and almost no pain at all; he finds he must send a dozen or two to our school to learn Osteopathy or be talked to death.

For the good of the stranger who may desire some knowledge of why a Doctor of any school or rank thinks or presumes to reason that Nature can throw off its burdens and be free from all diseases and enjoy good health again, which questions are wisely sent forth from the cautions man or woman, we will say Osteopathy only means a knowledge of the "on" and "off," the "in" and "out of place;" when speaking of curing diseases, Osteopathy cures no disease —no, not one; a skillful and wise Osteopath proceeds to see if every bone is in its place; if he finds it is not, then he knows it is *out* of place; he sees what mischief is being done by that condition and his duty is to stop and search abnormal mischief. He adjusts everything to its normal position only and leaves the work of curing to be done by the physiological power to heal.

June, 1899

The Still Institutions are Not to Leave Kirksville.

Rumors have been rife for several weeks to the effect that the American School of Osteopathy was shortly to be moved to one of the prominent western cities. Dr. A. T. Still, president of the institution, wishes this impression to be corrected. It is not true that any agreement has been made looking to the removal of the School or Infirmary. Several cities have made overtures to Dr. Still, offering considerable bonuses to secure the American School of Osteopathy, but they were not accepted. The school is making every arrangement to increase its accommodations and equipment for the fall term ; a large incoming class is regarded as a certainty; and patrons may rest assured that Osteopathy in the future, as in the past, will be taught best at its birth-place—Kirksville.

Dr. Still gave out this statement June 7th through the Kirksville papers :

"To the Citizens of Kirksvillle and all others concerned : Kirksville is my home. I have no intention of leaving the place. My interests are here for life so far as I know now. Let this answer all questions or rumors. Do your part and I will do mine.

A. T. STILL."

* * *

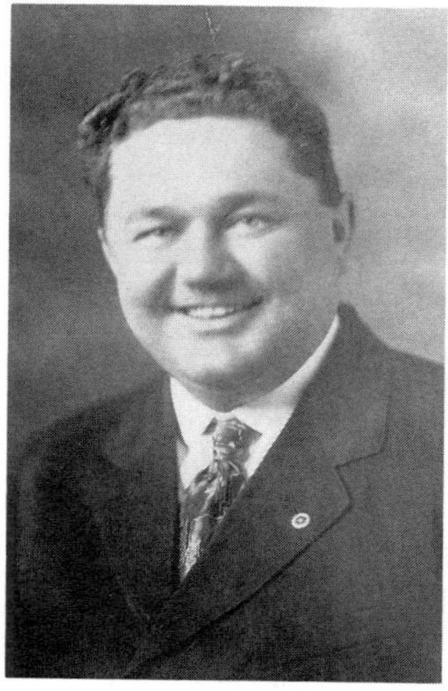

George A. Still

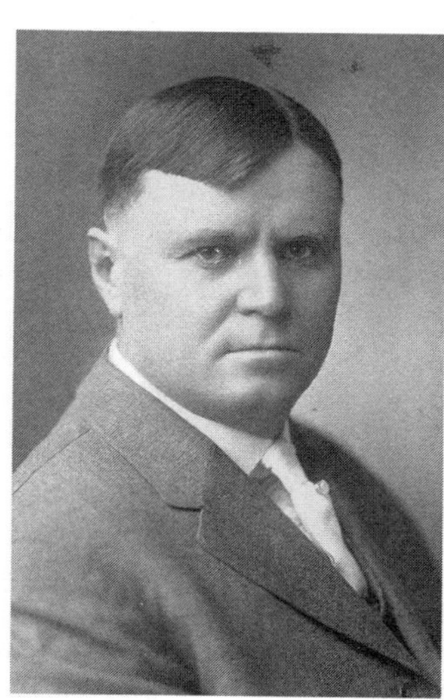

Harry M. Still

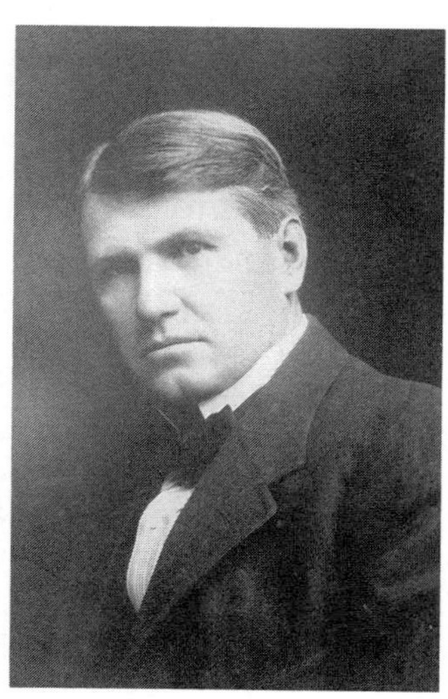

Charles E. Still

July, 1899

Consumption.

CONSUMPTION, I believe, will soon be with the things of the past, if taken and handled by a skilled mind, one that is trained for that responsible place. He or she must be taught this as a special branch; it it is too deep for superficial knowledge or imperfect work. Life is in danger, and can be saved by skill, not by force or ignorance. He who sees only the dollar in the lung is not the man to trust your case with. It is such men as have the ability to think and the skill to comprehend and execute the application of Nature's unerring laws, that obtain the results required. We believe the day has come and long before noon the fear of consumption will greatly pass from the minds of the people. We have long since known and proven that a cough is only an effect; if an effect, then a wise man will set his mental dogs on the track which is effect, to hunt the skunk, which is cause. He has all the evidence by the cough, location of pain, tenderness of spine, neck and quality of the substances coughed up to locate the cause, and to know when he has found it, how to remove cause, and to give relief will grow more simple as he reasons and notes effect. We do not think this result will be obtained every time by an average mind, unless he have a special training for that purpose. He must not only know that the lungs are in the upper part of the chest and are close to the heart, liver and stomach, but he must know the relation all sustain to each other, that the blood must be abundantly supplied to support and nourish three sets of nerves, sensory, motor and nutrient. If the supply should be diminished to the nutrient nerves, weakness would follow; reduce the supply to the motor and it will have the same effect, thus motion becomes too feeble to carry blood to and from the lungs normally, and the blood becomes congested, because it is not passed on to other parts with the same force that is necessary for health of the lungs.

At this time the nerves of sensation become irritated by pressure and lack of nutriment; we cough, this is an effort of Nature to unload the burden of oppression that congestion causes with sensory nerves. If this be effect then we must suffer and die, or remove the cause, put out the fire and stop waste of life without which all is lost. Nature will do its work of repairing in due time. Let us reason by comparison. If we dislocate a shoulder, fever and heat will follow; the same is true of all joints of the body. If obstructing blood or other fluid should be deposited in quantities great enough to stop other fluids from passing on their courses, Nature will fire up its engine to remove such deposits by converting the fluids into gas. As heat and motion have much to do as remedies, we may expect fever and pain until Nature's furnace produces heat and converts its fluids into gas and passes it through the excretories to space and allows the body to work normally again.

We believe consumption causes the death of thousands that it should not. We must not let stupidity veil our reason, and we are to blame if we let so many run into "consumption" from a simple hard cough. The remedy is natural and we believe from results already obtained that seventy-five per cent of the cases can be cured if taken in time. What we call "consumption" begins generally with a cough, chilly sensations and this lasts a day or two, sometimes fever accompanies the cough. The cold generally relaxes in a few days, lungs get loose and much is raised and this continues for a period, but the cough appears again and again with all changes of the weather and lasts longer each time, until it becomes permanent—then it is called "consumption" because of its continuance. Medicines are administered freely and often. but lungs gradually grow worse, cough more continued and much harder, till finally blood begins to come from lungs with wasting of strength. Change of climate is suggested and taken, but with no change for the better; another and another travels to death on the same line. Now the doctor in council reports "hereditary consumption" and with his decision all are satisfied and each member of the family feels that a cold and cough means a coffin because the doctor says the family has "hereditary consumption." This shade tree has given comfort and contentment to the doctors of the whole past.

If you have a tiresome and weakening cough at the close of the winter and wish to be cured, we would advise you to begin treatment with warm weather, then the lungs can heal and harden against next winter's attack.

As I write I will say I have never written a word on consumption because I wanted first to test my conclusions by long and careful observations on cases that I have taken and treated successfully. I have kept this from public print until I could obtain positive proof that "consumption" could be cured before I would so state. So far the discovery of the causes are of but little doubt and the cures are a certainty in a very great number of cases. An early beginning is one of the great considerations in incipient consumption.

For fear you do not understand what I mean by "consumption" I will have to write on a descriptive line quite pointedly. I will give start and progress to fully developed consumption. We often meet with cases of permanent coughs, with expectorations of long duration, dating back two, five, ten, even thirty years, to the time when they had the measles. The severity of the cough and strain had congested even the lung substance, and a chronic inflammation was the result. If we analyze the sputum we find fibrine and even lung muscle. Does all this array of dangerous symptoms cause an Osteopath to give up in despair? It should not, but on the other hand he should go deeper and deeper on the hunt of the cause; he may find trouble in the nerve fibre of the pneumogastric, in the atlas, hyoid, vertebrae, rib or clavicle—these may be pressing on some nerve that supplies the mucus membrane of the air-cells or passages. A cut foot will often produce lock-jaw, why not a pressure on some center or branch of nerve fibre cause some nerve division in the lungs that governs venous circulation to contract and hold blood indefinitely as an irritant, equal to cause perpetual coughing?

This is not the time for the brainy Osteopath to run up the white flag of defeat and surrender. Open the doors of your purest reason, put on the belt of energy and unload the sinking vessel of life. Throw over-board all the dead weights from fascia and wake up the forces of the excretories, let the nerves all show their powers to throw out every weight that would sink or reduce the vital energies of Nature. Give them a chance to work, give them the full nourishment and the victory will be on the side of the intelligent engineer. Never surrender, but die in the last ditch.

Let us enter the field of active exploration and note the causes that would lead us to conclude that we have found the cause that produces "consumption" as it has ever been called.

Begin at the brain, go down the ladder of observation, stop and whet your knives of mental steel sharp, get your nerves quiet by the opium of patience. Begin with the atlas, follow with the search-light of quickened reason, comb back your hair of mental strength, and never leave that bone until you have learned how many nerves pass through and around that wisely formed first part of the neck. Remember it was planned and builded by the mind and hand of the Infinite. See what nerve fibres pass through and on to the base, center, and each minute cell, fascia, gland and blood-vessel of the lungs.

* * *

July, 1899

The Buzzard.

"FROM the sublime to the ridiculous." God made both man and the buzzard. To open up the subject of the buzzard, I will say to my companions, (if I have any) let us halt, clean out and load our pipes with the best and most powerful tobacco of reason, puff a few times, and get coolly down ready to take up the subject of the most loathsome and filthy of all known fowls on the face of the earth. His odor is so obnoxious that no human can endure him even for one minute without turning sick and throwing up the contents of his stomach. It would look as if the wisdom of God had been exhausted to show how filthy he could make his created beings. When we read that "cleanliness is next to Godliness" and smell the buzzard we feel like the boy who says "how is that for high?" When God has made the most filthy that the genius of heaven could produce, when we read of purity and witness the most filthy of all in a bird and he turned loose above us to pollute the air that we breathe, and such birds spreads all over the earth by countless millions; why not fill the sky with sweetest roses with their odor to comfort his children in place of filling the space above us with filthy birds and the ground with stinking snakes, skunks, and thousands of offensive animals, bugs and reptiles. It does look as though Nature had tried to be filthy in general and particular.

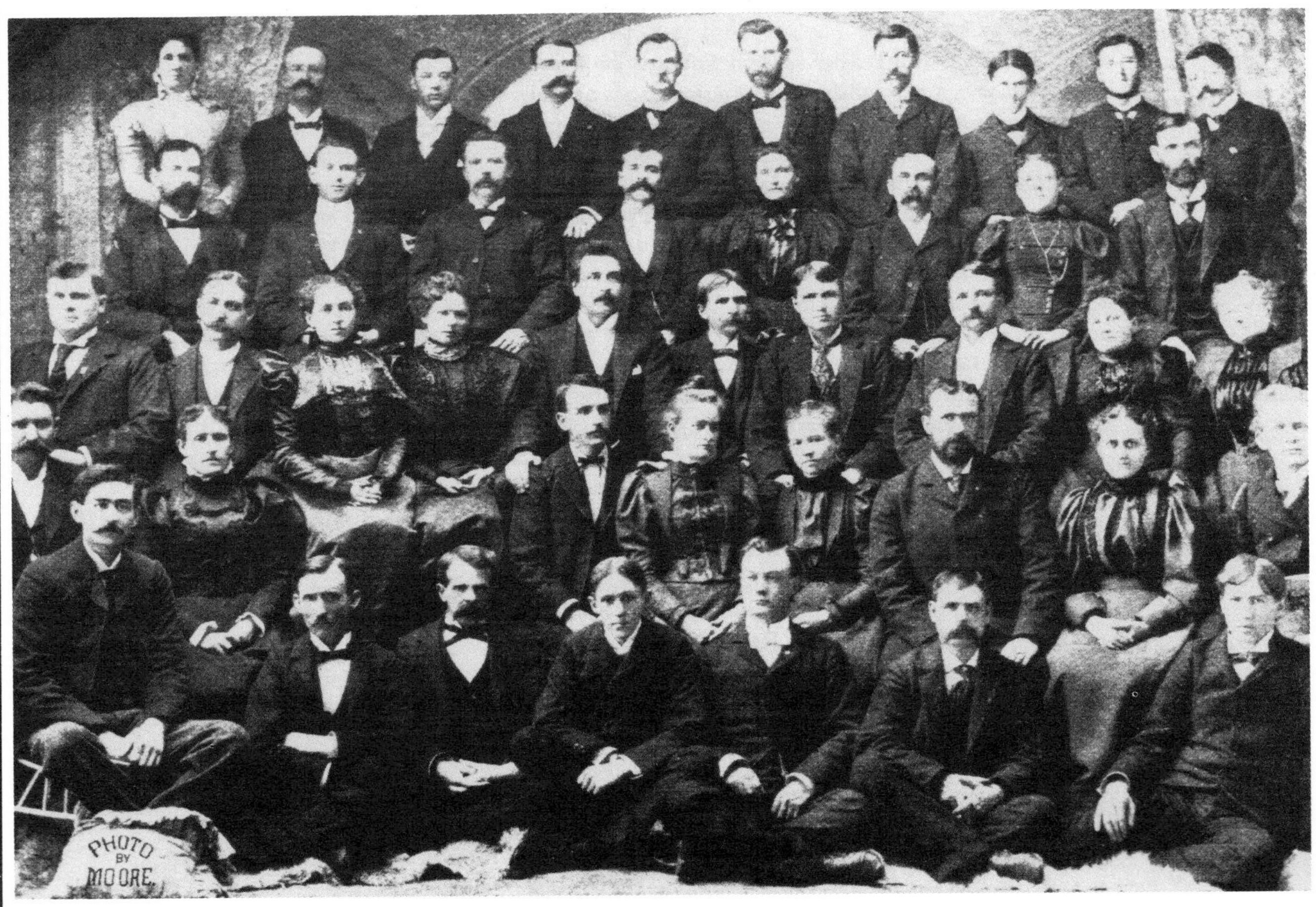

Graduating Class of 1898, February

is only a question of pounds of sulphur and magnetic action that keeps the lesser away, but when two worlds of equality in all respects run near, a union would surely occur, thus disease that has overcome one man can so do all men. Is it not reasonable to suppose that virus could take possession of a body whose living force is inferior to its own? Thus the disease that does kill the human is stronger than the resisting force of man and will grow in him as grass will flourish in the soil of the earth. Thus the odor of diseases fall on and take root and grow because of their power to prevail over the weaker and leave us only to see the effects of the cause in motion; we judge cause by its work to save the organs

Come boys, let us shake the ashes out of our pipes, clean the stem and fire anew and make the best we can of the filthy odors. We will have some music (not operatic) and see if we can enjoy ourselves better this congress than at the last—when all Nature seemed to be a sea of filthy beasts, birds and reptiles. I feel better now, our pipes smoke good; I seem to fall in deep love with all Nature's work.

When I think of the musk of the buzzard and all the reptiles, and fishes of the sea I see the wisdom and kindness of God is all his work wheresoever found by man. Had I been acquainted with the object of Nature I never could have been induced to think that God could have made a better buzzard—one that could eat the putrid flesh and not been so offensive in his own smell, which is so much worse than that of the worst putrid flesh that the nostril of man ever smelled; it is so much worse that the smell of all dead beasts is pleasant when compared with it. I see suns of beauty now where I could not even see a star in the mists of my mental sky. I feel that that the pen of man could spend an eternity in and with the laws and uses of odors.

Did you ever think for a moment that odors are living powers and that one can overpower and destroy another? Thus if a buzzard should stop and eat a man who had died of small-pox, that odor cannot overcome the effects of the odor of the bird and plant the bacteria of small-pox in him and kill him. Did you ever think how wisely Nature has fortified him against putrid poison? He freely eats of the horse that has died of the deadly glanders and no harm comes to him. Can you not sing or chant "Praise God from whom all blessings flow?" I feel that the gates of heaven are open to him who will behold and read the laws and uses which Nature put there in place and motion. I speak of the odors of fruits, vegetation and animals hoping by so doing other and wiser persons may be able to give us more light on the subject. I am of the opinion that by the laws of odor-force disease is often conveyed from one person to another, thus contagions are carried over the earth. If a person should take up the odor of small-pox, why not kill the microbes by the natural odors of a healthy person? Why not a lesser world side up to and be in company with the other? Reason would say the greater world would have greater magnetic force and repel the lesser, thus the health and safety of both are preserved. It of the body in at least working order or enough so as to begin repairs after the fire of the pox has been extinguished by exhaustion of all igniting substances of the body. It surely has taken much wisdom to arrange and make a channel that would and could take and dispel the dead and dying fluids of the body completely and leave the body purified. All offensive musks and odors have labored to save life by pushing such dead matter out of the system and in so doing, tear away parts of the skin in order to make openings to pass out the dead matter—thus we see the pox.

(These articles are published by request and are taken from the manuscript of Dr. A. T. Still's system of Independent Philosophy—which may be published in the near future·)

* * *

Something New Or Nothing At All.

STALE habit and imitation and quotations from the honest though ignorant dead will not be tolerated in this school any longer than I can ascertain the Osteopathic instructor who will come before the class with lists of quotations from medical authors who hate Osteopathy in their bigoted way. I wish no books with such productions presented to the honest seeker for Osteopathic knowledge, and I advise the student who reads any book abounding in quotations to take it to some competent Osteopath who will probably tell you how badly the author has missed the object and how unwisely you have spent your money.

A. T. STILL.

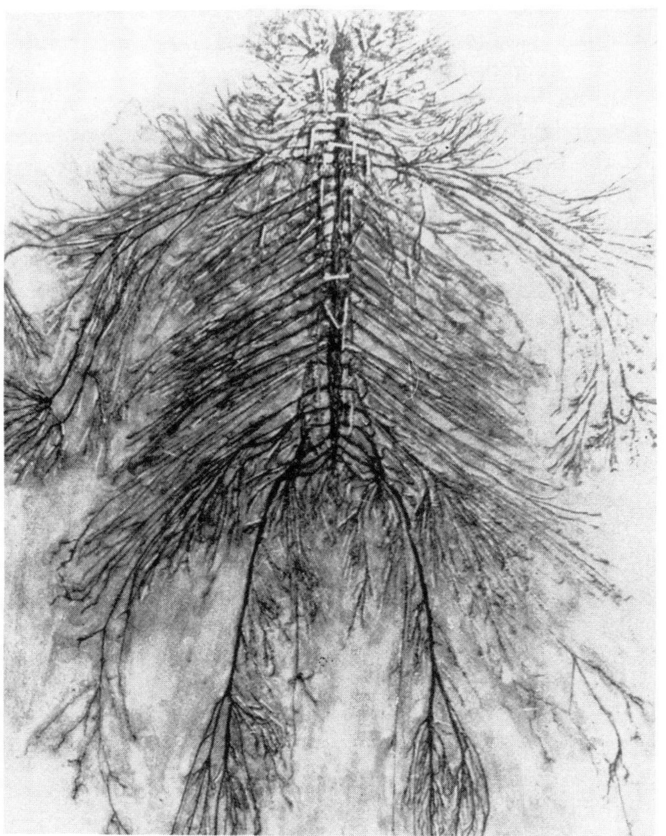

Nerve system of the human body

August, 1899

DR. A. T. STILL'S DEPARTMENT.

(Copyrighted)

Value of the Study of Anatomy.

LONG experience and experimenting with the human body has convinced me that there is but one way to comprehend and simplify the subject of healing. We have to look upon man whose deformities we wish to cor-

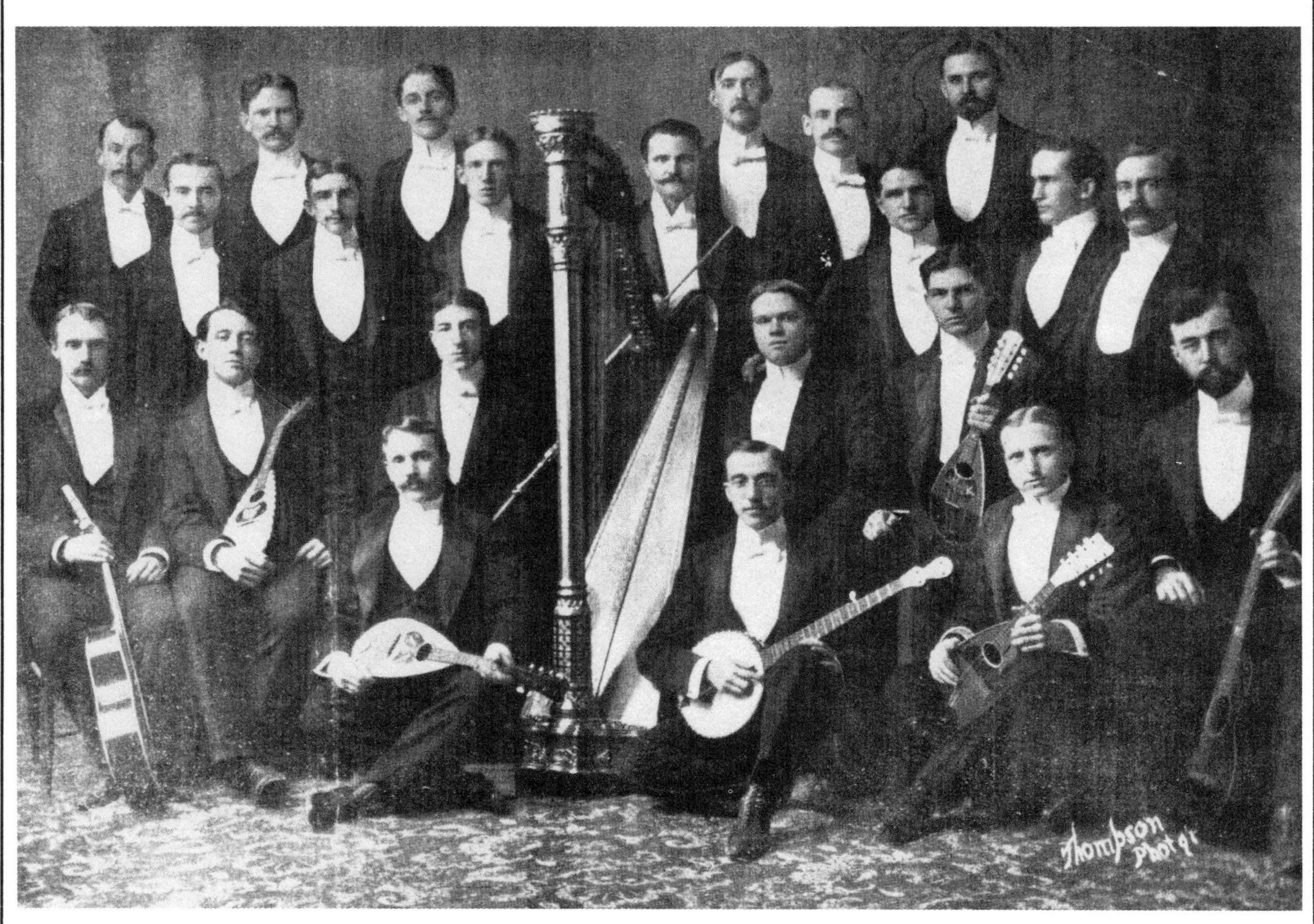

A.S.O. Glee Club and Orchestra

rect as a machine, of which all parts must be in a condition to do their part of the service necessary to producing and maintaining a healthy condition, and with this conclusion I have settled down to this method of reasoning, and that is, that all parts of the anatomy of man must be normal in size, strength and principle, to maintain health. I have decided that any other study than that of the human body—or the study of anatomy—is of but little use to him who would approach and find a body in an abnormal condition with a view of causing to return to the normal—he can only hope to do so by his knowledge of anatomy, which will skillfully conduct his mind from place to place to observe any variation of the system from the normal. Thus anatomy is his morning, his noon and his setting sun of light. One asks—would you not use physiology in the healing art? my answer is yes—and that physiology is a part of anatomy as much so as osteology is of anatomy. Another asks—of what use is histology? A ready answer to that question is that histology only draws the mind's eye to observe the very finest work and machinery known by the study of anatomy A third one asks—of what use is chemistry in this court of investigation? A proper answer to this question comes in so many words—it is only a witness to prove that chemical work going on in the works of Nature known as the physiological part of anatomy—therefore it is useful. Another asks—of what use is symptomatology? We answer that by asking this one question —of what use is a gauge cock or glass tube to an engineer but to mark the condition of the steam and water in the boiler? When I say this I do not mean the old and unreliable system of guess work that begins with—"I suppose so" and winds up with "however" and has the credit of being called scientific symptomatology, but I mean that kind of symptomatology that can and does tell what condition the engine is in by unnatural sounds, hissing, sizzing, "chucks and clucks," heats of boxing, journals and so on of his engine. I mean that if an Osteopath does understand his anatomy and is trained to observe—he can tell when the system is out of order and what causes the failure of a part or of the whole engine when he inspects it anatomically, for anatomy is what you want first, last and all the time, in your head, in your soul and in your hands in particular, because man is the engine and is the pattern of all engines.

For conveniences' sake the study of anatomy has been divided into several divisions or lessons for the student. He commences with the bones—their forms, and their uses which we call osteology. Lesson number two comes when the student learns to tie the bones together. In lesson three he learns the forms, places and uses of the muscles. His fourth lesson deals with the blood supply and the vessels formed for that purpose. His fifth embraces a knowledge of the use and quality of the nerves which convey vital forces. His sixth lesson teaches him where and how the blood and other fluids are prepared in the chemical laboratory that is found in the human body, this lesson is called physiology and is a very important lesson; It should be pointed and impressively taught, and be as little voluminous as possible for the practical Osteopath. With this lesson it is necessary to have a good rudimentary knowledge of chemistry and that knowledge for the light it throws upon the physiological laboratory that is playing in the human body all the time.

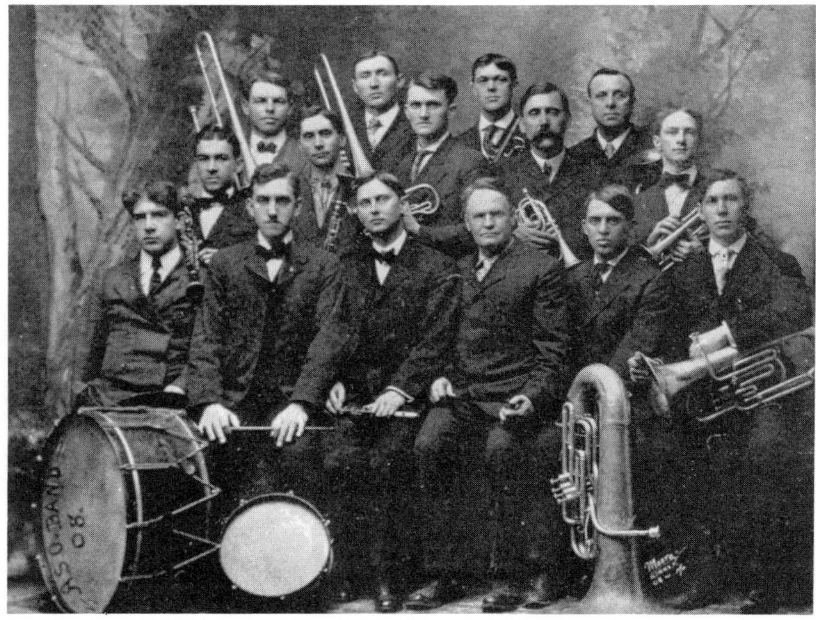

1908 A.S.O. Band

I AM often asked this and similar questions: "Dr. Still, what caused you to study out the great truths of curing the afflicted without drug remedies?" As you have asked me that question, I will give you this as a partial answer: First, I tried the ability of drugs, as taught and administered by Allopathy, then noticed closely the effect from the schools of Eclecticism and Homeopathy; I concluded all was a conglomerate mess of conjectures and experiments on the ignorant sick man, from the crown to the heel. I learned that a King was just as ignorant of the nature of disease as his coachman, and the coachman no wiser than his dog. I had passed through measles, whooping cough, and the full list of contagious, climatics, and diseases of the seasons. I was raised by a graduate of medicine, who trained me to observe the start, progress and the two endings of disease. The one to get well despite drugs and disease; the other to die amidst pills, prayers and all human efforts. I was familiar with the word "God" from a child up. My father was a good man (or tried to be.) He gave me castor oil, rhubarb, gamboge, aloes, calomel, lobelia, quinine and soap pills, then he would ask God to bless the means being used for my recovery. When I grew older I followed in his foot-steps all but asking God to bless the means and poisonous filth I was using in my ignorance of cause and effect. I thought the filth I had given would kill or cure if it was its nature to do so, and in time nature's scraper would scrape out the system and the patient would get well.

I began to look for a God of truth who did not guess at all things. I learned to believe that there was a reliable God at the head of all things—one who did not use morning bitters to tone him up for the coming day's work. I began to learn that all his work when done was placed above criticism or even a suggestion of criticism. I concluded I would prove him and see if he was as wise as I thought he was. I put his work on the race track of reason and experiment. It got the purse of victory every time and all the time.

I got ready to attend the fall races. I got up in the judge's stand where they ring the bell to "go." Nature's little pony came out on the track. He was not much bigger than a goat. He sided up by the fine steeds of drugs, and at the word "go!" he started out at full speed. I was afraid the fiery steeds would run over him. The race grew more interesting each quarter-post he passed, and he won the prize in fall diseases, because he depended upon Nature's law. The horses of much ribbon and big saddles tried their very best; they broke gait, ran and plunged in wild confusion, determined to pass Joshua, but he got the purse, blue ribbon and all, in the fall races.

They found that Joshua had nothing to do with jockey racing. He went on into winter and spring diseases; he commanded them to stand and they did stand.

When the races were through and the fiery steeds found there was no use to measure speed with "Joshua" they made many suggestions. That, as Osteopathy was a great truth discovered and demonstrated by Joshua, it could be made a great money scheme; that millions could be made out of it; that its literature should be placed upon all news-stands because of the anxiety of the people to know something of the pedigree of this little horse of so many victories on all race tracks, where the speed and efficacy of remedies should have a fair trial and the ribbon be awarded to the successful contestant; that the notoriety thus obtained will give in favor of Joshua the lever by which we can make countless millions, if we use it.

Joshua stopped and looked at the sun and moon which he had commanded to stand. The order had been obeyed at once, and while looking at those wonderful planets he said: "I will go into no jockey races, combines or organizations by which one dollar or cent can be taken unjustly from suffering humanity. Fame and money are not what I want, unless it be given me at the tracks where the ribbon of merit is awarded to the successful horse, without jockeying or collusion whatever."

Osteopathy is not the outgrowth of printer's ink; but of what it has been able to do for the afflicted when all other methods had failed to give relief. The mouths of the once afflicted and now well are the oracles through whom the growth of this science has been made great and world-wide famous. It is the cures, not paper stories.

* * *

ANATOMY AND OSTEOPATHY.

ANATOMY well understood and wisely applied for the alleviation of diseases is what should be meant by Osteopathy. Disease means some abnormality of the anatomy and the Osteopath must find and correct that condition to the true line of Nature's wants or he is only worthy of the name masseur or is a superficial blank. Nature is a large field with rivers of pure thought and he must drink and drink freely if he would succeed. The ways of Nature are pleasant beyond comparison; she from her kindly breast gives only milk that can feed and nourish the mind—that milk can make us see worlds of beauty where we failed to see even a shadow.

Osteopathy is Nature trying to vindicate itself by building anew all parts of the body from its own laboratory in which substances are prepared from crude material. Anatomy helps us to know and to judge when we are normal or when we are abnormal in all of the parts of the body. Anatomy is not simply a knowledge of each part of the body but treats of their use, either in a general or a special way. Chemistry has an important place to fill by way of proof that in man the most wisely arranged system of chemistry is at work all the time, and to be familiar with that is to know that life is a power and is wisely sustained throughout all Nature.

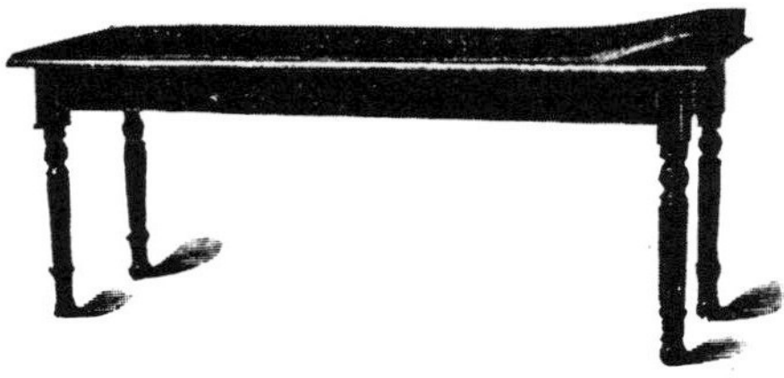

September, 1899

DR. A. T. STILL'S DEPARTMENT.

IN answer to the questions of how long have you been teaching this discovery, and what books are essential to the study.

I began to give my reasons for my faith in the laws of life as given to men, worlds and beings by the God of Nature, June, 1874, or began to talk and propound questions to men of learning. I thought the sword and cannons of Nature were pointed and trained upon our systems of drug doctoring. I asked Dr. J. M. Neal of Edinburgh, Scotland, for some information that I needed badly. He was a medical doctor of five year's training. He was a man of much mental ability and would give his opinions freely and to the point. I have been told by one or more Scotch medical doctors that a Dr. J. M. Neal of Edinburgh, was hung for murder; he was not hung while with me. The only thing that made me doubt him being a Scotchman was that he loved whiskey, and I have been told that the Scotch were a sensible people. But I will quote John M. Neal in this story; he said drugs were the bait of fools, that the drug system was no science, but was only a trade and only followed by the doctors for the money that could be obtained by it from the ignorant sick. He believed that Nature was a law that could vindicate its power all over the world.

As this writing is for the information of the prospective student, I will continue the history by saying that in the early days of Osteopathy I sought the opinions of the most learned, such as Dr. Schnebly, professor of languages and history in Baker University, Baldwin, Kansas, Dr. Dallas, a very learned medical doctor of the allopathic faith, Dr. F. A. Grove well known in Kirksville, J. B. Abbott, Indian agent and many others well known. Then back to the tombs of the dead, to better acquaint myself with the systems of medicine and the foundations of truth upon which they stood, if any. I will not worry you with a list of the names of authors that have written upon the subject of medicine as remedial agents. I will use the word the theologian often uses when asked whom Christ died for—the answer is universally—all. I will say all intelligent medical writers do say by word or inference that drugs or drugging is a system of blind guess work and if we should let our opinions be governed by the marble lambs and other emblems of dead babies that are found in the cemeteries of the world, John M. Neal was possibly hung for murder, not through design but through traditional ignorance of the power of Nature to cure both old and young, by skilfully adjusting the engine of life so as to bring forth pure and healthy blood, which is the greatest known germicide, to the mind that is able to reason and that has the skill to conduct the vitalizing and protecting fluids to throat, lungs and all parts of the system and ward off diseases as Nature's God has indicated. With this faith and with this method of reasoning, I began to treat diseases by Osteopathy as an experimenter, and notwithstanding I got good results in all diseases of climate and contagions I hesitated for years to proclaim to the world that there was no excuse for a master engineer to lose a child in cases of diphtheria, croup, measles, mumps, whooping cough, flux and other forms of summer diseases, peculiar to children. Neither was it necessary for the adult to die with diseases of summer, fall and winter and on this rock and my confidence in Nature I have stood and fought the battles and have taken the enemy's flag in every engagement for the past twenty-five years.

As you contemplate studying this science and have asked to know the necessary studies I will say, and wish to impress it upon your minds that you begin with anatomy, you end with anatomy, a knowledge of anatomy is all you want or need, as it is all you can use or ever will use in your practice, although you may live one hundred years. You have asked my opinion, as the founder of the science—yours is an honest question and God being my judge, I will give you just as honest an answer. As I have said—a knowledge of anatomy with its application covers every inch of ground that is necessary to qualify you to become a skillful and successful Osteopath when you go forth into the world to combat diseases. I will now define what I mean by anatomy. I will speak by comparison and tell you what belongs to the study of anatomy. I will take a chicken whose parts and habits all persons are familiar with. The chicken has a head, a neck, a breast, a back, a tail, two legs, two wings, two eyes, two feet, one gizzard, one crop, one set of bowels, one liver and one heart. This chicken has a nervous system, a glandular system, a muscular system, a system of lungs and other parts and principles not necessary to speak of in detail. But I want to emphasize that they do belong to the chicken and it would not be a chicken without every part or principle; these must all be present and answer roll call, or we do not have a complete chicken. Now I will try and give you the parts of anatomy and the books that pertain to the same. You want some standard author on descriptive anatomy in which you learn the form and places of all bones, the place and uses of ligaments, muscles and all that belong to the soft parts. Then from descriptive anatomy you are conducted into the dissecting rooms in which you receive demonstrations and are shown all parts through which blood and other fluids are conducted. So far you see you are in anatomy. From the demonstrator you are conducted to another room or branch of anatomy called physiology, a knowledge of which no Osteopath can do without and be a success. In that room you are taught how the blood and other fluids of life are produced and the channels through which these fluids are conducted to the heart and lungs for purity and other qualifying processes before entering the heart for general circulation to nourish and sustain the whole human body. I want to insist and impress it upon your minds that it is as much a part of anatomy as a wing is a part of a chicken. From this room of anatomy you are conducted to the room of histology, where the eye is aided by powerful microscopes and made acquainted with the smallest arteries of the human body which in life are of the greatest importance. Remember that in the rooms of histology you are only studying anatomy and what that machinery can and does execute every day, hour and minute of life. From the histological room you are conducted to the rooms of elementary chemistry, in which you learn something of the laws of association of substances that you can the better understand what has been told you in the physiological rooms which is only a branch of anatomy and intended to show you that Nature can and does successfully compound and combine elements for muscle, blood, teeth and bone. From there you are taken to the rooms of the clinics, in which you are first made acquainted with both the normal and the abnormal body, which is only a continuation of the study of anatomy. From there you are taken to the engineer's room, (or operator's room) in which you are taught to observe and detect abnormalities and the effect or effects they may and do produce, and how they affect health and cause that condition known as disease.

* * *

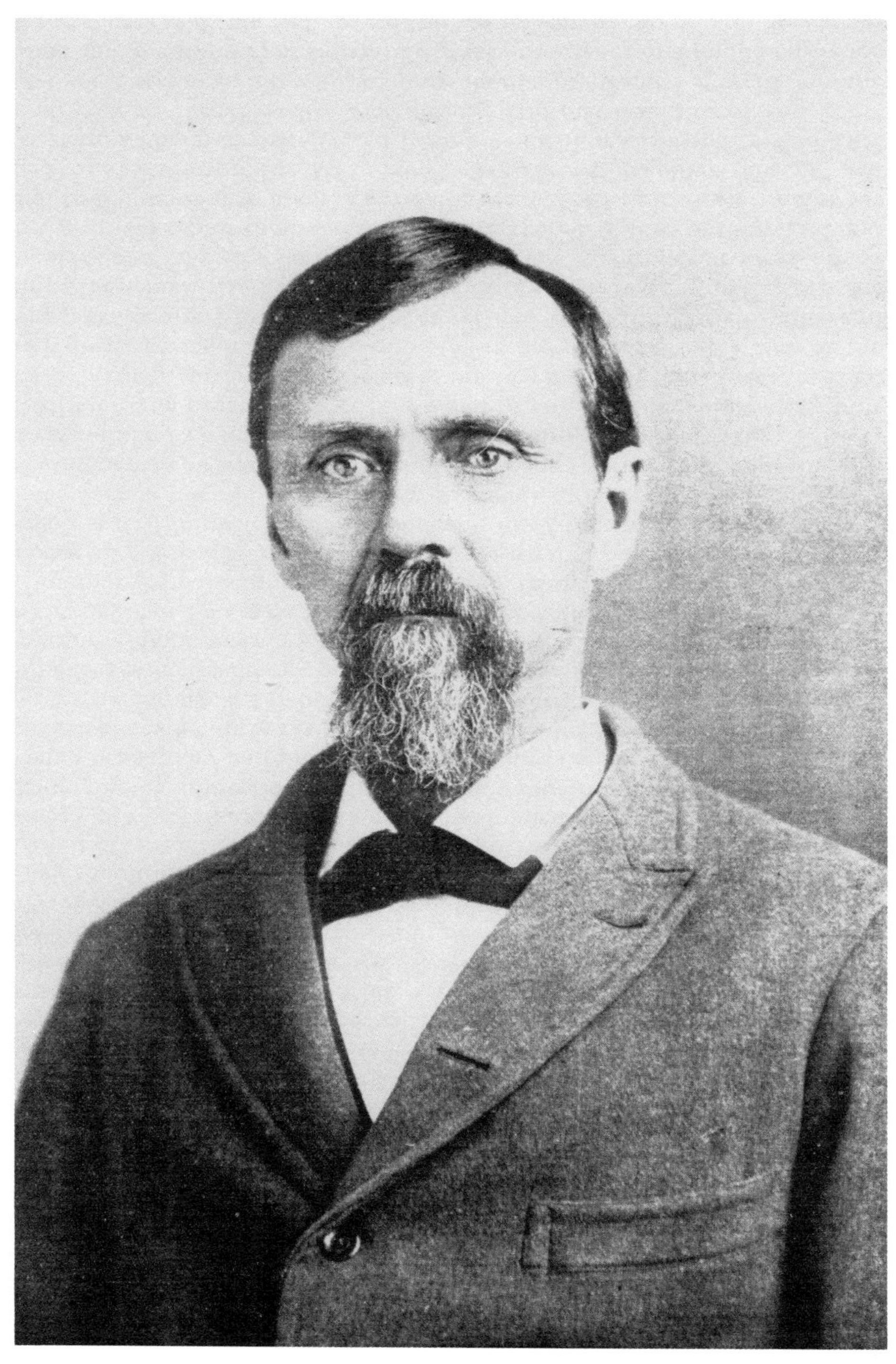

DR. A. T. STILL.

September, 1899

Consumption.

IN a former number of the Journal I spoke of lung diseases. I would let the subject drop had it not been for the light which I think has been offered by Osteopathy, in my effort to know more of the causes that would probably produce feeble action in the nerve systems, that should keep the lungs pure and strong to throw off all matter before it could accumulate and produce deadly deposits in such quantity as to suspend the natural flow of blood, lymph, air and the fluids of life and death. I have reasoned about so that each nerve of motion, sensation, nutrition, voluntary and involuntary must act their parts, and be able to do them well or such failure would be sufficient cause to mark one defect to each. Thus would not feeble sensation allow accumulations without sufficient irritation of the lungs to produce a cough which would or could blow out the accumulations of albumin, fibrine and such other substances that have become hindering deposits? Then again, if motion should be diminished by any cause, say from a partial or complete dislocation of some rib or spinal articulation, which would interfere with the action of the motor nerves of the lungs the power to cough and by that method discharge foreign substances, the air passages would be overcome and the deposits left in air passages and obstruct the action of the oxygen to the lungs to the degree of asphyxia or death of blood corpuscles. Then we will suppose that sensation and motion are both unobstructed and the action of the nerves of nutrition suspended from any cause whatever, the result would be atrophy of one or both lungs. Then should the nerves of the voluntary or involuntary system be disabled and all other nerves of the lungs normal, have we not caused them for the process of accumulation to go on and load down the lungs by congestion to the degree of suffocation? Now as the Osteopath is supposed to be finely posted in anatomy and physiology, should he take up the subject of consumption, has he not great cause or reason to believe one or more of the nerves belonging to the lungs are interfered with by muscular or bony disturbances either in the neck, ribs or spinal articulations? I do not wish to appear presumptuous nor leave the inference that I am the bright philospher of the day, but I want to tell the students and graduates of the American School of Osteopathy a few well known truths by the way of mental refreshment. For fifty years or more I have been in possession of the teachings of a well furnished medical library. My father was a medical doctor; I was born in the midst of cough drops, squill-syrup, with or without chloroform, laudanum, honey, pepper and alum cough syrup, hoarhound, onions, sweet milk, salt, black and red pepper cough-drops, inhaling tubes, blisters of all kinds, an occasional bleeding a pint or two at a time, blue mass pills for breakfast, castor oil, turpentine and sugar for supper, and on and on with prescriptions for something to take in the stomach for the cure of the lungs, and before I forget it I want to tell you that with all their syrups and drops they died; also I want to tell you once for all that in hunting up the opinions and "say so's" of the writers of the last four hundred years added to the previous four thousand five hundred there has been nothing said except to tell us what to take. If you doubt my word pull down from your medical authors from the days of "Why are not my daughters healed" and "Is there no balm in Gilead" and I think you will be surprised to find that in all your reading there has been nothing said that would be of any interest to an Osteopath, one who has been thoroughly trained in recitation, the clinic and operating rooms upon the great importance of a good knowledge of the nerves that rule and govern the lungs, which nerves are dependent for their well being on the nerves of the skin, the fascia and the whole viscera with all nerves thereunto belonging for healthy action of every organ, part and principle of the whole body if we expect the lungs to be normal in their action. One would say—this is much talk,but where is the sense? I will answer the same by asking a few questions. Have the lungs a nerve of sensation, one of motion, one of nutrition, one voluntary and one involuntary? Can they do duty with blood that has been detained below the diaphragm until it is diseased or dead before it enters the heart and lungs? Can blood be healthy for the lungs with a neck so badly twisted or strained as to cause the hyoid bone to be pulled back upon the pneumogastric nerve by the constrictor muscles of the neck? Use your brain, your knowledge of anatomy and your powers of reason. Answer such questions yourself. Throw your cough-drops to the doctor, not to the dog. Buckle around your waist the red belt of no quarter for what must I take or what must I give for lung trouble.

* * *

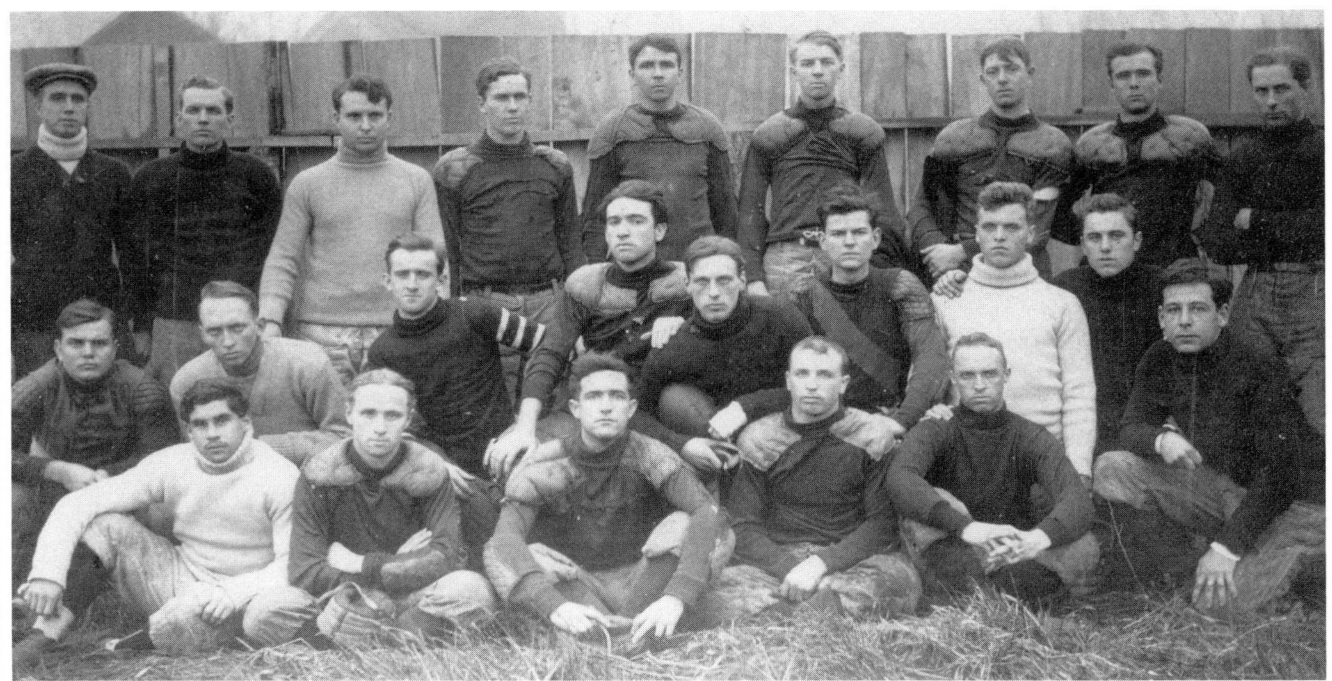

Undefeated 1911 A.S.O. football team

Dyspepsia or Imperfect Digestion.

IN our physiologies we read much about the hows and whats of digestion We will start in where they stop; they bring us to the lungs with chyle fresh, as made and placed in the thoracic duct, previous to flowing into the heart to be transferred to the lungs to be purified and charged with oxygen and otherwise qualified, and sent off for duty through the arteries great and small, to the various parts of the system. But there is nothing said of the time when all blood is gas, (if ever) before it is taken up by the secretories, after refinement and driven to the lungs to be mixed with the old blood from the venous system. A few questions about the blood seem to hang around my mental crib for food. Reason says we cannot use blood before it has all passed through the gaseous stage of refinement, which reduces all material to the lowest forms of atoms, before constructing any material body. I think it safe to assume that all the muscles and bones of our body have been in the gas state while in the process of preparing substances for the blood. A world of questions arises at this point. The first is where and how is food made into gas while in the body? If you will listen to a dyspeptic after he has eaten, you will wonder where he gets all the wind that he rifts from his stomach, and keeps up one or two hours after each meal. The gas is made in the stomach and intestines; we are led to think so because we know of no other place in which the gas can be made and thrown into the stomach by any other tubes or other methods of entry. Thus by the evidence so far, the stomach and bowels are the places in which this gas is generated. Now comes question two: As I have spoken of the stomach that generates and ejects great quantities of gas for a longer or shorter time after each meal—this class of people are called dyspeptics. Another class of the same race of beings stand side by side with him but without this gas generating; he too, eats and drinks of the same kinds of food without any of the manifestations that have been described in the first class. Why does one stomach blow off gas continually, while the other does not—this is a very deep, serious and interesting question. As number two throws off no gas from the stomach is this conclusive evidence that the stomach does not form gas continually? or does his stomach and bowels form gas just as fast as number one and the secretories of the stomach and bowels take up gas and retain the nutritious matter and pass the remainder of the gas by way of the excretory ducts through the skin? If the excretory ducts take up and carry this gas out of the body by way of skin and he is a healthy man, why not account for stomach number one ejecting gas by by way of the mouth, because of the fact that the secretions of the mucous membranes of the stomach are either clogged up or are inactive for want of vital motion of the nerve terminals of the stomach. Another question in connection with this subject: Why is the man whose stomach belches forth gas in such abundance also suffering with cold feet, hands and is cold all over the body generally, and number two is quite warm and comfortable, with a glow of warmth passing from his body all the time? With these hints I will ask the question:—what is digestion?

* *

September, 1899

A QUESTION:—Why is he too fat and she only skin and bone, while a third is just right? If one is just right, why not all? If I get fat by a natural process, why not reverse that process and stop at any desirable point in flesh size? I believe the law of life is simple and natural in both respects if wisely understood. Have we nerves of nutrition to carry food to all parts, organs, glands and muscles? Have we channels to convey to all? Have we fluids to suit all demands? Have we brain power equal to all force needed? Is blood formed sufficiently to fill all demands? Does that blood contain fat, water, muscle, skin, hair and every thing to suit, each division, organ and nerve? If so, and blood has builded too much muscle, can it not take that bulk away by returning blood to gas and other fluids? If yes be the correct answer then we can hope to return blood, fat, flesh and bone to gas and pass them away while in gaseous condition, and do away with all unnatural size or lack of size. I think it is natural with Nature to build and destroy all material form from the lowest animated being to the greatest rolling world. I believe no world could be constructed without strict obedience to a governing law, which gives size by addition and reduces that size by subtraction. Thus a fat man is builded by much addition and if desired can be reduced by much subtraction, which is simply a law of numbers. Turn your eye for a time to the supply trains of Nature; when the crop is abundant the lading is great, and when the seasons do not suit the crops are short and shorter to no lading at all. Thus we have the fat man and the lean man. Is it not reasonable as a conclusion of the most exacting philosophy that the train of cars that can bring loads of stone, brick and mortar until a great bulk is formed can also carry away until this bulk disappears in part or all? This being my faith I will say that by many years of careful observation of the work of creating bodies and destroying the same that to add to is the law of giving size and to substract from it the law of reduction; both are natural and both can be made practical in the reduction of flesh when found too great in quantity, or we can add to and give size to the starving muscle through the action of the motor and nutrient system, conveyed to and appropriated from the laboratory in which all bodily substances are formed. Thus the philosophy is absolute and the sky is clear to proceed with addition and subtraction of flesh.

September, 1899

(I approve the above article. The D. O. in the definition of Osteopathy was left out without my knowledge or consent, and was added as soon as I noticed the omission. We want no M. D. O. in our school—for the American School is strictly Osteopathic—and D. O. means just what it stands for, Diplomate in Osteopathy.)

A. T. STILL.

October, 1899

I want to say to the students and graduates of the American School of Osteopathy one and all, that I have tried for a quarter of a century never to camp two nights in succession on the same ground. My motto has been onward and upward, try to grow wiser and more effective in this science every day of the year. When I found that I had to labor very hard to set a hip or any other joint of the body and was too tired to talk at the end of the day's work I would think a part or all of the night following how to save my strength by an easier and better method, which I followed and taught to others, until I could make another advance, and on and on as a practical engineer would do to hoist, lower, advance or back his engine. I considered Osteopathy a system of engineering, and in teaching, my object has been to make thorough engineers, not to only unload fever but all other kinds of lading known as disease. I have labored to qualify each student as he goes out to take charge of and wisely conduct his engine, and before I affixed my name to any diploma I believed the receiver of said parchment had had an opportunity to learn all that we could teach him to the date of the receipt of this parchment. Not only that, but that he was worthy and well qualified to go out in the world and do good service whereever he might be, provided he had done his duty in studying his lessons and being present at all roll calls. He who has done his duty surely is prepared to think and make many advanced moves hitherto unknown by him. He knows if able to reason at all that Osteopathy contains the propelling force in great quantities of producing thought, reason and progress. As I have said in previous numbers of the Journal that when I think I have discovered any new method I will make it known at once, if I think it will be any advantage to the student or operator. I have solved many questions during the year 1899 that I did not understand in 1898, many in 1898 that I could not solve in 1897, and so on back to my childhood;so have you; you have been given carefully the basic principles of Osteopathy without reserve, according to the year in which you entered, from the baby to the present mammoth class. I will say that I have been greatly encouraged with the success and sober business conduct of at least 98 per cent. of all classes that I have tried to instruct. I have but one object and that is to know more of natural law and impart it as soon as obtained.

A. T. Still.

* * *

November, 1899

DR. A. T. STILL'S DEPARTMENT.

(Copyrighted)

THEN AND NOW.

TWENTY-FIVE years ago I was alone in all the work. I had no one to help, but many to hinder. But a change has come; I have a fully equipped school with those whom I have trained to lead the classes as teachers and operators; this has taken the burden off in that line. To have lost my trained anatomist at the beginning of my school would have been to lose all. There are others now that can and will take the place of him or any one who may sicken or choose to leave; we miss them but a few hours, for just as good stand in the ranks as led the last charge. Their drill has been to prepare them for all places, more so of late than in former years. If I should die or absent myself for a time my place would be filled. Each year we are stronger and better qualified. This school is no one man institution, that would fall if "Pap, Tom or Jim" should die or go off. You must remember that each year brings to the school just as good men and women as leave with their diplomas to battle with disease. Good operators and teachers have gone out each year. The question has often been asked me what I would do if he or she should leave; what would become of the school? I tell the enquirer this—I can fill the place, with just as good or better. I am often glad to have a chance to fill places made vacant. I have never been egged for my bad choosing. Some are not good instructors, though they may be good operators, and should be where nature fitted them best to go. Remember, I always have the best interest of my school at heart, and will try to keep the best instructors, those who are up to date.

In the clinic rooms of Osteopathy the order has always been that all systems of drugs with their teachings should be expunged, and that order must be respected and obeyed to the letter. I have spoken this by publication that the reader may know just how my school stands. On this line I have fought all previous battles and taken the flag in each engagement.

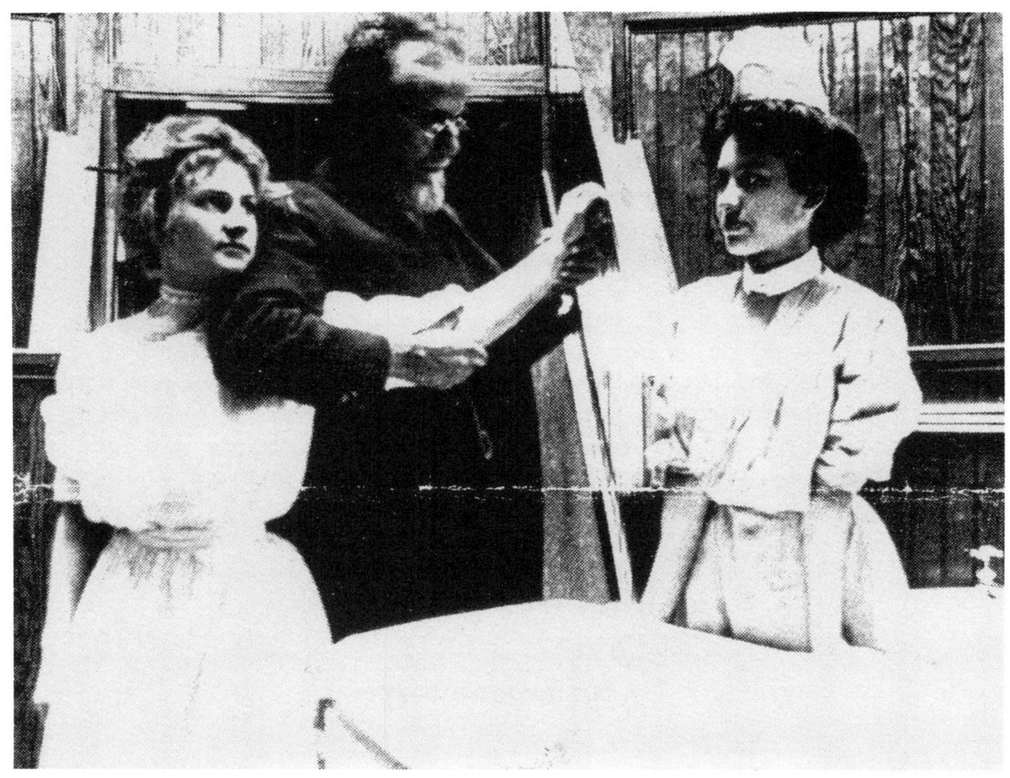

A. T. Still demonstrating a manipulative technique

WORK NOT TALK.

IT is not a question of how many patients an operator treats each day, but a question of how much sense he shows in the many difficult and "hopeless" cases that come to him. It is not how good a talker the doctor is, but what his work proves him to be. What good is talk when the patient has been nearly talked to death, and his back is still in the same shape that it was from one to three months ago, with just as much pain as ever. You must get your patient well; he wants work, not wind and smiles, he wants his hip put into the socket; he can and will do all the good talk if you set his hip into its place, stop his pain and send him home sound and well from head to foot. Then you will get truthful and thankful talk from him whom you have cured. He is the one to sing your praise; give him the job, he will do the talking.

I will say as a general rule a big gab is a poor operator. I would advise the world to take gab like the Indian said "much big gab much big fool, he scare game off with mouth, too much howl." I know you can do good work when you leave, and want all of you to roll up your sleeves; do good work to-day and better tomorrow, and let your patients talk for you. Never tell how smart you are; if you have brains the world will find it out by your good work only.

I am asked by my students how I worked up so much interest, and so large a business—if I advertised much, and so on; my answer to all has been, that I depended wholly upon my work. My motto has been to do good work and do it as quickly as possible and send the patient home well, and be ready to treat and cure the next bad or worse case and let them advertise for me. I have no use for "write ups" in papers because they all sound and smell fishy.

What I have said here is not an order for my students to follow, but to tell you that gab is not work, and that good work is what makes you famous and loved by the afflicted.

December, 1899

DR. A. T. STILL'S DEPARTMENT.

Exploration for the Cause of Consumption.

LET us begin with the supply train of life, the heart. In it we find the first motion of blood. From the heart to the lungs the road is direct, and if all functional demands are executed on time and with force and motion that will put the oxygen in quick union with the feeble corpuscles, then we can look for normal combustion of dead fluids of the lymphatics of the lungs. But if the heart has not the power to feed and keep up the vital action of the four systems of nerves of the lungs, then we have four causes for lesions in the lungs. If the heart should fail to feed well the motor nerves of the lungs we will find them too slow to drive blood fast enough to generate gases in the lungs by friction and union of oxygen with carbon, phosphorus and other substances, that are taken to the lungs to be converted into gas and blown out by the motor power of the lungs. Then if the heart does not feed and keep the sensory nerves normal, a filling of muscles, fascia and lymphatics will follow, and cut off the vital action of air while in the lungs, by its stupefying bulk. Thus the great use of the sensory nerves to be fully normal. Then we find that just as much depends on the nerves of nutrition as either the sensory or the motor nerves. Just the same demand of the normal powers of the voluntary and involuntary nerves, as all other nerves of the lungs. The heart must keep all nerves well fed and strong, or a functional failure will follow. Thus the Osteopath must know that a feebly supplied heart cannot keep the lungs from deadly deposits. So we find the human race dying by the millions from decaying deposits that have found their way into and stopped the lungs until by time and fermentation a condition known as inflammation sets up a process of waste of the muscles

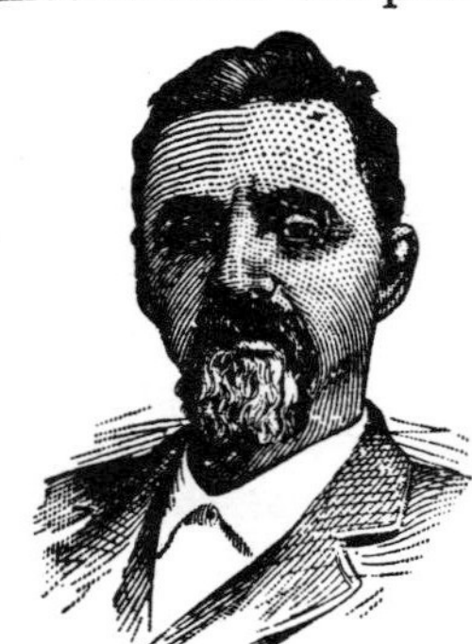

and other lung substances to such extent as to ruin all power of the lungs to purify and keep them builded to the normal standard, so that it can keep blood pure and healthy, that when sent back to the heart for general distribution it will meet all demands that nature makes on that food, by which the body is forever kept normal and ready to fill all its functions in the great economy of life. What and why does the heart and diaphragm have to do in allowing lungs to fail and give away under such burdens of waste matter that has not been consumed nor thrown off by combustion and the excretory system? At this time we will take up the heart for examination in this discussion.

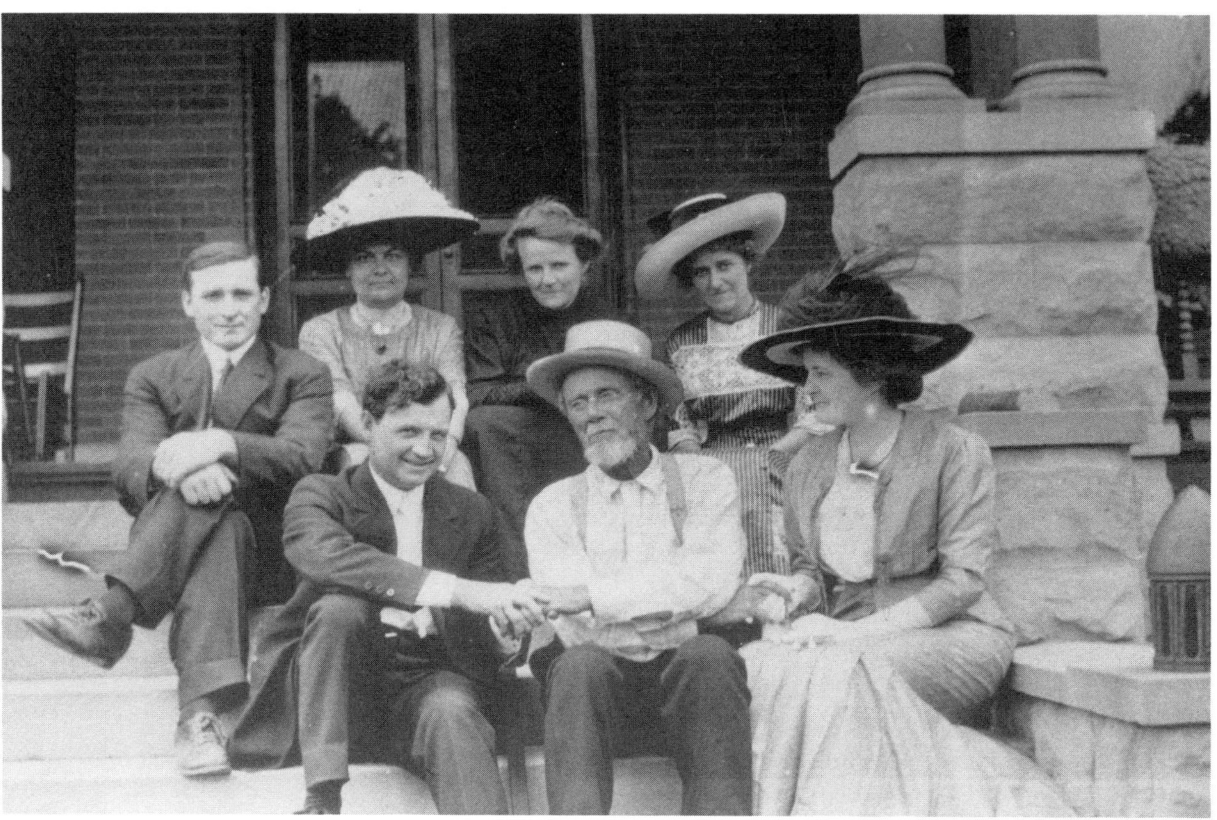

A. T. Still and students, c. 1915

We must not blame the heart with all who have died with wasted lungs, which disease is generally known as consumption. Suppose we give the heart a gender, and call him to the witness stand to answer. Court: Mr. Heart, state if you know how you are made, or supplied with blood? Mr. Heart: Well, I will state that before I do any supplying of blood for any part of the body, I provide for my own needs first by throwing out coronary arteries whose duty is to keep the heart normal in size and all functions; you see my demands are absolute and first to be supplied. Then as my duties are numerous I must be full of power so I can force the blood with power and speed enough to meet the oxygen and cause combustion by union with impurities of the blood of the lungs, and send such from the blood, by chemical union and action, and leave the corpuscles of life fitted for their every place. Thus I must provide for myself first or a failure will follow such shortages. If I am weak as an engine of blood the general supply will be in the same ratio, will it not? As I am general quartermaster of the division of life and am summoned before this court-martial which I esteem as a court of justice, and am charged with the murder of countless millions by my criminal neglect, in vindication of justice I will turn state's evidence, and "tell the truth, the whole truth and nothing but the truth, so help me God." First I am not guilty of a single case of murder that I am charged with, and as I am general quarter-master I have ordered in all cases that the inspector general shall feed nothing to my whole army that is not of the purest and most wholesome kinds. My inspector general's name is Mr. Lung, and you will please ask him to take the stand as he and the diaphragm may be more to blame than I am by this court of inquiry. I want to say in vindication of my innocence that I do deliver all blood to the lungs and all other parts of the body, just as it comes to me good and bad, but I will say there is great complaint in the report. He says so much dead or bad matter comes to his quarters for inspection and when examined and the bad left out that there is not enough good blood left to sustain the body in a healthy condition. He says he finds that all the chyle he receives for inspection is badly decayed when it arrives at his quarters, the lungs, to be separated and purified, and as the order comes from the Heart who is the quarter-master general is perfect purity, that when that order is obeyed but little blood canbe sent to the heart to deliver to the thousands of camps of the army of the living man. He has reported that he thinks the inspector general should send a commissioned officer to the camp of the diaphragm, and learn why all chyle sent from that great manufacturing region is badly damaged before it arrives at the quarter-master general's office. Will the court call the diaphragm to the stand and have him give reason why all provision passing through his gates has to be condemned by the inspector general?

The court calls Mr. Diaphragm to be seated. Mr. Diaphragm, state if you know why all provisions made in your shop and delivered by the hands of the thoracic duct are decayed and not fit to be eaten by the four laborers of life, sensation, motion, nutrition, voluntary and involuntary nerves. Well, to tell the truth, the whole truth and nothing but the truth, I will say I have done the best I could to get the goods to Mr. Heart and Lungs on time, but I have been squeezed by big dinners, by big suppers, big drunks, pressed up and pulled down or out and puckered out of all shape by the falling off of the ribs from the backbones from the top to the bottom, by falls, lifts, feet slipping on the ice, kicks from mules, gored by bulls, butted by rams, strained by vomits, purged by shovels full of pills, falling off houses, down wells, out of apple trees, running against clothes lines, plowing in roots and stumps and being tossed over the beam when the plow hit a root as big as your leg,—do you think it is any wonder that I squeeze the sour into my receptaculum chylii or pancreaticum "whum bum" or my "domen" when I am pounded by the heart to get the blood through my old rag of a diaphragm when it is held down by twisted back and lapped crus, till I am more twisted than a tin roof that has been blown off a house in a cyclone, and pounded against trees, houses, fences and stones, until there was not an inch of square tin in fifty feet. Now, Judge, you know I cannot do straight work in such shape, and if it were so you could take a ride through the little thoracic duct that conveys the chyle through me you would be old and toothless when you reached the heart to be sent to the lungs to have the dirty dirt washed out, and when it was washed out you would be so small that you would be of no use to feed the hungry millions of corpuscles that must have good food or die, which do keep the powers of the lungs able to separate the impurities from the blood, and thereby save life. When the Judge had heard all the evidence that came so earnestly from the diaphragm's honest face, he said: "This court is pleased to give you an honorable acquittal, and let you go, believing you have been the greatest martyr to man's ignorance that has ever been summoned before the court in ten thousand years, and you should have had a chance before the flood to say why man dies of consumption and no man knows your innocence and worth as well as an Osteopath.

Court: The reader will see at a glance when he has carefully studied the evidences given him by such able witnesses as have testified before this court, that at the wisely conducted inquest both previous to and post mortem, the heart has been clearly proven to be innocent of the charge of criminal neglect in receiving and delivering all chyle and other substances to each and every station of life both great and small as established before this court by all books belonging to that system of freightage.

It has lived fully up to the most exacting requirements of the commission, which bears the seal and signature of the hand of the Infinite. Equally so has the lung been vindicated and acquitted before this court. Then on the most crucial examination the diaphragm has proven its innocence of the charge of death of countless millions by consumption of human beings by not delivering chyle before decay had done its ruinous work.

Then you see by the same impartial court that the lymphatics are found to be equally innocent, with heart, lungs and diaphragm. But the spinal column has not yet reported whether for or against in this case, further than that his report will be to the point on the whys and causes that have given birth to the deadly effect known as consumption, which report will appear in the January number of the JOURNAL in which we will endeavor to give cause and cure of consumption by Osteopathy in all curable cases.

December, 1899

Fits, Convulsions and Spasms.

IN listing them by name we can say by our books of symptomatology "that twist is catalepsy, this twist is epilepsy, that face and eye with spine pulled back is hysteria," and on to a full list. At this time the book closes, and the pill box gaps its mouth wide open, with tongue of poison run out that is worse than four kinds of fits all put in a wad and run down the patient's throat at one dose. We all very well know that a spasm is not a turkey or a wolf, and we do know that we will have to go to some other than our medical books to learn the difference between a cow and a spasm. We have been left lamentably ignorant of the cause of spasms, why one person falls daily and one never falls with fits. Let us try and reason just a little by the rules of Osteopathy, and see what effect it would have on the motor nerves to stop the fluids in the spinal cord. Let us see if a broken neck might not be an irritant to a few nerves, such as sensation, locomotion, mind and even cause paralysis of half or even both sides of the body. Would a lumbar when pulled or twisted out of place or off sacrum be normal? Would a fit be normal to a broken neck? Can a fit live without a twisted spine? If all fits mark a pressure of a bone on some nerve of supply from medulla oblongata, middle or lower division of spinal cord why not close the pill box and open the brain box, get a new Osteopathic chain and compass of the very best make, and find and straighten up all corners, miles, sections, townships and range lines and stones as placed there by the surveyor general. Would it not be wise to look over the field-notes?

The subject of spasms becomes more serious to a medical doctor, or any other doctor when one or more of his family become the subject of his care. If his own should be his patient then we know his treatment will be to cure, because of his love for his child. We may say that the doctor works for money, but that view wont apply in such cases, but just the reverse; in this he is in earnest beyond all chance for doubt, he wants to cure, does all he can for his child, fails, calls council, he reads old and new works on the disease, follows remedies, but fails just as often. Not content to abandon his child he tries change of climate, hot, cold, wet and dry, he hunts up Faith-cures, Magnetic healers, Christian Science, and every thing he can hear of; he has time enough to use them all as his daughter has had fits for almost twenty years, and has been under the most skilled treatment, but with all his love for his child and all that has been done, the fits still continue.

We all know that man and beast are both subject to fits. We have all seen the sights, we know how horrible they look. We know some are harder than others. We know they will fall to the ground, down a well, in a fire or any place of danger as well as a place of safety. We know all about fits, we know he or she is totally separated from mind and motion. We hate to see them, we dread them, and so far our pills and prayers have failed to give relief—yet all have been tried. I know it—you know it, but we as human cannot give them up—we want the conscious reward of feeling that we have done all we could to banish the malady. This has been the custom for all time until Osteopathy began to explore the dark seas with its search-light of reason. And before its ship had recorded many knots it cast anchor at the neck for the purpose of noting the facts of active life that pass over the neck to and from the brain to spine, nerves and organs of life through the body. Soon after casting anchor we saw commotion in the veins of the neck; they were very full of venous blood that was in agony to get to the heart to be driven to the lungs to exchange carbon for oxygen. We saw that river of venous blood rise to fulness and overflow all lands that lived by the blood of life. We saw bridges torn up in the brain by this swollen river of drainage. At first we reasoned that we were in a land of beavers and they had surely builded a dam across the river, and that was the cause of such great inundation. We hunted for beaver by day and by night, we found none nor any sign of such dams as they build. Then we looked up and down the river to learn if the bank had fallen in and filled the channel. Soon we found a great stone had fallen into the channel and stopped the water on its way to all lands below that stone. Just so with the wise or skilled Osteopath; he too will find bones pushed in and across the blood channels of the neck and spine that will cause fits, convulsions and spasms.

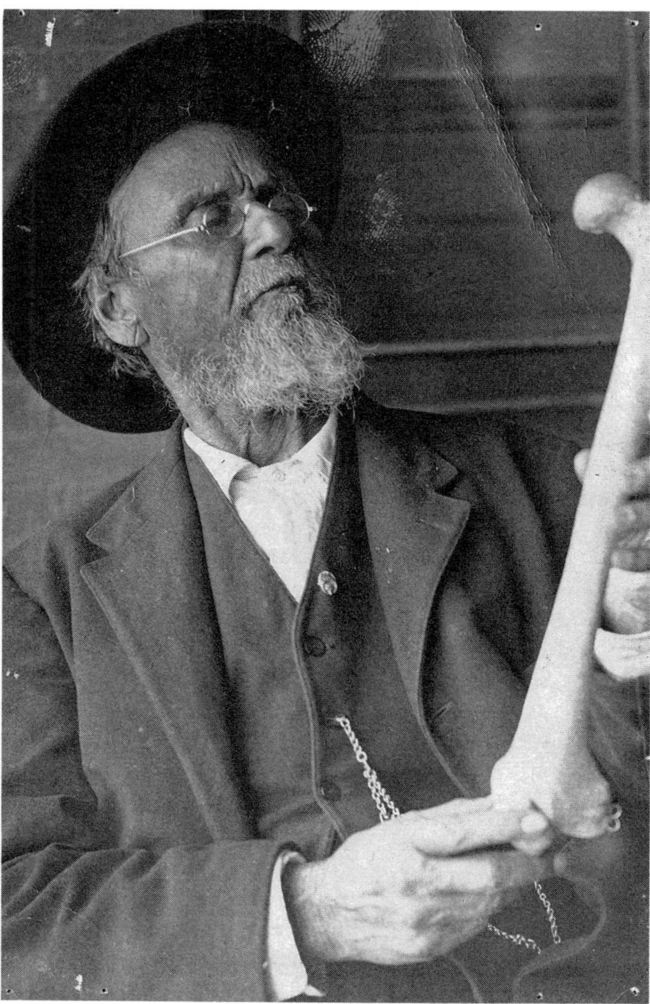

A. T. Still, c. 1907

January, 1900

DR. A. T. STILL'S DEPARTMENT.

(Copyrighted.)

CONSUMPTION, CONTINUED.

JUDGE: Court will now proceed with the prosecution of Mr. Spinal Column and wife, Mrs. Spinal Cord, as found in the indictment by the grand jury, whose verdict reads thus: A true bill of murder has been found against Mr. Spinal Column and Mrs. Spinal Cord conjointly, as being the cause of all the deaths now and in all periods of past time, by a disease of the lungs which is universally known by the name of pulmonary consumption.

Judge: Let your duty guide your investigation, and if you find the accused guilty of the charges as reported let your report read thus:

We, the jury, find after the most crucial examination that the defendants (Mr. Spinal Column and Mrs. Spinal Cord) are guilty of murder in the first degree, and are the cause of all delays in keeping up the purity and abundant supply of all fluids of human life. Let your search go far and deep into cause and effect, ever remembering that effect follows cause in all cases.

Judge: Mrs. Spinal Cord, you will please take the stand. You are charged of murder in the first degree of millions of beings by your neglect to do your duty in supplying force plentifully to all organs, glands and stations of life. You must now show your innocence by such truths as will prove that you have done your duty from start to finish, or you will have to suffer the penalty of the law which is death.

Judge: Madam, state if you know why you should not suffer the punishment as provided by law.

Madam: Well Judge, you say "state if you know," I will state that I do know what my duty is. I know my orders for they are all written with the red ink of life on the face of my commission. I know full well every inch and every thousandth part of an inch I am ordered to supply with blood.

Madam: Judge, I know something of your duty and will state if I know "and what I know." I do know that your oath when you took your seat was to do justice equal and exact to all without prejudice. And will ask you to examine the plan and specification of the spinal column, the house in which I dwell. I have certain duties to perform, which are to eat, drink and keep myself in the best of working order as when nature formed and finished me, and gave me the keys of the long bony house that reaches from man's head to extreme sacrum. I was given and required to study carefully both the plan and specification of the house in which I was to dwell as foreman and master mechanic. I was required to take charge and conduct all works of the chemical compounding of the laboratory of animal forms, and in all rooms see and know that all fluids were infinitely correct in weights and kinds, previous to making any compound substance to be used in forming brain, blood, bone, muscle, hair, skin, veins, arteries, secretory and excretory vessels with their associate system of nerves. I was not only given orders but was commanded to make and keep a full supply of chemically pure blood, with this caution heavily underlined: "*Pure blood*" means a perfect machine throughout, with all its parts free from all hindrances from perfect work. The machine must be true to the line and plumb, with space to suit its action. Then it can and will furnish all the power necessary to run all divisions to produ ce all forms and sizes of the body, to make and fit all atoms to their various places.

Then we will see that part or division of purity do its work of washing the body from all waste before its seeks an exit by other channels.

Madam: Judge, have you ever made an intimate acquaintance with the spinal cord and its duties? Do you know that by the forces passing it that the machinery that builds the brain, eye, heart, lungs, bones, long and short, bent or straight build to suit? Do you know that the blood that makes a bone cannot make an eye? Or the biood that makes a liver cannot make a bladder? Now suppose my husband, Mr. Spinal Column, should get on a "bender" and force the gall department to unload some gall fluid in the vats that make and keep the lungs strong and active, would you hope to have power in such lungs to separate and keep blood pure for its own use, or any other organ or atom of the system?

The command given to me is to keep all pipes free from interfering with all others or I will see disease, tumors, cancers, consumption and death as a result of such neglect.

The Osteopath must remember that no consumptive can show a normal spine from the first tickling cough to the end of his or her life. No spine can be normal with ribs tangled in muscles and held so by misplaced fibers, gotten so by some fall or jar that pushed bone and ligaments from their normal position, and caused the lesion that did the work of death from start to finish.

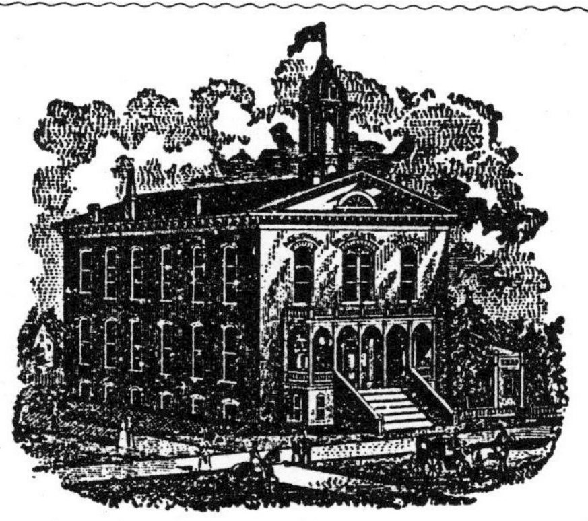

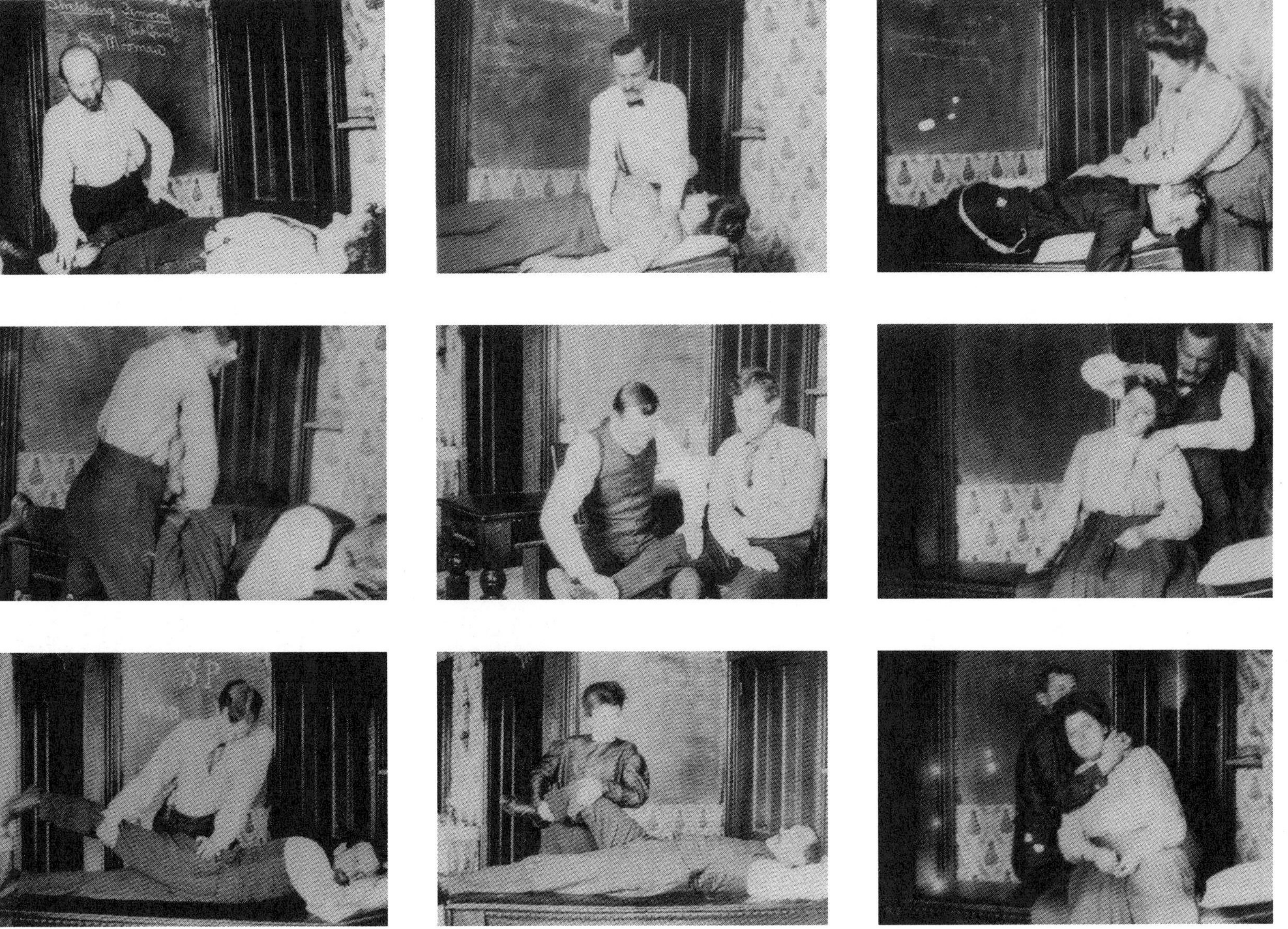
SP

ACT OF JUNE 27, 1890.

3706

No. 189004 UNITED STATES OF AMERICA Original.

DEPARTMENT of the INTERIOR

Engraved and Printed at the Bureau Engraving & Printing

BUREAU OF PENSIONS

It is hereby certified That in conformity with the laws of the United States, Andrew T. Still who was a Hospital Steward Cass County Mounted Missouri Home Guards, is entitled to a pension under the provisions of the

ACT OF JUNE 27, 1890.

at the rate of Twelve dollars per month to commence on the thirty-first day of May, one thousand nine hundred and four.

Given at the Department of the Interior this tenth day of August, one thousand nine hundred and four, and of the Independence of the United States of America the one hundred and twenty-ninth.

Thos Ryan

Acting Secretary of the Interior.

JKK Countersigned.

Commissioner of Pensions.

Certificate showing A. T. Still's Civil War Pension to be $12.00 per month.

March, 1900

DR. A. T. STILL'S DEPARTMENT.

BEFORE handing to you your diplomas, which you have earned by faithful and hard study, having passed satisfactory examinations in all branches:—It has been ordered by the trustees of the A. S. O. who have been constituted and legally authorized by the state of Missouri to issue certificates of qualification to all who shall have passed such examination. Such certificates are usually called diplomas.

All diplomas have local and significant values. Local because they cannot extend beyond the jurisdiction of the grantor. Instance: A diploma granted in the state of Missouri has no power to go beyond the boundary of said state. But by courtesy and the rules of reciprocity a diploma issued in the state of Missouri may be respected in the State of Illinois and other states of this Union. A commission or diploma issued by the U. S. goverment is only good within its jurisdiction.

By many who are ignorant and jealous of this system you will be advised that you should attend some medical college for the purpose of learning the use of drugs. When such advice is given, remember you have passed a rigid examination in all branches taught in medical colleges, as is shown on the face of your diplomas. No doubt your qualifications have made you competent to teach 75 per cent of all such persons for twelve months. I would advise you to examine them and if you find them professional blanks close the conversation and pass on.

Osteopathy has no use for drugs as remedies, but a great use for chemistry when dealing with poisons and antidotes. It recognizes and has a useful place for surgery, in both of which you have been well informed.

I will now draw your attention to the significant value of the diploma. If you have any power of reason you must know, and I will say you do know, that only by comparison can we arrive at an absolute knowledge of the difference in value of all things.

In speaking of the significant value and the comparative difference and moral force existing between two diplomas, one from a long and well established institution of learning that has the wealth to furnish all things necessary to a finished education, which school has been very careful in selecting experienced persons to fill the chairs in all departments, and the graduates who have completed their full course in all the branches necessary to that profession, be it law, medicine, sculpture, or any of the skilled arts, and whose graduates have gone forth into the world and proven by their work that such school or schools had the ability to give the necessary and useful information. Now in order to compare we will take a diploma from a school whose character has not been established, would you not arrive at the conclusion by comparison that there was a difference in the significant value between the two documents?

With due respect for all others we will take one from the world renowned medical university of Edinburgh, Scotland, whose thoroughness in all branches, is to-day established beyond doubt or inquiry. Wouldn't your judgment say, give me my diploma from an old established institution.

This comparison has been between old and established medical institutions for the purpose of bringing before your minds a foundation upon which you can decide whether you want established merit or prospective merit. As the American School of Osteopathy is the oldest and best prepared to teach the principles of Osteopathy, I believe that your diplomas will best sustain you in any part of the world. Because it has been as carefully guarded as any mother has ever guarded and cared for her children, morally, intellectually and justly, for one purpose only, which was to unfold the principles whereby life and health could be sustained by natural law, which requires no assistance but rest and nourishment, when all parts of the human system are in their natural position.

On this foundation Osteopathy has stood for twenty years, and successfully combatted disease of all kinds, without the aid of drugs. To the intellectually strong; the principles of Osteopathy will crown you with success, provided you adhere to them, while the wavering man will fall by the wayside.

American School of Osteopathy

Know all men by these presents, that
William Smith, M. D.
having attended a full course of Lectures on, and Demonstrations of Osteopathy, and having, after due examination, been found fully qualified to practise the Art in all its branches, is hereby conferred by me with the title
Diplomate in Osteopathy.

Given at Kirksville, Missouri
this, the 15th day of February 1893

A. T. Still.
President

April, 1900

Osteopathy, Not Drugs.

WHY NOT combine Osteopathy with drugs? is quite a common question and should be kindly answered. We will try and give our reasons for not wishing to associate the two methods of combatting diseases:

First—We will offer as an objection to such union that medicine has proven by time and long experience that it is a gigantic failure, not only when administered by the ignorant doctor, but equally so when administered by the most learned philosophers, that do or have ever depended upon drugs, as a life saving agent amidst diseases, and stands today so acknowledged by a universal vote of the gray haired jurors of sad experience. They long since have been convinced, that it, the practice of medicine, is not a science, and say the world would be better off without a drug or a drug doctor in it.

Second--If Osteopathy is a failure and without a scientific foundation, of what use to the sick would two failures be?

As Osteopaths we only claim a place for this method of healing upon its power to demonstrate the truths of its success in relieving the afflicted. Relief is what he wants, and has asked you to give when he is burning up with fever. He wants that destructive fire put out. His house of life is on fire—a self generated fire. He asks you to so adjust the machinery as to generate water, and pour it freely on the raging flames that are fastly consuming his body, and burning out the living man that dwells therein.

The Osteopath has this stone to place his foot upon: That man was made by the rule of perfection, in the shop constructed by the intelligence of deity; and in the construction can be found all the machinery necessary to his comfort and defense, both in sickness and health. Therefore he has something to start on. Knowing that the lymphatics do contain water, furnished by the action of the lungs upon the atmospheric air, they being assisted by nerves and other methods which generate water, and pass it through the wisely arranged channels, and keep them full enough of this fluid to put out the fires of all fevers.

As the Osteopath is well informed on the structure of the whole human body, and very well informed on the functions of the various parts, he can wisely give his attention at such times to the sensory, motor and nutrient nerves, that have been shocked by change of weather, from dry to moist; and a change of temperature from hot to cold, and from cold to hot, to that degree of abnormality found in the physiological action of the body, to cause this condition, which is simply the effect of imperfect functional action.

Our successes directed by this line of philosophy have been so satisfactory both to ourselves and our patients, that we are perfectly willing to trust to the dictates of nature.

After long years of experience, disappointed all the time, and never encouraged by any known good results coming from drugs, I will say to the drug, and the drug doctor, that I have no use for the drug, nor your counsel. Not because I consider you dishonest, but I do think the theory and practice of medicine is dangerous to be taught. Their effects upon the whole world have a tendency to breed drunkards, opium eaters and so on, and make the children of men cry for bread. Away from us with such theories.

Too Much Talk.

OF WHAT use is it to try any longer to make an American or any other sensible person believe that you have wisdom when like a parrot you can toot out a few words in Greek, Hebrew, Latin or a few Indian words from some extinct tribe? When man listens to man he listens for profitable wisdom only. In America men want facts, not words—time to us is precious. We want to know so we can act. Our American language is extensive enough now to express minutely anything, on any subject man wishes to discuss, thus what I want to impress is the great use of pointed brevity in our text books, and teachers. Look where we have drifted in law, religion and the sciences. Blackstone set forth the facts in law, and even his writing could be abridged much. I doubt not a lawyer now must have books by the thousands to be a man of legal ability of any note at all. What does his ability consist of? is the question. Is it to be able to give a great number of opinions on what justice is? If so why not give it to the world in good plain language. All truths are given for man's good. If so is it reasonable to suppose that it would help us to understand a principle more wisely to give such truths in a language or system of phraseology that would take ten years of hard study to even partly understand? Our professors who claim to be Greek and Latin scholars, I fear would be objects of pity as teachers in the school of the countries in which Latin, Greek and Hebrew are mother tongues. Why ape that which you are not when you have a language that is far better for your house?

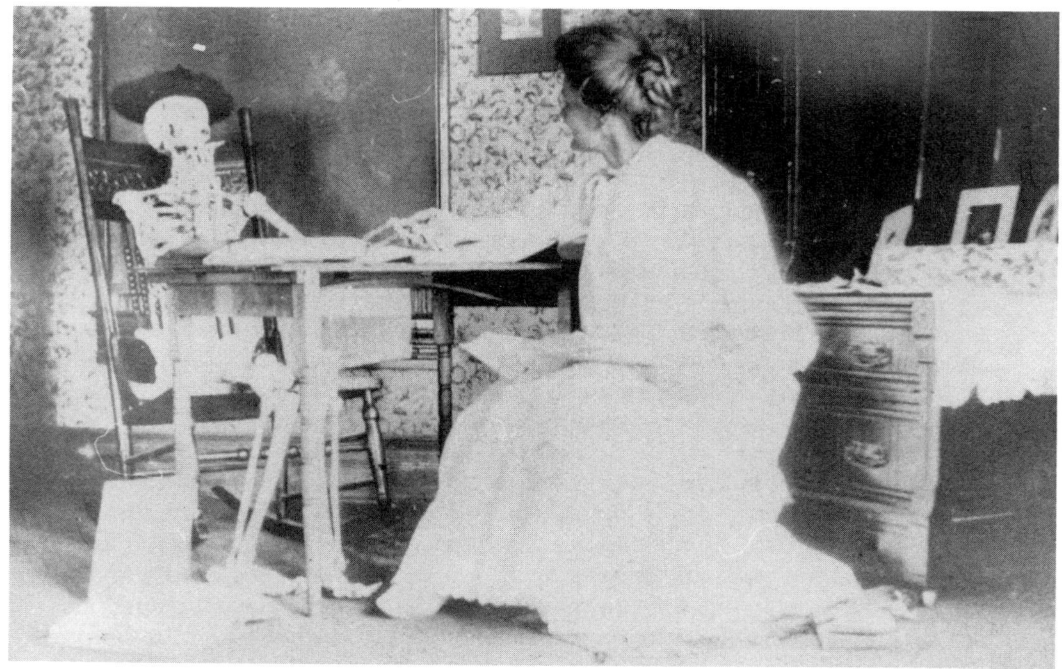

Taking the pulse of a skinny boyfriend

Osteopathy has no patience with graphophones running around on two legs. We want no more words than just enough to tell what color a black horse is with four white feet, a bobtail, blind in left eye, kicks, balks and runs away, and no good in any way. We do not think a history of the horse back to Babylon would do us any good. We want a horse that we can use.

Moral.—Osteopathy is a practical knowledge of how man is made and how to right him when he gets wrong. This school was made to study and learn what man is—and not humdrum your brains out with old theories that are of no practical use to man or beast. Be patient, you will soon be where theories will give place to demonstrated truths. I suppose Christ's drinks ofwormwood and gall were only a few old religious theories and intolerances boiled in the dirty waters of the rivers of superstition. Our school will soon have a finefilter that will never allow stale theory to pass through to be drunken by the seeker of wisdom.

March, 1900

LET Osteopathy speak once for all time. It has no relations on earth. It is a new book to us. It teaches curing by adjusting the body for all cures of climate and seasons. Anatomy is its training school. Osteopathy studies the bones of man to know how many he has, where they belong, and for what use they were formed. How, why and what they are broken up into so many joints for? If of any use seek that knowledge and not stop at pictures, dissection nor theories, but educate your head to hope for but little help from long stretched pages that are written by the yard to sell. The theorist never changes, because he is too cowardly to launch out on the open sea of defiance, on which none but free men cruise and catch the fat whales of everlasting truth.

The time has come to send forth this declaration. When Osteopathy first launched out as a cruiser it had fully made up its mind to be an independent one, for a better method of combating diseases than had ever been recorded to the year 1874. It was wholly and sorely disgusted with the failures made by him who confided and trusted in the efficacy of drugs. It took nature for its guide. It took the dead man's bones with the determination to quiz nature until an intimate acquaintance was made with the dry bones. Then with the knife ploughed through the flesh of man to find how one bone was attached to and held fast to another bone, and from there back to the surface. Osteopathy camped many long years to make an intimate acquaintance with muscles, tendons and ligaments. With the intermediate fascia, which contained lymphatics, nerves and cells beyond computation.

From there the inquiry led us to the blood supply, on which the whole system depended for its nourishment: with an intimate acquaintance sought that we might know how this fluid should be delivered to all parts both great and small without an exception. Thus a beginning at the heart must be the starting point to explore the hows and whys that fluid should be systematically distributed to the far off as well as to itself and adjacent organs and divisions of the body. Also the drainage system must be sought and found, which is so plainly demonstrated that without any further discussion we will say, that after the artery has supplied the system generally and the blood is of no more nutrient value, it is returned to the heart through the veins.

At this point one of the most important inquiries arises. Why and with what force is the blood conveyed to and from the heart? One could easily say by vital force, as vitality is one of the secrets that has never been delivered to man from the bosom of nature. Osteopathy feels willing to grant that to be a truth, and will simply speak of the universal accommodation that nature has made to pass all her forces by and through the nervous system. The Osteopath who has been in the service long enough to comprehend some of the functions of the machinery of life as found in the human body, soon learns that great and small variations from the truly normal, are what he must discover and adjust, to relieve the sick of disease and himself of doubt of the ability of nature to do all that can be done for the relief of suffering man when stricken down with disease.

We want to exhort you that this knowledge is obtained by the skilled mind of observation and the ready hand of application only. We want to further admonish you to treat theories with due respect, because many of them have been written with an earnest desire to educate the anxious seeker.

In conclusion we want to tell you that theories are not food for the American minds, to us domonstrated facts will be received and none other. This is the object of the American School of Osteopathy.

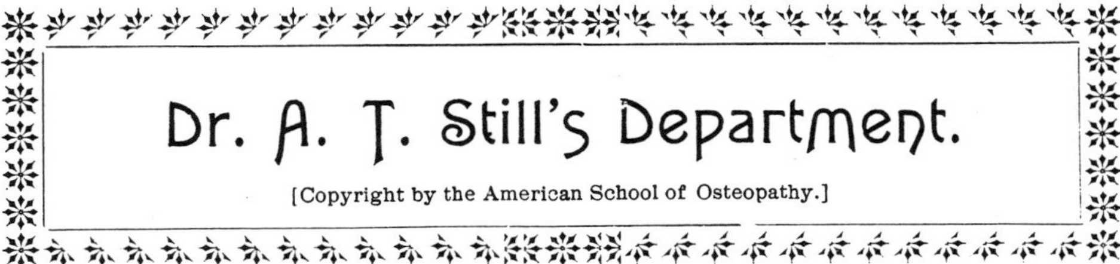

INDEPENDENCE.

AMERICA as a nation has said that in the course of human events it became necessary to separate herself from other countries, customs and governments, declare her independence and live accordingly. She lived and labored to put that thought into form and execution, though it cost much money, time and life to obtain that independence. For one hundred years we the posterity of our forefathers have enjoyed the blessings bequeathed to us by them. Today we are a powerful nation; wealthy in our great and fertile fields, and in our colleges of law, literature and skill. Once we were despised. Today we are respected, first for our intelligence, next our wealth and lastly as the defending champions of the seas; not the tyrants but the true friends to all that are manly. We have two methods only of commanding respect of monarchies and despots. "Liberty and equality to all mankind." If that does not call forth the respect of the world our fleets of both land and sea speak in such tones that monarchies say by both word and deed, that America has the men, intelligence and the skill to demand and obtain respect for its flag and country.

With Osteopathy the same condition is now before us. We have felt that we as a scientific branch of the healing art have discovered useful truths, that the world needs, wants and should have. But the "Czars" of medicine have said, you must die and be wiped from the face of the earth. Legislatures have been sought and asked to assist in putting to death the schools of Osteopathy, with more or less success crowning such efforts. They have said that the world should not choose for itself the kinds of help in sickness that he or she thought best suited to his condition.

If Osteopathy has scientific merit and carries no bottles of poison that would produce death and destruction of human life why should medical schools ask prohibitory legislation? Why not let the people choose from all schools of healing arts?

At this point let us enter a protest against prohibitory opposition, declare our independence, raise our flag and give to the world literature of our own production. Have we to be led to the altar condemned by their rules of symptomatology, which is only a poor system of guess work, and be drenched by the poisonous compounds of their schools of pharmacy? Are we to be prohibited by such schools from studying and applying the healing art as we find written in the book of nature? Does an American have to say "my lord" may I think a little? Or will he say as he has said for one hundred years just passed, that all men are free and equal. I will think, I will write, I will speak, though the smoke of roaring cannons of opposition should accumulate around me so densely that it could be cut with a knife.

We object to your literature being used as discipline; we claim the prerogative to abridge, substitute, amend, or reject all books from any medical school, or literary department, until Osteopathy shall have formulated such books and literature as its progressive demands have called for in thunder tones, and has never been answered outside of chemistry and anatomy, From now on be it known that we have graduates from the American School of Osteopathy who have never had a taint of the old system of drugs to bias their judgments by preconceived prejudice, or veil their eyes from the enjoyment of the beauties and healing art of nature. Their pens are abundantly able to furnish the needed literature.

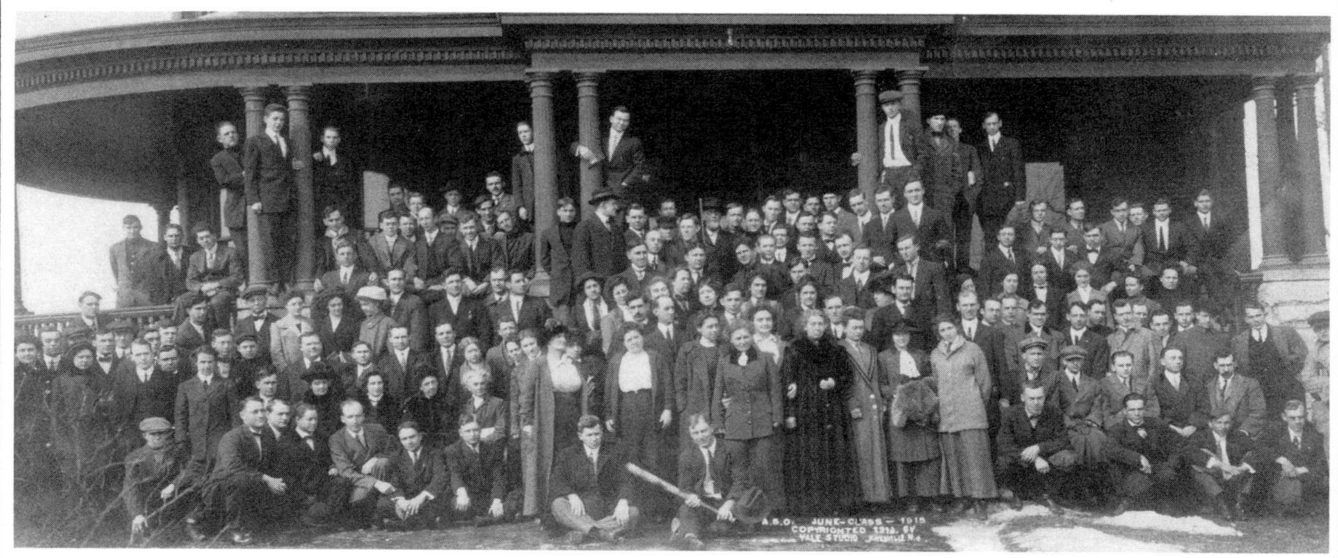

June Class of 1915. A. T. Still in the middle

CAUSE.

EACH person to get good results and improve from day to day must hunt for cause, then operate with a view to change the cause that has produced such condition, by change of currents of blood to nourish and wash away such accumulated bulks, by correcting bones and giving easy discharge to venous blood, that it may absorb and carry off deposits from joints, muscles and membranes. A goitre is only what blood has failed to be used by the nutrient nerves. Conditions not symptoms are what an Osteopath has to contend with. When he goes to a patient he asks for knowledge of conditions; he starts in with pictures of a body in healthy condition in his mind, and searches for variations from that standard. Thus an arm on one side when compared with the other arm must be the same in size, strength, motion and temperature, with the same color. A cold arm, blue in color and much larger than the other arm would present a condition that would be unnatural in form, motion, blood and venous action. Thus we see and feel a condition that is grave in its effect on health and motion. We must reason for cause, why this blood did stop and swell a part, and why it does not go on and reduce such swelling to its original size. At this time reason would take the exploring eye and searching hand to the bone structure, feel, look and compare all joints, in search of slips or variations from centers of actions; also search closely for impacted, twisted or overlapped and crossed muscles or ligaments, that would press on or across a nerve, vein or artery, and stop their normal work.

The Osteopath has the condition before him all the time; also all symptoms, but the cause is the mystery that has produced the condition, and when found he will find a mechanical cause for all the trouble he is likely to meet. Would we be safe in saying all diseases of climate and seasons with contagions are the results of local causes? When we meet fever have we not found a condition with cause in fermentation of fluids, of lymphatics of the whole system and those of the superficial fascia more than the deep seated, because of contact with atmospheric air? Then as we know the condition why not enter the combat at once, and remove cause of suspension, and labor for restoration of normal action? First by arteries, next the veins, then the excretory system.

The Osteopath's acquaintance with the nerve and blood supply, their local and general uses are sufficient guides if wisely conducted with that attentive perseverance that is due in treating diseases, which is nothing more nor less than the conditions produced by confused and perverted nutrition and renovation. Thus symptoms banish in quick succession from distress to recovery. We would admonish the operator to give attention to conditions, this is all important to his success. His eye and hand are very trustworthy as his microscope and thermometer, and more so and more useful in the sick room than all artificial appliances. Nature has provided and armed us with all that is necessary to explore for and locate cause, and successfully treat all diseases of climate or any season of the year. I have spoken thus freely to draw the student's and practitioner's mind to more attention to conditions, and treat accordingly; and less attention to our customary routine of name hunting before treating according to the rules laid down in authors on symptomatology.

A condition not normal is found in all diseased persons. That condition may have many symptoms common to other diseases, which would require much care and long acquaintance with books and observation to classify the name properly the disease according to the rules of popular symptomatology, which often fails to know smallpox from chickenpox, measles, scarlet fever and on through the many thousands of blunders made in giving names and treating according to such rules. Thus the importance of an operator dealing with conditions when he would wish to know the cause, and treat by the more safe rules of reason. A limb, organ or division of the body cannot show an abnormal condition without the producing cause being close by. The same law is just as true of pneumonia, flux, typhoid and other fevers; you find the patient in a condition and you have been called to get him out of such condition, your duty is to find the cause of the bad condition, seek and know where .the cut off is and what will relieve that person: You are not any wiser to know the Latin, Greek or Choctaw names for such and such diseases, unless you are a pill doctor. Symptomatology leads you straight to a drug store. Conditions, point you to cause hunting and finding, and just what to do to relieve the sufferer in the hour of need. Let the subject of conditions be your universal starting point and not hunting names. We should honor symptomatology because it is a relic of the visions of the stupidity of the kinds of literature that legislatures are called on to protect from deadly shots of bitter truths, that have come to stay and abolish unsound theories from the earth.

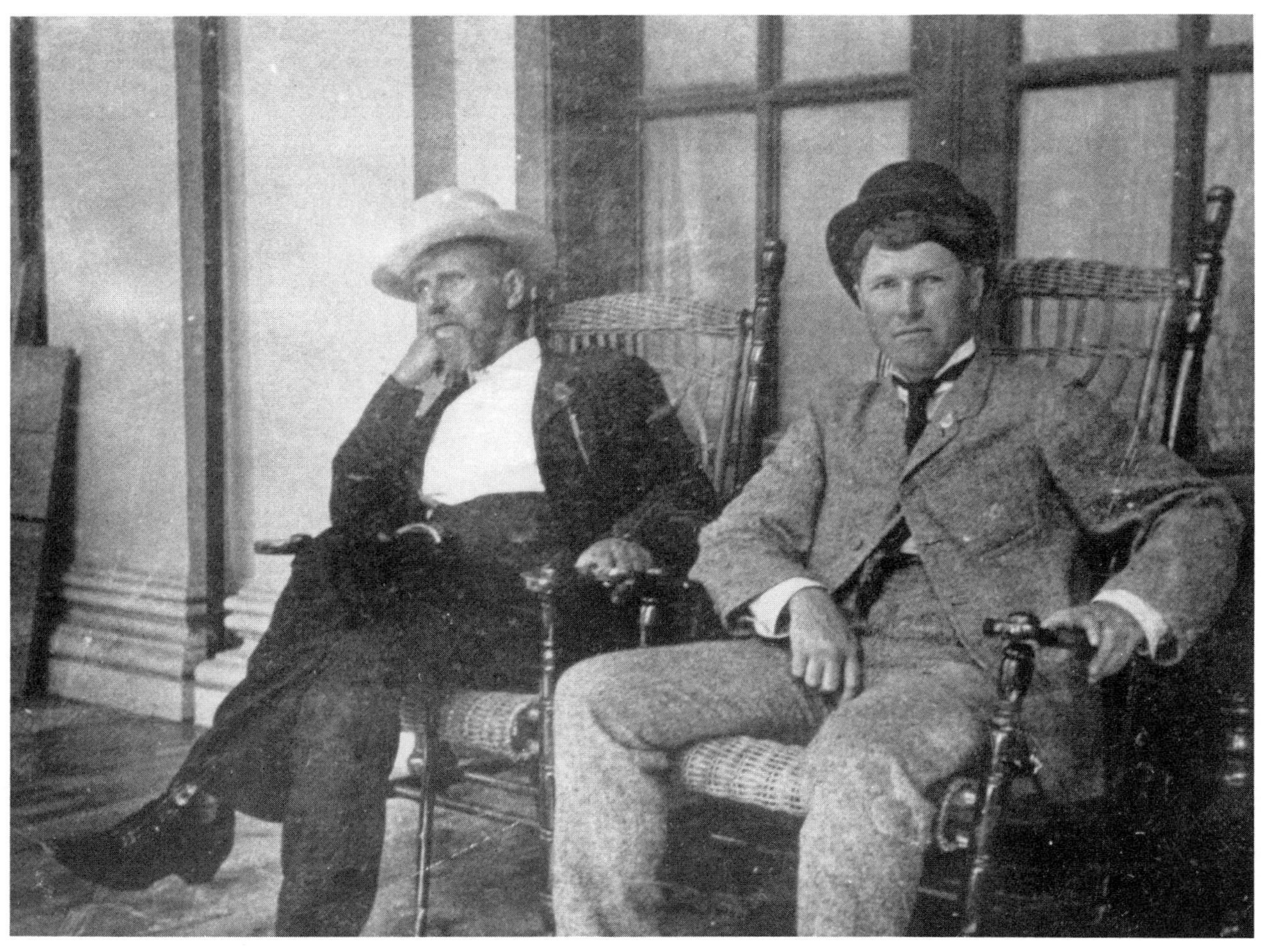

A. T. and Charles E. Still, c. 1905

GOOD ENOUGH.

WHEN a pen is taken in the hand of a writer for the purpose of giving the readers of the JOURNAL OF OSTEOPATHY something to read and study on, after it has been read, I will suggest that the writer confine himself to write what he knows or what he thinks he knows. His opinion is what we want, his observations are good enough. It is the writer's opinion written in the American style, and words from the American language. Why not use the American language? It surely can tell anything an American wants to say. An American should be proud of our institutions of learning and our dictionaries. "He should be boldly proud of our liberty of speech, press and pen. Then why should an American hunt up what old authors have said, and offer such quotations and piles of paper and book stories as his article? If I should give my opinion on some subject by telling in a nice scholarly manner what Edison, Franklin, Lincoln and a thousand other witnesses have said, what court would listen to such testimony? Any judge would laugh and say, Mr. Wart please tell what you know in this case, if you know anything, if not please retire. It is what you know that the court wants of you, not what John Doe never did know. It is easy for anyone to write on the subject of Osteopathy, and give us something to read that is new and fresh from the writer's pen. I want to kindly open the pages of the JOURNAL for original productions, minus quotations, from old books of howevers. You and your word are good enough for me; give us your own, long or short, and to the point in about one or two thousand words, or less if you can tell all in such limits. But few persons will read ten, fourteen and twenty pages in the JOURNAL on any subject. It is brevity wisely used that we like.

June, 1900

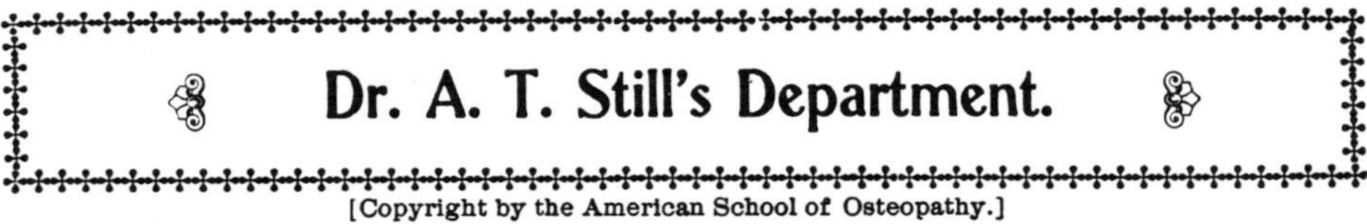

Dr. A. T. Still's Department.

WHY SHOULD A SCHOOL OF OSTEOPATHY TEACH CHEMISTRY?

LET us reason on that question. Does Osteopathy claim or teach that the doctor of Osteopathy must use the compounds produced by the medicine chemist as remedies? If so, then the study would be imperative. Then if the Osteopathic doctor does not use medicine to cure the sick why should he go through the hard study of chemistry? Because he could not understand physiology, a very important branch of anatomy, which embraces animal chemistry, the greatest chemical laboratory known to the mind of man. Whilst we do not expect to ever know more than that in man's organization the finest chemical products are produced at every stroke of the heart, why and how that work is so perfect when seen by the eye of man is what man has sought to learn, and today the mystery is just as great as it was a thousand years ago. We do not know how to make one drop of blood, urine, sweat, saliva or fat. We know an artery is different from a vein, and a piece of liver is not a part of a lung. In all our labor to learn the hows and whats of physiological action we only read the records of what man has seen after nature's machine has finished a tooth, an eye, ear, muscle or bone. He hears the music but fails to imitate. All he has learned to date is that something is wrong in the wheels of life when we are sick, he has tried all remedies of compounds poisonous and innocent but fails to relieve the sick. He takes counsel and obeys his preceptors, and witnesses the deaths of just as many when he returns from wise Europe, and writes his prescriptions in the oldest and purest Greek, French and Latin, as the most ordinary savage medicine man does with his weeds and antediluvian cures. The Osteopathic doctor's only hope is that nature will do the work, or it will not be done. All he can do is to line up the body, and his success as a doctor will book him to the degree of his ability to detect and adjust all physical variations to the normal, and leave his work in the hands of the chemist of the laboratory of animal life.

As doctors of Osteopathy a knowledge of physiology is of but little use to you when in the sick room, further than to know the locations of the organs of the body, their functions and their connections with the nervous systems, lymphatics and blood supply. Then there is but one more lesson to learn, and that is that no delays can be tolerated in nature's work. Then by all methods of search, find the cause of delay and remove at once, then his work is finished. For this reason he should know something of elementary chemistry before he can comprehend that natural chemistry does all selecting and combining; first of atoms, then proceeds to unite by its definite law corpuscles, and on to construct the parts of man by its atoms. He must keep the roads ever open to receive and forward the needed supply, nature will do the rest.

It has not been my object to place a low estimate on physiology; but on the other hand to make a more valuable use of that branch of anatomy than we have had for centuries back. It is not the lack of value of that part of anatomy that I object to, but I do think the writers of physiology are too voluminous in words, and too meager in useful and pointed truths to be of much use to our system of healing. When we have learned all that is written in any book to date we only read a book of supposable truths. I would like very much to find the author on physiology who would boldly say what he knows and can prove by demonstration, and not feed the anxious student with long lessons of other men's experiments, that abound with quotations from other men who have experimented and are only able to tell us that they too have failed to find a truth that is, has and can be demonstrated on man. We read all about dead frogs, doves, cats and dogs, we know they have killed the live dog but failed to wake up the dead dog. We want a book that we can learn by its pages how to help the sick dog and the sick man. We want knowledge. Americans are too progressive to be bored with trash that is being poured into the heads of our students from year to year, and sends them out after four to six years' hard study, with no more practical sense than a mule.

The requirements of Osteopathy in teaching are so very different from all other schools that have to heal the sick as to its object of teaching, that it is almost impossible to find a half dozen lines in a book of one thousand pages on physiology that would be suited to give the instruction that the doctor of Osteopathy needs in his training. His training should be that of a machinist, an engineer, who should know all the parts in both the normal and the abnormal form. He must know if he has any reason at all that all living beings during life are only shops of construction and repairs, and that his highest attainment when obtained would be an engineer, wise as an observer of the truly normal, and any variation from that condition. He should be skilled in detecting and correcting any variation from the normal, and should learn that beyond that point he has no stone in truth to stand on.

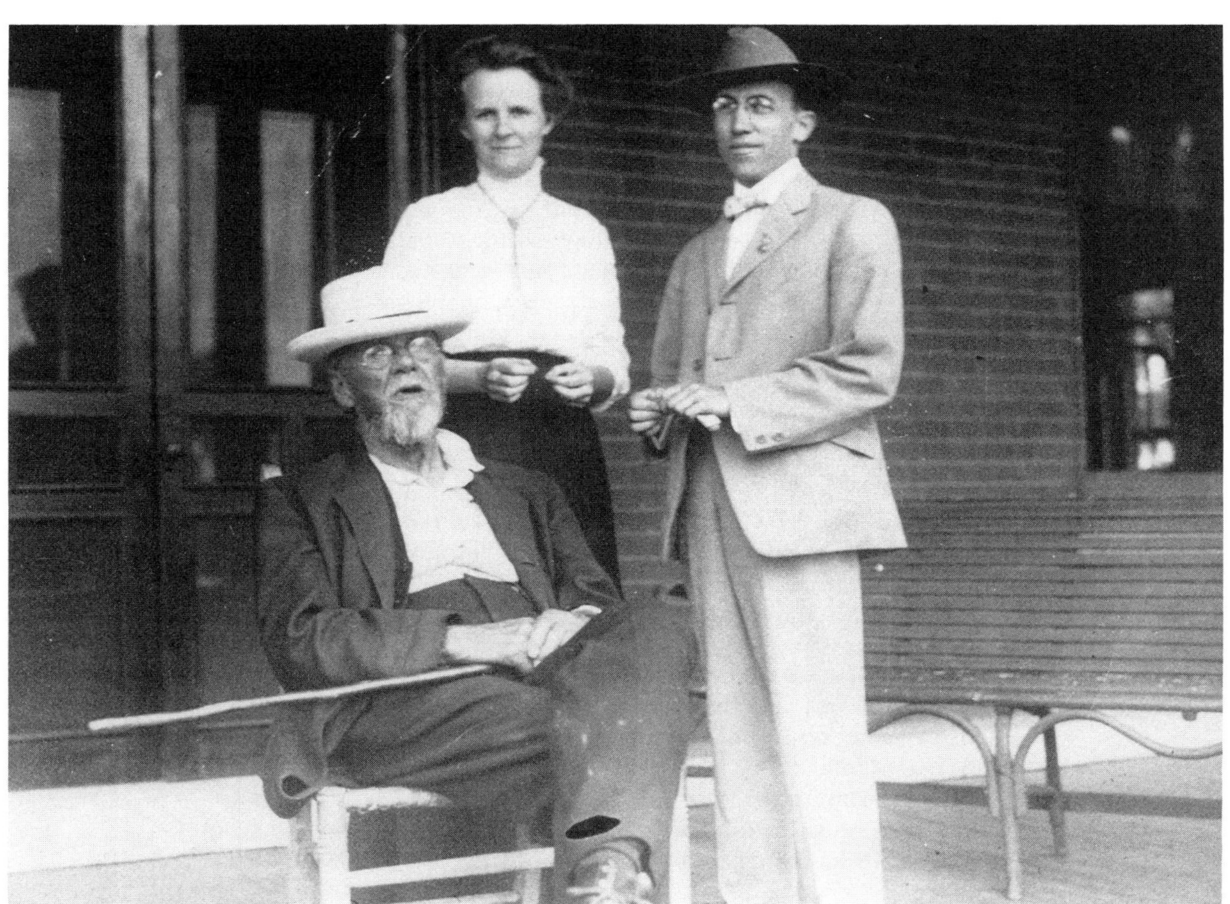

Blanche Still, Asa Willard, A. T. Still, c. 1915

This Year.

IN CLOSING this school year I feel that the friendly readers of the JOURNAL would like a few lines of history of a school that had grown from sixteen pupils in 1893, to a class of seven hundred in 1900. The reader would naturally ask why such rapid growth? What is there in Osteopathy as a healing art that would call the wise, and all grades of minds to investigate its merits, give it the most hearty support and work for the spread of such knowledge without money or without price? I feel much embarassment as I take my pen to answer such kindly asked questions. I think I can truthfully report that all the fame Osteopathy has or would claim is that of merit above old systems. It has long since been an acknowledged truth that medicines have no claim as scientific. It is now felt by the whole world to be blind guessing at what is the cause of disease, then a more dangerous system of guessing at remedies. What to give and how to keep that dose from killing the patient before the disease would get in its deadly work, if at all. In council the more doctors that are called in the greater the danger of the patient, is too often the case. Osteopathy has quietly followed the dictates of nature, and in each case studied and treated. Each effort has been to get a crumb more of knowledge to add to those we have taken by treating previous cases. We have been well rewarded when we have worked and trusted nature to heal by its own nourishing rivers of life. It is not my object to make war on doctors, but point the reader to the fact that I have found to be indisputably true, that nature has never lost sight of natural law in making worlds and beings. Then what claim has man to take that work from the hand of God and begin his work of cut and try? What has the doctor to encourage him when he fails at every effort to save life? He knows such is the case. He knows that the people have long since learned that medicine is only a trade, not a science.

My object in writing at this time is more for the purpose of giving the reader such information as I think would naturally arise in his mind in the way of inquiry. One *question* would be something of this kind: what is there in the School of Osteopathy that is so wonderfully enticing to ladies of wealth and refinement, and of those of less wealth who are seeking some honorable vocation by which they can make a living for themselves and those dependent upon them? The enquirer says I see about two hundred and fifty to three hundred ladies in the classes of the American School of Osteopathy, all seem to be hopeful and industriously applying themselves to their studies. To the surprise of the stranger who may choose to visit the classes he or she at a single flash of the eye will see that the ladies of all classes present great brilliancy of countenance and very much to the surprise of the listener those ladies answer all anatomical, chemical and other questions pertaining to a scientific knowledge of Osteopathy and its application as a healing art. The success of the lady graduates who have gone from the American School of Osteopathy has been so satisfactory to the afflicted, wherever they are or have been, that they have been given much praise and have been financially remunerated, to such degree that she not only feels proud of her profession but her independent ability to receive and lay up something to lean upon in old age. I have never heard any lady groan, or repine, that she had suffered privations for two years with hard study, in our school, but hundreds of ladies, I say hundreds because hundreds have been pupils of this school, all with sparkling eyes say "I am proud of my profession, and my alma mater, the American School of Osteopathy." The same brilliant light has fallen upon the gentlemen who have graduated in our school, and gone forth into the world to labor and do good. Without a single exception all have reported "blessed be the day when we entered the American School of Osteopathy."

 Dr. A. T. Still's Department. 

The Heart.

THE heart is to this system of cures of universal importance, as the first evidence of life and motion is found at the heart, and all bones and softer parts must obtain all matter entering their form and kind. Then it is only in keeping with reason that to explore the arterial system of blood supply for cause of disease would be to begin the search at the heart. If you stop at the heart, the headquarters of blood supply, you will see a division, or set of arteries going toward the head and arms, and the other going down toward the abdomen and legs, these two divisions comprise all. We know all failures to supply blood will be justly charged to one of these divisions, and we can hopefully hunt for cause of variations, and in proportion to our knowledge of anatmy we will locate the cause of such lesions.

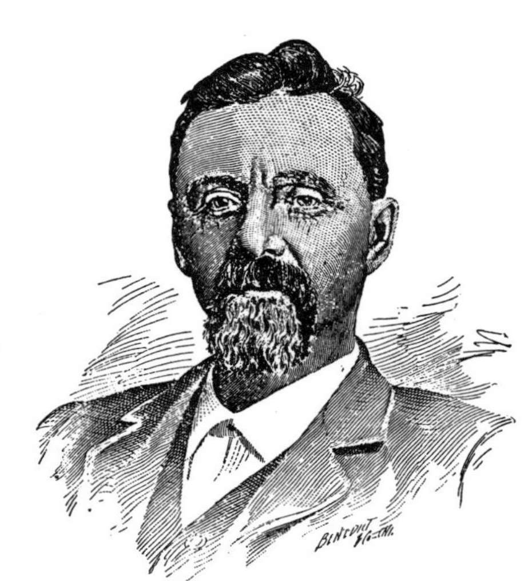

DR. ANDREW T. STILL, FOUNDER OF OSTEOPATHY.

* * *

Obstetrics.

HOW and what to do in all cases of parturition is the query of the young doctor when he has finished his school days. I think a little advice may be acceptable to him. Two objects line up and demand his cool-headed attention. The life of a woman and child are placed in his charge for his safe delivery. How and where he must deliver the two safely are the questions of weight and importance to the man with theory only, and no experience. He begins now to feel that the lack of experimental knowledge is the veil that clouds his sky. I will offer a few words of what I know to be good advice to the beginner in the responsible duties of the doctor at this time. First, keep cool until you think a few moments; there is a large body that has to come out of a freight depot; stop and take another cool breath, ask yourself if there is a door to the depot that is as large as the package that is to be taken out, if so, then when is that package to be rolled out? When he finds the fruit must stay on the tree until ripe and ready to fall off, then is the time to roll the package out; then he has settled the point to be patient till the time for birth has fully come. How may he know when that time has come in the case before him? He must shut his eyes and memory to all bugaboos, bones and deformities that he has seen in books on midwifery that he has grown to almost believe he has to meet every time he is called to attend a case of obstetrics. He should remember that he may meet one bad case of pelvic deformity in one thousand times that he is called to attend. He should study well the use of the forceps and other instruments that he may have to use in delivery in badly deformed women. But he must remember that his hand is far better in ninety-nine cases out of every hundred than any instrument that man has or ever can make. Osteopathy says you must not come bulging in to such places with an arm full of carpenter tools, the sight of which is enough to scare a woman into a spell of paralysis of the womb, and stop all action or power of the whole system to deliver the child by natural expulsion. I think the most foolish thing a doctor can do, is to act so as to cause a woman to feel that she has nothing to do in the delivery of her child, and her only hope to be delivered is to let the doctor pull her child away by brute force. You must teach her that the God of nature had formed her for that purpose, be patient and trust to nature and ninety-nine women in a hundred will have no trouble in the safe delivery of her child. Has not nature formed and given power to her muscles to deliver her? What do we find but wisdom in her formation? We find strong sphincter muscles to hold the womb closed from conception to the hour of birth, then they cease to act as constrictors till the expelling muscles have forced the contents of the womb out to the world. Don't be too anxious to assist nature artificially with your constipation pills, your vaginal douches, and what she should eat when pregnant; if she wants a few apples let her do like Eve of old just shake a tree and eat. Let her alone, she sometimes has more brain than the doctor that has been called in.

Often mothers have what is mistaken by the young doctor for labor pains, such pains often occur two to four weeks before natural labor comes. Remember that to bring on or cause labor prematurely is abortion, and you may by such hasty imprudence cause the death of a healthy woman and child. You cannot use too much caution with your advise and work at such times. This is written for the Osteopathic beginner in obstetrics. Iwill close by saying that all deformed cases should be advised to go to some lying in hospital where assistance is plenty, and where they have the best of surgical skill and experience.

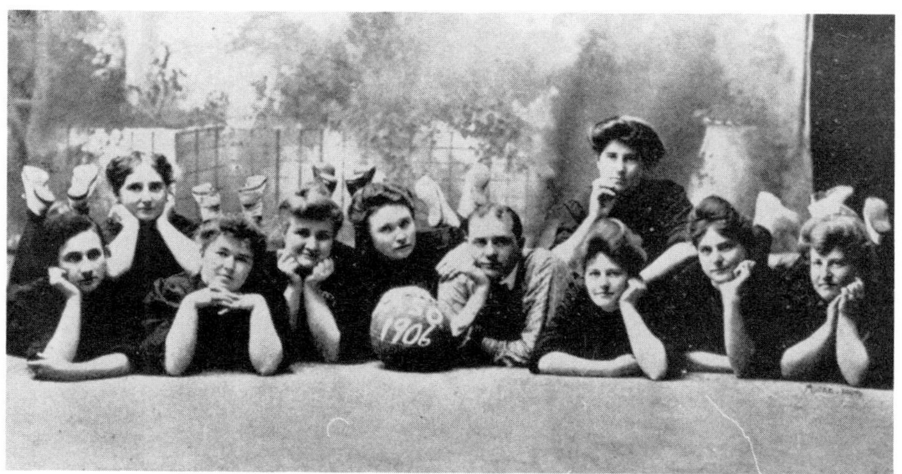

Women's Basketball Team of 1906

July, 1900

Old Theories.

OLD theories give but little if any useful knowledge for our day and generation. They are mostly like a last year's drunk would be to this year's happiness to an Irishman's stomach. They may have been good for old drunks but they are too tedious and tasteful for our boys and girls. I tell you they were old drunks and very poor drunks too. They were watered to death by talk, with no object but to talk old theories, and like peacock tails they look well in the spring of our lives, but they fall out feather at a time, babies pick them up feather at a time but lose them just as fast, even babies know they are too long, that is American born babies. Why should we bother with the dead theories? Why call the student's mind from his study? Hasn't he got the bones in his hands? Let him look, reason and adjust till he finds he wants help, then do so if you can. He calls you to tell the place and use of some bone—-tell him and show how and why a bone has such shape, don't drop him into the quagmire of old theories. Man is a machine and must be studied to know how and why it does its work. You should and must ever remember that Osteopathy is a science that pertains to active, healthy man, and to know him you must acquaint yourself with his form and motion by study and contact. How much would an engineer know of an engine by theories drained from Thomas Benton, Henry Clay and Lewis Cass, for and against Morse's telegraphy, or Fulton's steam engine delivered in congress. These great men asked the great statesmen for wisdom and help, they were insulted by blackguarding and being called fools. The stone they stood on was individual knowledge.

* * *

Our Farms, The Tables of God.

ON THEM is found the food, wisdom, raiment and wealth of the world. By their successes we prosper, and by their failures all nations wither and die. On farms wise men and women are born. From the farm all of America's wisest generals, presidents and statesmen came. Our greatest men have only to look over their shoulders to see their fathers and mothers toiling with grain and herds. None but fools would fail to love the honest mother's grave who lived and died on the farm. On the farm is not the place to look for thieves, liars and hypocrites. Farms are the places and homes to find well posted men and women. One farm will grow more reformation than the oldest city. In cities and towns are the places to find idiots born, not on the farm. The farmer's wife has something to eat and wear, and the pure blood of herself and husband keeps corruption away from her children Her children are ignorant of the asylums, gallows and skeleton keys of a sneak-thief. The farmer's hand is rusty, so is a diamond, they are the jewels of the world, they shine when well dressed paupers have failed to be called even dim-lights. When I see a town woman fail to speak to a farmer's wife and family when they meet in town I wonder if that woman has not been a kitchen girl some time in her life. I pity the shoulders that carry such weak heads. Let us close and say, give due respect to merit without asking are you from a farm or the orphans' home, where the city sends the children of sotted fathers and heart-broken mothers.

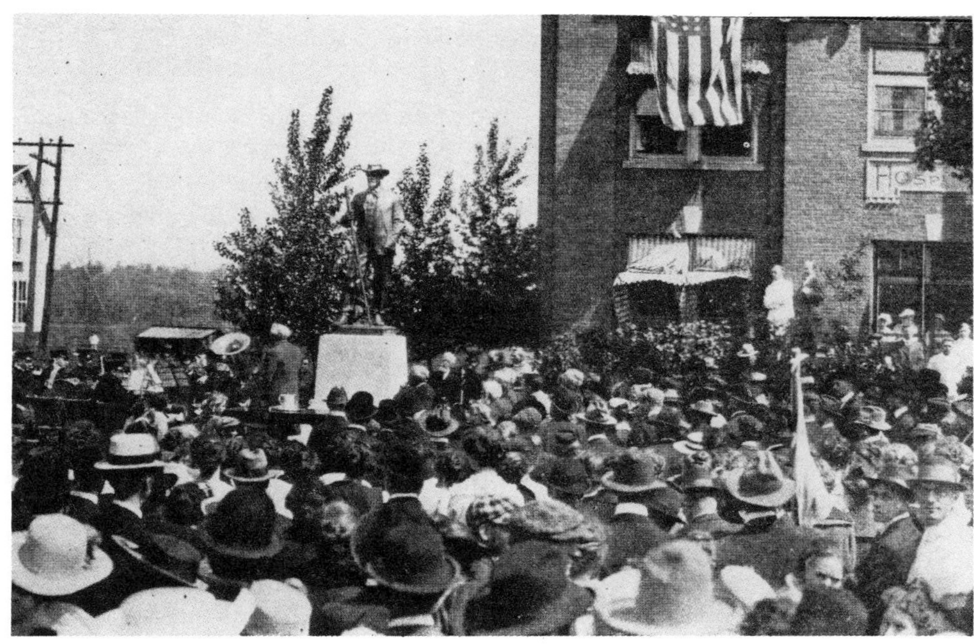

Dedication of the Still statue, June 1917

Dr. A. T. Still's Department. 

Yes, I Said So.

YES, I did say that nature's laws were as old as eternity and as true as God. And I believed in that law was the true chart and compass that pointed to the fountain source—manufacturing, delivering and building all parts and principles that belong to man's form, motion and mind, both vital and material. I did say the more a person knew of the human body and how perfect all the works were, that he, as an honest juror under oath, would say that Nature's God had in mind to do a perfect job, when he said "Let us make man." Since I have spent my whole life in the study of the form and functions of man, both dead and alive, I have reasoned that such a proclamation as "Let us make man" being issued from God, meant, "Attention worlds, I, the God of the universe do proclaim to all coming ages that I will make the greatest being of creation by the rule of known perfection, and it shall stand as a living test of my ability to do and build a living, self-moving being, endowed with mind, motion and matter, which represents all substances that can be found in the universe, mind and life included." I do and have believed for many long years that when God proclaimed that he would make man, that he was fully able to do what he proposed, that he did do the work and do it in such perfect order that no anatomist of ten thousand years' learning could find a single flaw, lack or failure in the osseous design; no machinist could suggest a single change or addition to a bone, ligament or muscle, that no bone in its entirety under the most crucial examination suggests any lack or shortage in all that is meant by the word perfection in design or place, planned and executed by the divine architect, than whom none is higher nor better supplied with intelligence, experience, force and material. He, who has qualified himself, by his learning in anatomy, by his exploration with knife, microscope, chemistry and otherwise, who has obtained the best acquaintance with the physiological and chemical actions, driven by that force known as animal life, has not been able to the present date to obtain light and wisdom enough, to suggest any variation whatever from the original plan and specification, as found upon the trestle board on which all the designs of animal life have been written with the red ink of eternal truth.

Having found the construction and workmanship perfect from the least to the greatest parts of the person and being, forced by all methods of reason to grant and acknowledge the perfection of the architect and builder of man, can we not trust that the same wise, thoughtful and honest builder did think, provide for and place all of the remedies and safeguards to ward off or cure diseases as man's condition might require, during his natural life?

Let us count the above remarks as something of a prelude, or an apology for what may follow. At this point I will ask the attention of the kind student of nature to go into camp with me and partake of such fare as we will find on the table, which food for the philosopher is abundantly supplied to suit all stomachs that may wish to camp by and feast in the rich valley and fertile lands that are situated below the diaphragm to the lowest point of the bones of the sacrum. Hitherto mysterious diseases of the human have come and done their deadly work, swept away countless thousands of our race, despite the remedies of the best known skill of this and other known ages.

I will begin abruptly with assertions which I believe on further investigations will prove to be philosophically true. To date our best authorities are blank as to the cause or causes of gall stones, bladder stones, fibroid and all grades and kinds of tumors, that have appeared and have done their mysterious work of constructing tumors, generated deadly fluids and destroyed life. Their mystery today, if popular writers are to be believed, I repeat, the mystery is just as great today as in any time of the past. When he has written his thousands and tens of thousands of pages, he lays his pen down in despair, and says in the most emphatic terms in word and deed that he does not know the cause, and in his ignorance he resorts to the administering of various kinds of drugs, hoping that some one of them may contain the quality that would diminish and remove such bulky deposits, either of the fluid or the flesh. He seems to have never asked the question, nor suggested to others that the cause might be traced to strains, partial or complete dislocation of the innominates from their normal position on the sacrum. I have never seen nor known the question to be asked nor answered with any degree of intelligence of the cause of hysteria, bright's disease, diabetis, constipation, dysentery, abnormal monthly conditions and on. Have we ever read after any author that he believed by falls, jars, strains and otherwise that the pelvis might become deformed, that the sacro lumbar articulation might be so much disturbed as to produce lymphatic and venous congestion, which would likely terminate in tumefaction and on to the whole list of diseases above named?

* * *

July, 1900

ONCE A YEAR OR OFTENER.

ONCE a year or oftener we should report the progress of our school, it is new. The first few years I devoted to the study of anatomy I had dish rags and close the doors to all such vampires of comfort that would eat you out of house and home without even a thank you, take a scholarship in the American School of Osteopathy, spend two years and use the same mental and physical energy to obtain a knowledge of this science that you have used to please and comfort those lazy drones, that you will obtain an honorable diploma from this school which will say "dear la ly you have a commission to fill and that commission is to go into the world heal and comfort the sick and receive a compensation that will sustain you and yours with the comforts of life, and lay by something on which to depend during your declining days." These are facts that any lady that has gone from this school will endorse as true and very true, as she has prov en since she received her parchment from the American School of Osteopathy.

I would like a letter from every lady graduate with her experience for and against. A. T. S.

* * *

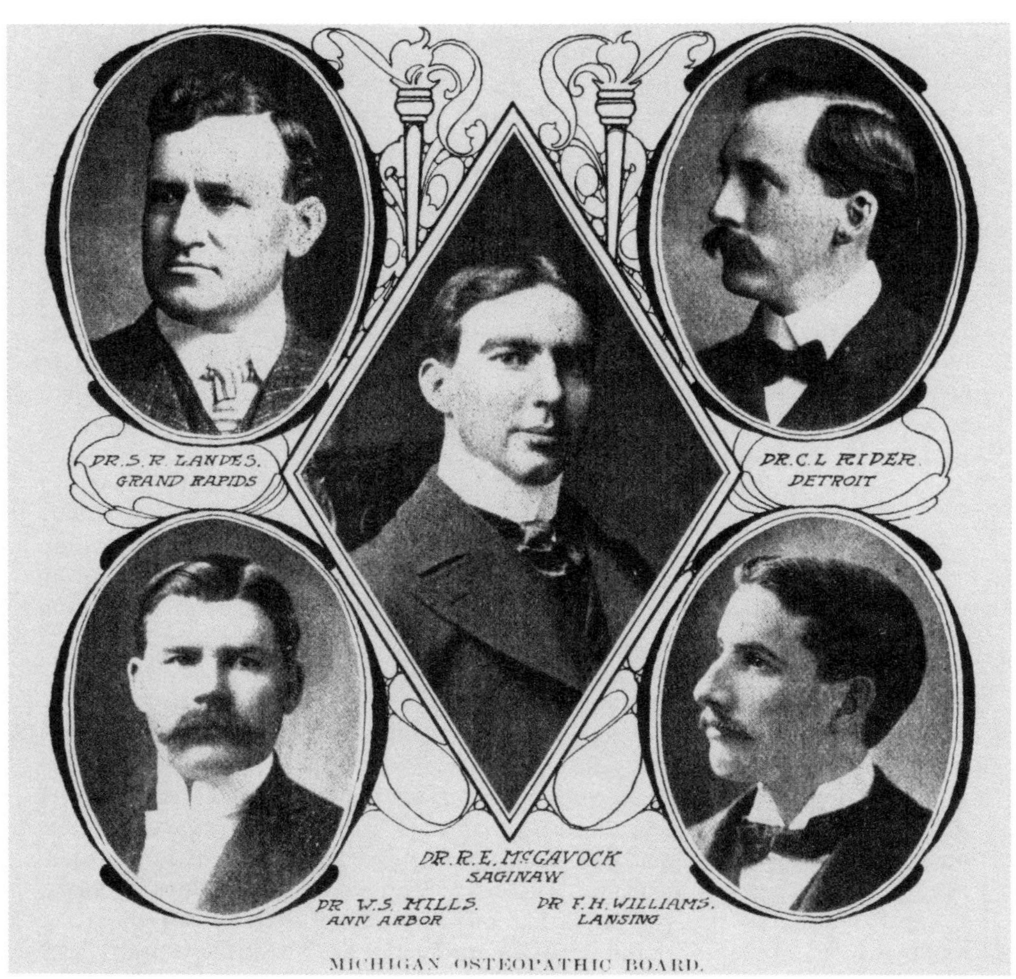

MICHIGAN OSTEOPATHIC BOARD.

July, 1900

Woman.

I THINK it right to give her credit for what she is. I think the world has been too slow in giving her the words, and I will say the words of thankful kindness that are due her. She toils from early dawn until late bedtime for the good and comfort of those with whom her lot is cast. She is not a servant, but for the comfort of family and friends she willingly fills the place of one, and does the work that two or three should have divided among them. She does it all with tired limbs and aching back; all without a murmur or complaint. When we look back over the past years of our short lives we find she has filled the place of something like a "Sunday slave" who has to scratch her head and think fast, whether she has plenty or little of what she will have on her table for those that may accidentally drop in from church and other places. She freely divides of such as she has, often and too often she feeds a half dozen unthankful gad-abouts only to be told by those whom she has fed that they don't see how she gets along without servants.

Now, ladies, I have told you the truth, and you know it to be the truth, and if you will permit me I will tell you another truth, one that I have told other ladies for the last ten years, and that is if you will throw down vour least to the greatest parts of the person and being, forced by all methods of reason to grant and acknowledge the perfection of the architect and builder of man, can we not trust that the same wise, thoughtful and honest builder did think, provide for and place all of the remedies and safeguards to ward off or cure diseases as man's condition might require, during his natural life?

Let us count the above remarks as something of a prelude, or an apology for what may follow. At this point I will ask the attention of the kind student of nature to go into camp with me and partake of such fare as we will find on the table, which food for the philosopher is abundantly supplied to suit all stomachs that may wish to camp by and feast in the rich valley and fertile lands that are situated below the diaphragm to the lowest point of the bones of the sacrum. Hitherto mysterious diseases of the human have come and done their deadly work, swept away countless thousands of our race, despite the remedies of the best known skill of this and other known ages.

I will begin abruptly with assertions which I believe on further investigations will prove to be philosophically true. To date our best authorities are blank as to the cause or causes of gall stones, bladder stones, fibroid and all grades and kinds of tumors, that have appeared and have done their mysterious work of constructing tumors, generated deadly fluids and destroyed life. Their mystery today, if popular writers are to be believed, I repeat, the mystery is just as great today as in any time of the past. When he has written his thousands and tens of thousands of pages, he lays his pen down in despair, and says in the most emphatic terms in word and deed that he does not know the cause, and in his ignorance he resorts to the administering of various kinds of drugs, hoping that some one of them may contain the quality that would diminish and remove such bulky deposits, either of the fluid or the flesh. He seems to have never asked the question, nor suggested to others that the cause might be traced to strains, partial or complete dislocation of the innominates from their normal position on the sacrum. I have never seen nor known the question to be asked nor answered with any degree of intelligence of the cause of hysteria, bright's disease, diabetis, constipation, dysentery, abnormal monthly conditions and on. Have we ever read after any author that he believed by falls, jars, strains and otherwise that the pelvis might become deformed, that the sacro lumbar articulation might be so much disturbed as to produce lymphatic and venous congestion, which would likely terminate in tumefaction and on to the whole list of diseases above named?

* * *

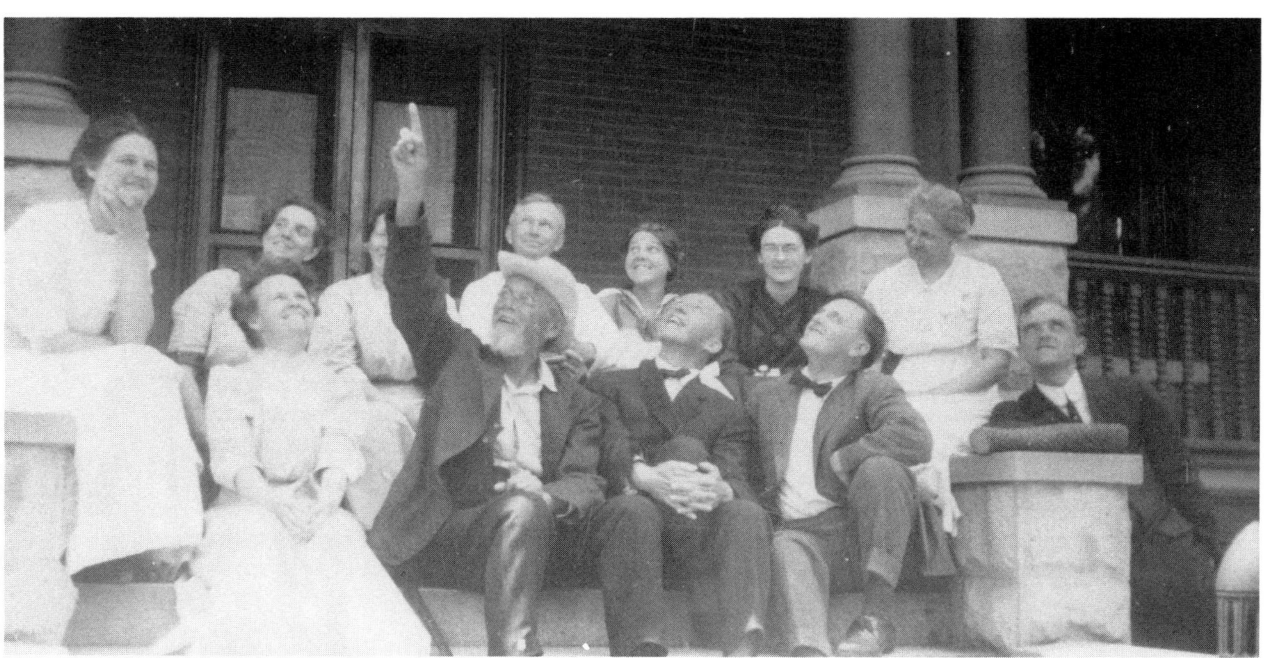

On the front porch steps of the Still home, c. 1913

ONCE A YEAR OR OFTENER.

ONCE a year or oftener we should report the progress of our school, it is new. The first few years I devoted to the study of anatomy I had dish rags and close the doors to all such vampires of comfort that would eat you out of house and home without even a thank you, take a scholarship in the American School of Osteopathy, spend two years and use the same mental and physical energy to obtain a knowledge of this science that you have used to please and comfort those lazy drones, that you will obtain an honorable diploma from this school which will say "dear la ly you have a commission to fill and that commission is to go into the world heal and comfort the sick and receive a compensation that will sustain you and yours with the comforts of life, and lay by something on which to depend during your declining days." These are facts that any lady that has gone from this school will endorse as true and very true, as she has prov en since she received her parchment from the American School of Osteopathy.

I would like a letter from every lady graduate with her experience for and against.

A. T. S.

* * *

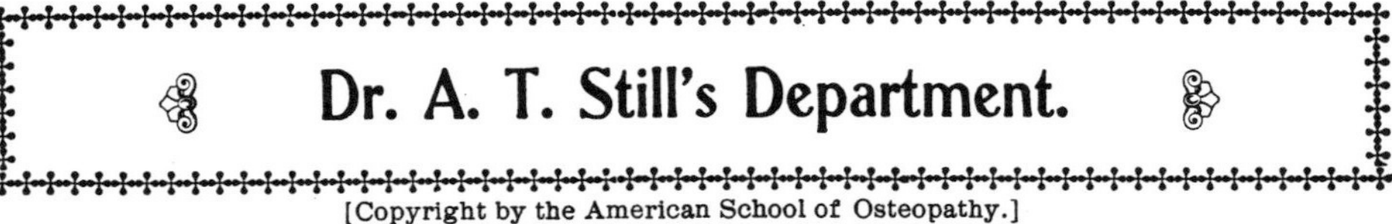

The Scientific Medical Doctor.

I WISH I could believe that the medical doctor was scientific. I have tried to believe him sincere. I could do that, but when I would ask him to prove that medicines of any kind could demonstrate their scientific usefulness either in a general or specific manifestation when administered to diseased persons, right at this very important moment he says, his profession has to use great caution in selecting and administering drugs to suit the person more particularly than to match and successfully combat the disease with which he is invited to conduct. He will tell you that there is no known specific for any disease. He will tell you that quinine is as universal as a specific for malaria as any drug known to the profession to the present date. Then he brings in that good old reliable word "However," which means all you want or nothing at all, and informs us that many cases of malaria are met in our practice which resists all known remedies, and only yield to change of climate. Then we ask this sage of experience if he knows of any specific for any disease of country, climate or season? If he knows of any specific that he can recommend under oath that will put to flight such diseases as cholera, smallpox, summer complaints, diseases of the lungs, brain, liver, kidneys and bowels? He will tell you he would not like to swear in favor of any specific's power as a remedy; that some drugs seem to be the very essence of relief to one person, and death to others suffering with the same class of disease, either of contagion, or other kinds. He winds up his story to the enquirer for truth by saying, that more depends upon the practitioner's knowledge of what kinds of persons he must administer large doses of sedatives to in order to control their nervous system, and what class of people would die under the influence of such sedative treatment. What class or kind of blue or black eyed, red, light, black haired people die if they did not in his judgment have alcoholic or stimulants, such as fly blister, mustard plaster and so on, and when he has talked to you he says "I am in honor bound although old and gray in the practice of medicine to say to you that my experience for lo these many years has been crowned by heart-rending disappointments. I do not know how many I have killed with drugs if any. I do not know how many I have cured by the use of drugs if any at all." Then that mighty friend comes forward,

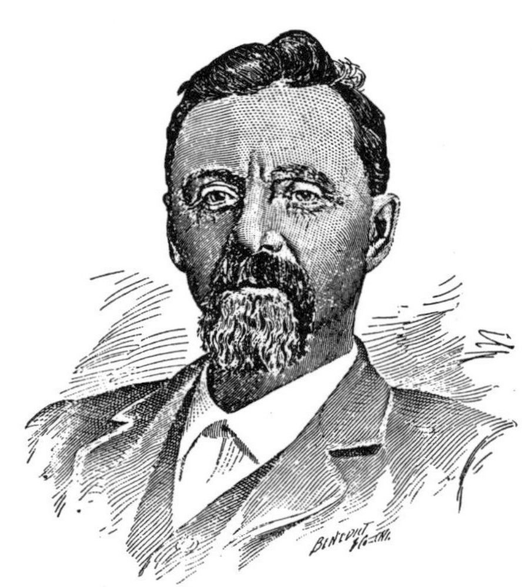
DR. ANDREW T. STILL, FOUNDER OF OSTEOPATHY.

that good old "However" and he says "It is my trade, by it I make my daily bread and must be satisfied to conform to established usages (legalized ignorance.)"

This is the kind of unreliable information that the seeker for truth does now, and has received when he cruises on the ocean of time for that kind of knowledge that he can use and apply, and know he will get the desired results as a reward for his labor. He knows that our machine shops can make an ax, a saw, square, auger, compass, plane or any tool known or used by the mechanic; and he knows that the mechanic can get the result or results once or many times. If he wants to bore a hole he knows that by the assistance of the auger he gets the result. When he wants two pieces of wood to connect either at side or end that his square will indicate the proper place to saw, and when the two ends are brought together if sawed by that rule they will fit, notwithstanding one was squared and sawed in London the other in New York. He knows if skillfully done that all will come together, fit closely and prove the reliability of the square.

This same rule of certainty is just as good with ten thousand instruments when used skillfully for the purpose or purposes for which they were designed.

All of the mechanical doctor's remedies do get the desired results, of which he is proud. The medical man's remedial agents are used and applied, all fail because the medical carpenter has no square by which he can work.

* * *

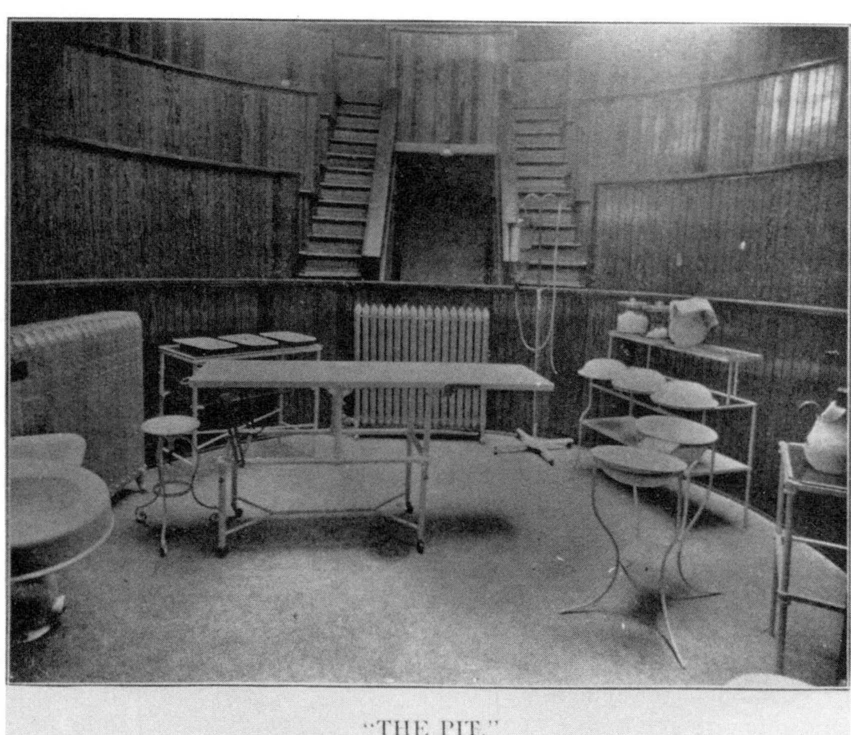

"THE PIT."

September, 1900

Diseases As Wounds

AS PRESIDENT of the A. S. O. I want to make a few bold statements of what I know to be true of Osteopathy, which has one and but one plain meaning, and that is if there be any faults or failures in successfully treating such diseases as come under the claims of Osteopathy, that there is but one known cause that the honest and most competent searcher has found or is liable to find, and that is ignorance of anatomy, and what that body can and will willingly do. I believe we today are only beginners. I believe every day of two years in anatomy has only made us able to see that old theories outside of strict attention pertaining to the forms and functions of the parts of the body is time lost. Ages have been blindly wasted, and theories that are devoid of truth as to what move the "healing man" or doctor should make. I am sure the doctors of all ages have had the blind staggers, they have been blind to the fact that God had put in man a mind to direct him in all business undertakings. That he gave to flesh the power of wisdom and locomotion, he associated life with it. He did place in flesh a power to heal and repair wounds, broken bones and on, and no power has yet been found as a substitute for that endowment bequeathed to the flesh of man or beast. That quality is the surgeon's only hope when he has performed his work. He trusts in that great nurse, and leaves knowing that the case is in the hands of the living God, the only trustworthy trained nurse of all hospitals. He has learned this great lesson by his knowledge of anatomy with what he knows of the healing powers of the body in a surgical line, I was led to go farther with the inquiry and try and ascertain if nature went farther with the healing art than to consider all diseases as wounds and treat them accordingly. Thus if fever is a wound of the lymphatics by strokes of heat or shock of cold, would the patient have to go by the laws of repair to healthy blood, the same as from a wound from a knife or saber? The answer came slowly, and then only when I learned to seek and detect lesions that indicated the obstruction that would stop blood long enough to ferment, and cause such disease. I have given much time and study to find a term that would apply to all diseased conditions, either of contagion, location or seasons. I believe I can show by reason that the word wound would express more fully all conditions known as diseases, general and specific. What is small pox but a general wounding of the nerves and machinery of life located in the fascia? We have said wounds because of the deadly shock the nerves and glands just beneath the skin have received. It matters not how gentle the stroke at the time of conception, the effect has proven the wound to be a confusing jar to the nerve cells and glands of the whole system, and the pox is only the failure to receive vital fluids to save life and throw off impurities as fast as they were deposited. Then it would be natural to try to leave the body by decomposing dead blood, and form gas and expel water while in the gaseous form. In him we have a wounded man; he has been hurt by the explosion of nature's effort to form vaporous gas and drive that out by way of the excretories. Is not all this trouble the result of the shock to the nerves and glands? Let the Osteopath consider that he is a surgeon, remove all hindrances to the normal continuity of all forces and fluids, and trust to nature's trained nurse who does all repairs by nutritious blood. The surgeon with knife and saw knows that to hope to restore his patient any other way than from pure blood he would be branded and known as a fool. I hope by this time that the student knows what I would try to draw his mind to by calling all diseases surgical wounds, coming in as many ways as the number of all diseases, cuts, jars, shocks mental or physical, heat, cold, eating too much, loss of sleep, property or friends; all are shocks to the nervous system, and the case is a wounded person, and the doctor must treat accordingly.

* * *

IT WAS my good fortune or bad fortune to introduce Osteopathy in its swaddling clothes a quarter of a century ago in North America. It was a good sized boy baby, with strong lungs. It has talked to the people of the beauties of the discovery that it had made, which are a few of the principles that govern animal life, which, no doubt, are as old as the days of eternity. After twenty-five years of close investigation, I have made no discovery of any defect whereby I could suggest an amendment. I have used freely the scalpel, the microscope, and the chemical laboratory; made a free use of the opinions of all philosophers with whom I could consult; at the end of each season of investigation the conclusion has universally been that the laws bear upon their face absolute evidence of perfection, and are so taken and accepted by the learned people who have time and desire to investigate the truths of Osteopathy.

While I have taken no pains to give this science notoriety by publication, it has been more or less known for ten or fifteen years in the capital of the United States, and today is known, more or less, in every town and village in the states and territories, and is also known in foreign lands.

I will say for those who desire to know more of this science that whenever you see a diploma from the American School of Osteopathy, you will find the possessor qualified to give you the necessary information and to demonstrate the facts of the science by his or her skill and ability which they have obtained during long months spent in obtaining a thorough education in the American School of Osteopathy at Kirksville, Mo.

My signature only goes to those parchments after long acquaintance in the school room with the receiver thereof, and the signature of the trustees and faculty of the school is all that is necessary or that we can do by the way of recommending as to character and qualification. As I know all have had a good opportunity to become well qualified for the duties of a healer, I will make mention of no particular name or person more than to say that without merit these diplomas would not have been issued to the persons now possessing them, and for me to say who is good or who is bad would be a contradiction of what I have already said—that he or she has our highest recommend on their diplomas.

THIS school has grown to its present dimensions by the founder doing other work than dosing and instrumental surgery; he has by proving to the world that fevers of all kinds can be stopped by changing the motion of blood from quick to slow caused man to see that blood moves fast or slow just in proportion to the amount of force or energy that is given to the nerves of motion from the brain. The nerves move fastly when irritated by causes that would excite electricity to become more active. Surely electricity has much to do in heat and motion, and motion must precede friction, then it is natural to have friction before we can have heat. Thus we say fever heat, but we can just as easily say that heat is only electricity in quick motion. Motion and friction the cause, heat the effect. The Osteopath can modulate nerve action either to reduce or increase heat if he knows his anatomy and the functions of the nerve and blood systems, he need not guess but know how and what to do to get results desired. A. T. S.

October, 1900

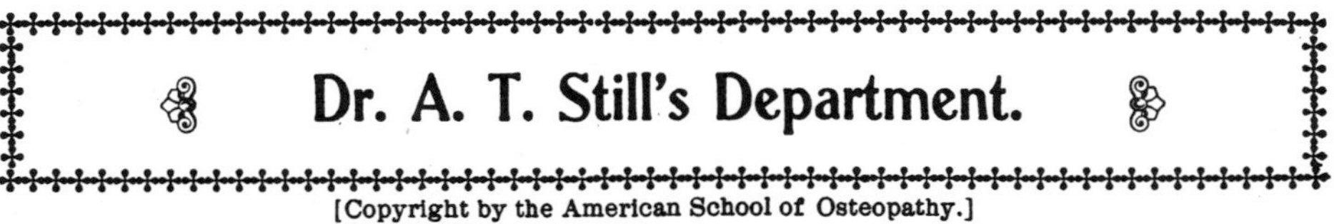

Remember you are an Osteopath, not an M. D.

AN OSTEOPATH has said he is not a medicine doctor. The M. D. gives his hospital report of classes of diseases, say fevers, eruptions, contagions, and so on. He reports the name, symptoms, and remedies, names the kinds, quantity and the hours of administering, gives a daily report for weeks and months and all changes of the disease and changes of medicine, to recovery or death; tells much of the effects but fails to give any reason why he gives a sedative, purgative or stimulant more that said drugs are very popular in France, Germany or Austria, and was very highly recommended by Dungleson and very, very many of the doctors of the Royal Staff, but gives no reason why they piled in such poisons; finally a big However come to report that the same doctors have abandoned its further use because of too great mortality in Her Majesty's Charity Hospitals.

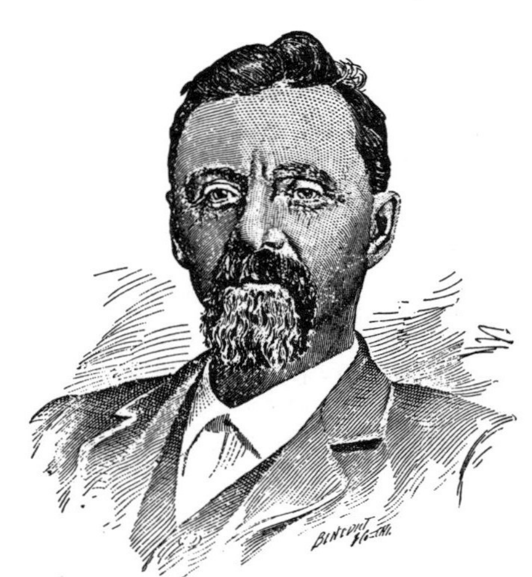

DR. ANDREW T. STILL, FOUNDER OF OSTEOPATHY.

You can read such jumping, changing reports a thousand years, and do as they do, and all you can say is that you have acted and treated your patients professionally.

An Osteopath must give reasons why he treats here and there, or he is only another professional imitator. If you treat the neck or knee for eczema, sneezing or colic, tell what nerve element you want to act on, give us reason to think that you are after the fire of fever with water found in the lymphatics, or breaking constructions that are causing the blood to halt in the brain, lungs, bowels, kidneys or any other place. Tell us why you spread the kidneys apart in typhoid fever, flux, pneumonia and so on, and not tell that you treated the great and lesser splanchnics, but tell why you should and prove your powers of reason by the results.

If you do not, you have both feet in the old medical ruts of cut and try. An Osteopath can and must reason why he does his work because he has his compass and knows his landing if he follows his needle.

* * *

Inhibition.

THE physiological definition of inhibition by Webster is a stopping or checking of an already present action, a restraining of the function of an organ, or an agent, as a digestive fluid or ferment, etc., as the inhibition of the respiratory center by the pneumogastric nerve; the inhibition of reflexes, etc. Inhibit is a word much used by Osteopaths. Many words convey the same meaning, such as move, motion, action, thenqualifying words such as quick, fast, faster, slow and on. In Osteopathic practice inhibit simply means to temporarily stop the flowing of arterial blood; then if we change to the vein we stop or inhibit the venous flow, the same rule of pressure will stop the current of electric, magnetic or vital fluids between the brain, heart, lung, bowels, womb or limbs. Inhibition is natural when any pressure is great enough to put a rib or any bone on a strain that would stretch or strain a ligament enough to cause the bone to move from its natural place or position one thousandth part of an inch. Here at the bone you should learn your most valuable lesson, when you see that all muscles and ligaments originate on one bone and insert into some other bone and that thousands of finest nerves mingle and pass with and from spinal cord to vivify and be fed from that great trunk of supply, then you are prepared for your first time in life to know what is meant by that Latin and other words, "Inhibit," "stop," "suspend," "prohibit" and on to the end of synonyms. The great object of Osteopathy is not to inhibit but to prohibit farther delays of blood to the wounded parts, which failure is directly traceable to the bony frame-work of the system. Remember that the brain is the chief source of vital force, and that all of the brain and spinal cord is enclosed in bones, no ligament, bone, muscle nor organ can get an atom of force or motion from any place but from within the bony parts. Thus we must seek a thorough acquaintance with the powers of life therein contained, and that changes of temperature, seasons and conditions do reach the constrictor nerves at periphery and center, and cause muscles to contract all the length of the neck and spine, so powerfully as to pull one spine against another or to cut off the intercostal nerves by forcing ribs to spine by such constriction that they are found under the hand of a well trained observer to be abnormal in position, and off transverse process at costal articulation with the spine, then we have great pain in pleura and lungs by venous blood. A question: What stopped the blood, or why was it impeded in the veins of the lungs and pleura while on its way to the heart? Was it by constriction of muscles around veins? If so, what part of the spinal cord was impinged on by such strictor muscles? Then if the trouble is from a loss of nerve force to reach lungs, pleura or any other organ would it not be wisdom to unbolt the gates at the neck and spinal cord and flood the parched fields with the waters of life? We speak much about stimulating and inhibiting and think as the masseur does, that he has found a sine qua non for all diseases, until he gets better acquainted with the bones, what is in them and how to get that current out without hurting his patient. I will say like Sampson of old, give me the bone and I will slay the Philistines of disease, even though it be the bone of an Ass.

* * *

CRITICISMS.

MEN go to schools to learn that which they do not know. They run a great risk of losing their time and money in any school that is not responsible financially for its contracts with its students. Suppose you pay me $300 or $500 for two years schooling, you have filled my demand, now what have I done for your safety in the contract? I have your money and if I do you justice I will give you bonds to do as I agree, or you are left at the mercy of my honor. I would advise all persons to know that any school that they enter for Osteopathic instruction is responsible for all contracts, and has shown its honest intentions by its bonds deposited in some bank for the faithful performance of said contract with you.

* * *

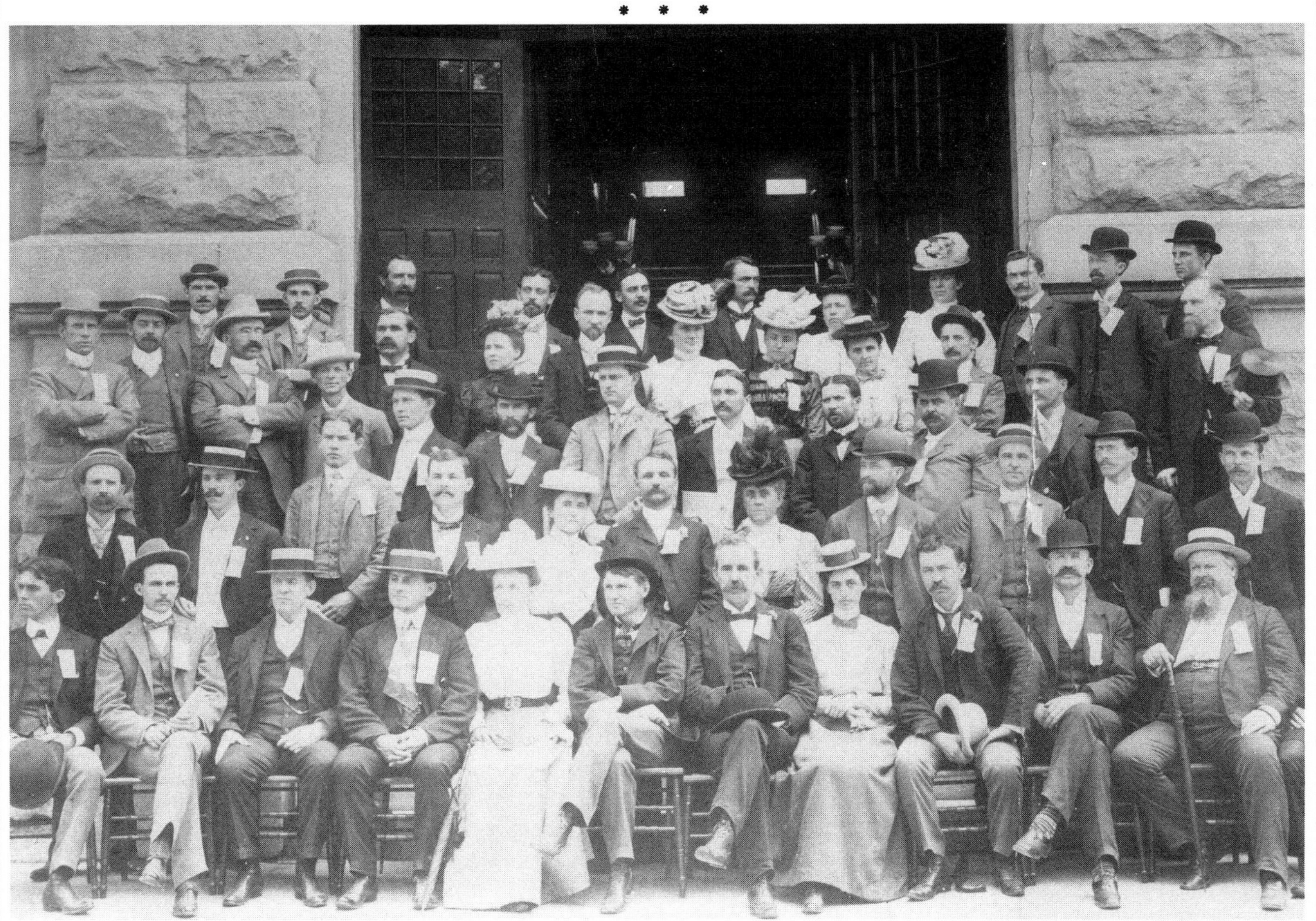

1899 A.S.O. convention at Courthouse in Kirksville

October, 1900

ANSWERS TO DAILY QUESTIONS.

How extensive are the demonstrated claims of Osteopathy as a healing science ? Does it succeed with acute as well as with chronic diseases? Would medicines or drugs be of any assistance to Osteopathy? What are its claims or does it claim to offer a substitute for surgery to any degree? if so, how much? What are its claims as a better method in obstetrics than older systems?

QUESTION 1. How extensive are the demonstrated claims of Osteopathy as a healing science? For a quarter of a century it has met and combated in open fields the diseases of summer, fall, winter and spring. We are glad to report that the diseases of the four seasons yield more readily to Osteopathic treatment than to medicinal remedies. As you are well acquainted with all diseases of the summer season we will not list.

QUESTION II. Does it succeed with acute as well as with chronic diseases? We are ready to answer yes without reservation. I will state that with all the summer diseases none excepted, that Osteopathy has succeeded beyond the shadow of a doubt in saving far above 90 per cent who have been attacked by bilious fever, chills and fever, congestion of the brain, lungs, liver, kidneys, stomach and bowels, as can be verified by the books of our clinics and practice. The universal reports are the same of the graduates of the American School of Osteopathy who are practicing in all the states and territories of the United States, also Canada and Europe. The doctors of Osteopathy have and do continue to report cures by the thousands and deaths by the ones.

QUESTION III. Would medicines or drugs be of any assistance to Osteopathy? To this question I will give an unqualified answer, No, and will insert a protest to the employment in any acute or chronic disease, any man or woman who claims to be an Osteopathic doctor and knows so little of the science as to betray his ignorance by even suggesting that the wise God of the universe ever intended to make a slop pail of the human stomach, to receive the poisonous compounds that ignorance has given to the world, hoping that some accidental illegitimate child will be produced in the stomach, rise, go out, conquer and be the monarch of conquest. No Osteopath has any use or place for any drug or drugs.

QUESTION IV. What are its claims or does it claim to offer a substitute for surgery to any degree? We want to book ourselves emphatically that we do recommend the use of the knife when the wisest Osteopathic methods have failed. By Osteopathy I think I am safe in saying that seventy-five times out of one hundred that the knife is used in the so-called appendicitis that the Osteopath could relieve the patient of his malady and save him from a torturous operation, the death list of which is appalling. In tumefaction, abdominal tumors, enlarged liver, gall-stones, bladder stones, Bright's disease, diabetes and dropsy, the Osteopath is worth more to ninety-five patients in each one hundred than all the knives and skill of the best surgeons of the whole world, provided he has a reasonably fair start with the disease. The knife has an honorable claim to a place which we willingly grant and concede as meritorious.

QUESTION V. What are its claims as a better method in obstetrics than older systems? We will answer this question by saying that the skilled Osteopathic accoucheur, the well balanced head of an Osteopath who is worthy of the name of his profession, long before he graduates and receives his diploma does learn that the Architect who planned and constructed man and woman had an object and worked to the same, and he made that object to wisely work as he intended, and that he had so constructed the womb that it would naturally deliver its contents at foetal maturity in all women who had escaped accidental pelvic deformities. The science of Osteopathy carries before the operator the search-light of reason and success, from the first indication of labor to the completed delivery of the child. Relaxation and natural forcible expulsion can easily be conducted by the informed Osteopath, and the average time of labor from twelve to eighteen hours in five hundred to seven hundred cases reported and now on record show less than two hours duration. Hemorrhage after births by his skill ceases at once. We teach the use of instrumental delivery that he may be well armed for anything that may come before him in the way of pelvic deformities. Such deformities may never appear to the operator but he should be posted and ready to act under any emergency.

A. T. STILL.

October, 1900

Dr. R. H. Williams, of Nevada, Mo., graduate of the A. S. O. Feb. Class 1900, and Miss Grace Wright of Macon, Mo., were married Sept. 19th.

Dr. Wilderson and wife are now visiting their friends and relatives, also the school of which he is a graduate. He has for the past two years been practicing Osteopathy in Memphis, Tenn. He reports a good run of practice and good results with his patients. Many of his Tennessee patients write of his skill and good luck both in chronic and acute diseases. He is one of the many finely skilled mechanics, that I consulted on Osteopathy, or the fact that man was a machine from start to finish, and should be the object of the machinist's deepest thought. He was then able to ask "If man is a machine of perfect construction why not treat accordingly?" As soon as he could close out shop in Nevada, Mo, he moved to Kirksville, and entered my school, the A. S. O. He began at the bone and quit at the soul of man. He is an honor to the profession. I can heartily recommend him to all the afflicted, as a genius, a safe council and a good operator. We have sent out hundreds of operators, of whom we can speak kindly and will ever so speak if they stick to Osteopathy; a few have slapped this school in the face by dabbling in drugs. Such an one is to be pitied for his native stupidity. "But while the lamp holds out to burn, the vilest sinner may return."

I make special mention here of this fact. I have been constructing a chair, seat or table on which the patient may sit or recline while being treated, and as Dr. Wilderson and I have spent many days in his workshop and knowing his ability as a machinist and his scientific knowledge of Osteopathy, I took him into my private room in which I keep my device, rolled it into his presence, showed him the beneficial claims I had for the machine. After he had treated several of my patients, he gave his opinion in the following words: "To say that it is a complete success is drawing the term mildly."

A. T. STILL.

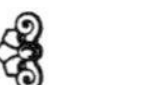 Dr. A. T. Still's Department. 

What Killed the Baby, the Little Boy and the Little Girl Also?

OUR doctors said it died from the effects of diphtheria which ran into malignant sore-throat and tonsilitis of gangrenous nature.

Our doctor is a mighty good man, he did all he could for sister, he said he wanted to save sister and in consultation with two doctors that he had summoned from Boston and New York, he did all he could to save her life; they used all remedies both new and old, they had swabbed her throat with costics and given the most powerful throat washes known in Europe and America, and all the simple family remedies, and even put a tube in sister's wind-pipe to let the air into the lungs, but she died in spite of all that could be done or thought of.

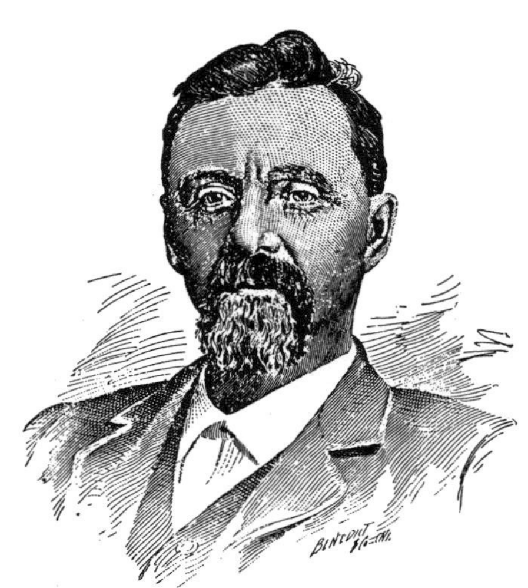

DR. ANDREW T. STILL, FOUNDER OF OSTEOPATHY.

Now the baby, boy and girl are dead; the disease was called "diphtheria, a very dangerous and contagious disease" and so reported to the board of health, who ordered flags as warning to others to keep out. This has been the practice and treatment for lo, these many years. Who has ever questioned our sages and our systems of reason and treatment in colds and diseases of the throat, tonsils, and glands of the neck and the air passages? Did we ever halt and reason that the white patches found in mouth and throat were put there to guard the parts against coming injuries that hurried breathing, cold air, food and drink might produce?

Did we ever ask why God put such covering over such exposed surfaces? When we remove such natural guards to life, have we not flatly disputed the wisdom of nature?

If we are justified to remove such and do no harm, would we not under such rule of reason be just as wise in removing the bark off our fruit trees and expect the trees to do better without the bark than to let it stay where nature put it until the tree grew its wood and fruit and dropped its old bark, when it had made new and was prepared to part with the old that was of no further use to the life of the tree? Would it not be wisdom for a few times in our practice among sore throats, to let the bark stay where nature had formed it till it had done the work for which nature had formed it?

A word from long experience in disease of the mouth, throat and neck of the young. We have given much more faith to local symptoms and local treatments, than we should; because the best we can say of such is that it leads us into a system of routine work, which is followed by the school the doctor of medicine hails from.

Forty years ago I began to let throats alone, by keeping all kinds of washes out of sore throats. For sore spots I gave the baby boy or girl starch gruel, the white of egg, gum arabic or some pasty drink to cover sore spots. Give such often till soreness leaves the throat.

I am proud to report that I have lost no case of croup, sore throat, diphtheria or tonsilitis since I quit the unphilosophical practice of washing and swabbing children's throats, which I think kills seventy-five per cent of such patients who have died from infantile throat disease.

Give your patients sensible Osteopathic treatment and keep washes out; give them plenty of gruel to eat and cover sore spots, and you will have but few dead babies on your list of throat diseases among children.

* * *

In talking on diphtheria and other throat diseases to the students of my school, I do so with the knowledge that I am before men and women of learning, and that you are fully posted in the very best of American literature, which is equal to the very best of the most advanced nations of the earth. I know too that you did not come here for any foolishness nor child's play, at a heavy loss of time and money. You came to this military school for drill that you could be better prepared to combat with the great army of diseases that is dealing death to the human race all over the earth by the millions annually. I know you mean business and I propose to talk business to you during your sojourn with us.

Our medical doctors are only men of our race, and they have bravely fought for the lives of our children; they have used the best weapons they could plan and build, they have failed to batter down and take the forts of the enemy. The enemy has guns and ammunition of better strength and longer range, he has made the most skilled generals of medicine run up the white flag of surrender, and the blue flags of danger, which means to keep out of range of diphtheria, small-pox, and on to the full list of contagions and infections.

Who ever run up a white flag but he who knows he has no power to resist longer nor hope of victory? What has the doctor done but multiply his drugs and chronicle defeat? He knows and says that drugs are strong compounds of which he is just as ignorant as a boot-jack. Like a rhinoceros he sees and fights only the smoke of the gun that throws the deadly bullets that tear asunder his frame and lets the life out. Thus he ends with his little book on symptomatology, doses and kills babies now just as fast as any time for a thousand years.

He knows his practice is not trustworthy; he cuts and tries and does not know whether a tree will do better or worse if he skins the bark off the babies' throats. He swabs, bobs, and daubs and tries to keep up with the last antitoxin fad and then turns the dead baby over to the deacon who labels all babies for heaven, and tells us that "The Lord giveth and he taketh."

Then the hunter sets out on a hunt for more quails, he shoots on the wing only, but he gets a heap of quails, and asks all legislatures to give him a good quail law and keep out all hunters but him and his kind.

December, 1900

I HAVE concluded to write an article on smallpox which will contain a history of the most deadly and loathesome disease that has ever visited the human family. It is my intention to give from the very best authors on smallpox a carefully prepared description of how the disease is taken up by the human system and give its daily progressive steps from start to finish of smallpox. As I have come in contact and treated the disease and never taken it, have often been vaccinated without any effect, I believe that during the last twenty-five years, pondering upon the question of why I was exempt from the disease and vaccination, I have obtained truths and enough of them to come to the conclusion, that we have a more powerful germicide than the germs of variola, which I will try and present in the JOURNAL in the January number, for the consideration of the readers, historians and philosophers of the world.

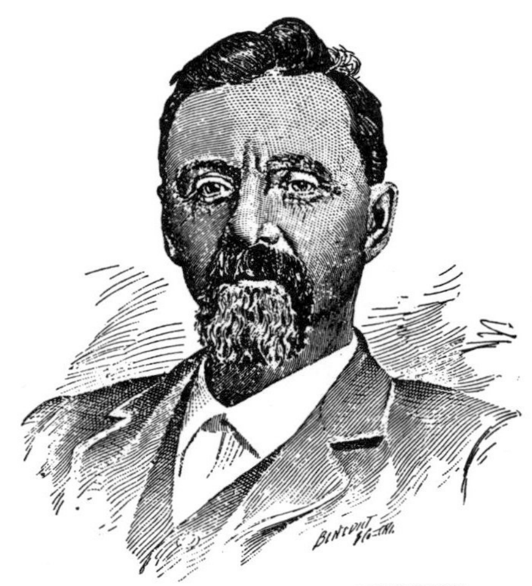

DR. ANDREW T. STILL, FOUNDER OF OSTEOPATHY.

* * *

PATIENTS AND DOCTORS.

WHEN a patient enters my Infirmary for osteopathic treatment he should be told by the doctor who examines him about how soon to look for a change. If patient should be a case of general debility, a few physiological facts should be told in plain words that can be easily understood. Explain to the patient who has been medicated for months and years that he or she has a compound disease, composed of the disease itself and the effects of the drugs that have been taken and are still in the system.

Patiently listen to the patient's story, when first his health began to fail, and for what he had been treated and how long he was under drug treatment, what school the doctor was of; then after you have summed up the points that would be of value to you, tell the patient that you would like to examine the case, to learn if it was the result of a fall, strain or anything that had caused disturbance of the nerves by partial or complete dislocation of bones of the neck, spine, limbs or ribs. When finished the doctor can give a few similar cases and about how such cases terminated. Be patient with your patients, for in one way they are not all patient. They have been doctored out of patience long before they came here and your work is to get them well or on the mend, then you will have smiles from faces that you have given hope to by your work and skill.

Tell your patients to obey you and do as you direct and you will try and get them well. Tell them if they come under your care and advice that they must come and be treated just as often as you say and no oftener, or go home. Your business is to cure; tell your patients that you must be "boss" and not ask every person on the street to give them a treatment; tell your patients that too much treatment is injurious and tell them why; convince your patient that you are fully able to run the case, and you have the full confidence of the heads of the Infirmary or you would not occupy the responsible position which you hold.

* * *

EXPANSION.

NORTH AMERICA has just closed out a big political campaign. One of the questions was: shall we "expand" our commercial and other kinds of trade and pursuits or will we contract our business?

The vote was cast and counted and expansion carried by an overwhelming majority. Thus we have said we want to expand. Will we as osteopath students expand our knowledge of anatomy, physiology and the functions of all organs of life for four years to come or will we sleep like Rip Van Winkle for the next four years, and wake up and bore our eyes to see that while we slept, boys had grown to be men and villages to be large cities? I am proud to see that the students of our school have the very best of intellectual steel in their make-up; they are high up in all their classes, can kick foot balls sky-wards, 16 to 6, and I am sure they will make the best of score with all the games of head as well as foot. Our lady students are all expansionists, they are up in all their grades in all branches taught here and other places. I believe expansion is, has, and will be the everlasting watch-word for the A. S. O.

I cannot leave this most important subject of expansion without begging you with the greatest anguish of my soul to remember that all from the greatest to the least pupil, professor, sexton and all must expand all you possibly can on Thursday of this week, which will be the biggest expansion day of this year. I saw sixteen turkeys in one pen yesterday all for Thursday's expansion. Our gobbler is dead and the minister will be at our house Thursday. He is small, but can expand awfully. Amen.

December, 1900

Treatments.

HOW AND WHAT I MEAN BY TREATMENT.

One writer will say you must stimulate or inhibit the nerves here for constipation, there for lost voice, and here for weak eyes, there for sore throat, and this set of nerves for coughs, that set for caked breasts and so on. I wish to emphasize to the student that when I say you must treat the neck for fits, sore throat, headache, dripping eyes and so on to the whole list of troubles whose causes can be found in slips of the bones of the neck between the skull and the first dorsal vertebra, I mean, if you know what a neck is, to treat that neck by putting each bone of the neck in place from the atlas to the first dorsal and go away. You have done the work and all the good you can do. Reaction and ease will follow just as sure as you have done your work right. Begin at the head and start at the top bone of the neck and don't guess, but know that it fits to the skull properly above, then see and know that it sets square on the second bone, then go to the third, fourth, fifth, sixth and seventh or last bone of the neck; now go up that neck with your fingers and push all the muscles of the neck to their places, then blood and nerves will do the rest of the work of repair. Follow this work once or twice a week, and don't fool away any time fumbling to stimulate and inhibit.

Let the nerves and blood loose that have been cramped and kept away by twists of the bones of the neck. Professors must get off of words and lead the students by showing him how to find a small or large slip in all the bones and how to put them back to where they belong, and why the patient is sick, and why and how they will get well when treated right.

If the student is not well trained so as to make him know the extent of the curing powers of osteopathy by the professors who should train him how to detect causes of diseases in slips great and small, that can and do cause diseases, that student is liable to want to go to some medical school, magnetic healer, physical culture, or any other school to learn something. Keep your money until you need it.

A. T. STILL.

★

Instructors.

Instruction should never be given to a student on any branch of osteopathy with any other object than to give or teach him how to get a knowledge of the normal frames first, then bring in the abnormal position on the frames or bodies of patients; compare the truly normal frames with the abnormal, teach him both conditions and the difference between the two, and how to move the bones of the abnormal to where they were in time of good health. Take the students hand and put it on the normal frame and show him why it is normal or abnormal. Talk more to his hand and less to his head.

It is not theory that teaches him; it is work done by his own hands that convinces him and starts him to see and feel and know what is meant by the word treatment. The object of teaching anatomy in osteopathic schools is to get knowledge that can be useful to the osteopathic doctor when he has need for it. Men must be handled like babes, when they start to search for variations from bone centers that would cause variations from normal health. Many of those slips and twists are so small on the spine and ribs, that an old operator has to use all his caution or he will fail to observe one, and many times is at a loss to know why his patient gets no better.

If he is a feeble-minded osteopath he will send for a medical doctor and let him kill or cure. Then the cub is off to some medical school and gets into the swim as he calls it and he feels safe then to go on with his ignorance and give another dose of anti-toxin, feeling that a patient dies better under the medical ass than by an osteopathic fool. Let the osteopath try and if he fails let him try again, and keep on till he finds the cause of the disease and the remedy also.

A. T. STILL.

January, 1901

Dr. A. T. Still's Department.

SMALLPOX.

WITHOUT any apology whatever, I have taken my pen to record and give my opinion to all who have ever been students of the American School of Osteopathy on the subject of smallpox, as a disease, and some of the remedies which have been used by the human races of all nations on the face of the earth, China, Russia, Italy, Germany, France, England, Ireland, Scotland, Spain, Sweden, Norway, the islands of the seas and North America, which is my home; under whose flag all men are free and equal to speak. On this soil we tip our hats to no crown nor gown, government, statute nor national edicts, neither do we ask the privilege to express our opinions for or against the custom of our own government, nor the habits of others upon the face of the earth. We respect truth and justice to all.

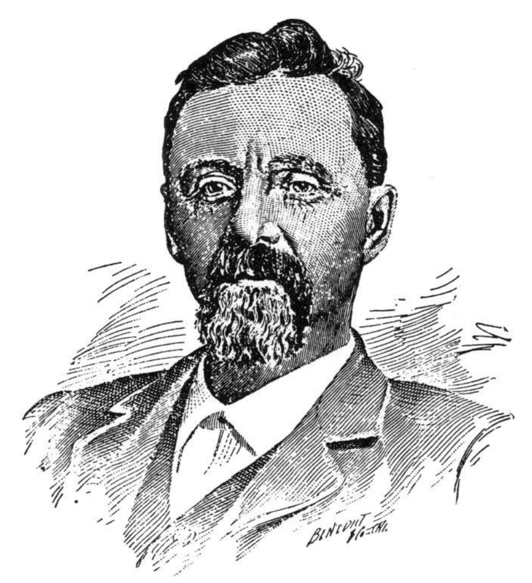

DR. ANDREW T. STILL, FOUNDER OF OSTEOPATHY.

To begin, will say, smallpox is a very loathsome and deadly disease. From history and statistics we have no positive evidence that smallpox has ever been conquered or even modified in its ravages and destruction of human life by any method of treatment; in the wigwam, the dwelling house, the pest houses of any village or city at any place on the face of the earth.

China and other nations have inoculated with the virus of smallpox with the result of increasing its spread only. The people of other governments have also thought favorably of inoculation and have inserted the poisonous matter into the bodies of those who did not have the smallpox at the time of its insertion, spread without modification was the result.

An eminent scientist by the name of "Jenner" with whom all historians are familiar as the discoverer of vaccination to whom we should give all honor to his memory for even trying to combat so deadly a scourge, notwithstanding vaccination has long worn the black garb of mourning because his theory and practice have fallen to rise no more, it having failed to conquer the deadly enemy as hoped for by him.

Vaccination is not only believed to be a gigantic failure but is believed to be the cause of the spread of tuberculosis and many other incurable and most loathsome diseases, such as leprosy, syphilis, cancer, glanders and all of the horse and cattle diseases, being injected into and retained in the human body, which was healthy all days previous to vaccination, the effects of which have caused deaths up to many thousands, if history with statistics are reliable.

I am now talking to the graduates and students of the American School of Osteopathy whose charter reads thus, to "improve our present system of surgery, obstetrics and treatment of diseases generally." I want to draw your attention to one very serious truth that should forever be before the mind of every graduate and student of this school, and that is the meaning of the word

Osteopathy, which means to improve on other systems of the healing arts. Let us as practitioners in Osteopathy live up to our obligation, and let our motto be from the rising of the sun to the setting of the same ''eternal vigilance'' with the word ''improve on'' and not imitate past theories, unless they have been weighed in the balance and not found wanting. You are not warranted nor safe in vaccination unless you do know that such person is made immune from smallpox by it and is as safe from the contagion after as though such disease did not exist upon the face of the earth. You must know that the virus you are about to put into a healthy child's arm is free from tuberculosis, syphilis, leprosy, glanders, erysipelas, cancer or any other loathsome disease of man or beast, and know that it will immune your patient from smallpox and leave no bad effects as a future annoyance, without which you are not justified to imitate the teachings of the arts of this or any other government. Before you act, halt and ask this question, where is the improvement and how may I know there has been any improvement in ten thousand years in combating smallpox? Know you are right and go ahead or hands off forever.

Do not consider me as combating the effort to cure or relieve the human race from smallpox, but I do combat most emphatically the idea of vaccination because other persons have done so. I most sincerely hope that we some day will solve the problem, meet and conquer smallpox in the open field.

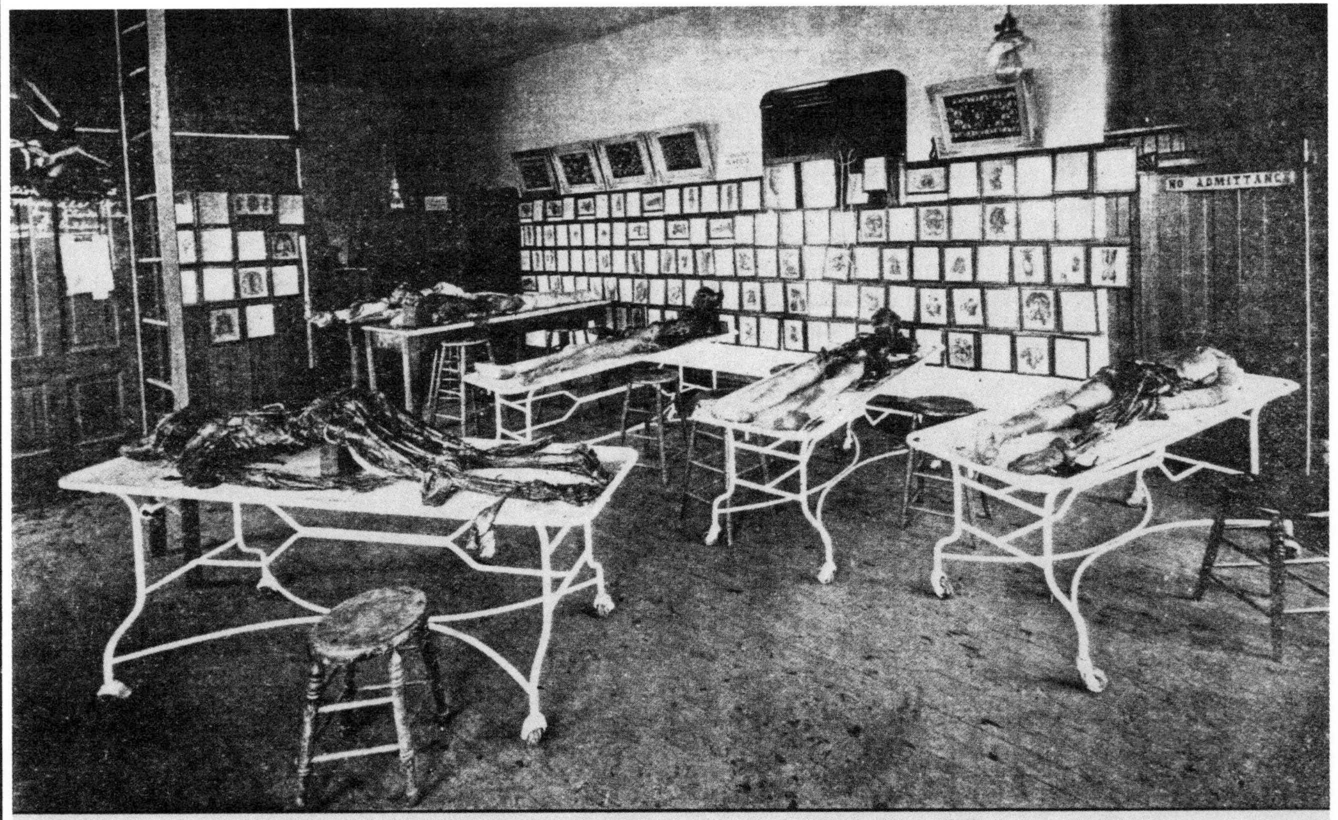

DISSECTING ROOM.

For twenty-five years and upwards I have looked on smallpox as an infectious disease, which requires about ten days from its contact with the human body to begin to show its furious upheavels on the skin of the body. It has long since been proven that its seeds when breathed into the lungs will gestate and develop from day to day and take full posession, also by inoculation.

Under my school charter I took on myself, not you, not they, not them, an obligation to improve on existing methods of healing the afflicted. I am personally responsible and not you, they, nor them, for what I may say in laudation or condemnation of any measure or method which is or has been used for the relief of suffering humanity. Self evident facts well proven by demonstration all have a friendly welcome by me. Like "Jenner" I want to relieve human suffering, but that does not say that I am competent to get results that would render the necessary relief to the afflicted and mental joy to myself. Right here I will report my own experience, I have been vaccinated many times in my arms just the same as other persons, possibly twenty times in all. I have used the vaccine quills, bones, the dry scab and the fresh matter from the living arms, all to no effect. I have been exposed and in close contact with genuine confluent smallpox, not varioloid nor chicken pox but variola pure and unmixed, and treated them for such disease. I have not been affected by either that or vaccine matter,

For many years following my exposure to smallpox I was in a quandary why I was immune from both. In talking to my mother on the subject she said possibly she had blistered all of the smallpox out of me when I was a child, at which time I had a long spell of white swelling, caused from a fall on my right hip, which resulted in inflammation of the superior crest of the right ilium, out of which a number of pieces of bone an inch and less were taken. She said she kept the fly blister active and running for six weeks. Some years later a very large swelling appeared in my left groin from the saphenous opening down the thigh about four inches. My father being an M. D., ordered the blister over the swelling, which was kept up a week or ten days, at which time the pus was let out with a lance and healed nicely. Five or six years later I was attacked with pleurisy of right side from the 8th to 12th ribs, my father bled me a quart from the arm, then ordered a blister of Spanish Fly about six by eight inches. I am now and have long since been of the opinion that I have been immune from vaccine and variola from the effect of cantharidin which was absorbed in my system during the times that I was blistered to allay the above named inflammations.

I will now proceed to tell you in the fewest possible words how smallpox proceeds after it appears on the skin, to death or recovery; also I will give you the visible appearance of the blister fly from contact to recovery or death. The first appearance of smallpox is thickening or reddening of the skin. The Spanish Fly raises the skin and reddens it, it makes a blister on the outside of the skin. Smallpox begins with a blister, eats down into the skin; cantharidin also eats down into the skin, it creates a high fever, headache, backache, suppression or stoppage of the urine, unconsciousness, convulsions and death. Variola eats down into the skin, creates a high fever, much headache, much backache, suppresses or stops the urine, produces unconsciousness, convulsions and death. Both are diseases caused by infection. Cantharidin is capable of acting from seven to ten days quicker than variola. There I think is our opportunity to start the work of the cantharidin after we have been in contact with smallpox, and let it get and hold possession of the body as an infectious disease and prohibit gestation and development of smallpox.

Sixty years ago when a man was blistered for all aches and pains, which was the popular remedy in those days, we heard and knew but little of smallpox. I have wondered for lo these many years if so much blistering as practised then had not been to a great extent a preventive to the ravages of smallpox. I would like to have a report from physicians from sixty years and upwards with their observations on the line indicated. I am very much of the opinion that the potato beetle and Spanish Fly will hold possession of the human body and hold it against infections, smallpox in particular, long enough if properly used for smallpox to disappear from any village or city.

If osteopathy can see or invent any method that can abate or abolish smallpox then we can joyfully report to the world that we have improved on other systems. It was not my intention in writing the above to write a prescription of how to prevent or treat smallpox, that will be a future matter.

* * *

Post-Febrile Paralysis.

I wish to be understood as addressing the pupils of the American School of Osteopathy on the question of why so many persons who have passed through typhoid and other kinds of fevers, leave their beds with paralysis of one or both lower limbs.

Let us coolly reason as we seek for the cause that would likely produce the effect, known as post-febrile paralysis of the limbs.

I do not wish to tire you to sleep with pages clipped from some little nor large book written on symptomatology, you men and women of all classes in this school know what fever is, just as well as I do, you know that fever makes you hot, and hot all over, you know that in a day or two that will cool off, or keep hot, get well or die. You may lose the use of a leg, arm, eye, voice, hearing and on through the list. Now you are out of the sick bed, but no legs to walk with, the doctor tells you that you have paralysis of the limb or both limbs, he often fails to detect the head of the femur out and above the (acetabulum) or below which would account for lost power of motion of the limb, by pressure of femur on sciatic nerves; or tell you that the nutrition for the nerves had been shut off by a partial dislocation of one of spines, before or during the attack of fever. Or that mercury, belladonna or some of the drugs you had taken could drain the nerves of all nourishment, and for lack of such support that the nerves of motion had failed to perform their functions. Thus the importance of close hunting among the bones of the spine and limbs to find and adjust all variations from the perfectly normal fittings of both limbs and the spine from head to sacrum. Remember that any joint of the whole spine if partially or completely off may and does effect the paralysis of both lower limbs. If you fail to find the trouble in the spine then your next place to look is for medicinal poisons, they are to be found in hundreds of kinds, beginning with calomel, bluemass, zink and on to the full list of minerals, also the vegetable remedies that are being used daily are capable of producing partial or complete paralysis of any part or organ of the body, or derange the functions of nutrition and all that pertains to health and motion.

In conclusion I wish to draw your minds to a few facts in all fevers. Generally a tired, sore and stiff feeling prevails for a few days, previous to a time that a cold or chilly spell sets in for a few hours, with pain in head, back and limbs, after which fever sets in for a short or long time, which generally goes off with profuse sweat, then patient feels relief from all previous effects but very much exhausted.

At this period we find the patient changing for the better or on a stand, with thirst, pains returning, a chill, followed with high fever, dry tongue, sick at stomach, often vomits gall, no desire to eat anything offered and goes into a long spell of fever and prostration. Now we begin to hunt ourselves, or inquire of our doctor for names for the fever so we can dose accordingly. By this time the doctor has witnessed great commotion of the brain, heart and nervous systems, motor, sensory and nutrient, with the lymphatics of the entire system filled by congestion, straining and pain equal to fermentation and inflammation of the lymphatics of all parts as results of the great nerve and blood commotion. It is but reasonable to suppose that the blood vessels that should feed both motor and sensory nerves have been overcome by the poisons generated by fermentation whilst in the struggle to empty the lymphatics, but could not while stupified by opiates, and the system laboring to complete prostration in an effort to throw off large doses of mercurial and other debilitating poisons. Thus you have Post-Febrile Paralysis.

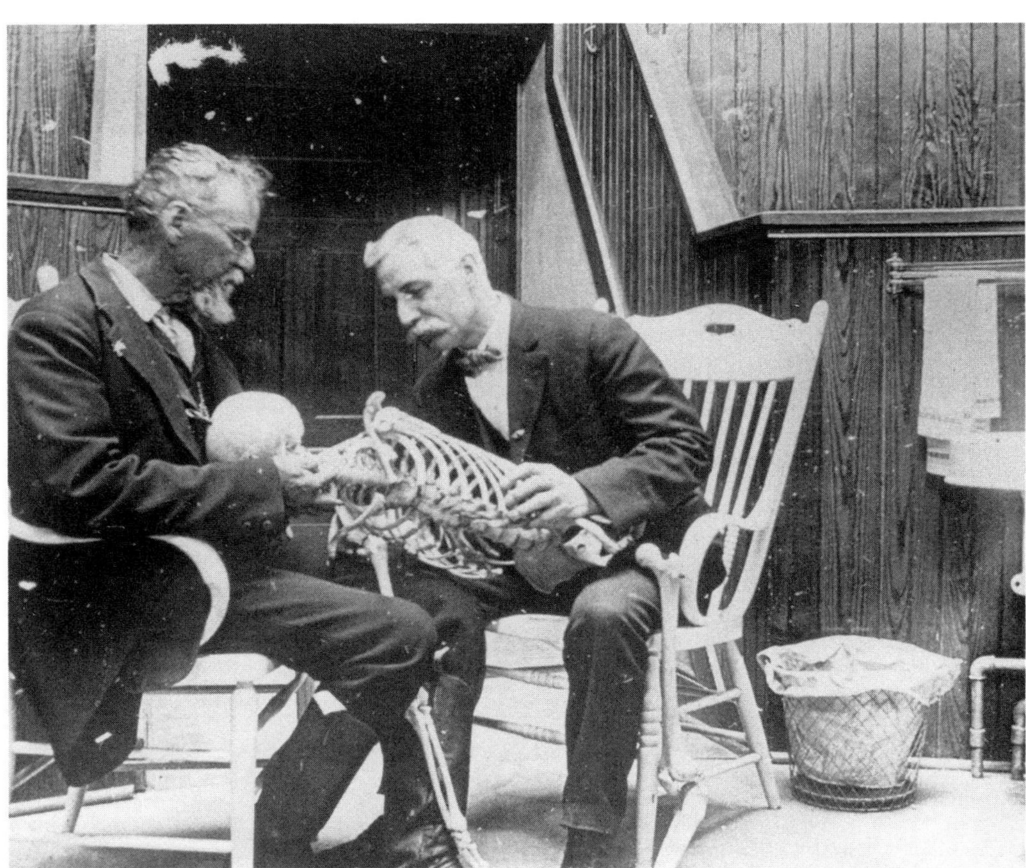

A. T. Still and colleague, c. 1913

A LETTER FROM A. T. STILL

To the Graduates and Students of the A. S. O.

Once a year at least I think the graduates and students of the A. S. O. should have a statement for their own information as to how this school stands in comparison with other schools bearing the name of Osteopathy. When I gave my consent to open a school for the purpose of teaching what I believed to be a true science, I knew a few things were necessary to establish a school that would stand before the learned critics of the world, and that one indispensable article was money to employ talented teachers. Then it would require money to purchase material and apparatus to show, by demonstration, that which would be useful to the practice when the student was out and needed its use as a D. O. Knowing such to be the case I at last gave my consent and opened a small school, with about a dozen in my first class. All went along nicely, they learned well and closed in the spring. I took the summer season to rest and attend to my usual routine business. When the fall season came we thought best to have another winter term in anatomy, chemistry, physiology and other branches that would help to a more useful understanding of how to cure the sick, not as medical cures but as engineers of skill, that could run the engine of life, so as to keep it strong and well, by its own laboratory which comes with all men, and from a competent source. On that rock I have stood and successfully combated the disease of climate and season. I have taught in all the classes that the more a man knows of anatomy and physiology the less confidence he has in drugs or remedies. Once in a long time I found a student who held to the drug phantoms up to and after he had graduated, and went into the world with pills in one hand and the name of Osteopath in the other. For the sake of truth he is to be pitied, he was weaned when the sign was in the bowels, not in the brain. I have kept an eye on his success and he has proven to be a failure, as far as I can learn. A few who carry diplomas from any school get drunk and disgrace themselves. I would say, pass them by, a drunkard is not to be trusted. A few times I have been deceived and employed drunken professors but all such were put out promptly.

Osteopathy has been tried before the most exacting courts of the world; it has been weighed and never found wanting. It calls for and stimulates man's reason. It pays better than any other profession. It feeds both mind and body, and feeds them better than the most sanguine could expect. While other schools that started wrong have died out this school has grown from a feeble child to powerful manhood.

Financially, the trustees are now and have always been fully able to make all contracts with the stndents good, or pay any damages to the student for the loss of time and money if the school should fail to live up to its contract in any particular. Thus I assert that our word and contract with you is a sacred obligation, and as such we will live up to it. We ask that you examine the records and learn that these statements are true before you spend one cent with us.

Some schools offer to pay the graduates of my school so much a head for each student drummed up and sent to such schools. If a student of the A. S. O. has that little sense you can set him down as a business fool, to recommend any school to be better than his Alma Mater.

If he has as much reason as a rat he will go around all such traps. If you take a few dollars for sending a student to any school but the A. S. O. that school will send one of its graduates to your town and take the business and bread out of your mouth. Then when letters of inquiry come asking if you are a prudent Osteopath we can easily say, that by your past acts you are not. We commend all true A. S. O.'s and cannot recommend a cheap man to any sick person.

Your Alma Mater stands to-day far ahead of the whole list of Osteopathic schools. We can do more for you than all combined. A diploma from this school is more valuable because it is a recommendation from the head of the science, and it is known and acknowledged to be solid all over the world. We offer nothing to any one to drum for us. I have tried to be just to all and attribute our growth to being above trickery.

This paragraph will be devoted to answering parents, and other persons who are seeking for information whereby they can select some trade, business for themselves, their children or friends, when they shall have finished their education in home schools. To your first question I will say that Osteopathy offers more encouragement to the graduates than any other profession I know of. First it takes you, your son and daughter into the very best society. Next, there is a great demand for skilled graduates of the A. S. O., there are thousands of places seeking such services as a graduate of this school can render, with good living remuneration for attentive skill. You know as well as I do that many other professions are over stocked; such as music, painting, telegraphy, book-keeping and so on. I know that thousands of places are calling aloud for help without drugs. Every diplomate that has left the A. S. O. kept sober, attended to his own business reports success both in curing and financial matters. There are plenty of good places now open and ready to receive you so soon as you are qualified. Long before we hand you the parchment with the seal of the A. S. O. thereunto attached we are asked by persons and letters to send Osteopathic help, with the assurance of patients to begin with.

I will close this letter with kind regards.

A. T. STILL.

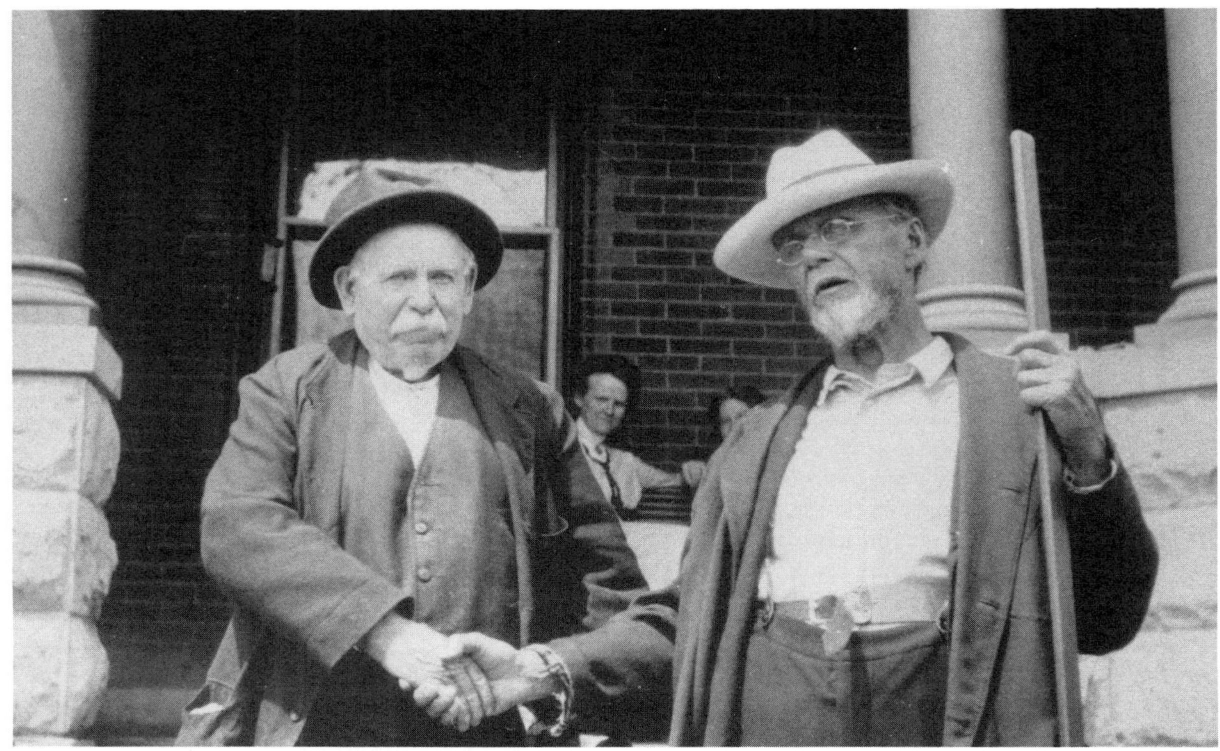

A. T. Still and his close friend Robert Harris, c. 1912

February, 1901

Dr. A. T. Still's Department.

PROCLAMATION.

IN THE year 1874 I proclaimed that a disturbed artery marked the beginning to an hour and a minute, when disease began to sow its seeds of destruction in the human body. That in no case could it be done without a

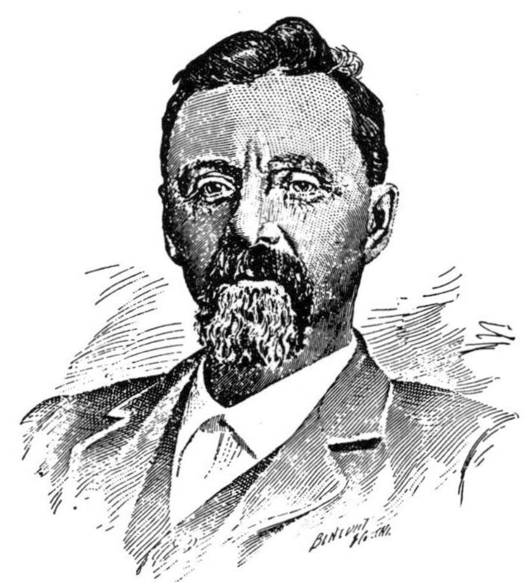

DR. ANDREW T. STILL, FOUNDER OF OSTEOPATHY.

broken or suspended current of arterial blood, which by nature was intended to supply and nourish all nerves, ligaments, muscles, skin, bones and the artery itself. And he who wished to successfully solve the problem of disease or deformities of any kind, in all cases without exception, would find one or more obstructions in some artery, or some of its branches. At an early day this philosophy solved to me the problem of malignant growths and their removal, by reproduction of the normal flow of the arterial fluids, which when done transfers the blood to the venous circulation for return and renewal after the process of renovation is completed, by the lungs, excretions and porous system. Fevers, flux, head-ache, heart and lung trouble, measles, mumps and whooping cough and all diseases met and treated since that time, have proven to my mind that there is no exception to this law. That the rule of the artery must be absolute, universal and unobstructed, or disease will be the result. I proclaimed then and there, that all nerves, sensory and motor, depended wholly on the arterial system for their qualities, such as sensation, nutrition and motion, even though by the law of reciprocity they furnished force, nutrition and sensation to the artery itself. And further proclaimed, that the brain of man was God's drug store, and had in it all liquids, lubricating oils, opiates, acids and anti-acids and every quality of drugs, that the wisdom of God thought necessary for human happiness and health. On this foundation and by its teachings, I have unfolded nature's system of mid-wifery, which would blush and be ashamed of its ignorance, for a diplomate of this science to ever be guilty of acknowledging so much stupidity and ignorance of the laws of parturition, as to take into the sick chamber of a normally formed woman, the brutal forceps which is death to the child, torture and laceration to the mother. When I see all over the land those pitiable objects called mothers, ruined for life, I often wonder if that man has the heart of a brute, or the brain of a human, that has inflicted such torture and left her in a condition to go under the surgeon's knife and deadly "ether," a far more dangerous operation, with but little hope of benefit. Such are the teachings of the prevailing systems of mid-wifery all over the civilized world.

Osteopathy says, if this be civilization and skill, what would be brutality and ignorance? I often laugh when a young osteopath says, I have taken up osteopathy, at the point that I found it had stopped in the "Old Doctor's hands" and have made many new discoveries. I am proud to know that the Rip-Van Winkle in him had gotten his sleep out, and found his old gun had been by his side for twenty years. He did not learn in school what was there for him, which he would have learned had he not left in hunt of the shining dollar before he had absorbed the juice of reason, that always comes after twenty months' close drill in the philosophy of the arteries. Nothing is newer than this philosophy as shown by any one up to date. Its applications may be more thoroughly understood, but the philosophy is eternally the same.

March, 1901

Dr. A. T. Still's Department.

Dehorning Bulls and Other Cattle.

In the course of human events, with the accumulated power to observe and reason, it has been thought to be an act of wisdom and mercy to dehorn cattle, though it may be a little severe on the animals at the time. But for the safety and good of the people, to stop unnecessary torture and death of weaker cattle, horses, sheep, human beings and so on it has been thought best to take their horns off. The result has been good, in many ways very satisfactory, and is now adopted and recommended.

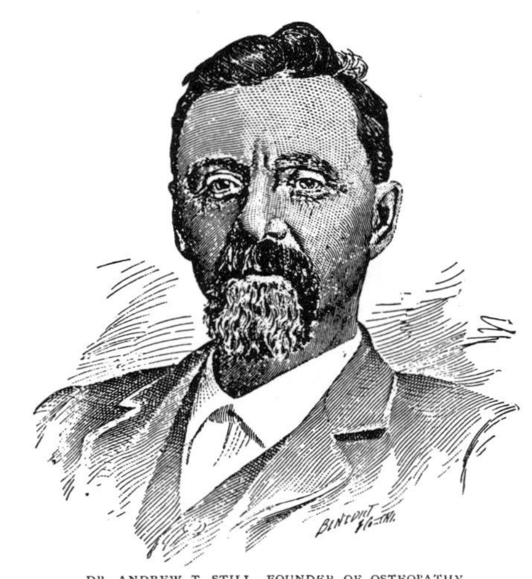

DR. ANDREW T. STILL, FOUNDER OF OSTEOPATHY.

Twenty-five years ago when first I took up Osteopathy I went out into the open pastures of nature to view the cattle of a thousand hills. I had not traveled very far until I saw scraping and heard bellowing, it was a warm day and I traveled to a shade tree, sat down to rest and converse with the gentleman who was with me. Soon I saw three or four burly old bulls, the champions of many victories coming toward the tree. I felt safe enough as I had been raised among cattle, until they approached close enough that I could see their eyes were green with rage, so my life's safety and that of my friend was to climb the tree without delay. One of them seemed to be endowed with the power of speech and entered into a conversation with me. He asked me what my profession was. I told him it had been in the practice of medicine. He asked me why I had abandoned so great a profession. I told him because it was not worthy the name of a science, and the most that I could say and speak honestly of it, was, it is simply a system of guess work, "cut and try." I spoke a few words, tried to point him to a higher and more Godly system of relieving diseases, a more rational system. He got into a rage, pawed the ground, pitched his horns into the tree in which my friend and I were situated, and we thought it a god-send that we could climb a tree. Soon the other two began to bellow, scrape and paw, their voices became dangerously shrill. The old one who could talk said to me, "You must get out of this pasture and never appear again or we will horn you to death." He went back roaring at the top of his voice, which was much stronger than any fog-horn used to proclaim the danger of one vessel meeting another in the seas of Newfoundland. In a very short time he was surrounded by hundreds of older and younger bulls, big and little bulls, lank and fat, they seemed to be greatly under his influence and control. He turned his voice toward us and with one single bellow many thousands of angry bulls from all over the United States seemed to fly around our tree of safety, which was a sturdy oak. My friend was very much agitated, he asked if I was not afraid those bulls would kill us. I told him we were perfectly safe as long as the tree stood. He asked if I was not afraid of perishing for the want of food. I told him that I believed according to history that one man had fasted for forty days and nights. While we were meditating upon horns, starvation and death, away from water, under a temperature of 110° in the hot days of July, a very angry cloud appeared in the west, we could see in it much lightning with the appearance of hail. My friend was afraid it might be a cyclone and would shake us down among the cattle. I told him to sit still as a cyclone or hail storm always had the effect to drive cattle to hiding places. After a few loud cracks of thunder the bulls began to look one at the other, they seemed to have some intuitive power that govern wild beasts. They became restless, quit roaring at us and seemed to be in a quandary what to do. At this time a very hard and terrific clap of lightning struck an old tree close to us and tore it all to pieces. My companion says "My God, we will catch it next." Said I, "My friend, be easy, see that hail falling thick and fast, look away back there, we are safe here in the tree, the foliage is thick and will protect us."

I called him "Joshua" I said "Josh, be still, mother nature is going to scatter the cattle." It pelted, rumbled and pummeled them and in five minutes' time there was not a bull in sight. I said, "Now, Josh, jump out and let us go." Josh said, "Pap, did you think about dying and all such things as that, while you were up the tree?" I said "No my son, I thought I would get a rope and saw and would dehorn bulls until they would eat grass and attend to their own business."

In 1784, I began the business of dehorning medical jerseys, durhams, herefords and every other name and shade. If you will just listen to the report of this and other states that are trying to pass laws to prohibit dehorning, you will be very glad that "Josh" and I stayed up in that tree during the storm, instead of coming down and being hooked to death by those bulls.

Moral:—Osteopathy like any other important science seeking adoption has had to contend with the bellowing of ignorance and intolerance.

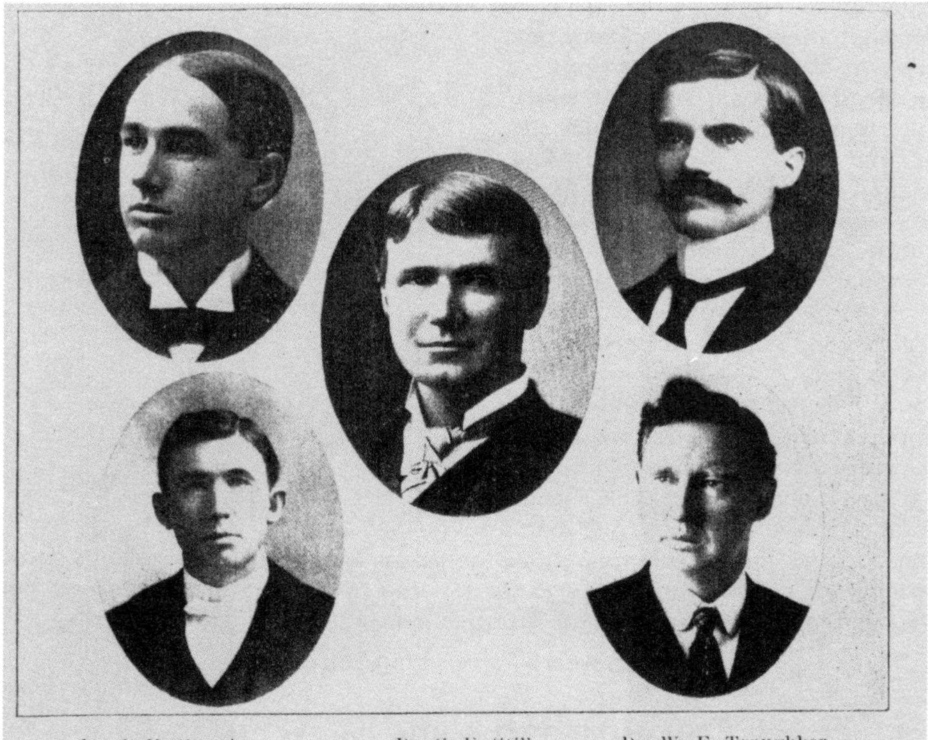

Dr. J. H. Crenshaw. Dr. C. E. Still. Dr. W. F. Traughber.
Dr. Chas. E. Boxx. Dr. A. L. McKenzie.
MISSOURI OSTEOPATHIC BOARD.

March, 1901

SURGERY.

How much surgery should be taught in an osteopathic, school is a very important inquiry, and should be answered positively to the point. We claim under our charter to teach surgery, and if we fail to teach that branch we have not lived up to our promise, and we have failed to honor our obligation to the student. We have a chair of surgery filled by a professor whose learning and practice have made him an able judge of the importance of this branch.

In answer to how much surgery the Osteopath should have taught to him we will say, that he should be armed with a general knowledge of operative surgery to the degree that the physician when in ordinary practice will always be ready and sensibly qualified to meet all emergencies in common practice; such as setting dislocated shoulders, elbows, wrists and fingers, then the hip, knee, ankle, foot, and bone or bones of the arm and leg. He should know how to adjust fractured ribs and bandage the body to keep such fractures in place until the bones unite. He should be taught to explore and note all dislocations of the spine from the head to the coccyx; and how to adjust and keep in place the many divisions of the spine, the neck, the dorsal, the lumbar, the sacrum and the innominates. He should be and is taught to do all operative surgery, with or without council, that is generally done in small villages and in the country; such as amputations of a toe, a foot, a leg or thigh. How to operate to relieve watery and other deposits of the abdomen and the chest. To remove external growths that appear upon the body at any place, that is done by the ordinary surgeon in general practice.

Then in obstetrics we teach thoroughly and impress good training in the use of instruments in that branch of practice, as we wish him particularly trained for the responsible duties that an hour may throw on him. We teach the use and the administration of anesthetics, and how to proceed in gunshot, knife, saw and other wounds. In short, our school is prepared and intended to qualify its graduates when called in council or to lead, that they may have the necessary information at that time so they will not be handicapped nor embarrassed.

* * *

OSTEOPATHY.

LISTEN to me !

I, A. T. Still, created or coined the name Osteopathy way back in the eighties. I had worked and tried to reason that a body that was perfectly normal could keep man in the full enjoyment of health just as long as the body was perfectly normal. On that conclusion, I worked first to know what was normal in form and what was not normal; then I compared the two in disease and health. I found my hard study and experimenting that no human body was normal in bone form whilst laboring under any disease, either acute or chronic. I got good results in adjusting these bodies to such a degree that people began to ask what I was going to call my new science.

I listened to all who thought I ought to name my baby, so I began to think over names such as allopathy, hydropathy, homeopathy and other names, and as I was in Kansas when the name Osawatomie was coined by taking the first part of the word Osage and the last part of Pottawattamie and the new word coined represented two tribes of Indians. I concluded I would start out with the word os (bone) and the last part of pathology and press them into one word Osteopathy, and I was like the Dutchman when he named his boy, he went out of his house to his barn and filled his lungs full so that he could talk loud then he began to call at the top of his voice, "Oh Yockup! Oh Yocup!" and said, "Dat poy vas named now already, and I don't care vat others call de poy, I like Yocup best."

I wanted to call my boy Osteopathy and I don't care what Greek scholars say about osteo, osteon, osmosis, exosmosis or endosmosis, I will call my science Osteopathy.

I give the students this bit of history that they may know from me why and when I coined the word. Pathology is a system of treating disease, and the bone is my guide in treating disease, thus bone or osteopathology—Osteopathy.

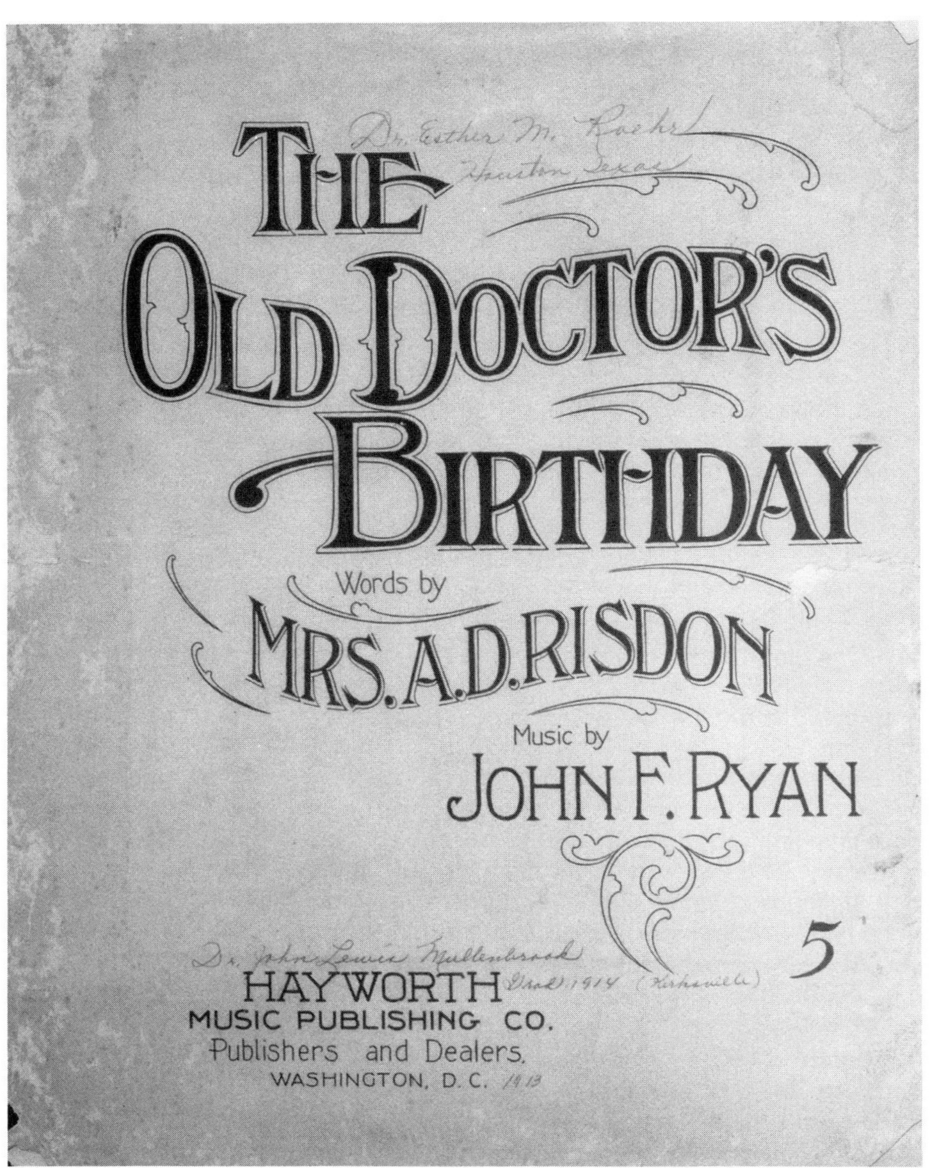

Music written in honor of A. T. Still, 1913

Dr. A. T. Still's Department.

War, Successes and Defeats.

Nations often go into war when friendly and wiser methods fail to adjust the differences of opinion as to rights that should be freely conceded and enjoyed by all. There are many reasons why measures of justice are withheld from the masses by the few. One of the most positive reasons is that men of all ages have arrived at the conclusion that possession was wisdom and all else was to be set aside. They have held fast to the rulings dictated by the possessors, and people were forced to obey all edicts of the power held by the lords of possession. Nations often unjustly oppress their own subjects and extend their unjust tyranny over other nations because of the power of wealth and resources to enforce obedience to such demands.

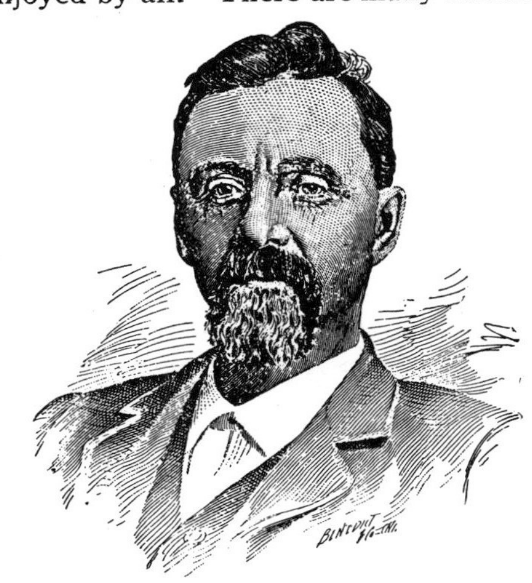

DR. ANDREW T. STILL, FOUNDER OF OSTEOPATHY.

In course of time man grows wiser even under the hand of the tyrant's brutal ruling who hates the God of justice, but as necessity is said to be the mother of invention, the seeds of justice are planted deep in the minds of the oppressed. He begins to drop a few wisely matured words to friends whom he can trust, men who would die rather than to betray. Some say we ought to ask for mercy, but such cries have long since been handed to our rulers with effect to be oppressed the more. To rebel is death to all who oppose or assist in the struggle against the usurpers of the power that know nothing but to kill all or rule by the old tyrant whose children have been educated to hate the words or thoughts of justice. Thus the fear of worse forms of torture holds the oppressed to continue in anguish of mind for the future of themselves and all who should be free. Thus ages roll on and on.

In mind war is long seen before it is proclaimed. A deliverer begins to enter the nightly councils of the caves and jungles. He cautiously enters the anxious crowd and after entering into the council, after testing the firmness of all, he takes names and organizes the few into a company, sworn to die before betraying another person, then sends men to other places to feel the sentiments of a few more. He desires to move slowly and find out if others feel the tyrant's lash bitterly enough to join and fight to the death for the joys of humanity; sets a day or night to report and council to move and do accordingly. Thus a wise man moves on and on and counts his host, and makes ready for a crushing blow at tyranny. His last words of counsel before his declaration of war is, "Let us enter all forts and arsenals, know the number of guns and other arms, the caliber range, and energy of their explosives, because this is a fight of greatest magnitude. The enemy has ruled so long that they think right is divine, and they will fight to the hour of death. They have been lords so long that they will lose rivers of blood long before they run up the white flag of surrender to their oppressed subjects. Thus we must use caution well matured. We must be sure that we choose men to lead in all parts of this army who have manliness and brains enough to conduct all divisions to success. Never allow a man to conduct any division who does not know whether he is an osteopath or medical doctor."

As a foundation, I give the reader about the usual process of procedure. How they come, why they come; how they succeed and establish new and better governments. I had to do this to show by comparison why the best and wisest government or any school or science can be ruined in its greatest and most useful days by lack of such caution. As I have told enough of revolution; to tell how they succeed to throw off the old and make the new and more human system of government. I will say a few words of how such good government generally fails and finally falls; here is the dangerous cause. The new rulers forget that had not the wisest council been used in all the meetings and preparations for such revolutions that all the leaders and many of the rank and file would have been put to death. In this medical revolution no less caution was safe. As I had been at the head of the revolt, I tried to use just as great caution after as before the battles were won, and to-day I have to keep an eye on all books that are admitted as text books.

I think to keep our science in line of progress and to let the world know that osteopathy is a complete and wholly independent system of treating diseases of all shades and kinds that we should not rely nor depend on old medical books to sustain its philosophy. I have caused the board to create a chair of literature for the purpose of inspection, who will provide such books as are written according to the philosophy of osteopathy from start to finish in all branches. I want to emphasize that no book clipped and copied from old systems of practice can find a place as a text book in the A. S. O. We cannot recommend their teaching and be consistent in the eyes of the world and claim to be an independent science.

* * *

May, 1901

Poisons And Antidotes.

A WORD OF ADVICE TO STUDENTS AND GRADUATES OF THE A. S. O.—HOW I WOULD PROCEED IF I SHOULD BE CALLED TO TREAT SMALLPOX.

First, I would put on my left arm (I am right-handed, so my left arm would suit better)—I would put a fly blister on my arm at the usual place to vaccinate, about as large as a half dollar, and let it stay until the arm gets quite red. For a lady, about the size of a quarter of a dollar, a child, about as large as a dime. Two to four hours is generally long enough to get the skin quite red and hot, then take blister plaster off and dress with a wilted cabbage leaf, or milk and bread dressing.

Blister ointment can be found at any drug store. Renew blister every three or four days until the smallpox has left the city or country.

To prevent persons from taking the smallpox blister arms of people who have been exposed and renew blister three or four days apart until disease leaves the community.

Be careful with children and do not let the blister stay too long. Take plaster off as soon as the skin turns red and dress.

When you have blistered your arm, you can go on safely and treat your cases osteopathically who have small pox broken out.

June, 1901

Dr. A. T. Still's Department.

THE DRAGON OF IGNORANCE

APPEARED from the muddy waters of that ocean whose surface never sustained a compass by which reason was pointed to any shore. This dragon of tyrannical stupidity closed his eyes and ears to the panorama of the eternal beauties in form, paintings and decorations of color.

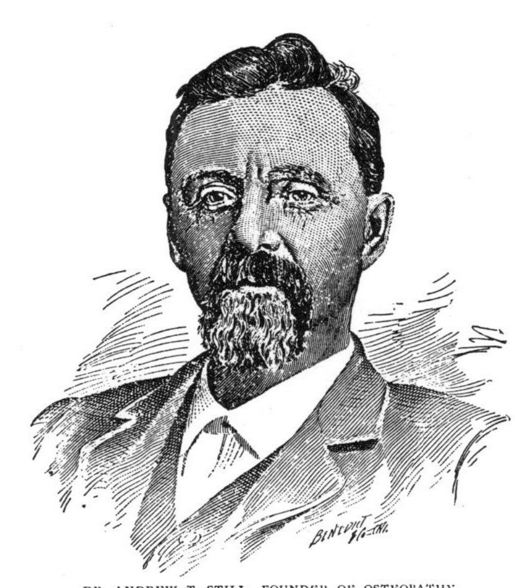

DR. ANDREW T. STILL, FOUNDER OF OSTEOPATHY.

This dragon hates and dreads reason and would sacrifice the child of thought upon the altar of his selfish-ambition. He seeks and labors to dwell under the dark clouds of fog. The black smoke and deadly gasses are his breath and happy dwelling place. He hates and would kill the child whom he finds sitting in the bright light of the ascending sun of progress. He hates the mother whose body gave that child birth, who unbosoms her breast with milk and love to nourish and encourage that child whose choice is light in preference to darkness. His amusements are the groans, shrieks and moans of that child's loving mother. That dirty old dragon has prostrated nations that were flowered and perfumed with learning, prosperity and progress. He has burned the manuscripts and books of the literati of the world. Like a blood-hound no foot-prints of intelligence can grow too old for his ability to keep on their tracks. He makes hideous gods who are minus of all that is good and lovable; strengthens their arms that they may destroy all that do not love such gods. He was never known to create a god whose love extended beyond the personality of a brute. In his god making he left out every principle of kindness, intelligence and love except that of his own foolish dogmatism. He would destroy all who sought to acquaint themselves with that God who creates and qualifies all his beings to live and labor for personal and universal comforts. He is always busy traveling from nation to nation. He is very fond of whisky, beer and wine. He is a successful general; he attends to but one business and that one business all the time. He dynamites, shells and destroys every fort in which he finds liberty and reason. He hates man and all men whose day-star is intelligence, whose eyes observe, minds comprehend and tongues speak the beauties of nature. He hates that God in whom reason dwells. He is never so happy as when he builds and armors a fort and knows it is well officered with well drilled bigotry; he knows such generals will make and keep him happy. He is so jealous of man's happiness and brotherly love that he will destroy the usefulness of the assembled statesmen with his drunken bitters, and is never more happy than when he receives the tidings that his chief executive is on a drunken spree.

June, 1901

"Medical Osteopathy."

Many uninformed persons are asking themselves the question, should drugs and osteopathy go together? Those who ask this question are of the class but little posted in the science of osteopathy. If drugs are right osteopathy is all wrong; if osteopathy is anything in the healing of diseases it is everything and drugs are nothing. This may seem a bold assertion but there is not a true osteopath living who will not back up the assertion. The man who pretends to be an osteopath and at the same time uses drugs wants the dollar and is neither an M. D. nor an osteopath. If he must depend upon his drugs at all, why not be honest and depend on them wholly and not attach D. O. to his name in order to draw custom.

Osteopathy and drugs are so opposite that one might as well say white is black as speak of medical osteopathy. You can no more mix medicine and osteopathy than you can oil and water. The man or woman who has this science deeply imbedded in his or her heart and head, who understands its principles, would blush for shame to be called a "Medical Osteopath."

Nevertheless there are certain schools which pretend to teach medicine and osteopathy. They are said to be the Medical Osteopathic Institutions, which like the bat are neither bird nor beast, and have no classification. They are mongrel institutions, snares, set to capture the unwary and unthinking. The man or woman who pays his money into such institutions gets neither medicine nor osteopathy, but a smattering, enough to make a first class quack.

I have so often laid down the law that osteopathy is hostile to the drug theory that it seems almost superfluous to repeat it here. Every man and woman sick and tired of drugs, opiates, stimulants, laxatives and purgatives has turned with longing eyes to this rainbow of hope. It has been held out as free from whiskey and poisons, and yet these medical osteopaths are trying to paint this rainbow with calomel and perfume it with whiskey.

No osteopath can believe in medicine, the very evil osteopathy is to regulate. If one wants an osteopath to treat his ailments he wants a true osteopath and not one who is half and half. If one wants a medical doctor he will secure a graduate from a real medical college, not some half and half who is nothing.

If you are going to be an osteopath don't be a sham, but a genuine osteopath. Put all your time on the study of the science in some reputable school and when you have graduated have a diploma of which you will not be ashamed and which the law will recognize and give you its protection.

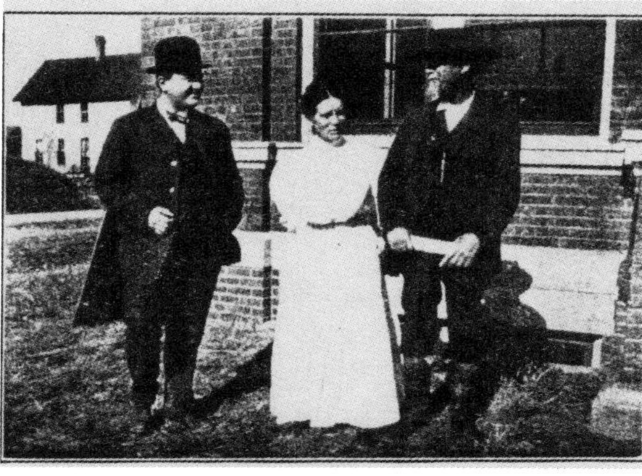

July, 1901

Dr. A. T. Still's Department.

EACH year as time rolls around to the anniversary of handing the graduates of the American School of Osteopathy their parchments, which are tokens of our greatest confidence that you, each and all, have filled the laws of our school charter and the rules of our school so manly and lady-like that no heart could feel other than love as parent, sister and brother for all of you, at all times and places. It has been the effort of my life, soul and body, to make you wiser and happier than you were or even hoped to be when you entered the school and had to stem the privation of two years from home and loving friends, to learn that man was carefully planned and wisely joined as mind and matter by that great law giving power of vast eternity whom no man has ever solved and only partially learned by sight and reason. You have learned to love the laws of life by the sublimity stamped upon all bones, their forms and uses, then as your eyes open and see how that same law has bound all bones to others, then added rivers of living blood to feed bones and form muscles, sinews and nerves, and unite all and give them a brain of power to move all, and mind to govern the harmonious action of each body of man, beast, fowls and fishes. He has endowed all with love to suit its peculiar kind and life. I know you have willingly done your duty to us and yourselves, then why not live to love and be loved by all? I will kill the ox and together we will eat the meat and bread, and drink pure water, the best token of sober and fathomless love that I can think of for the students of the A. S. O. Leave your long faces all behind, give and take the everlasting greetings of love in meeting and parting. I am in deepest love with all, I believe you have done us honor and yourselves justice by attending the best osteopathic school to date. I believe when all schools will cry what must I do to be saved? that you will say I wisely chose salvation when I matriculated in the American School of Osteopathy.

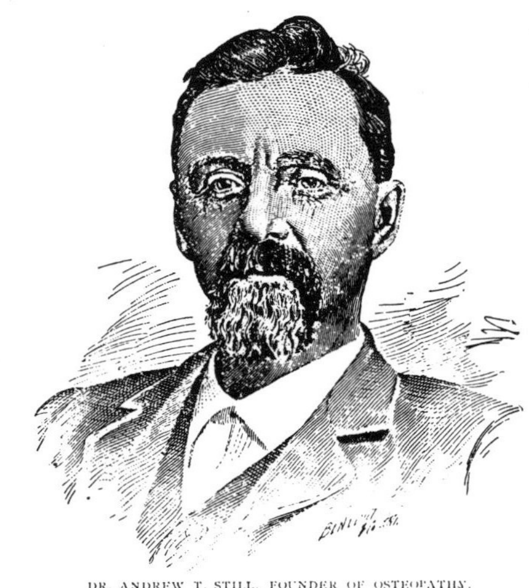

DR. ANDREW T. STILL, FOUNDER OF OSTEOPATHY.

God bless you all. Eat, drink and be happy, and come and see me next year.

A. T. STILL.

* * *

July, 1901

WHY NOT?

Why not speak a few words of kindness of our first, second and third termers? I was taught that the sins of omission were just as bad as those of commission. If so, I do not expect to be tried before a court for either sin. In a separate place I have sounded the dismissing doxology to the fourth and graduating class, and in that doxology I felt that soon many miles would separate all of us, for longer or shorter periods, and possibly forever. Then in my saddest hours I thought I would tame my emotional sea with music, not operatic squaking, but with those good old hymns, "How Tedious and Tasteless the Hours," "Am I a Soldier of the Cross?" "I Am Bound for the Promised Land." So I would be in a good mood to say to those left behind, "Well done thou good and faithful" we too will soon be fourth termers. A. T. STILL.

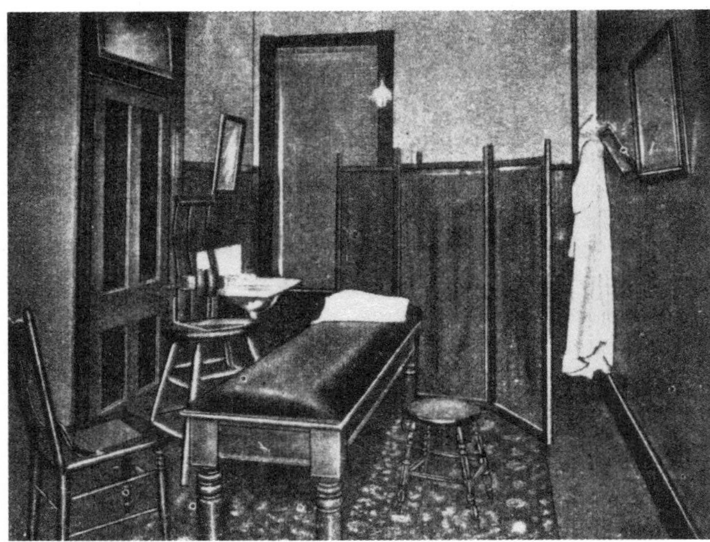

Interior of one of the Treating Rooms at the Still Infirmary

August, 1901

Dr. A. T. Still's Department.

GYNECOLOGY

AS TAUGHT and practiced by schools of medicine is of but little importance to a school of osteopathy, further than to show the student and the reading world how much ignorance and brutality have gone hand in hand for *many thousands* of years in the name of obstetrics. Such books are very vo-

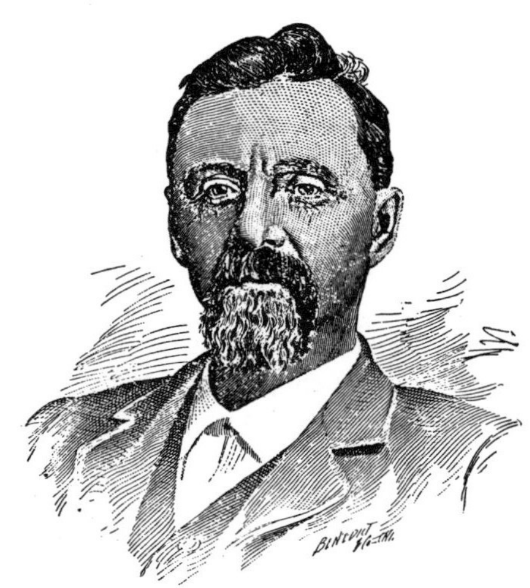

DR. ANDREW T. STILL, FOUNDER OF OSTEOPATHY.

luminous, extensively illustrated, that is they have pictures by the hundreds showing how lacerations look. It is horrible to even look at them, then follows the heart-rending thought that the mother has been ruined for life, while in the hands of ignorant doctors from schools of medicine, who have not added a single beneficial truth to discoveries for a thousand years. Not a single book on obstetrics or gynecology to date has been written under the electric lights of reason by any of them.

I am ashamed to see even a few doctors, let alone a majority, so brutally ignorant and stupid that they do not know that their stupidity and lack of knowledge necessary to safe delivery of mother and child is the cause of all of this torture, maiming and crippling of the mother, and that morally he is to blame and should suffer the penalty of malpractice for her second course of suffering under the surgeon's knife. He does not know how to pilot the mother safely or he would start with a sound woman and take her from start to finish through all periods of delivery without a rent or blemish. Is he a fool? Her condition after delivery says he is. It says he is an ignoramus. Perhaps the doctor is not so much to blame as the school in which he graduated. They teach him but little in midwifery that he can use. Books on obstetrics are full of deformities. He sees them so much and long that he goes out of school believing that he must have a car load of tools to be successful as an obstetrician. He has had so little of the normal taught that his ideas of nature's delivery are totally lost, and when he is called to attend his first ten or more cases and the child is born while he is asleep in his chair or on the lounge, he wonders why some one did not wake him up to see nature help itself safely even though the doctor did not have time to get his valise open and get his forceps out in time to insert and make a five inch laceration.

In the course of a few months, anxiously looking for cases on which to use his finely silvered $200 case of obstetrical instruments, he thought that perhaps nature is the best midwife among all beings and will do all work well that is to be done by nature's laws. He soliloquizes that he has been badly deceived by his school and picture books. He feels sheepish to learn after attending the birth of fifty children that nature let alone would and had done all its work long before a doctor was born. I do not want to allow any part of the old school theories to be taught in my school. My reason is about this. Many years before I consented to teach osteopathy, I had proven the theories of medical schools to be untrue, I proved them all to be false, unreliable and at the head of the column that was ruining our whole world by drunkenness, opium fiends and opium fools who persisted in their ignorant, ruinous habits until both doctor and fiend were almost imbeciles, and I now think such teaching is the greatest calamity that ever befell any nation on earth, and for that reason I will not tolerate any professor to teach from any old book on midwifery, gynecology or theory and practice. I do not want any part of such stuff taught in the walls of my school. I want all of my professors to teach what they know to be in strict conformity to nature. The world has no further use for the old trash taught in medical schools. They have nothing that we want or need, and I want, insist, and order all professors to kick old trash out of their lectures or trot at once. We do not want nor need old midwifery. Not a bit of it. We do not need nor expect to use their rot and ignorance in gynecology. We ask nothing and would only get bundles of trash not fit to make sow beds if we did ask.

I want to say and emphasize that the dread of having instruments used in confinement and the dreadful torture and tearing of the flesh of the mother by those instruments that are uselessly displayed in books written on midwifery and gynæcology is the cause of so much abortion. There is but little trouble for a woman to find some old murderous brute that ought to be hanged for murder ready to produce abortion, kill a child and mother both for ten dollars. No wonder life is a misery to the young married ladies. When she sees books on midwifery full of the most torturous pictures of instrumental delivery, then to add to her dread of motherhood every boy who graduates in a medical college brings a box full of instruments, calls all his neighbors in, spreads out his cases of tongs, knives, saws, hammers, chisels, forceps and says, "I expect to make female diseases a specialty." Our school has for its object to simplify all its work, follow nature, develop reason. Do better work each day and let that work prove the skill of the genius who did the work. We pay men to lead; we pay men to charge all forts and retreat from none, use the new guns or go. We want no battle-axe leaders at the head of our column.

* * *

The Lonely Philosopher.

The lonely philosopher loves company. Why not? Before he can reason and prove his theory by facts demonstrated he must be well filled with a loving soul. He must love nature and all of its products, thus he naturally loves his fellow-man. His soul hungers for the most ardent rivers of love that flow in the breast of man. He loves his mother dearly, if alive, if not her memory in the cold grave with eye-blinding oceans of briny sobs of a child's sweetest love. If he should possess the powers of an accepted philosopher, he knows he owes it all to the silent ashes of his mother, and when his mind drifts from her sacred tomb to other forms of nature he goes with silent engine of love fully charged into new fields as an explorer for new truths. He could not succeed, did he not love mother nature with all his mind and strength with the very sweetest emotions of every throb of his heart. Many persons feel that he is not a companion to be sought, that he is devoid of love and only a cold machine of cause and effect. He learns that he must be a man of one subject at a time only. He often weeps bitter tears because he is left alone to travel from first mile posts to all others, alone without a kind hand to even touch his burning forehead or drop a word of approval of his labors of day and night for months and years. He too very often feels that all his friends have long since been the silent occupants of the mossy graves of deserted lands while he has been plowing deep in the stumpy lands of the forests to plant a few sprouts from the tree of life and knowledge, he must be patient even though he grows gray.

When he measures space and counts and measures the great world and truthfully reports what he has seen and knows of the wheeling and counter-wheeling in space, all in obedience to the laws of love, even mighty worlds many million times larger than our earth, let him rejoice and be exceedingly glad that his lonely hours have turned loose rivers of joy to millions of men of his day and generations to follow. Be merciful on the poor lonely philosopher, he loves you but has not the time to give in words what his heart feels for you. He has given you all from the dug-out to the steam monsters of the sea, he has given you the law of loving government, he has taken the lightning's furious power, tamed it, made it grind your bread, cook the same, and made by his cool head a mouth that can be heard many miles away. He has lighted your cities, turned his search-light on the ocean wave, that you can see friend and foe. He has made all you have, that is joyful mentally and physically. Honor his day, thank him for his mental worry—all his sleepless nights given for your comfort. He, too, could be a giddy sport and drift with the animals of his race and day. With his powerful mind given with all his native powers to animal pleasures, he could excel even as a man of that class, but he could not be untrue to his convictions, and thus he left off the pleasures of his day for that, which would stand the tests of all days and leave to us that everlasting legacy—wisdom.

Often he soliloquizes when alone "Am I singled out and coldly deserted by all." Yea, even the beasts of the field seem to shun my presence, as though I were the chief of cold-blooded tyrants." I am not, I love them, because God gave them a place to fill, both in time and space. I am in deepest love with their form and being, without them, nature's decorations would be a mourning blank. This thought came as a consoling friend in my hour of wailing and it gave me words of cheer. "That he who can reason must learn to be happy in seclusion just as much so as in the mirthful throngs," conscious that he feeds the hungry by his genius, clothes the naked by his skill and gives rest to the weary.

Why not count the silent philosopher as among the first to be joyful, when his mind soars aloft and dwells among the mysteries of the starry heavens.

* * *

WHAT DO THE DICKEY BIRDS SAY
Name the baby
OSTEOBLAST.

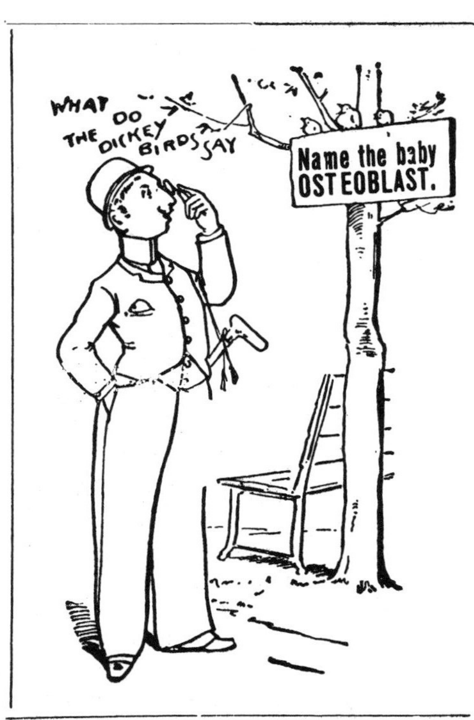

August, 1901

SMALLPOX CONTINUED, BY A. T. STILL.

TO THE students and doctors of our philosophy: I think it is necessary to continue the subject of smallpox and its prevention as the disease is so very prevalent all over the world. I have written twice before on this important subject. It occurs to my mind, that while the Spanish fly blister bids fair from results already obtained, to take the place of vaccination and render useless that dangerous system of multiplying other diseases which are inserted into the human body with its seeds of syphilis, cancer, leprosy and an innumerable host of diseases, that can be and are inserted into the human body, many of them never disappearing until death claims its victim. Then another important question comes up this time. You must remember that you are in the enemies' country; I mean you are surrounded by medical men who are now organized to combat and banish osteopathy if possible. You have only to think of the venom that has been manifested in the Legislatures of a great number of the states to cause you to be very cautious in the selection of the purest and best quality of cantharidin. Know that it is chemically pure, because the fly if not pure, if it has gone into a state of decomposition or eaten up by the fly mite or the parasite that is found in poorly preserved cantharidin, or should the cantharidin moulder into deadly decay you cannot depend upon its effectiveness. Remember this one very important thing, and I desire to make the impressive caution, that unless you have all reason to believe that the blister ointment is chemically pure the certainty of good results is debatable and doubtful. We will suppose a case that is not at all impossible. Suppose you should send in a prescription for a blister one inch square to some drug store, and behind the counter a doctor should sit whc is a deadly enemy to your school of osteopathy who might incorporate a small amount of antimony, arsenic, sulphate of copper and other poisonous drugs, into the blister ointment, and a serious ulcer should follow for months and years at the point or place on the arm to which you had ordered the application of the fly blister, then you are in the condition to be arrested, prosecuted, fined or imprisoned for malpractice. In order to make you perfectly safe and place in your hands the ointment to be used as a preventive to smallpox in place of "vaccination" I have through my chemist who is capable of analyzing any substance for its chemical purity, selected from the very best manufacturers that which is chemically pure. I have just received a small amount and can ship to the order of the graduates of the A. S. O. with instructions how to apply and treat, to prevent you and your patients from taking the disease, and how to successfully treat those who have the rash broken out when you are called to treat them.

This is not by order of the school, therefore address me personally.

A. T. STILL.

* * *

August, 1901

WORDS ARE ONLY LABELS FOR THOUGHT.

All such labels should be chosen to represent some quality belonging to the package manufactured in the mental work shop. Thus the mind manufactures a package of ideas on any subject, then the person names or labels his compound; he tests and if his ideas prove to be true, then is ready to label with a name to notify the reader what kind of compound is contained in that package, thus all our words are ideal labels. The short words are found in all truths, the long words are used by fools only.

* * *

A. T. Still at 50th anniversary reunion of the first Kansas Free State Legislature, 1907

August, 1901

WHAT IS MIND?

"Mind" is a term used when we talk or that associated force whose qualities are endless in both numbers and effects, unlimited in all spheres of its action. It creates by association; it destroys by disconnecting adhesions; it is the motive power of all atoms, all worlds, and beings. It is to itself a perpetual mathematician, a master architect. It is so far above the being in which it dwells, that the being can obtain no knowledge of how and why it acts. Thus we have its use. It acts beyond man's mental vision in its perfection in its work. It does faultless work. How? We know not. It never tires, does its work once for all time. We ask in deepest reverential soliloquy: Is mind a chemical compound? Does it exist independent of all else, as electricity, and occupy all space at the same time? Is mind a power that must go with all nature both to plan, to construct and guide all works of motion to each design? It acts with equal care with atom or world. It builds the tree, the planet. It cares for its own welfare as it does for the delicate mite. It gives us love, joy and pain. All with the same cool head. Our joys and misery effect it not. It plans its works. Its only duty is to act. Listen and obey that great law-giver which is itself, the monarch of all. We know its power by what it does, only.

* * *

I am as proud as a lord with a new hat and a Prince Albert coat and have been so ever since the A. S O. barbecue on June 22, 1901. It was given by friends in honor of June 22, 1874, the birthday of the discovery of osteopathy. I think fully 10,000 attended the feast. I never saw as many happy men and women, old and young, in our day as then. Car loads of people came as guests, and wagons full by the hundreds. All were happy. They ate, drank, all got full of joy. I only want to tell you one and all, that it was a pleasant time long to be remembered by me, and I hope to see all of you often in future days.

* * *

CANTHARIDIN VERSUS SMALLPOX.

I HAVE to report that very satisfactory results have been reported to me from osteopathic graduates who are all over the U. S., Canada and other countries. Hundreds have been immuned to smallpox by the blister fly or cantharidin in different localities. In all, when added up would run into several thousands now reported. I am not so anxious to report great numbers who have used the fly blister to prevent smallpox as to prove that it is virtuous in all cases as a preventative. I am fully convinced that after a fly blister has been on the arm long enough to draw a good blister it will hold that person free from smallpox, "Cuban itch," chickenpox, mumps, measles, varioloid, scarlet fever, and I hope to see leoprsy, succumb to it as a germicide. I promise to report monthly on the results as observed and reported to me.

A. T. STILL.

August, 1901

THE OLD DOCTOR AROSE THEN FOR HIS FAREWELL.

You are going out, he said, as volunteers, who wonder like the soldiers where they will camp at night. With a soldier the saddest time is not when he is suffering with his wounds, but when he gets his discharge and must say farewell to the comrades who have shared his trials in the campaign. I want to see many of you next year.

I WANT YOU ALL TO WRITE TO US.

Explain your meaning simply when you write, and when you talk to patients use plain English so they will learn what a sensible, reasonable thing osteopathy really is. Attend strictly to your own business. Let politics go, and let the medical doctors also go. Do as I did, and take the obligation to improve. I have improved on surgery, mid-wifery and have conquered smallpox too.

I give you your discharges but I invite you all to come back and I will help you. I am now only 73 years old and

I EXPECT TO LIVE TO BE A HUNDRED.

Prune your profession of all that is obsolete. Cultivate your sense of touch.

After the Old Doctor finished he handed diplomas to each of the two hundred graduates and shook hands with them. If there is any man on earth for whom the students have a kind regard it is the founder of osteopathy, A. T. Still.

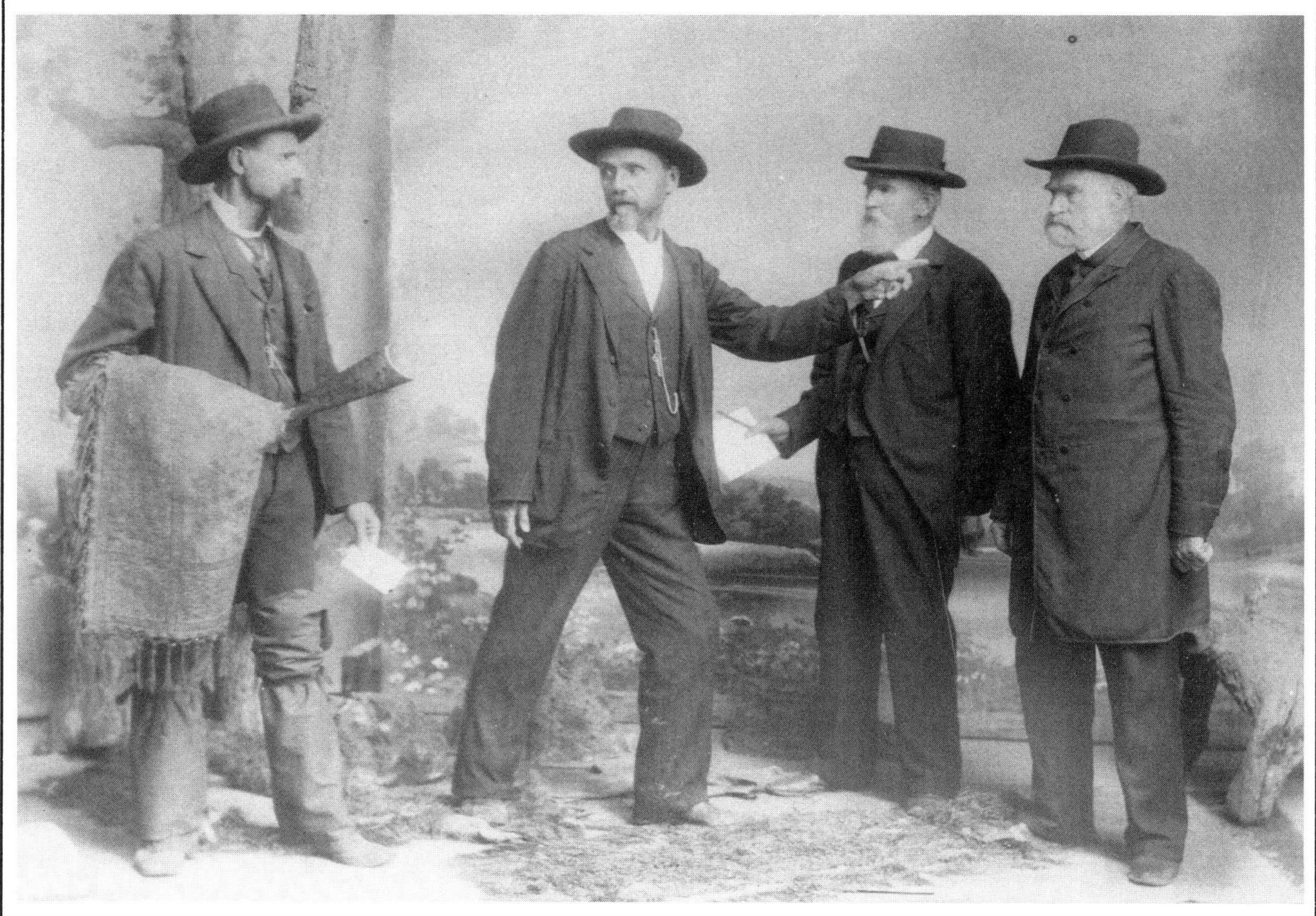

A. T. Still, in the center, with friends of the first Kansas Free State Legislature, 1907

My Lecture or rather
Social conversations, have
not been given to teach you.
but to rather encourage you
to dive deeper and deeper till
you are fully masters of your
profession. it is pleasing to
know that the law of life is
absolut. it needs much and
generates of such kind as
is needed to form nerves veins
arteras and such vessels as
are necessary to contain the
blood and distribut in
such quantities and kinds
as wanted. now back of all
this wonderful machinery
you find yet a more wonderful
power called life. Self
Existing infinite in kinds
and wholy incomprehensi

it moves on and to to perform the wonders of motion to construct and move the machinery of all animal bodies. now as we know nothing of any Substance in our bodies we must be content to try and keep our bodies adjusted, bone replaced that may be much or less off from normal centers, as all your physical comfort and mental happiness depends on the truth. Muscle and bones at the place to give you a long and happy life.

A. T. Still's handwritten notes

Previous to a great move in nature a calm takes possesssion. Instance: before an earthquake, a volcanic upheaval, a storm on the sea, great storms of rain, snow and wind, a great common calm seems to take possession of the elements for a longer or shorter time. The upheavels, storms, cyclones, down-pouring storms of rain of unusual quantities and force in proportion. We could reasonably conclude that nature had finished the preparation and turned the further action into the channels that run into forces of delivery. All nature has been laboring with all its might to complete the work. When it has completed and stopped we have a calm or rest in forces. The philospher, being a child of nature, labors to solve some important problem, when done his mind goes down to rest; he feels that something has deserted him, possibly his health will retire from his person and leave him a lifetime invalid. Thus he feels lonely and speaks of spells of despondency, commonly called "blues." It seems that his nature is being accommodated to a season of rest, which is vastly important for his health, mentally and physically, to be kept up to full normal condition. in order that he may wrestle successfully with other problems as great or greater than the one he has just disposed of. Thus considered his spells of despondency prove to be a natural course to preserve his health and strength.

A. T. STILL.

***

And the Governor proclaimed and said, let us pray on a certain day and hour for rain to fall upon the face of the earth to develop and mature the crops. This custom has been practiced since time has made it's records by the pen of man. To date we have no records, sacred nor profane, that the God of nature has thought to listen to his subordinates and change the course of his army of clouds, winds, rains or anything he does. In all honesty and justice to God would it have been an evidence of greatest wisdom in him to change the time of delivery of the quantity of rain and so on according to the requests of the rank and file, be he saint or sinner? Before we should egotize to ourselves the prerogative of instructing God when and where to send a cloud of rain would it not look far more humbly intelligent in us to recognize and acknowledge by our words and deeds that nature is far better off to furnish its own plans and specifications than to ask instructions of us the most hypocritical bigots that ever lived in animal form? The cool headed man sees wisdom in a drouth and the burning sun, in the destruction of cabbage, apple, cherry, plum, and corn worms, chinch bugs and a thousand other good things coming from a drought and hot-days. I want all osteopaths to remember that the God we worship and respect is good in anatomy, physiology and chemestry and knows how to prepare and distribute the fluids of life through all nature. He will do with mathematical exactness, always has done, always will do all his works on all things else as he has done in the construction of man.

A. T. STILL.

***

Dr. A. T. Still's Department.

A Plea for Americans to use the American Language More and Dead Languages Less.

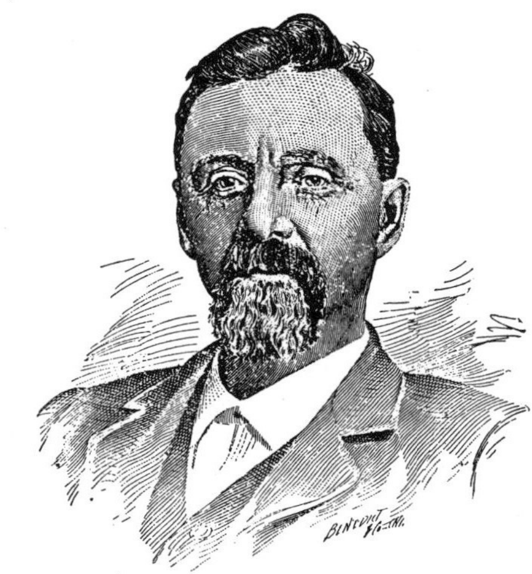

DR. ANDREW T. STILL, FOUNDER OF OSTEOPATHY.

We surely have at the end of four hundred years found the kind of words to make our people understand what ideas we have on any subject, scientific, religious, political or secular. To-day we have praise-worthy laws, and we are proud of them and pleased to defend and live under their protective and just dealings with all. They are all written in plain Americanized English. Our America has been known of by the commercial world for at least three hundred years. Some persons of all nations have left their old homes and joined hands with the proud, free and ambitious Americans to help build one of the wisest systems of loving justice. All have been kindly invited to join in what is called the "push." All Americans have been invited to speak freely on all subjects and labor to get the very best. That meant to adopt the use of words of the shortest and deepest meaning from the languages of the whole globe. Thus an invited and willing freedom to speak has been before the inhabitant of America, the few and the many, and as we ask to be considered brothers it became necessary that we should formulate a language that could be used to express this united kindness and brotherly love.

About two hundred years have passed since printing was introduced into America, although at first, rudimentary it has been one of the chief methods of educating the people to understand the meaning of all words and phrases of the brotherhood. Thus we have printed and made common property of the choice phrases of the whole world. Many very choice phrases now in common use in America have German origin, also French, Italian, Spanish, Greek, Hebrew, Latin and the various tribes of Indians of this country, no one of the languages could be used and universally comprehended by the new brotherhood. Thus small dictionaries began to appear with definitions short and comprehensive, easily spoken and easily remembered. Very few of the words contained more than three syllables, so they saw wise to adopt words of one, two and three syllables. Sample: man, horse, earth, tree, crop, fruit, with an extensive list of one syllable words. Then two syllables, such as wagon, timber, water, heaven, then when we enter words of three syllables we began to compound and say, shoemaker, navigate, hesitate, religion and so on.

The reader will see that at the end of four hundred years we have selected choice words from all and made the American language which is undoubtedly one of the best languages in use. The scientist has no difficulty in describing minutely any principle that he wishes to hold forth and explain, it matters not what science or skilled art he may choose. The words of the American dictionary are ample and ready for his use, and the American reader will comprehend what he has said when he has reduced his ideas to written publication.

The American School of Osteopathy is an American institution. The American emblem floats at its top. The American language with its ability to describe and answer all questions intelligibly and fully is the language chosen to be used by all the instructors of this school, which has been chartered, organized and is in full motion for teaching the new philosophy and practice of healing, which is based upon a comprehensive knowledge of anatomy, physiology, chemistry and the producing causes of diseases of climates and seasons, and the remedies to be found in nature's store, the human system. Its claims on surgery, mid-wifery and general practice and its method of causing natural cures are all peculiar to and must be well understood by the successful practitioner of osteopathy. Therefore the demand and use that the American language be used in all branches taught and in giving instructions how to exchange deadly effects and thereby give the laboratory of life an opportunity to heal with the vital fluids therein provided as under the hand and wisdom of God himself.

We have no professor that wishes to whitewash his ignorance with the deadlime of defunct Latin, Greek or any other tiresome and inappropriate phrases. He would much rather show his intelligence as an American thinker using our own language.

* * *

Tic Douloureux.

We give place for a definition by standard authority "Dunglison" whose authority is acknowledged by all English speaking people, also the popular diagnosis and treatment by standard writers. I am aware that in all past ages that the doctors of medicine have found much difficulty in curing or giving relief further than temporary. All remedies that the genius of man could produce have been freely used, all with failing results. All doctors hate to meet a case of "Tic" because all cases previously treated by the best medical remedies have been recorded as total failures on the lists of cured diseases. Now at the end of twenty-five years' treatment by osteopathy we have to say, though it may seem strange to persons who know nothing of this science, that no case has ever failed to be cured by it to date.

Dr. Laughlin: What are some of the causes of lumbago, Ashcroft?
Ashcroft: Exposure to cold and drafts, or a treatment by Daniel.

Dr. Gerdine: Are there two Murphys in this class?
Murphy: Yes, sir. One is sick and in the hospital.
Dr. Gerdine: Which one are you?
Murphy: I'm the one that's here.

JOHN R. MUSICK DIED APRIL 13, 1901.

I remember John R. Musick. I lived close by him many years, kind words for all came from his lips as rivers supplied from mountain springs of purest water. John R Musick was company for the man who sought green pastures of reason. He was not the man of yesterday but a man of up to date today, and saw far into the morrow and was always ready at the gate to give the new-comer a welcome- God made him and he tried to keep God's man in line with progress. I loved John because he loved himself and tried each day to be more usefnl to his race. I loved him because he never spoke foolishly, by his study and industry he did make a great and good man of himself. He was a deep thinker, a fine writer, the products of his pen have a good cause to claim love and respect for him as an author. I miss him more today than any man I know of. He was my counsel and comfort in compiling two books, he was a wise counselor to me for four years. I feel his loss and mourn that his hand is cold and silent forever. I say I miss his wise counsel. I am now at a point that wise counsel is at a premium with me, I am ready for him to compile another book, "A. T. Still's Complete Work on Osteopathy." I call, he answers not as of yore. He dropped his pen to pick it up no more.

A. T. STILL.

S. T. Furrow.

As we say, "*died*" Aug. 15th, 1901. No, he is not "dead". Many years will come and go before he is dead in the minds of many who live in Kirksville and other places where he has lived. I have known the man for 28 years. Kindness and justice to all persons was the motto of his soul. To the unfortunate in business life his kind hand went out to help—he said "be of good courage, hope and work." He was better often to others than he was to himself. He will be very much missed by his many friends whom he had helped in the hour of greatest need and I wish to be listed as one who will ever bless him for kindness to me. I feel that he leaves thousands behind that feel as I do—and will close by saying to his bereaved family that we too, one and all, extend to you the deepest sympathy and sorrow in his loss. He has been a true friend to osteopathy ever since I landed the science in the town. He and his good wife gave me my first dinner after I raised my little flag in Kirksville, Feb. 1875, which, with their kindness then I can never forget and hope never to while life lasts. I speak for our school and all its friends and associates.

A. T. STILL, Pres. A. S. O.

Dr. A. T. Still's Department.

MASONIC SECRECY.

MASONIC secrecy seems to be a fat, fearful bugaboo or spook. I have been a mason for forty years, I took no obligation that I would be ashamed to take before God or man. I took no obligation of disloyalty to God or government, none to be fouud in a saloon drunk. I took no obligation to hate everything but masons because they did not see as I did. I took no obligation to meddle with people's religious views, but I did take or promise to be a good citizen with all that means. We have a few signs and words of recognition. In free America that is our privilege under the personal privilege granted to us in the constitution of the United States. In masonry we get no right to persecute the catholics nor any religious divinity because they are not masons, we are quite well pleased to grant to all sects and individuals the right to choose and live with the religious, political or scientific organization of their own choice. Churches have signs such as a kiss, cross, baptism, breaking of bread, drinking emblematic wines and many things that masonry does not have. We say nothing of such because part of masonry says do no wrong to any person and we feel we would be out of our places to meddle with other people's business. Masonry does not ask you to become a mason, you must ask and work or forever stay out. If my brother wants to be a catholic he has the right and would be a coward not to use his freedom. I think masonry is honorable. Here is a masonic charge I will tell you although I may be expelled for divulging it, this charge is to young masons as they go out to mingle with the world, never allow your zeal for masonry to get you into argument with ignorant and uninformed persons. The merits of masonry may be very limited but it suits many persons of all nations. It has lived many centuries, the world could have lived without it, just so with any organization now existing. The sun would rise and shine just the same. It is much to be hoped that we will some day have something better than masonry, and that the churches from Mahomet down will give way to something better, and all rally around the flag on whose face you read "Love thy neighbor as thyself."

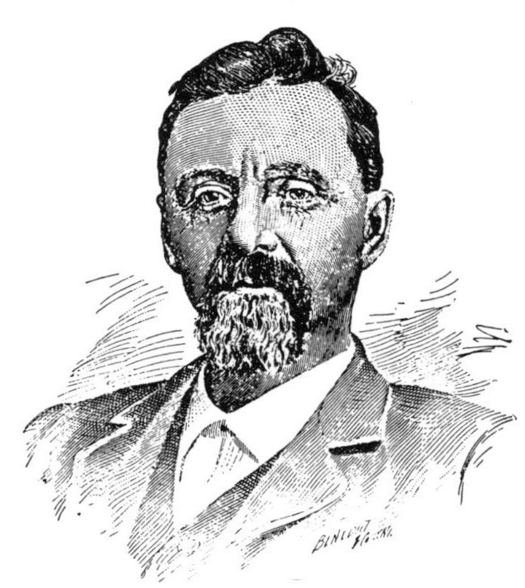

* * *

PRAYER.

O LORD, we ask for help quick. Since life is so short and man's days are few and full of sorrow, we ask that we get some more brevity in our school books. Lead us not into temptation to make our "text books" big. Thou knowest if we do that they will have to be made by clippings from old theories that begin with "as I remarked in my last lecture to the owls, that this and that theory was quite popular with Cæsar's coachman, however the wife of Pythagoras said, she saw no sense in the theory that the earth was four square but would say nothing to antagonize the theories of our schools as there was no harm in them, only they were uselessly consuming time." O Lord, we do feel to try thy word and promise, that if we ask in faith we will receive. Now Lord, we ask Thee to either add twenty years more to our days on earth or teach brevity to the professors in all institutions from which we are supposed to receive practical knowledge and useful education. Thou knowest, O Lord, that long prayers come from the insincere, therefore, I do want to see thine arm bare and thy fist doubled and see Thee pound the stupidity out of the heads that do not know that he who would show wisdom by quoting from others is born with a great degree of native stupidity. Therefore, O Lord, break his pen, spill his ink and pull his ears till he can see and know that writings are a bore to the reader and only a vindication of a lack of confidence in himself to tell the world anything that is profitable and practicable. Amen.

Dr. A. T. Still's Department.

Tradition.

Tradition should never have any claim whatever on our religious, political, scientific or literary opinions. Truth does not come from tradition. Tradition is a stranger to knowledge. It is a stranger to genius. It has been the everlasting parent of tyranny. It is an enemy to God, peace and prosperity. To act by the tenets of tradition would stop the revolutions of the planets, thus heavenly bodies seek and obey the harmonious law of absolute truth. Should the moon be older than the earth, why should the earth revolve and travel through space with the same motion and velocity that the moon does when her velocity would not succeed in retaining the designed functionings of the earth? Thus a velocity and a different orbit would be demanded by the size, form and function of the earth. If the earth was the same as the moon in all particulars then without tradition it would act in time and motion as the moon does. The philosopher begins an ignorant man, knows this to be his condition and uses the many methods that occur to his mind to better his condition by a knowledge of demonstrated truths. Thus he seeks demonstrations, satisfied that they will never lead him astray. Thus he is content to labor days and years with the hope of the reward of demonstrated truths; and when he has received a satisfactory demonstration he adds this to his store of knowledge, until that quantity has accumulated to the extraordinary degree of being sought by men of similar desires as their instructor, by giving the benefit of the truths he has received; thus he is considered and received as a careful and trustworthy philosopher upon cause and effect. He has no more respect for tradition than the web-footed bird has for the traditions of all the geese and ducks that ever sat upon the face of the water. They act upon the self-evident fact of demonstrated truths; why not man?

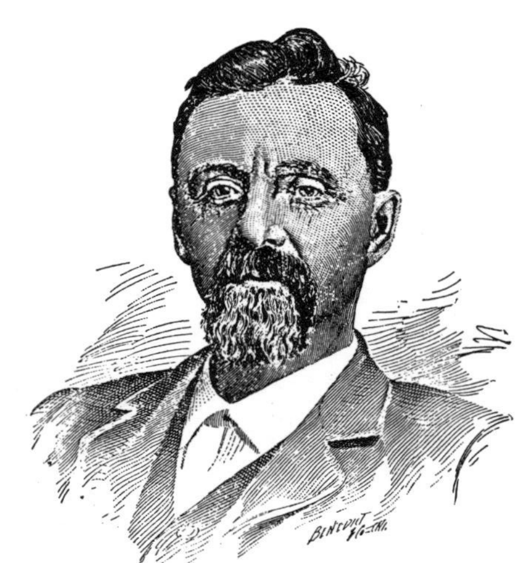

The scientist is only an ignorant man well fed with experience. A history of the experimenting of others is beneficial to the historian, but lacks the practical part, which experience can only afford. Another reason why the customs of tradition should slumber in the tombs of the past is, that with the velocity of time useful demands of a different nature appear and multiply so fast that we do not have the time to devote to the accumulation of traditionary knowledge, when that knowledge would be of no benefit to us now.

Each day and generation has by its philosophical powers to bring forth new truths suited to the wants of the present day. Thus the reader will see that navigation handed down to us by tradition would be of no benefit to us.

When two or more soldiers meet, visit and tell their many exploits they are dealing in realities that have existed with themselves. A great many of them have been dangerous adventures, some have been laughable things that afford great pleasure and satisfaction to the narrator and his fellow comrade;

but when his day and generation has passed away it would simply be useless tales of tradition for his children to rehearse what he had said about the war; how he ate, took chickens from the enemy and so forth. The young man belongs to a new day, a new generation, he becomes a part of the government and a system of customs that has to be formulated and adjusted to suit his day, with no place left in which traditionary customs could be used.

In old methods of war and in preparations for the same would only be a useless expenditure of time, labor and means to be lost by defeats. With time and acquaintance intelligence grows. The skilled arts take the places of the clumsy methods of war in preceding generations. "Each day must be sufficient for the evil thereof."

The great generals Napoleon, Alexander, Washington and all great warriors who have led successful armies a half century previous to this date with the attainments that have come up in arms, military skill, explosives, etc., such great generals would be forced in this day to surrender sabers and armies to a 4th corporal, thus the hope of good coming from that line would be a failure.

Our theologians are our most devoted specimens of tradition, no two of them know or worship the same God. Their traditionary life seems to be a desire without a compass.

Our colleges come under another heading, that is very little if any better than the blunders of tradition. They talk much, demonstrate but little, they are theorists in place of time saving philosophers.

Our great and useful men and women are those who have been content to wrestle from morn till night with the stern realities of cause to produce any or all natural effects. Our best painters are not theorists but practical men. Our chemists, machinists, architects, great ship builders and on through the wonders given to us, navigating of both land and sea, and constructing the useful machinery that the whole world enjoys—such men are the hard-fisted, determined successes of the world's present day triumphs.

Tradition has its good effects. The oral part is good if for nothing but pleasant pastime. Much of the talk of the ancient struggles of the human race to elevate its standard of useful knowledge is of but little use for our day, and but little use can be found for these productions, either in their philosophy or practice. Civilization has become so extended that time gives a premium on brevity. We have to learn so much more now to be practical than then that we cannot afford to spend years on theories of the infant past, when all that is useful in a thousand pages of traditionary theories can be written in more intelligent form on a single sheet of foolscap.

Why write any more, when you have said all you know. We read and philosophize for knowledge and should use some healthy brevity when we talk, as instructors. A theory may do for today and be a clog to the foot of progress tomorrow. Then to use such theories would be foolish procedure for any man born above the condition of an idiot. Our school wants long strides towards brevity in all branches. When a house is on fire who would stop to read how the city of Sodom burned and what kind of goat skins was used to "tote" water in to quench the fire. Keep away with dead theories of record or the tongue of tradition unless they be demonstrated truths.

"When Did Man Appear Upon The Earth?"

Did he exist for many millions of years as a mite in protoplasm before he got for himself a "brainless form" that was neither man, beast, reptile nor fish? Or were all the substances in a shapeless condition that compose man, beast, mineral, vegetable and animated nature with all the material substances as found in strata, such as coal, stone, metal, oil, vegetables, fruit, and of each being that was to inhabit the earth, with the substances that would take the form of the being, tree, fruit and cereals, such as corn, wheat and rice? I say, or wish to be understood as asking the question, was not the earth going through a chemical preparation to make men and all material forms whilst in the gaseous or nebular condition?

I will ask, how is a cloud formed from gas? How is rain formed from gases? How is iron, gold, copper, oil and each substance formed which is found in the earth? Is it by material affinity of gaseous conditions?

We see no reason why we should not allow the arm of nature guided by its own store of knowledge of how to prepare for a great event and momentary change, the change from the gaseous condition to a globe (the earth.) It is formed of many strata, all different in kind. All the results of the perfect law of affinities.

Since our earth has ceased to act as a world of gas as under the law by which the change from the nebular life to organic beings of reason and individual actions, I will say to him of the protoplasm theory to allow twelve months, or twenty years to change from the gaseous condition and allow man's life, mind and material form to appear as a result of the law that gave the great change from the nebular to the organic beings for the first appearance of man in form and life, with powers of future propagation of his race.

Let us grant that Nature is law, wisdom and motion, and that motion is life's proof of its universality with all visible and invisible actions. A nebular display of gaseous matter appears in space, visible to the astronomer, and a change appears each year. Is that change by chemical additions to the nebular laboratory? When chemical with definite union is complete we can well look for magnetic action, and a new globe appears where a nebular spot has vanished. Thus as men of reasonable observation will see when we cut into that new globe (or earth) we would expect to find strata of stone, mineral and matter selected and deposited by affinities, and all wisely done to a completed world, with man and beast, with fruit and grain for the animal stratum on which to subsist, and continue life and species of animal and vegetable for all time after nebulative mother has handed the earth over to the male and female law given to man to continue his race. He was given full size when our nebular mother closed the door after nebular birth. Thus man and beast were conceived and formed in our nebular parental action and man is the result.

Question. If the nebular theory be true of all worlds, when will mother Saturn throw off her nebular veil, and open her bosom and say to the beings she has given birth to whilst in the nebular state, that from now on man and beast, fowl and fish, tree and grass, and of the whole globe shall bear seed after its own kind, be fruitful and multiply as the earth does since she threw off her nebular veil?

* * *

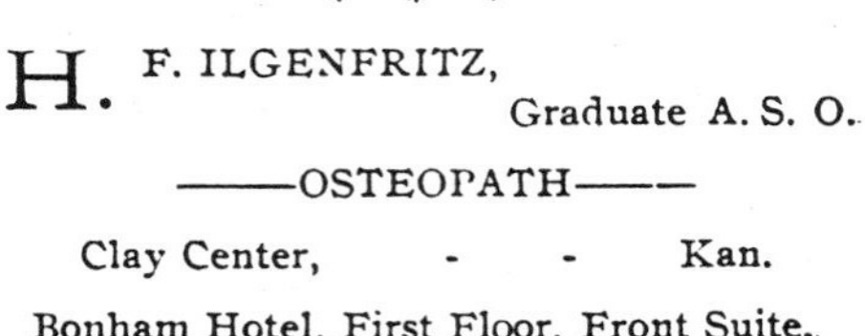

November, 1901

What is God? What is the eternal genius of nature? What is life? Is it that calm force sent forth by Deity to vivify all?

Man has tried for millions of years to solve the mysteries of animal life. At the end of all efforts to know and answer the question, "What is God?" "We know not." God to-day is just as near man's comprehension as when the sun turned her light upon the earth the first time. Of God man has learned nothing; of his works but very little. He says in humble soliloquy, I am the effect, but where and what caused man to appear? When I behold man, I halt in the open field of crushing amazement. I feel that man is the work of the most exalted mental genius, that man, is also a secret, that no finite mind can even approach for acquaintance. While man is not the creative being as conjoined and sent forth, he is just as hard to solve as his author, God. He, the man, begins and ends in a perpetual soliloquy. How did I come? Who or what is the cause that gave man form, life and mind? Man is only a mite of creation, but he is an astounding mystery. How he came we know not. He is formed for many uses, and has power of reason sufficient for them all. A few generations of his ancestors he knows of by history, and no further. He reasons from his form, life and attributes, that he is the result of great wisdom. He thinks much of the cause of his being. One believes that his being, wonderful as it is, came by a law of "spontaneous production." Another mind thinks there was great work done during seven days by God's own hands. Another thinks he sees the mite that was to progress through many millions of years in protoplasm and appear as man. One guesses that when the earth was in the nebular or gaseous condition that it was a female world, covered and surrounded with protoplasm in the gaseous state, and the harder parts condensed and formed a placenta which was enveloped by a covering from the condensed gas that surrounded the earth, as the womb surrounds the placenta, and formed a sack that gave life and growth to man, beast and all vegetation at that time only; then the earth ceased to give life as the nebular parent or mother, and left further propagation of species to be from the beings that had taken form and size with such endowments as each required. This philosopher thinks while the earth was in the nebular condition that the laboratory was mixing life, mind and matter for the seven days of creation, and that the mental effort to make man from this gaseous condition to a living being with all his endowments, could be no greater effort than to make a stratum of coal, or of stone. He thinks no more mystery would appear in making a stratum of animals than there is about making a stratum of coal. No matter how we look at the subject, one is just as mysterious as the other.

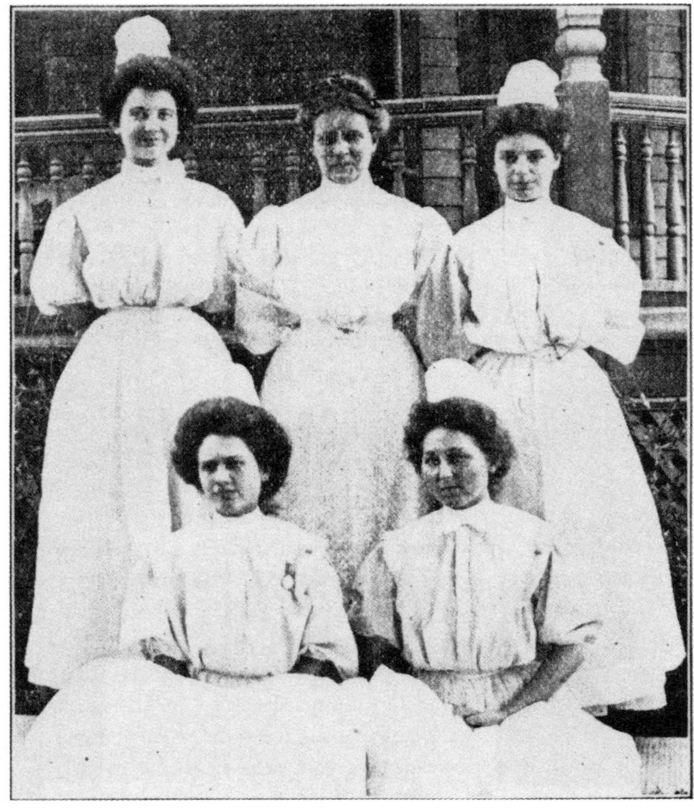

NURSES AND CHIEF.
Left to right—Top row—Miss Ammerman, Dr. Mary Walters, Miss Morais.
Lower row—Miss Schreve, Miss Smith. Photo by Samuels.

December, 1901

DON'T MIX.

THEY begin with "Osteopathic School" and "Infirmary," then comes the kite tail tied to osteopathy. We are up-to-date; we give suggestive treatment; we teach suggestive therapeutics, water cure; we teach how and what to eat; we use salt water and olive oil baths; we think all these doings "*help osteopathy.*" All persons know that if they do not wash the dirt off once in a year or twice that they will stink a doctor out of his office. Osteopathy supposes that cleanliness is common. It makes me ashamed to read in any sanitarium journal or school catalogue claiming to be osteopathic to be so far off as to poke in a lot of cheap trash and say it will "help osteopathy." Such may come from old medicine fossils, but will not come from an up-to-date osteopath of brains. The trouble comes from genuine ignorance of anatomy and physiology.

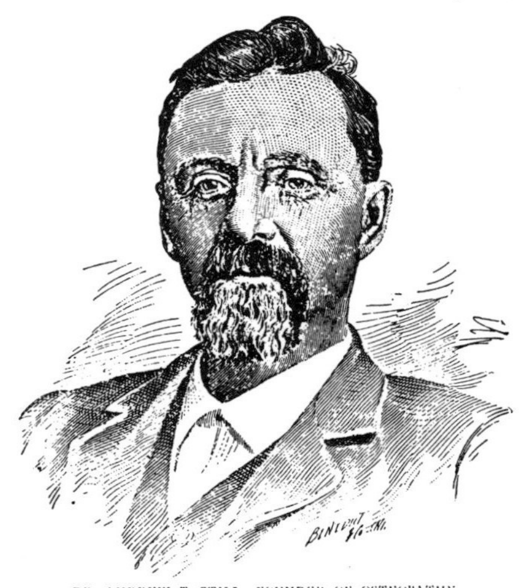

DR. ANDREW T. STILL, FOUNDER OF OSTEOPATHY.

He who knows only a smattering of osteopathy is just the man to substitute water cure, suggestive therapeutics, mesmerism, salt, oil and all kinds of systems, old and new, brag up osteopathy and use the name in big letters to catch customers and fleece their pockets. Osteopathy is a complete science and is not dependent on allopathv, homeopathy, eclecticism, suggestive therapeutics, christian science or any system or school of philosophy. But its own philosophy of surgery, midwifery, and general treatment are complete and defy refutation, and pronounces all conglomerates to be traps baited with flattery and deception to deceive the afflicted, to obtain their money. I repeat that such writers do not know the first principles of the philosophy of osteopathy or their pens never would betray their ignorance by their weak productions such as I have read in journals claiming to champion a school of osteopathy. I am proud to find no brainy graduate of the A. S. O. guilty of any such shortcoming. The successful osteopath knows his business and sticks to it.

* * *

Inhibit: Inhibition.

Much stress has been laid on the idea of inhibition of the nerves as a remedial agency. Allow me to say that inhibition is almost universally the cause of disease. Dunglison defines inhibit—to restrain or suppress—stimulate, to goad; that which excites the animal economy.

For the student's benefit, I wish to refresh his mind on anatomy, that he may fully understand what I wish to present as a truth, to guide him while treating his patients, and to point him to the dangers of doing more harm than good by pushing, pulling and kneading the abdomen, with the idea that he inhibits the nerves or excites them to greater energy thereby helping nature do the work of restoration of the normal functional action of the organs of the abdomen.

I will say after forty years' observation and practice that no good can come to the patient by pulling, pushing and gouging in the sacred territory of the abdominal organs, but much harm can and does follow bruising the solar plexus from which a branch of nerves goes to each organ of the abdomen. Upon that center depends all the functioning of the elaborate work of the abdomen. I say, hands off. Go to the spine and ribs only. If you do not know the power of the spinal nerves on the liver to restore health, you must learn or quit because you are only an owl of hoots, more work than brains. I want the student who wishes to know the work that is done by the organs or contents of the abdomen (the viscera), that he is also to know the danger of ignorance and that wild force used in treating the abdomen cannot be tolerated, taught or practiced as any part of this sacred philosophy.

You must reason. You can reason, I say reason, or you will finally fail in all enterprises. Form your own opinions, select all facts you can obtain. Compare, decide, then act. Use no man's opinion, accept his works only.

* * *

December, 1901

Whites, Leucorrhœa.

A FEW sensible Americanized questions and answers such as, What is the disease you call leucorrhœa or whites? Why do you call it leucorrhœa? Does luco mean something that is white? Why do you give nothing but big names and leave out causes. Why does she waste off or out that white compound? Our old authors have never told us a word that would point the student to the cause of such wasting of the bread and meat of a woman's life. Is not her blood the bread and meat that sustain her life? If so, what effect would be natural to take away her life support? How high up her back and how low down on her sacrum will the student find nodes or clusters of lymphatics, glands, blood supply, fascia, muscles, membranes, cells, secretions and excretions, venous drainage and arterial supply? In a word, why are we summoned to learn how to cure an affliction that you cannot give us any light on its cause? As this is said to be a school of philosophers, where is the philosophy you have to offer the anxious seeker? When the pilot gets lost, then a committee of the whole is formed and suggestions are in order, from all or any one. A new pilot is sought. Trouble is in the camp, a remedy is demanded. The life of the old pilot will pay the penalty. A mutiny is in all the camps. A Moses must be found to lead. No old field notes will suit for guides. We have followed them to the letter. We are lost and to follow farther will be suicidal. Nature's compass must guide us is the report of the committee of the whole. Now let Moses tell what leucorrhœa is and its cure.

* * *

Osteopathic Surgeons.

FOOLS write what they have read, wise men write what they know, have learned and proven to be true. They write their successes for the good it may add to the books of progress. In America we get tired and sick of clippings and compiled trash called "treatise" on this and that subject. We have but little use for quotations from old authors on midwifery, female diseases, surgery and general diseases. We are osteopaths and have no time to spare to listen or commit to memory anything from old books that are obsolete, dead and out lived by all men. Our success in knifeless surgery comes from superior knowledge of the form and uses of the whole body. We learn the form, place and use of the many muscles, ligaments, blood fountain rivers that supply blood to each part. We learn the location and use of the nerves, motor, sensory and nutrient, and must learn how to assist them to natural action, both to build and remove wastes, or we will allow waste matter to be piled up. Then if we do not understand how to set the excretory nerves to carry off such trash "tumors, etc.," we will begin to cut into the body and slash our knives into sacred organs, destroy the physiological uses, "cure" a few for a time and kill or maim for life seventy-five per cent. An osteopathic surgeon with a knife in his hand is a very poor argument for the professor who taught him surgery. Surgery to us is a very serious subject and does mean to know enough of the human system and its power to keep us in form and function that we will not be deformed and diseased by growths and decay, if we keep the body perfect as nature gave the body to man. Then to learn surgery here does not mean to cut and saw, but it means to stop and carry away growths by adjusting the body from the variations to the original, normal condition. Our students must learn to keep between the knife and his patient, he must reason or he will fall into the old ruts of medical schools. I say in all candor that your finest powers of reason must be kept in trim or you will fail to cure, and may be meritoriously called a fool.

* * *

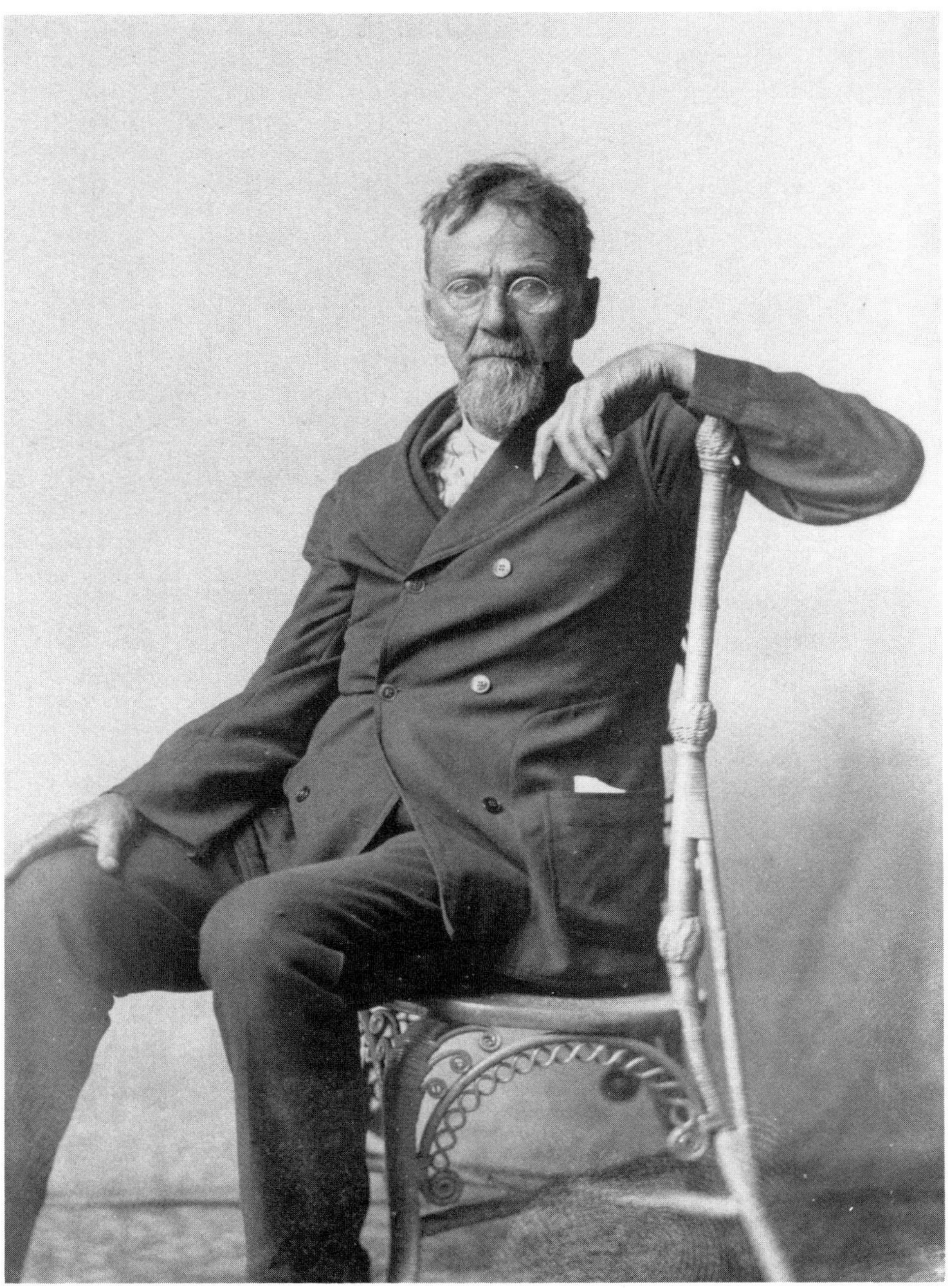

A. T. Still, c. 1903

December, 1901

Knowledge.

Knowledge is the result of our mental faculties being trained in the school of Nature. Knowledge is Nature understood and when wisely applied results appear in all material forms and actions. Thus he who knows the most of Nature is the wisest man, and his supposed powers are only Nature shown by his genius in conducting cause to produce results.

* * *

Engineering Skill.

The osteopath cures by his engineering skill, that skill is only obtained by careful study until the student has learned the parts and functions of the body by his anatomy. In descriptive anatomy he learns form and place of all the parts. By physiological anatomy he learns the functions local and general. By practice he learns to be skillful and he cures as Nature does when harmony prevails in the body. The doctor of osteopathy must acquaint himself with all organs, blood and nerve supply, their separate and combined actions and uses or he will fail in getting good results as he hopes to obtain. Thus his successes mark his scale of anatomical and physiological knowledge. A person may be very fluent in words and very foolish in practice, thus the great use of much practical training on the living patient in the school room. The more normal the better for the student; he must get normal in his mind, he must drop the idea of abnormal wisdom. Midwifery can never be learned from deformed pictures.

* * *

Confidence.

The osteopath who has not confidence enough in the science to implicitly rely upon it under all circumstances is not entitled to the respect and patronage of his patients, and should blush with very shame when he accepts the money from his patrons. In the hands of the qualified and experienced practitioner it can be depended upon in all diseases incident to this climate. Osteopathy will never be found united with saloons or combined with drugs.

January, 1902

DR. A. T. STILL'S DEPARTMENT.

The American School of Osteopathy.

The American School of Osteopathy raised the "lone star" in 1874, because it saw no use to continue with old systems of healing.

I felt that the world had been injured by the teaching and practices of what was called the science of medicine. I saw that the thinking people had

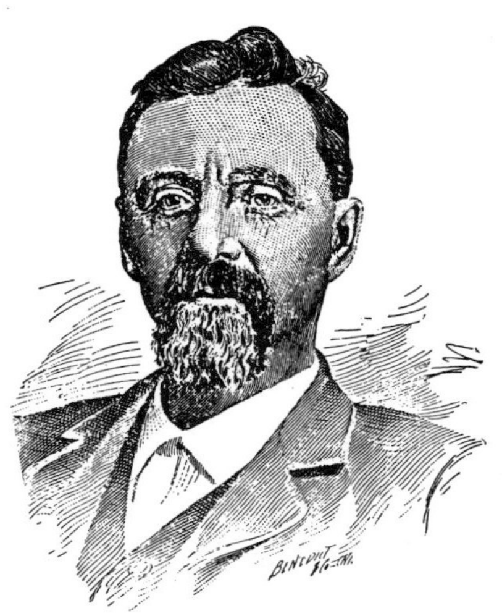

lost confidence in drugs and had good reason to complain against the fruitless promises that had been made and not fulfilled by the schools and practice of medicine.

The American School of Osteopathy is young. It has had the usual amount of worry that all truths have to meet and combat when being brought to light and proving by all necessary tests to be true and useful. That day has been passed by osteopathy. It stands before the world to-day as an established, useful and advanced science. The people, both the most learned and wise and the most humble and lowly call aloud that it be taught in its naked purity and given to them more abundantly than we have been able to do. Our school began the struggle without a penny's aid from the government, state or other outside help; worked from infancy to manhood by its own energy and its eternal devotion to truth, with but few friends that realized the truth in all its claims, which have since been proven greater than even its wisest advocates at that time dreamed or hoped for. It would be useless to speak more of the merits of osteopathy with which millions in America and Europe are familiar to-day. Our duty is to fence strongly against the poisonous effects of old theoretical medical trash; purge our school of such, and all dim lights that are not blazing with the oil of up-to-date reason and progressive osteopathic skill and the thunders of effective execution against disease.

Osteopathy has a system of surgery after it has exhausted all reason to save life or limb by nature's powers to reduce tumors by vital excretory activities, banish ulcers by bringing more good blood and repairing faster than the powers to waste can destroy. After exhausting those means then bring in the knife and saw. Osteopathy has but little use for the knife, but when no human skill can avail in the effort to save life or limb without knife and saw, then we are willing to use anything or any method to save that life or give relief, and will be bold enough to do so for the best, and hope for good results.

I want to impress on the minds of the students that we are not any part of a surgical trust that would cut open and kill a wealthy woman for her money and pass by a poor woman with the same kind of disease and tell her that she would likely die upon the table. That is too often the case in present day methods in the practice dignified with the title of "major surgery". Why is not the wealthy woman warned of the danger of death as the poor woman is? The five-hundred or the five-thousand must answer that question, "I think her money took her life." Remember that all cities of above 25,000 or thereabouts have surgical sanitariums or hospitals. Some are in the hands of surgeons of honor and trustworthy skill. Then there are others that neither have brains nor honor within their walls. Some surgeons care nothing for human life. They are worse than the murdering highwayman.

What osteopathy needs in Kirksville is a large surgical sanitarium of its own, to which the diplomates could send all cases needing surgical treatment. When we get that, then we will be complete as a scientific brotherhood. A person educated in a school of osteopathy should have protection by having such a sanitarium to which he could send or to which he could recommend his patients. It would be a protection for him. All that a doctor of osteopathy can hope for now if he sends a patient to a medical hospital, is that the medical doctor will tell the patient that the osteopath was not countenanced on account of his incompetence by the M. D's., not even allowed to see the operation, and all this after he had brought the patient for operation. In other words, he gets snubbed by the man with whom he has tried to be friendly. Probably the very surgeon to whom he has taken his patient could not pass forty on a scale of one-hundred, in a regular class examination in anatomy or surgery at the American School of Osteopathy. Still you have given him an opportunity to call you an acknowledged surgical ass. Such is often the case. The ethics of medical quackery is very exclusive bigotry and will make a hard effort to never show an osteopath any respect.

Thus, the demand for some reliable place to which our doctors of osteopathy can recommend patients requiring surgical attention such as the busy osteopath cannot accommodate, is urgent.

* * *

OSTEOPATHY is young and should be cautious and use good judgment. It was intended for and is the superior of any other method of healing that has ever been given to man. We are to improve upon the failures of the past and give the people a science of healing with a philosophy that will feed the minds of the thinker or even the casual reader. We are giving our demonstrations to the world daily. Under osteopathic management more cases are being cured and relief is given in more kinds of diseases in less time than any other form of treating disease known to man.

We began the search for truths that were not based on suppositions, taken or handed down by tradition for centuries, known not to be trustworthy and known just as well to be hopeless failures for many centuries. One of our problems was to avoid failing in our hunt for truth and not to make the criminal blunder of teaching that which we know is only honored and practiced for its age. We know that the so-called old system of medicine is only ignorance legalized and fastened upon the people by unthinking legislatures, nearly always toward the close of the legislative session at a time when members are tired and worn out by their hard labors and impatient to return to their family firesides. We have no knowledge that the people ever asked a legislature to make laws to regulate or legalize the hours or days of the week that the people should be dosed or vaccinated by any particular school of medicine. It is natural that the people should want wise men and systems to compete and allow the best of any mental production prevail, with the people as the sole judge and jury. It is a pretty good American idea and a pretty good one to follow, to give all systems an equal chance and give the sick man his choice of all. Our systems of religions, politics, inventions, sculpture, fine arts, music, navigation, astronomy, manufacture, commerce, literature, scientific publications, etc., are all so varied and too imperfect to be fastened onto the people by laws. It is a time to legalize when competition is no longer an incentive to excel and not before.

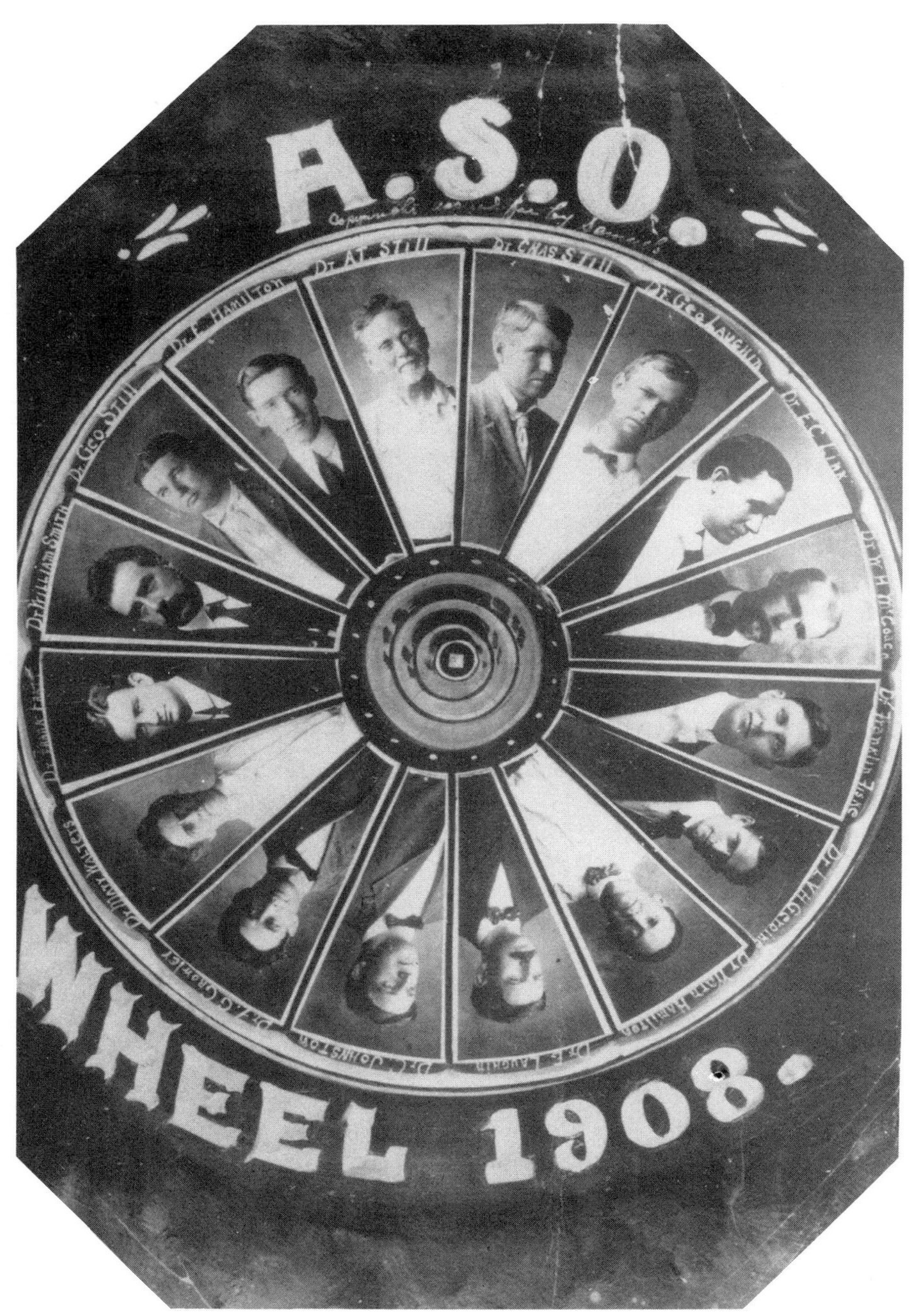
A.S.O.
WHEEL 1908.

January, 1902

Dr. A. T. Still's mail during the holidays was full of tender missives of greetings and well-wishes, from his legions of friends throughout the country. He is so busy that he feels that he will be unable to acknowledge them by personal letter and has handed to the Journal the following, as a general acknowledgment of the receipt of the kindly messages: "I wish, in my feeble way, from the depth of my heart, to thank my friends at home and abroad, for their many and various expressions of kindness and well-wishes to me and mine, for a good time during the holidays. I never relish good things alone, and I want you all to belt on the robes of comfort and good cheer and wear them every day until you land safely in Abraham's bosom. If you should find that all occupied, jump into 'Pap's' bosom, into his vest or pants' pockets and take out a few apples of love. There will ever be a goodly supply for all 'mine babes.' Affectionately yours, with wishes for a Happy New Year to you all.

"Pap."

February, 1902

DR. A. T. STILL'S DEPARTMENT.

With my fifty years of experience in treating disease in its great multitude of forms, I feel that I am competent to speak of the weakness of drug medication theories and the drug medication training followed in the so called "old schools of medicine" especially as I was a disciple of the "old school" for many years and among its most faithful practitioners, until a better intelligence and a better understanding of God's provisions for the cure of human ills in the body mechanism itself, led me to sever the ties that once held me blindly to drug medication.

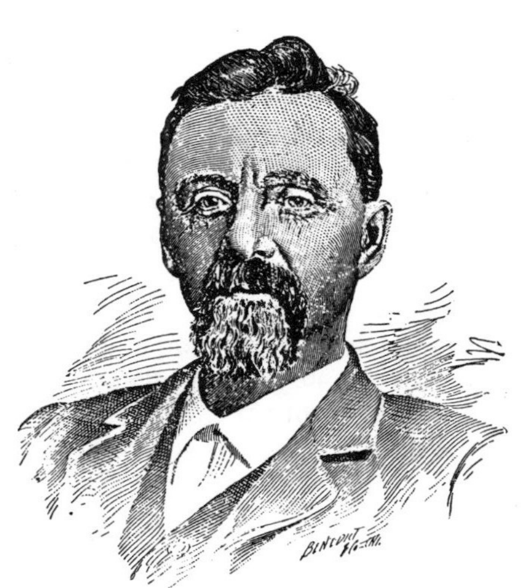

Typhoid fever, bilious fever, yellow fever, scarlet fever, mountain fever, hectic fever, and all other fevers known by various names, are simply effects with different appearances, but to seek and to know the cause or causes that produced the effects has ever been lost sight of by the doctors of the "old school." No attention or very little, if any, has ever been given to the parts of the body in a search for physical changes that have caused unnatural conditions in functions. They have been drilled in the faith that symptoms, well known, constitute a sufficient wisdom with which to open the fight. The drug physician finds some "heat" in the patient. He thinks that if he learns how "hot" his patient is, that he then is in a position prepared to open the combat. He feels for his "pig-tail thermometer" and lo, finds that it has slipped through a hole in his pocket and is lost. And the owner of the thermometer is just as totally lost.

The M. D.'s training is largely limited to observation of pulse and temperature. In the case of fever he has been loaded up with the importance of finding out how "hot" his patient is in the morning and how much hotter he gets at night, on through the days as the disease grows older in days and weeks. He is exhorted to keep a record of the degrees of heat, two, four, six, twelve and twenty-four hours apart and keep a similar tab on the pulse. He has been well drilled in the use of his "dirty" thermometer that goes into rectum, vagina, under arm and then into the mouth of a patient, but no thought is given to the physical changes of form or the functions of the affected organs of the body. Nor is the student of that school shown the causes of the change in temperature and pulse. His leading guides stick in their examinations and diagnosis to the pulse. He pulls out his watch and times the beats of the heart at 6 a. m., writes 83, at 6 p. m., 85; next day at 6 a. m., 84, at night 87, and so the record of gains or losses goes on.

He has learned to tell what his patient's temperature is each day for a week. How much head-ache, limb-ache, he has had, how body-tired and how sore he has been. How thirsty he was. How many times the bowels moved in twenty-four hours. How yellow, brown, red or furrowed the tongue has been on the first, the fifth, seventh, ninth and fifteenth days. But he has never been told by his school that these symptoms are only the effects and not the cause of disease.

"Now we have the symptoms and we will put them all in a row and name the disease," says the medical doctor. "We will call it typhoid, bilious. or by some other name before we begin to treat it. Now that we have named it we will run out our munitions of war and pour in hot shot and shell at each symptom." The command is given, "throw into the enemy's camp a large shell of purgative, marked 'hydrargyri chloridum mite.'" Then the order comes to stop that groaning and those pains. "Fire a few shots into the arm with a hypodermic syringe loaded with a grain of morphine" is the next command. Then one might add, "look the pigtailum oftenum and note the temperum till it reaches 106." But he is given no idea of the cause of the trouble on which to reason.

The above is given as an array of truths from start to finish. My object is to draw the mind of the student of osteopathy to the necessity of his thinking well as he reads books on diseases written by medical authors. One of the requirements of the old school and one on which so much stress is laid, is the knowledge of symptomatology by which they are first to name the disease, the name to give them a foundation on which to build the course of treatment by drugs. Their books generally begin by telling us that fever is an abnormal heat that shows a degree of abnormality beginning at about 98 degrees Fahrenheit and often running to 105 and 106 degrees. These effects are told and pointed out in detail, and if a certain amount of symptoms are found in a case that case must be called typhoid fever and treated by the sacred rules laid down centuries ago for the treatment for that disease. Still they tell us that "they are self-limited diseases." Then they take up other fevers whose symptoms are similar in so many respects that one is puzzled to know what name to give the disease. He does not find quite enough symptoms to warrant him in calling it typhoid fever. Then he is at sea without a compass and is left to do the best he can, even thongh boat and crew may be lost.

We are in the beginning of the twentieth century and the wisest doctors of all schools and systems of the healing art have said that typhoid fever is "a self-limited" disease, in the treatment of which "drugs are a total failure." This, in substance is the conclusion of them all, excepting the most bigoted, and we believe that the conclusion is an honest and a wise one. The old school physician is now saying, "keep out the drugs and bring in the nurses." And I will say, that they give to the world no more light on any other fever, and no more hope to succeed with drugs in the treatment of any other fever. I believe that they have turned on their very best search lights and ploughed through every possible sea in their hunt for the wise god of drugs, and all in vain.

I have been your leader for nearly thirty years but I have had no books to guide me excepting those on descriptive and demonstrative anatomy and those few in such crude form that they only suggest the wondrous provision that the God of nature has placed in man with which to ward off or banish the cause of disease if man were only studious and would only learn enough to detect the variations and readjust the deviations back to the normal. I have long since believed that an engineer of the human body was the sick man's only hope and to become a competent engineer the student must become masterly proficient in the knowledge of all the parts of that wonderful machine and the functions of all its parts. Not only to know the anatomical forms and positions of the parts, but to thoroughly know the entire system, the head, neck, chest, abdomen, pelvis and limbs with each separate function, and all functions in harmonious combination, free to perform their work as nature had planned for man's health and comfort.

February, 1902

OSTEOPATHY WITH THE LAW-MAKERS.

ADDRESS OF DR. A. T. STILL, PRESIDENT OF THE AMERICAN SCHOOL OF OSTEOPATHY, TO THE SENIOR CLASS OF THE SCHOOL.

LEGISLATURES are being constantly implored to choke off and drive out any new school of the healing art, by means of oppressive laws. We, as osteopaths, wish them to take notice that as Americans, we are seeking and will demand justice for our science, and no more. We ask for justice believing that we merit, before the law, equality with any other science in existence. As to our practice, before the people, we feel that we have demonstrated and will continue to demonstrate our equality, if not our superiority. We trust in the wisdom of our legislators and feel that they will be as ready and willing to grant us justice as we are to ask for it. It is certainly not un-American to labor and ask for equality. Should any member of a legislature raise his hand or voice against granting us equal and exact justice, he is to be pitied more than condemned. We propose to show that we will not only demand justice, but **that we will fight before the people, until we stand, before the law, side by side and equal in all things with all schools. We cannot afford to be taxed and not be represented. I thoroughly believe in that Biblical admonition, "Ask, and it shall be given you, seek and ye shall find, knock and it shall be opened unto you."**

We have never asked a legislature to protect us. What we do ask of legislatures is to meet us in fairness and deal out justice to all, to encourage the individual or the school of healing to meet in competition and endeavor to excel. Destroy that principle of competition and you shatter one of the bulwarks of the American people. It is the essence of our success as a nation.

As a school of healing, we should tell the law-makers what we want, as it is to them we look for just laws. We should tell them that we want laws recognizing, and fitting to our school of science, which has been reasoned out from more than an ordinary study of anatomy and physiology and their application to health. We should ask and demand that legislatures listen to men that are educated in the principles of the science of osteopathy. They are the only ones that are capable of giving legislators competent and reliable information on the subject. It is a well known fact that we have no patience with nor do we tolerate the beliefs of the medical doctors in the administration of drugs, often deadly, on which they pin their faith and their hope to cure the afflicted, and that, in the face of their admission, that they, "do not know the nature or the power of any drug, or the nature or action of any disease." We consider that their beliefs are old theories that have neither truth nor knowledge behind them, but are built upon the blunders of deadly conjecture handed down by dark and dangerous guess-work through the centuries. Can we hope or look for justice when such schools would dictate to legislators what laws shall govern our conditions and our methods? A thousand times, no. The medical doctor hates us. He hates everything and every method that cures where he has failed. His trade of mystery and guess-work is his meat and bread. He never will give us justice.

Go to your legislators and demand just laws, with a provision for a board of osteopathic examiners that is competent to pronounce upon our abilities in surgery and obstetrics and to treat any and all diseases. Remember that our science is thirty years old, with friends by the thousands in all parts of the Union. There is no need to be timid when the people are with you in your cause. They are fully as anxious, and seek and will demand just legislation in your behalf. When every state gives to osteopathy a board of examiners composed of osteopaths, before whom all persons claiming the right to practice the science will be obliged to appear and pass examinations before they receive certificates allowing them to practice, with heavy penalties for violations, then spurious work will cease. There are fakirs in the osteopathic field, as well as in others, and it is a true though sad commentary that the medical doctors encourage the "breed." When we get that justice, with osteopathic boards in each state, then peace and harmony can prevail between all schools of the art of healing, and competition to excel will enter the contest for the voice of public approval and patronage. All will then be placed on their merits and on their merits alone should they be judged.

A little history at this time will probably be useful. I will say that no more caution has been used in framing governments or plans for great business enterprises than was followed in framing the charter and constitution of our school, the American School of Osteopathy. We were guided by the wisdom and experience of the ablest lawyers in the state of Missouri. We consulted members of the United States Supreme court whose opinions stand second to none. All had acquainted themselves with our science by taking treatments themselves, or having members of their families who were invalided by disease, brought back to health by osteopathic treatment. We have treated here many United States senators, governors of states, congressmen by the score and state legislators; and in all of them, osteopathy has warm friends and supporters.

Why go into a state of restrictions that will not allow a man's qualifications to be used wherever and howsoever they may be required? Remember, that you have passed with high grades in all branches of study in the foremost school of osteopathy in the world, including descriptive anatomy, demonstrative anatomy, physiology, chemistry, urinalysis, hygiene, neurology, surgery, histology, pathology, bacteriology, gynecology, and obstetrics. The professors who have vouched for your ability by affixing their names to your diplomas were chosen by the board of trustees for their honor, learning and abilities to impart to and qualify the students in their respective branches. As to their abilities and characters, we court a comparison of the members of our faculty with those of the faculties of any medical school in the country.

With the diploma awarded you, you have a voucher of your merit that should be respected and recognized in any state in the Union, and I have no doubt that if you present your cause properly to the several legislatures, you will receive that recognition due you and you will be welcomed in every state, to practice your profession in all its departments, with restrictions on none. Your diploma says that you are worthy and well qualified to practice surgery, obstetrics, to treat and handle contagions and epidemics, and down through the list of all diseases in a general practice. You have the names of fourteen well qualified judges that have passed upon your qualifications. You have met all requirements to win your diploma and the respect of the educated world, and you should not be robbed in one single iota of the right to practice your profession in all its branches, by a misguided medical trust. And you will not be, if you go before your legislatures and present your claims in proper form. I believe that when many of our most scholarly and learned men, both of America and Europe, have passed upon a science and have pronounced it good and recommended its merits as scientific and useful, that it is high time that it receive the endorsement of legislators. But it should be presented to the latter class in the best possible way, by our leading and foremost men and

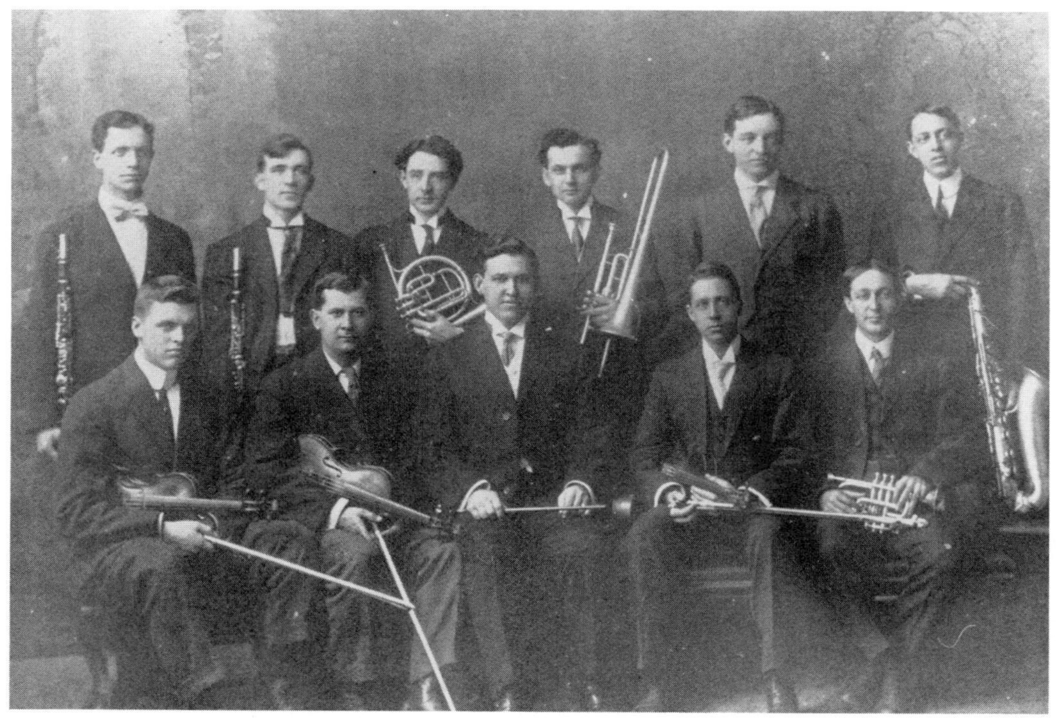

A.S.O. musicians, undated photo

instructors in our most advanced schools, and should be presented in its scientific truth. Then all that needs be done is to have a bill properly framed, introduced and a hearing obtained. Let your attorney present the reasons why it should become a law and with intelligent explanations given by competent osteopaths, that bill will become a law nine times out of ten. No sensible body of law-makers will drive a good school of the healing art out of their state. They cannot afford to. The reasons they cannot are too apparent for me to need go into them. Just to illustrate one of them. Before Iowa, our neighboring state to the north, recognized osteopathy to the extent of legalizing its practice there was expended here from out of that state, I will say between fifty and one-hundred thousand dollars annually, by patients flocking to us for treatment. Since they in part began to legalize osteopathy in Iowa, the amount has decreased and now Iowa is keeping that money within her borders, and that state is now preparing to give osteopathy complete recognition, with the practitioners allowed to treat any and all diseases, that all the states, I have no doubt, will in a short time give. They will see the error of their ways as has Iowa.

The American School of Osteopathy was not chartered to kill or destroy any school of medicine or any school of the healing art It was simply organized to teach a more rational system of dealing with disease, contagions and epidemics, obstetrics and surgical cases.

In place of killing, we have only asked and are asking to be given a chance to improve on old methods and do better work, to slay "fever" and cure more. We have felt that if we could do better work by our system, that less valuable systems would naturally become obsolete.

If other systems wish to kill osteopathy, they can do so by better work and not by prohibitory legislation.

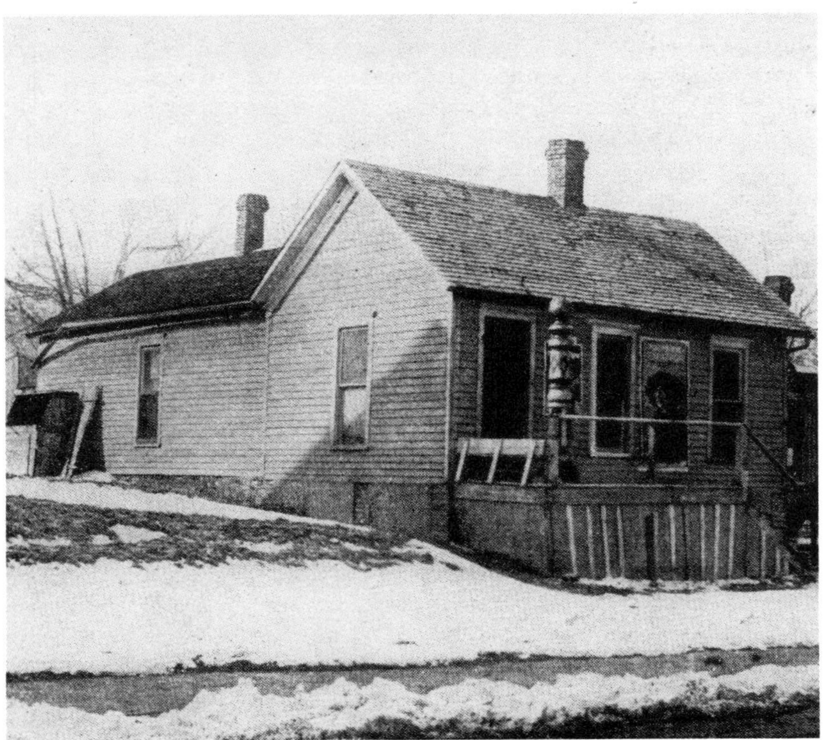

THE ORIGINAL SCHOOL OF OSTEOPATHY

This building has been partly wrecked and moved to make room for Dr. Laughlin's new hospital.)

A PROPOSITION.

Osteopathy has said to the world that it teaches and is a complete science. Thus, before the world, we stand committed to enter the general field of practice qualified to treat and handle contagions and epidemics, to meet and treat all diseases of seasons and climates, also competent to do surgical work skillfully, and to go to the mothers' rooms prepared to do the best and most skillful work in obstetrics.

Our school feels that when it says that the school of osteopathy is a complete science; it is competent to judge as to the extent and purport of the claim, and is prepared to meet in competition the most learned of other schools or professions of the healing art. We are able and willing to show why our system of therapeutics, osteopathic materia medica, surgery and everything pertaining to our science which has been masterly considered, applied and proven before being proclaimed to the world as a trustworthy science, is superior to other systems.

In our course of study we consume all the time on all the various branches, that we think is necessary for a good, practical knowledge for the graduate that is to be sent out into the world as a competent engineer to practice the skilled art of running the machinery of the human body, with all its complicated works, and regulating the functions of the physical parts in producing good or bad health. If other systems wish to insist that our time is too short, I will say to such schools that the American School of Osteopathy stands ready to meet them in a competition to determine the relative quality of the training received here as compared with that of any school that wishes to enter the lists with us. I will make the following proposition: I will take a team of six or ten or more students of our senior class and meet an equal number of the members of the senior class of any other school in America in a competition for excellence in examinations in anatomy, surgery, physiology, chemistry, theory and practice, and obstetrics.

(Signed.) A. T. STILL,
President of the American School of Osteopathy.

Kirksville, Mo., Jan 6, 1902.

February, 1902

SMALLPOX.

CANTHARIDIN AS A GERMIFUGE.

ADDRESS OF PRESIDENT A. T. STILL TO THE UPPER CLASSES OF THE AMERICAN SCHOOL OF OSTEOPATHY.

IN catharidin, commonly known as the Spanish-fly, I have discovered a perfectly harmless and effective germifuge, which I have subjected to every possible test during the past few years in all parts of the United States where smallpox has been rampant, and I have never found a single instance in which the trial has not proven my theory that the cantharidin will immune man from smallpox. You are all familiar with the results obtained in Kirksville during our recent so designated "smallpox scare."

All these years Jenner's discovery has been the single weapon that the medical profession has wielded in the fight against the dreaded disease, as far as a germifuge was used in the battle. Notwithstanding that the so-called preventative has in thousands upon thousands of cases proven worse than the disease smallpox itself, the doctors have been content to follow Jenner's teachings and there is not a single piece of evidence on record that any effort has ever been made to effect a departure from the long taught and faithfully practiced lesson of injecting the cow-pox virus with its hidden impurities into the arm of man, to immune him from smallpox.

The subject of smallpox has been a serious one for the minds and pens of the doctors of this and many centuries of the past. We have learned nothing of the origin, nothing of the action of the deadly poison which it contains, and when we sum up all that has been written for many thousands of years, we only learn that the doctor does not know what it is or what it does, more than that it has the power to kill the human race by the millions. From their pens, our wisest doctors know nothing more than the savage of no books, and thus, in the twentieth century we need not look back for knowledge from them. The field is just as cloudy today, for the doctors, as any period of the remotest days of man's history, when he thought that God had sent smallpox as one of his choicest plagues to punish the nations for some sin of disobedience to His holy ordinance. Man has tried many things to stop its deadly work, he has has prayed, sacrificed and dosed, but to no effect, to the hour of the coming in of the twentieth century.

My first experience with smallpox was in Kansas where I was associated early in my practice of medicine with my father also a disciple of the "old school." About the time that Kansas was opened to settlement, smallpox and all other eruptive fevers began to make their appearance and do their deadly work. Of all diseases man is heir to, I dreaded smallpox the most, for if it did not kill it left you disfigured for life. I had been vaccinated a great number of times but without effect, and should I contract the disease I felt then that I had little hope of living through it. Thus smallpox was my dread by day and by night. I was called to the sick a number of times not knowing it was smallpox until after entering the house. It was then too late to back down and I had to submit to the inevitable. I found frequently that I had well developed cases of confluent smallpox to treat but I generally got my patient through safely. Later I was again called to a supposed case of fever which proved to be confluent smallpox from which the man died. His wife claimed to have a sore eye and upon examining the eye I was surprised to find a pock of variola with which she had suffered many days. It was from that pock her husband had taken the contagion and died. Again I was in fear and agony that I would contract the disease from that family and die as I had no vaccine pock-mark to hold between myself and the dreaded coffin. At this time my anxiety was intellectually and very satisfactorily modified by a conversation with my mother, who said that possibly while a boy I had absorbed enough of the fly-blister which she had applied to my hip for a case of white swelling, as she then called it, to perhaps make me immune from smallpox. She had blistered and reblistered my hip for three months, many pieces of bone coming out of the superior crest of the ilium during the process, the marks of which are abundant to-day, both of the ulcers and the blisters. I have long since come to the conclusion that the cantharidin thus absorbed was the cause of the immunity that stood between me and the smallpox at that time in my practice, and I am also convinced that the cause of unsuccessful vaccination, the cow-pox virus having been inserted into my arm often from a child up to manhood, without effect, was also due to the cantharidin in my system.

I would not antagonize the popular belief in the efficacy of vaccination but would most emphatically combat the insertion into the human body of the putrid flesh of any animal. With this belief in reference to vaccination as a preventative to smallpox and with the chances to contract other diseases of which the cow and horse are subject so very possible and well proven by the great number of persons who have been vaccinated and crippled for life, I concluded that it was about time for the sons and daughters of America to take up

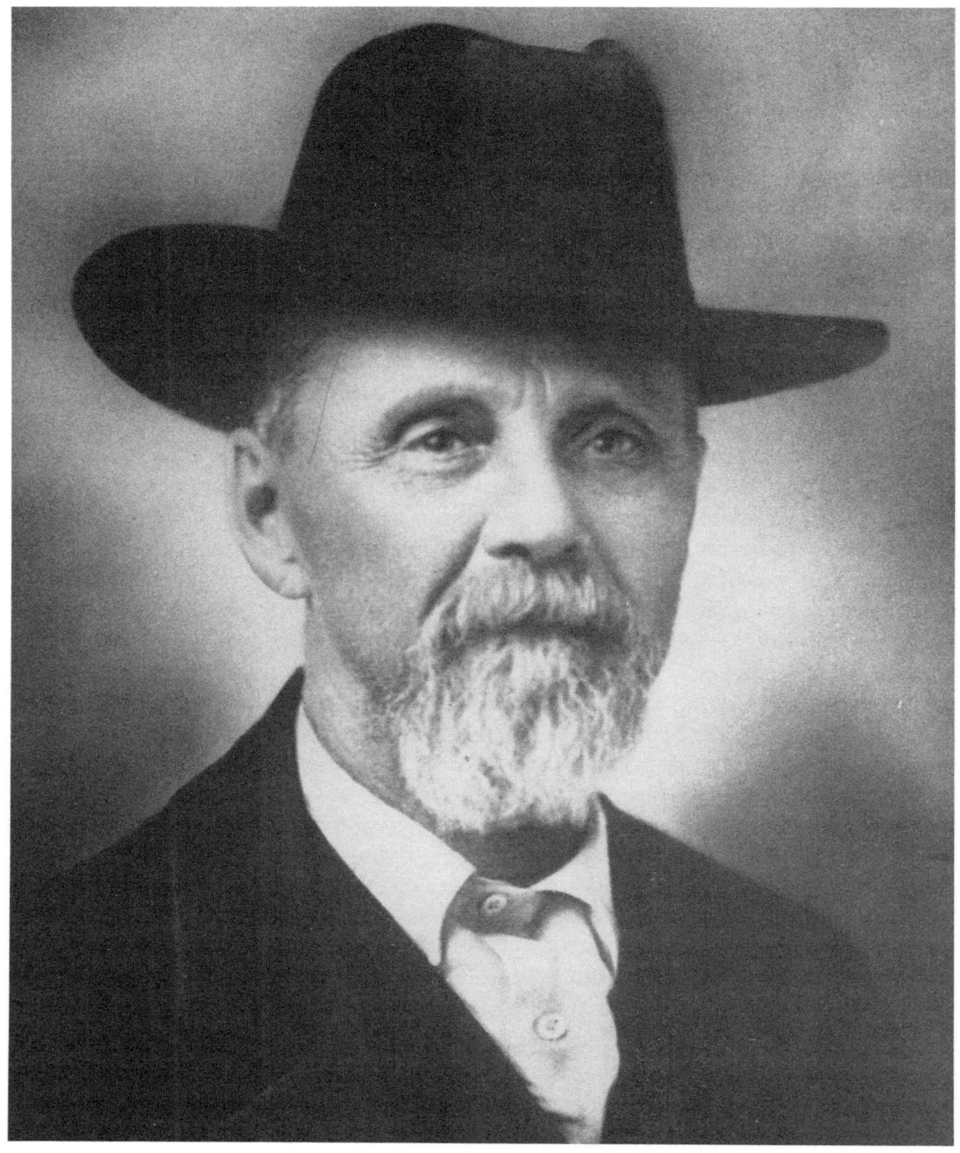

the subject of prevention and see how their skill would compare with that of Jenner of England. In the January (1901) number of the JOURNAL OF OSTEOPATHY, I published an article discussing the probable value of cantharidin as one if not the greatest germifuges of the world. I there gave my ideas of how to proceed. A Spanish fly-blister about the size of a half dollar when placed upon the arm will at once start an infectious fever, whose energy is in full eruptive blast in from four to six hours, or forty-eight times faster than variola which requires twelve days to reach its highest energy. *My theory is, that the first active occupant of the body by an infectious fever will drive off others and hold possession of the body until its power is spent* and the excretory system has renovated the body.

My philosophy is that the possession of the human body by an infectious germ, can only immune by germicidal possession. Thus we are immune by vaccination or any other infectious substance, whilst it is in possession of and effecting the machinery of human vitality, and no longer. Thus, we see that vaccination leaves the body, according to the belief of its friends and advocates, in from one to seven years, leaving a demand for repeated vaccination with its lurking dangers. The Spanish-fly blister may be used on the arm many times a year if necessary and act as a preventing germifuge without harm. I have solicited correspondence from doctors of sixty years of age and upwards, on the subject of the fly-blister's work in their early practice when it was used in any and all forms of disease. The correspondence has been exceedingly gratifying to me, for in every instance my deductions as to the value of cantharidin as a germifuge in smallpox where my correspondents could correctly answer my questions, have been proven correct. But what is more to the point, since my article appeared in the JOURNAL OF OSTEOPATHY last January the graduates of the American School of Osteopathy, who have been guided by my instruction, have reported thousands upon thousands of cases in which cantharidin had been used as a preventative to smallpox in the contagion, with the reported results of not a single individual whose arm had been blistered, contracting the disease.

I have often been asked, what are my ideas of vaccination? I have no use for it at all, nor any faith in it since witnessing it slaughterous work. It slayed our armies in the sixties and is still torturing our old soldiers, not to say anything of its more recent victims, whose number will run up into tens upon tens of thousands.

I believe that instead of passing laws for compulsory vaccination, a law prohibiting the practice, with heavy penalties for violations provided, would prove a wholesome experiment. Simply take the fifty cents out of the "dirty" practice and it would die out spontaneously with all doctors of average knowledge of the harm done by it. The philosopher must find something better as a germifuge, or by legal measures, hands off. I always believed that the wisdom of man was sufficient for the day of a successful hunt for an innocent and trustworthy germifuge for smallpox, and that it would be proven early in the twentieth century, if we would but work and reason.

I will not dispute or try to criticise so great a man as Jenner, but I will say that in all the histories of the man and in his own works, I do not find a single word of his philosophy nor any reason why he believed that the cowpock would fortify the human body against the entry of smallpox. He simply reported that a less number of milkers took the smallpox after they had had "sore hands" supposed to have been caused by getting the poison in some cut, scratch or broken surface of the skin of the hands. Since his day, the world has been content to hunt for that "stuff" that was on the cow's udder. No questions were asked, it was simply, "I want some of that stuff what makes folk's hands git sore." Jenner did put "rot" into his patients to keep the "rot" of smallpox out, so you see there was a fight for possession between the two great "rots" and the cow-rot is supposed to have hooked off the smallpox rot. That is all the immunity there was about cow-pock holding free from smallpox.

I believe that the discovery of Jenner gave nothing to the world excepting the history of an accidental cure or supposed preventative to smallpox. He gave no reason why one poison would immune the person from another poison. The doctors simply accepted, tried and adopted the supposed remedial power of cow-pox, sore or cankered heels of the horse. They gave us no caution or hint that the grease heels of the horse might be a venereal disease peculiar to the horse only. They told us nothing of the cow-pox, whether or not it was venereal in its nature. Like the adoption of most "remedies" the doctor uses or has used, it came to notice by accident.

I do not wish in the least to antagonize the efforts of Jenner. I believe that they were good, but I do think that more effective and less dangerous substances can be used than the putrid compounds of variola. I also believe that the philosophy that I present, can and will be found just as protective against measles, diphtheria, scarlet fever, leprosy and syphilis as against smallpox, and other infectious contagions. This is the twentieth century, our school was created to improve on past methods and theories; let us keep step with the music of progress. I feel certain that the time is close at hand when compulsory vaccination will not be necessary, for a better method, one that will do the work and leave no bad effects as is the case in vaccination with the cow, horse or other animal poisons, has been found. The dread of disease and death that follow vaccination, causes people to hesitate in having vaccine matter put into their own or into the arms of children by military force. When they learn that a fiy-blister as large as a fifty-cent piece will keep off smallpox in all cases, then there will be no fear or trouble about smallpox or vaccination.

February, 1902

HOW TO USE CANTHARIDIN.

IN answer to many inquiries on the subject, Dr. A. T. Still has furnished to the JOURNAL his instructions to graduates of the American School of Osteopathy for the application of cantharidin as a preventative to smallpox contagion. His directions in detail are as follows:

For an adult, take an amount of cantharidin equal to the size of two grains of corn. Spread it smoothly over a piece of coarse sheeting one and one-half inch square. It will cover the cloth. Press the plaster into the arm from three to six inches above the elbow, avoiding old vaccine scars. When the skin begins to look quite red, take off the plaster and dress with vaseline or mutton tallow on cotton. Allow the bandage to remain until the arm itches. Then take off the dressing if the cotton is loose. If not loose leave it on the arm a day or two to allow the blistered spot to heal. The work is then all done. For a child under ten years of age, use a plaster three-quarters of an inch square in dimensions. For an infant, use one about one-half inch square. Do not have a plaster on an infant over an hour. Take it off and after dressing it with vaseline, leave it a day to see if the blister has taken. If not, try again, but watch carefully and do not blister too deep. In all cases a single good blister will immune for a year at least.

The power of cantharidin as a germifuge has been proven, but it is imperative that only pure and fresh cantharidin be employed. Dr. Still has made arrangements by which he gets the very best direct from the manufacturers. He cannot advise the promiscuous purchasing of the ointment from old stocks. Time will kill the cantharidin and render it useless. Impurities may also get into the ointment. Dr. Still feels that the best way to supply the A. S. O. graduates is to keep the fresh and pure for their use and protection against old stocks. He is preparing to publish in pamphlet form a treatise on smallpox, cantharidin, etc., and with all orders for cantharidin which he puts up in $1.00 orders, he will enclose the ointment, directions for its use and one of his pamphlets.

Dr. A. T. Still's Autobiography.

NOW IN PRESS.

SPECIAL ANNOUNCEMENT.

Dr. A. T. Still's Autobiography will be ready for delivery in a few days. Those desiring a copy of the first edition should send name and post office address to Dr. A. T. STILL, (Book Department) Kirksville, Mo. Be sure in addressing to state explicitly "Book Department," so as not to confound the book orders with business connected with the School and Infirmary.

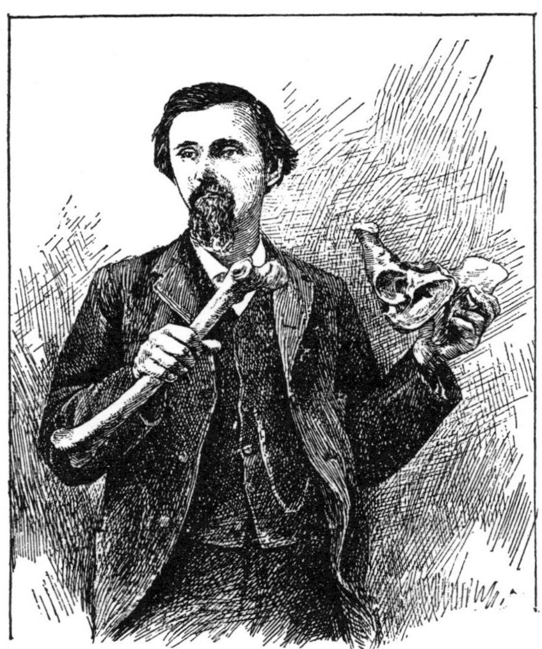

Motto: "Load to Suit and Shoot to Hit."

WHAT THE BOOK WILL BE.

Dr. A. T. Still's Autobiography will consist of about 500 pages of clearly printed letterpress, profusely illustrated by a large number of halftones and line engravings prepared especially for the work. It is written in the Doctor's own original vein and embodies many amusing as well as pathetic incidents in his life, and gives the first complete and authentic account of the discovery and development of the science of Osteopathy and many illustrations of its application to the cure of disease without drugs.

In ordering use the following blank:

DR. A. T. STILL, BOOK DEPARTMENT:

Kirksville, Mo.

I will take one copy of A. T. Still's Autobiography, price $5.00, and will send money for same when notified that the book is ready for delivery.

Name ....

P. O. ....

State ....

February, 1902

We Only Ask What We Would Give.

From a talk by Dr. A. T. Still.

If we are to fight battles in defense of our country, pay taxes, build public buildings, schools. work out our road taxes, and do our full duty in all things that our government requires of its people, why in the name of reason and common sense can't we expect the government to say, that you, and I, this, that and every school of the healing art, are to be equal in the sight of the law one with another? It doesn't step in and attempt to dictate to you or to me what religious principles we shall entertain or to what church we shall give our moral or financial support. Nor does it step in and tell us, "Here you walk around and vote the Democratic ticket, step up lively now." What a picnic there would be if such a thing should happen, for instance in Ohio. But would all this be more unreasanable than the laws on the statute books of many a state, conceived by an iniquitous medical fraternity that would dictate to the people how, when and where your child, my babe, ourselves, are to be treated when sick in body and sore afflicted. Think for a moment how they would curtail our God-given and man-fought for-rights. And the saddest thing of it all is that many of us have sat quietly by and haven't raised even so much as a finger in protest. It is high time that in a mighty chorus we join and break the bands that we have allowed legal measures to strap around us. Is man to have the privilege of calling in whom he will when he is ill, to choose any representative of any school that he may desire, or is a medical trust to answer the question in its own way and in its own time? I think I have said enough. There is often much in little, and I hope that there is in this the thought I wish to make clear. Osteopaths, I want you to always be considerate of the beliefs, traditions. ideas, etc., of other schools of healing. I want you to interest yourselves in politics to the extent of getting clean men in your state legislatures, irrespective of the party he may represent. Let a man's honor and abilities determine whether he is to get your support. In a few years we will have no red-nosed drug doctors meddling with our business or our profession, but in the meantime do your work in your profession and as American citizens and voters, to the best of your abilities and with ever a high standard of moral ethics as your guide.

Osteopathy Legalized.

Osteopathy is legalized and its practice regulated by legislative enactments in the following states: Vermont, Missouri, North Dakota, Michigan, Iowa, South Dakota, Illinois, Tennessee, Indiana, California, Kansas, Wisconsin, Texas, Montana, Nebraska and Connecticut.

DR. A. T. STILL'S DEPARTMENT.

WHO has been throwing the bomb shells of demonstrated reason and advanced thought that have been striking the camps and forts of old traditions and theories during the last century? Who or what has started such excitement and commotion among the doctors of medicine, clergymen, men of science and philosophies, engineers, mechanics, law-makers and justices, and down into the ranks of those in the more common and humble pursuits of man?

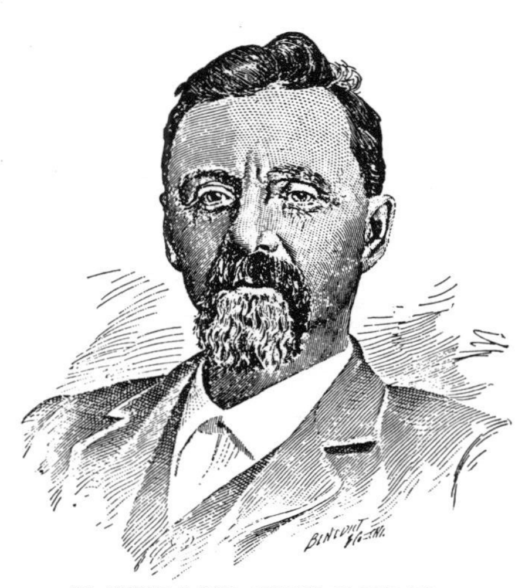

DR. ANDREW T. STILL, FOUNDER OF OSTEOPATHY.

The question is, "Who threw the bombs?" They certainly have created consternation all over the world to some extent and in the United States to the degree of a panic. There are many ways to answer the question. One would be that they forced themselves to the front under the laws of supply and demand. But the man or men who threw the terrific shells have not been the product of a day or of a generation. They are the culmination of mental effort to better and improve the old. In the single branch of the healing art, it has resulted in an improvement on the best known methods of human relief in the time of sickness and distress. Some minds have been able to harness the furious forces of electricity and turn them to man's benefit. Other minds have grown wealthy in the knowledge of the "hows" to plough the oceans, and why such forces could successfully be applied to man's greater benefit and with less danger to life. They have been able to almost annihilate the terrors of a seafaring life and of an ocean voyage, man now being able to travel from shore to shore in speed, comfort and safety. Other minds have been turned upon the successful navigation of the dry land with ever increasing speed and have been triumphant in the effort. Engineering has been the great and eternal study of the land navigators. With just as much reason for demand for great engineers to solve problems of ocean and land travel, there has been a demand for an engineer of a different kind for many thousands of years, one to plough through the black and bitter waters of disease. The living man and his form constitute the compass that points to and successfully delivers man from the sorrowful elements of sickness to the joyful land of health and repose.

Osteopathy is the name given to the engineering science that takes charge of the vessel of life, conducts and repairs the superstructure from birth to a rensonable day of longevity. The demand to live to a reasonable age has been with man since his first appearance on earth; we suppose no less so ever before than at the present time. It is no longer a question with most people, so widespread have become the truths of this great science and philosophy, what causes abnormal conditions in the parts or functioning of the parts of the human mechanism. It is known to be the effects of defects caused by mechanical injuries, climatic heats and rigors. It is no longer a question what the result is of readjustment to the normal. The universal answer is health.

Since the child osteopathy has grown to full manhood, it has received a hearty welcome, just in proportion to the capability of the intelligent man or woman to comprehend enough of the physical laws to know the reliability of nature, which vindicates itself in all grades of construction to health. The verdict of the people is "Welcome to the new school of philosophy. It shall have an equal chance with other schools to prove its methods and merits in relieving suffering humanity from now on, without let or hindrance."

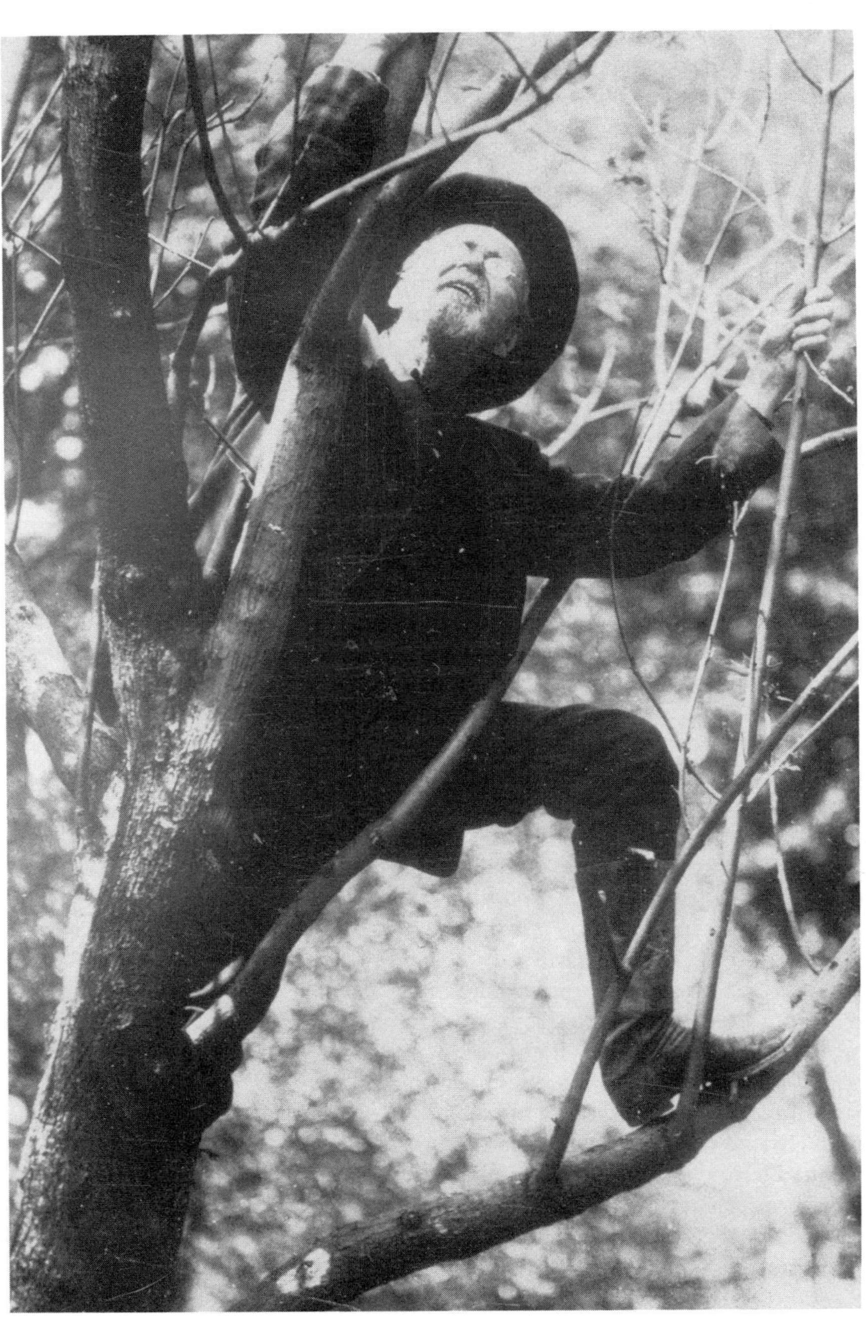

A. T. Still climbing pear tree in his yard

Henry E. Patterson Dead.

After an illness lasting only a few weeks, Dr. Henry E. Patterson died at Washington, D. C., April 10, of peritonitis superinduced by inflammation of the liver. The

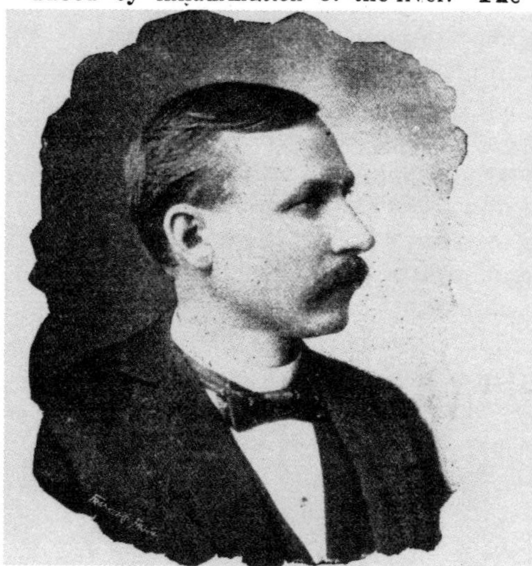

HENRY E. PATTERSON.

cause of the fatal sickness was an injury that Dr. Patterson had sustained while raising a heavy window in his office which had been lowered from the top. A large radiator stood adjoining the window and as he reached over it to raise the window, he wrenched his spine in the dorsal region. He thought little of the injury at the time and continued his work as usual. He suffered more or less inconvenience, however, and took treatment which relieved him temporarily only, for the the trouble returned upon any exertion on his part in his practice. He finally decided to close his office and with his family repair to the mountains to recuperate his strength. He was then suddenly taken worse and in spite of all efforts to check the course of his trouble, he sank rapidly and death followed a week later. The funeral services were held in Washington where burial also took place.

In the death of Dr. Patterson, osteopathy loses one of its most ardent advocates and ablest champions. His strong mentality, his masterly conception of the great principles of the science and his earnest devotedness to it, were a power which had done much toward giving osteopathy the place and the recognition it has before the world today.

Henry E. Patterson was born in Adair county, Missouri, in 1860. He was educated in the state normal school in Kirksville and later studied law. For a number of years he was in the real estate business in Kirksville. In 1882 he was married to Miss Alice M. Smith. Soon after Dr. A. T. Still had opened his school of osteopathy Dr. Patterson became interested in the science and entering the school he was graduated in 1895. He became connected with the American School of Osteopathy in the capacity of secretary, a position he held until 1898. In January of that year he went to Jacksonville, Florida, to spend the balance of the winter, and the following summer accompanied by his family he went for a season's outing to Mackinac Island. In the fall of that year he located in Washington, D. C., for the practice of his profession and he there built up one of the largest practices in the country. His wife, also a graduate of the American School of Osteopathy, will continue the business established conjointly by herself and husband in Washington and adjoining cities. Beside his wife one daughter survives him.

The following tribute to Dr. Patterson is paid by Dr. A. T. Still, who held Dr. Patterson as one of his closest and dearest friends:

"We join our friends as they mourn the loss of those who have been dearest to them. In the last year we have been called to grief over the loss of our friends many times and the last sting or wound was the news of the death of our great and good friend, Dr. H. E. Patterson, the man, who as secretary of the American School of Osteopathy, placed the school on a business standing. He was a graduate of the school he helped to form from crude material to a gem of finest polish. It appears that the last twelve months have almost turned our eyes to briny oceans of sorrow and grief over the loss of our loved friends who have been in the ranks or at the head of command in all our battles to hold osteopathy at the top of all banners that were run up as tokens of the healing arts. This sad occasion calls to mind the happy day that Dr. H. E. Patterson, John R. Musick and I ate a good dinner cooked by the hands of Mrs. Anna Morris and set on her kind table. All four of us ate with joy and kindly greetings and all feasted on the joys that came from the mingled reports of the good work being done all over the world. Patterson, the secretary of the American School of Osteopathy, Musick, the compiler of my two books, "Philosophy of Osteopathy" and "Autobiography of A. T. Still," and Mrs. Morris, the kind hearted amenuensis of both books. Let me love all, though three out of the joyful four are in their cold graves and I am left to eat alone with nothing but the waters of sorrow to wash down my grief. Let me say for myself, my household and school that we can mourn their loss but never can forget their good deeds. Many other friends have mounted the white horse of peace to mortality and gone from mortal sight, but our bosoms heave in grief that our hand can touch our loved ones no more in mortality, since the river of death stands between us and them. Let me say to one and all that love is much stronger than death and we will always love our sacred dead.

A. T. STILL."

June, 1902

ADVICE TO THE STUDENTS OF OUR GRADUATING CLASS.

BE ye always therefore ready, dear children. You are now about to give us the final parting hand. With well earned diplomas under your arms, you are going out into the world and I may never see you again. I would advise you to go to the surgical supply shop, lay in a large supply of all kinds of surgical tools for female and general surgical uses, such as speculums, sounds, endoscopes and above all be sure get an X-ray, machine, the most costly that you can find, because you may have some use for it the first year. You must not break down in your feelings when you enter your second year's practice and reflect that you have had an X-ray machine of the finest kind and you have X-rayed much and many times during the first year and have learned that it is of little use to an osteopath, whose hands are well trained to search and find the causes of diseases better with your head and hands than all the X-rays that have ever been made. Don't feel bad that you have had no use for your speculum, endoscope and probes, and have discovered that an osteopath's outfit of tools is his knowledge of anatomy conducted in such a manner as to give relief in almost all diseases by his skillful application of the mechanics of the science of osteopathy, which is as far from all other systems as the east is from the west. Don't do as I did, dear children, twenty-five years ago, enter the field of practice with no other surgical tool than a little four blade surgical knife, that I could carry in my vest pocket, which knife has been there and done all my surgery through all my combats with disease, and I have not had any use for it only occasionally to open a boil, felon or pick out a splinter.

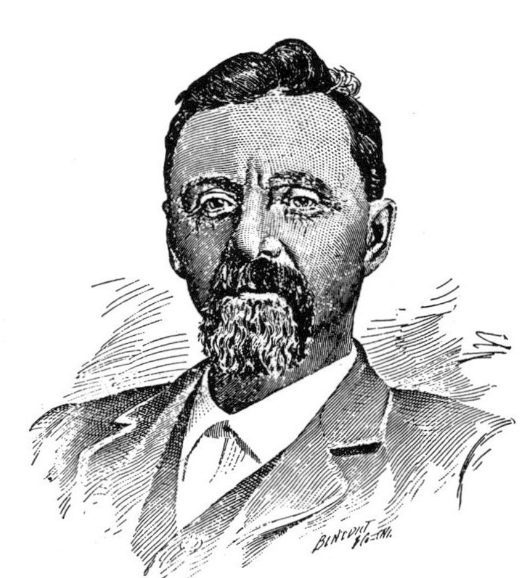

Now, ladies and gentlemen, don't fail to buy freely and rig up yourselves well for the first year, for that year will be the only twelve months you will feel inclined to waste with X-ray or surgical tools, as an osteopath. I say, don't fail to get them; mortgage your farm and property and everything else you have, but be sure and get a thousand dollars worth of tools. Get them, I say, if you have to give a note drawing ten per cent interest. Tie yourself down with debt, put your anatomy, physiology and chemistry, and books of practice and philosophy of ostepoathy in a box and nail them up tight for the first twelve months. I advise you never to examine your patient's spine nor limbs. Take a little book on symptomatology, another on physical diagnosis, the most voluminous old books on obstetrics and gynecology, written by the old schools of medicine to the highest scientific skill they know. Arm yourselves well with such literature for the first year. I think by the time you have wasted one year with this trash which you will discover to be trash, observation as a practical osteopath will fix upon you an everlasting disgust that will create in you an admiration for the mechanics of osteopathy, which your diploma does guarantee you to be worthy and well qualified to go into the world and practice as an osteopath and not as a medical however of cut and try.

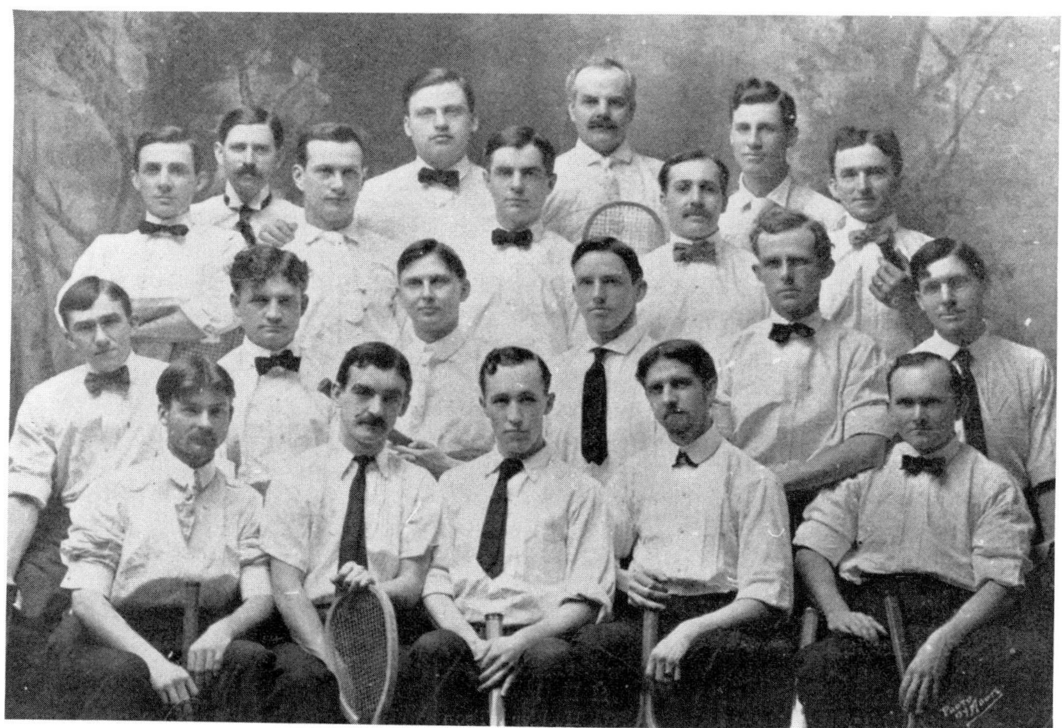

A.S.O. tennis team

Dr. A. T. Still's Department.

PAP'S DREAM.

I will tell you my dream. I have had another dream and I do not know who to tell it to. My wife says, "People will laugh at you for such foolishness." I know she is level headed, I would like to respect her judgment and retain her kindest feelings towards me. She has advised me wisely and very kindly given me many suggestions. But this dream I will tell at a venture. A very devout old darky who was present every Sabbath and oftener at religious services, if within his reach, when his soul would get full of "de love of de Lord," he would say, "amen," often and loud. Finally his master told him if he did not quit so much amening in church that he would have to whip him. So Pomp continued to attend church services and he got full of "de love of de Lord" and music. his soul could stand it no longer, he remembered that his master had promised to whip him, if he didn't quit it, so Pomp shouted out at the top of his voice, "Amen at a venture," so with kind regard and much love for my wife's advice, I will tell my dream at a venture. I dreamed that I was in a large congregation, how I got there I do not know, and it proved to be a watering place, a summer resort. In the mighty host I found medical doctors of all schools of the whole civilized world. I dreamed that they were very kind to me notwithstanding I was an old backwoods osteopath, they were very kind and gentlemanly to me. And they asked me what school of medicine I represented, I told them that I represented the American School of Osteopathy. Many of them arose to their feet to listen to what the chairman of the meeting would say when he asked me on what foundation was this new departure from the old and well established medical theories of the world. I asked the venerable chairman if he himself was an osteopath, and he said, "Nay, verily I am an allopath of the old regular system, which changes not, neither has it the semblance of change." I asked the chairman if they were bound by any obligation or oath never to change nor march with the mighty host of progressive thinkers and philosophers who navigate all seas, enter all ports, seek and use the very latest and best of all. The chairman told me that he was very choice and it was a principle taught in their school to associate with nothing but the very faithful. He said to me, "Why young man we have stuck close to and abided by the tenets of our profession which is to do and imitate our ancestors in all that we teach or do in surgery, midwifery, theory and practice, their wise teachings must be respected and lived up to. Should a brother stray off and be found in distant seas under any pretext, our discipline would have to surely expel him for perjury and infidelity to that obligation which is to be true and faithful to the teachings of our system of medicating and trust in the efficacy of the drugs, though it took all of the most innocent and deadly poisons under the hope that the poisons would be just as deadly to the disease as to the patient." He said he did not wish to be arbitrary and unkind to a stranger and asked me to come forward and state why I had become so attached to the theory and practice of this new system which he said that I just called "osteopathy."

After being introduced through the kindness of the president to the medical brotherhood, composed of all schools who use drugs as remedial agencies in combating disease, he asked me very kindly to make a statement of the

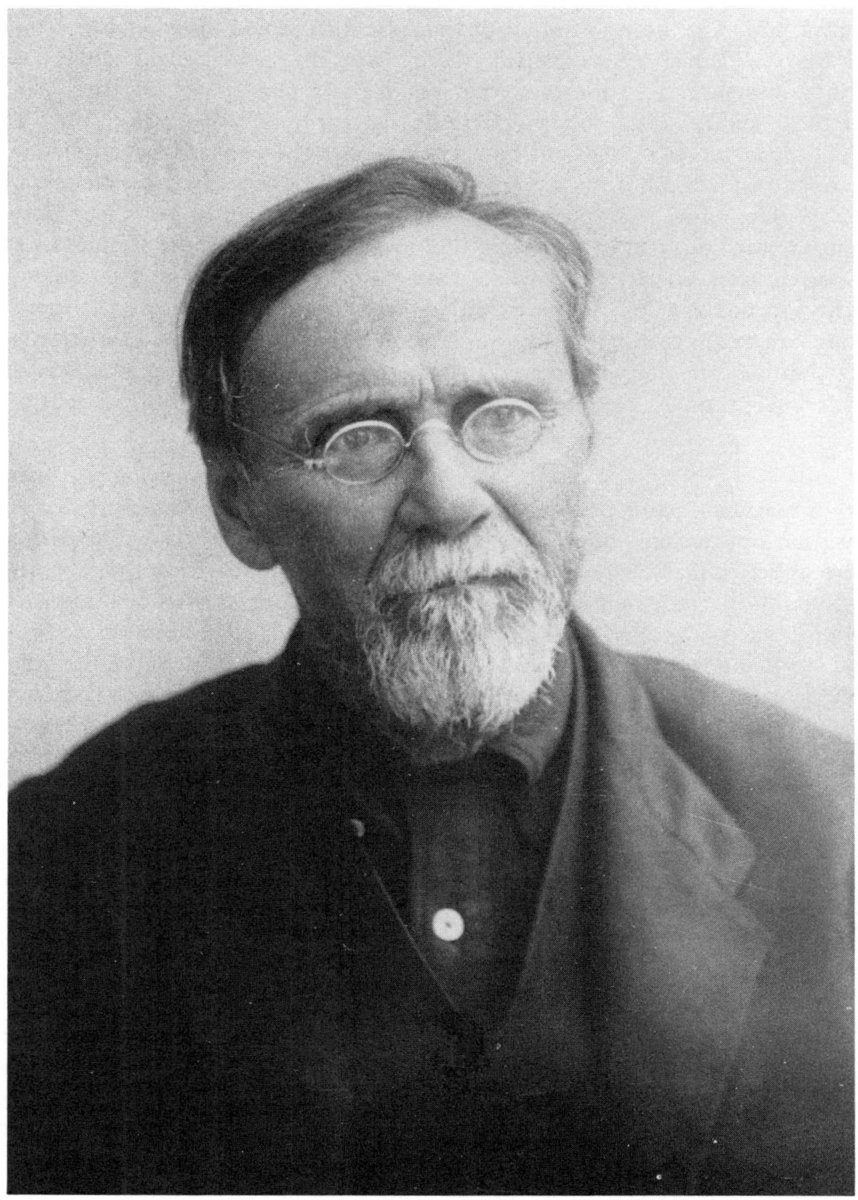

A. T. Still, c. 1909

principles of the philosophy of osteopathy on which osteopathy stood. I opened my subject to this mighty host by saying, "Mr. chairman, ladies and gentlemen, by invitation of your president I will say that osteopathy does not antagonize the idea of using drugs to combat disease, but on the other hand it does advocate the use of drugs. Right here, ladies and gentlemen, of the congregation, I will state to you that the osteopath does want drugs, he needs the use of them, but the drug that he seeks must be chemically pure, it must come from the laboratory of the Infinite; that drug must be selected, prepared and compounded in the chemical laboratory of the human organism which begins its preparation from crude materials in the abdomen and passes to the lungs to be finished to perfection. The substance is known as blood, the highest and most wisely compounded substance that has ever been prepared by any laboratory, which laboratory is coducted by the mind and energy of God himself." At this time the kind chairman asked me if I did not know that the schools of medicine had prepared and kept on hand chemical substances that would make blood, bone, tissue and all the substances found in the human body. I told him I was not aware of that fact. He said "Surely we do and you should so inform the American School of Osteopathy." I thanked him for the information of which he seem to be very proud and willing to make for my information and good. I asked him to bring forward his chemist that I would only be too happy to see the president or any other of his followers make one single drop of blood that I might take it back to the benighted osteopaths, that I would not ask for any great quantity as I simply wanted proof. I wanted one drop of fat, one drop of urine, one drop of gall and one drop of amniotic fluid or of bone, flesh, muscle or hair as compounded by the oath bound schools of medicine who are proud to say, as you assert, have stuck to the tenets of your school for ages so closely that no case of perjury has ever been booked against the faithful. I said, "Mr. President, with all kindness allow me to ask you, if you have ever produced in the best arranged laboratory of all your schools one drop of blood, bone or muscle." He seemed to grow angry at this point and said, "Any fool can ask questions." I said to him, "Hold your passion, Mr. President, it is information I seek, you have asserted and failed to bring one drop of blood or bone, I boldly assert and am ready to bring forward witness that the laboratory out of which the osteopath receives his drug is marked and known as the laboratory of the Infinite." These drugs are pure and effective, they have constructed, they do construct and keep in order the human body and all machinery of life." He grew a little more boisterous at me and spoke in sacred language, "Knowest thou not that we live by what we pretend and not what we do, with us it is meat and bread." By this time the old gentleman seemed and looked very red in the face and rubbed his head and said "I have the headache very badly; now, sir, prove to me what you have said and remove this headache, it comes from constipation." I walked up to him with the usual dignity of an osteopath, I shoved my fingers of both hands under the ligamentum nuchæ. I found some variation in the bones of his neck. I adjusted the bones and compressed the occipital nerves a little, told him to get upon the writing table in the knee and chest position. I adjusted the cecum and all signs of headache and constipation disappeared right there. And I asked the venerable sage and his congregation if they would not like to be osteopaths now, "Have I not demonstrated what I have asserted." And he said, "Comest thou again some time."

* * *

From the fullness of my heart my mouth speaketh. You of the graduting class now hold in your hands your diplomas. They are yours. You have well earned every line, word and all the signatures that are affixed to them. I speak what I know to be true of all of you. I know that you have had no child's play, nor lover's comfort to deal with, nor roses to smooth your paths. Many of you have had to use the best economy at your command to meet the expenses that naturally go with such a great undertaking. Many times your hearts have filled with longings for just a day at your old homes to be with your friends, but the joys have all been pushed aside that knowledge should be obtained. For two years you have worked with both body and mind to keep abreast with your classes. Many times your hearts and heads have ached with pain, but this day has proclaimed your freedom from the toiling of both day and night to keep pace with your studies. You are now men and women commissioned to go forth and do battle with disease, not as babes but as men and women who are well drilled in the arts of this great war. Whilst you may not conquer in all combats, I feel that you will bring many scalps as tokens of victory. You will go to all points of the compass. I will think of you from the rising of the sun till the setting of the same. My love shall ever follow your foot-steps whithersoever you go. Come and see me often. I feel when I give you the parting hand that it means all the day of mortal life for many of you. But I feel that my love for you and the cause will be the anthem of love sung in my tomb by my bones till time knows us no more.

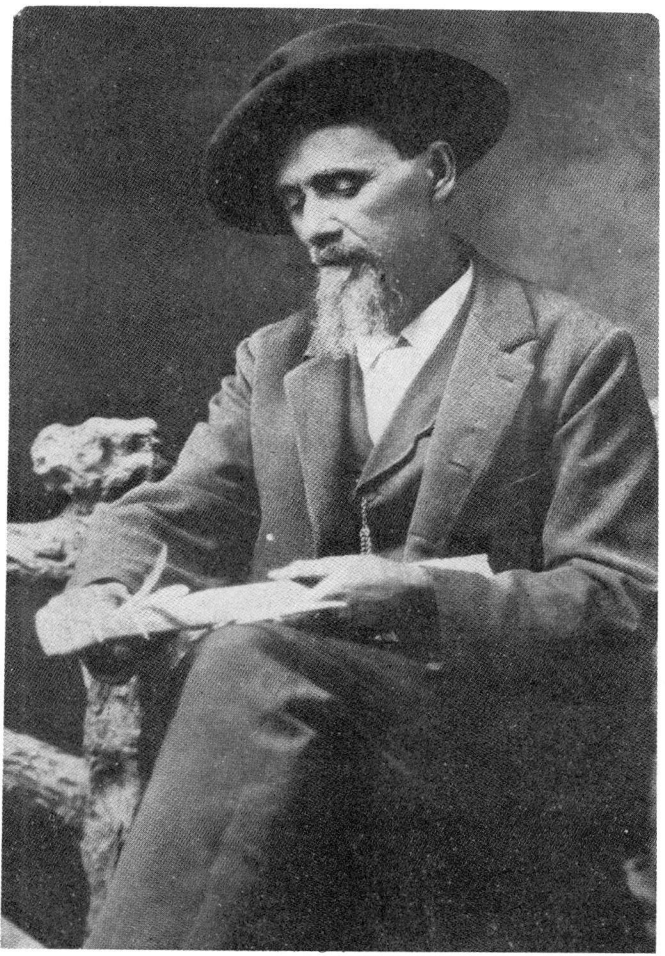

A. T. Still, c. 1910

August, 1902

The first requirement of an osteopath is a thorough knowledge of the human engine, all its powers, parts and principles. Thus armed, you are prepared to decide whether the trouble is in the boiler, steam-chest, wheels, valves, shaft or any other part of the machinery. Without this knowledge you cannot give a correct diagnosis, prognosis or treatment.—A. T. Still.

***

The osteopath who has not confidence enough in the science to implicitly rely upon it under all circumstances, is not entitled to the respect and patronage of the people and should blush with shame when he accepts money from his patrons. In the hands of the qualified and experienced practitioner it can be depended upon in all diseases incident to any climate. Osteopathy will never be found united with saloons nor combined with drugs.—A. T. Still.

***

Men go to schools to learn that which they do not know. They run a great risk of losing their time and money in any school that is not responsible, financially, for its contracts with its students. Suppose you pay me $300 or $500 for two years schooling. You have filled my demand. Now what have I done for your safety in the contract? I have your money and if I do you justice, I will give you bonds to do as I agree, or you are left at the mercy of my honor. I would advise all persons to see to it that the school that they enter for osteopathic instruction is responsible for all contracts, and has shown its honest intentions by depositing bonds in some bank for the faithful performance of its contract with you.—A. T. Still.

***

"Too much patent headache powders," caused the death of Joseph Hane of Marion, Ind. The verdict given by the coroner at the inquest, was: "I find that Joseph Hane came to his death as the result of taking too much patent headache powders, which acted as a heart depressant." David Gunion of the same city, had been in the habit of going to one of the hospitals for treatments. By direction of the doctor he was given a drink of whiskey whenever he arrived at the hospital. July the 12th one of the nurses had given him a drink and then left the room. Gunion then took a second drink from what he supposed was the bottle of whiskey on the shelf near by. He died fifteen minutes later. He had taken a drink of nux vomica from a bottle beside the one containing the whiskey. Another man died a few hours after the administration of some medicine. The coroner considerately found that death was caused by some organic lesion and that no "blame was attached to any person or persons." The columns of the daily press are full of similar "news" items. People with a blind faith in drugs and their remedial powers will continue to take them, never dreaming of the harm they do nor the danger that lurks in them, until fatalities such as these occur. Only a passing notice is given the subject even then. The majority of the people, still held in the bonds of superstition associated with drug medication, will go on doping, but gradually, day by day, the number is being decreased, as the people are being aroused to a realization of the truth of the claims of osteopathy.

***

The technical training of the osteopath skills him to detect mechanical faults in all parts of the body. He recognizes disease by the symptons manifested by it, but interprets these symptoms by tracing them to their real causes in the mechanical disturbances which produce them.

Here lies one radical difference between osteopathy and medicine. The diagnosis of of the disease does not stop with naming the symptoms of a certain disease; it goes further to diagnose the actual physical disturbances causing the disease.

Another radical difference is found in the method of treatment. The osteopath rights what is mechanically wrong, and leaves nature free to act. It is clear that he thus reaches the specific cause. His remedy is applied, not to overcoming the symptoms, but to eradicating the cause. The human system is a perfect mechanism, and it must be in perfect mechanical order that it may perform its various functions aright.

***

The practice of osteopathy rests upon the assumption that disturbed function is largely dependent upon disturbed structure, and will only be permanently corrected by the adjustment of that disturbed structure. When that is accomplished the inherent recuperative powers of the organism manifest themselves in a rapid mechanic, chemic and physiologic regeneration sufficient to restore to every organ its normal function. It is assumed that so long as every organ receives its normal amount of blood, lymph, nerve force, or other vital fluid, and so long as it is properly drained of the waste products of metabolism, health must follow as a logical necessity, and that whenever an organ fails in the performance of its functlon, that fact is prima facie evidence of some obstruction to the incoming or outgoing forces. In the case of an organ whose arterial channels are obstructed, that organ must of necessity suffer from the effects of a local anemia; if an obstruction to its venous drainage be present, the ill effects of a passive congestion are inevitable; if its channels for the propagation of nerve impulses are impinged upon, disturbance of the power of the organ must manifest itself. Hence disease is looked upon as a condition of an organ or of the organism in which function or activity cannot properly obtain because of some interference with one or more of these various pathways. The structures which produce the obstruction may be any of the tissues of body, but are found to be principally luxated bones, contracted muscles and strained or overgrown ligamentous or connective tissue material. With this proposition in view the osteopathic diagnostician is not content with a diagnosis of the location and condition of the organ, which he recognizes as important enough—but by methods peculiar to his system attempts to locate the disordered structural condition which is at fault in the production of the perverted function. Having by these methods determined the abnormal structural condition present, he limits his field of operations, to a large extent, to the reduction of such structural condition as far as may be done, or attempts by his special manipulative measures to render the organism such aid as will enable it to overcome or adapt itself to the changed structure. In his manipulation he does not depend alone upon his ability to force a mechanically abnormal part back into its place, but also upon the fundamental principle that as soon as structural parts are dislodged from their false positions and relations, the normal tension of immediately adjacent and related parts will tend to restore the condition of mechanical integrity. Hence is formulated the foundation principle that nature constantly tends toward a normal condition both of structure and function, and the province of the physician is not in seeking a healing power from without, but in assisting the organism to maintain its structural integrity, which animated by the vital principle is sufficient of itself to generate and distribute every element necessary to normal functioning.

***

Disease is the result of physiological discord. With this fact established in the mind of the doctor of osteopathy as a truth, he is warranted then in hunting the facts that would prove the position, that disease is the result of physiological discord in the functioning of the organs or parts of the physiological laboratory of life. Thus, as an explorer or seeker of the cause of disease he would naturally reason that the variations from the physiological perfection would naturally be found in disordered nerve connections to the degree of breaking or shutting off the normal circuit of nerve force from the brain to any part of the body that should be sustained by that force when normally conducted to any organ as the power necessary to its process of vital functioning. If this be true, there is nothing left in his procedure but to find the break or obstruction to the natural passage of blood or any other fluid that is necessary to a normal condition, which is health itself. Thus, the physician of any school of the healing art must know and act upon the philosophy that disease is the result of physiological discord. The cause of disease can be traced to bony variations from the base of the skull to the bottom of the feet, in the joints of the cervical, dorsal and lumbar vertebrae, the articulations with the sacrum, also the arms and lower limbs. Strains by lifting, jolts, jars, falls or anything that would cause any organ of the chest of abdomen to be moved from its normal to an abnormal position is cause sufficient to confound the harmony of natural functioning of the whole viscera, both above and below the diaphragm and be the cause of an unhealthy supply of nerve fluid and force of the limbs and the organs of the body both internal and external with the brain included. Thus, we have given about what we consider a short philosophical definition of what we mean by the word osteopathy. We use the bones as fulcrums and levers to adjust from the abnormal to the normal that the harmonious functioning of the viscera of the whole body may show forth perfection, that condition which is known as good health. A. T. Still.

***

EXTRACTS FROM THE INTRODUCTION OF DR. A. T. STILL'S NEW BOOK, THE MECHANICAL PRINCIPLES AND PHILOSOPHY OF OSTEOPATHY.

MY AUTHORITIES.

I quote no authors but God and experience. Books compiled by medical authors can be of little use to us, and it would be very foolish of us to look to them for advice and instruction on a science of which they know nothing. They are not able to give an intelligent explanation of their own composite theories, and they have never been asked to advise us. I am free to say that only a few persons who have been pupils of my school have tried to get wisdom from medical writers and apply it to any part of osteopathy's philosophy or practice. The student of any philosophy succeeds best by the more simple methods of reasoning. We reason for necessary knowledge only, and should start out with as many known facts and as few false theories as possible.

Anatomy is taught in our school more thoroughly than in any other school, because we want the student to carry a living picture of all or any part of the body in his mind, as an artist carries the mental picture of the face, scenery, beast, or anything he wishes to represent with his brush. I constantly urge my students to keep their minds full of pictures of the normal body.

AGE OF OSTEOPATHY.

In answer to the question, "How long have you been teaching this discovery?" I will say: I began to give reasons for my faith in the laws of life as given to men, worlds, and beings by the God of Nature, in April, 1855. I thought the swords and cannons of Nature were pointed and trained upon our systems of drug doctoring. Among others, I asked Dr. J. M. Neal, of Edinburgh, Scotland, for some information that I needed badly. He was a medical doctor, a man of keen mental abilities, who would give his opinions freely and to the point. The only thing that made me doubt that he was a Scotchman was that he loved whisky, and I had been told that the Scotch were a sensible people. John M. Neal said that drugs were bait for fools; that the practice of medicine was no science, and the system of drugs was only a trade, followed by the doctor for the money that could be obtained by it from the ignorant sick. He believed that Nature was a law capable of vindicating its power to cure.

I will not worry your patience with a list of the names of authors that have written upon the subject of drugs as remedial agents. I will use the word that the theologian often uses when asked for whom Christ died; the anwer universally is, "All". I began to realize the power of Nature to cure after a skillful correction of the conditions causing abnormalities had been accomplished so as to bring forth pure and healthy blood, the greatest known germicide. With this faith and by this method of reasoning, I began to treat diseases by osteopathy as an experiment; and notwithstanding I obtained good results in all diseases, I hesitated for years to proclaim my discovery. But at last I took my stand on this rock, where I have stood and fought the battles and taken the enemy's flag in every engagement for the last twenty-nine years.

Columbus had to navigate much and long, and meet many storms, because he had not the written experience of other travelers to guide him. He had only a few bits of driftwood not common to his native country to cause him to move as he did. But there was the fact, a bit of wood that did not

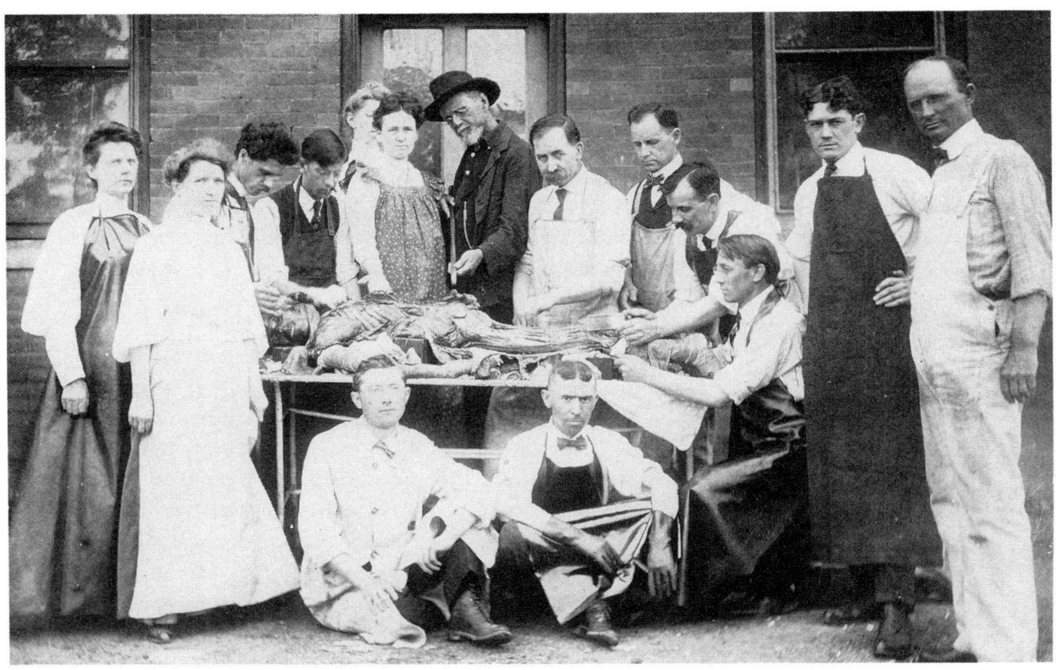

grow on his home soil. He reasoned that it must be from some land amid the sea, whose shores were not known to his race. With these facts and his powerful mind of reason, he met all opposition, and moved along, just as all men do who have no use for theories as a compass to guide them through the storms. This opposition a mental explorer must meet. I felt that I must anchor my boat to living truths and follow them wheresoever they might drift. Thus I launched my boat many years ago on the open seas, and have never found a wave of scorn nor abuse that truth could not ride and overcome.

DEMAND FOR PROGRESS.

The twentieth century demands that advances in the healing arts should be one of the leading objects of the day and generation, because of the truth that the advancement in that profession has not been in line with other professions. The present schools of medicine are injurious schools of drunken systems that are creating morphine, whisky and other drug-taking habits, to the shame and disgrace of the advancement and intelligence of the age. A wisely formulated substitute should be given before it is everlastingly too late. The people become diseased now as in other days, and to heal them successfully without making opium fiends and whisky sots for life should call for and get the best attention that the mind of man can give.

This work is written for the student of osteopathy; written to assist him to think before he acts, to reason for and hunt the cause in all cases before he treats; for on his ability to find the cause depends the success in relieving and curing the afflicted.

With the posted osteopath all the old systems of treating diseases are relegated to the waste-basket and marked obsolete. He must remember that the American School of Osteopathy does not teach him to cure by drugs, but to adjust deranged systems from a false condition to the truly normal, that blood may reach the affected parts and relieve by the powers that belong to pure blood. The osteopath must remember that his first lesson is anatomy, his last lesson is anatomy, and all his lessons are anatomy.

December, 1902

APPENDICITIS.

Extract From Dr. A. T. Still's New Book, The Mechanical Principles and Philosophy of Osteopathy.

At the present time, more than at any other time since the birth of Christ, the men of the medical and surgical world have centralized their minds for the purpose of relieving local conditions, excruciating pain, below the kidney in both the male and female.

For some reasons, possibly justifiable, it has been decided to open the human body and explore the region just below the right kidney in search of the cause of this trouble. The explorations were made upon the dead first. Small seeds and other substances have been found in the vermiform appendix, which is a hollow tube several inches in length. These discoveries led to explorations in the same locality in the living. In some of the cases, though very few, seeds and other substances have been found in the vermiform appendix, supposed to be the cause of inflammation of the appendix. Some have been successfully removed, and permanent relief followed the operation. These explorations and successes in finding substances in the vermiform appendix, their removal, and successful recovery in some cases, have led to what may properly be termed a hasty system of diagnosis, and it has become very prevalent, being resorted to by many physicians, under the impression that the vermiform appendix is of no use, and that the human being is just as well off without it.

Therefore it is resolved, that as nothing positive is known of the trouble in the location above described, it is guessed that it is a disease of the vermiform appendix. Therefore they etherize and dissect for the purpose of exploring, to ascertain if the guess is right or wrong. The surgeon's knife is driven through the quivering flesh in great eagerness in search of the vermiform appendix. The bowels are rolled over and around in search of the appendix. Sometimes some substances are found in it, but more often, to the chargin of the exploring physician, it is found to be in a perfectly healthy and normal condition. So seldom is it found containing seeds or any substance whatever that, as a general rule, it is a useless and dangerous experiment. The percentage of deaths caused by the knife and ether, and the permanently crippled, will justify the assertion that it would be far better for the human race if they lived and died in ignorance of appendicitis. A few genuine cases might die from that cause, but if the knife were the only known remedy, it were better that one should die occasionally than to continue this system.

ANOTHER VICTORY.

Osteopathy furnishes the world with a relief here which is absolutely safe, without the loss of a drop of blood, that has for its foundation and philosophy a fact based upon the longitudinal contractile ability of the appendix itself, which is able to eject by its natural forces any substances that may by an unnatural move be forced into the appendix.

I have treated many cases of appendicitis, probably running in numbers up into hundreds, without falling to relieve and cure a single case. The ability of the appendix to receive and discharge foreign substances is taught in the science of osteopathy and is successfully practiced by its doctors. In my first case I found a lateral twist of lumbar bones. I adjusted the spine, lifted the bowels, and the patient got well. I was once called to see a lady who had been put on light diet, by the surgeon, preparatory to the knife. She soon recovered under my treatment without any surgical operation, and is alive and well at this date.

MANY QUERIES.

To many, such questions as these will arise. Has the appendix at its entrance a spincter muscle similar in action to that of the rectum and œsophagus? Has it the power to contract and dilate, to contract and shorten in its length and eject all substances when the nerves are in a normal condition? And where is the nerve that failed to act to throw out the substance that entered the cavity of the appendix? Has God been so forgetful as to leave the appendix in such a condition as to receive foreign bodies, without preparing it by its power of contraction, or otherwise, to throw out such substances? If He has, He surely has forgotten part of his work. Reason has taught me that He has done a perfect work, and on that line I have proceeded to treat appendicitis for twenty five years, without pain and misery to the patient, and have given permanent relief in all the caaes that have come to us. With the diagnosis of doctors and surgeons that appendicitis was the malady, and the choice of relief between the knife and death, or possibly both, many such cases have come for osteopathic treatment, and examination has revealed in every case that there has been previous injury to some set of spinal nerves, caused by jars, strains, or falls. Every case of appendicitis and gall or renal stones can be traced to some such cause.

These principles I have proclaimed and thought for a quarter of a century.

Dr. A. T. Still's Department.

WE must remember that when we write or talk, we have asked the reader or listener to stop all pursuits and read or listen to our story. We must be kind enough to give him something in exchange for his precious time. We must remember that time to an American is too valuable to be given for hours to a long story that does not benefit him. We care but little for what queens, kings, and professors have said; it is what you know that we want. Man's life is too short and useful to be spent reading any undigested literature that amounts to nothing. Suppose that a farmer should write on stock or grain-raising, and his book informed the student just how Professor So-and-so planted, bred, and failed, and gave no lesson that did not close with a "however," or "I would remark, as stated before" and so on. Of what use would it be to the young agriculturist who read it, and if he had no other instruction, what would he amount to as a farmer? You know he would be a total failure in the profession until he learned to be governed by known truths. His success depends on what he knows, and not on being able to recite what someone had failed to accomplish.

Osteopathy.

What is osteopathy? It is a scientific knowledge of anatomy and physiology in the hands of a person of intelligence and skill, who can apply that knowledge to the use of man when sick or wounded by strains, shocks, falls, or mechanical derangement or injury of any kind to the body. An up-to-date osteopath must have a masterful knowledge of anatomy and physiology. He must have brains in osteopathic surgery, osteopathic obstetrics and osteopathic practice, curing diseases by skillful re-adjustment of the parts of the body that have been deranged by strains, falls, or other cause that may have removed even a minute nerve from the normal, although not more than the thousandth of an inch. He sees cause in a slight anatomical deviation for the beginning of disease. Osteopathy means a knowledge of the anatomy of the head, face, neck, thorax, abdomen, pelvis, and limbs, and a knowledge why health prevails in all cases of perfect normality of all parts of the body. Osteopathy means a studious application of the best mental talents at the command of the man or woman that would hold a place in the profession. Osteopathy has no time to throw away in beer-drinking, nor has it time to wear out shoe-leather carrying a cue around the pool or billiard-table. It belongs to men of sober brains, men who never tire of anatomy and physiology or of hunting the cause of disease. An osteopath answers questions by his learning. He proves what he says by what he does. An osteopath knows that to the day of the coming in of osteopathy the whole medical world was almost a total blank in knowledge of the machinery and functions of the abdomen of the human body. The medical man to-day, if we judge his knowledge by what he does, is perfectly at sea as soon as he enters the abdomen. He combats bowel disease by methods handed down to him by symptomatology. Beginning with chronic constipations, he reasons not on the causes. His one idea is to fall onto a successful purgative drug, which never should be used excepting with great caution. When the most active purgatives fail, with the aid of injections, to effect a movement (the bowels filling up and packing the abdominal cavity so full and tight that no organ below the diaphragm can act and all motion is lost, even to the blockage of arterial and venous circulation of the blood; with the stomach crowded with food, then on to vomiting of fecal matter and the vitality low all over the body) what is left for the medical doctor but surgical interference? And he proceeds with his instrumental skill with hope and doubt. The osteopath gets his success with such diseases through adjustment of the abdominal viscera, with the view of relieving the bowels of bulks of fecal matter, either hard or soft, that are laboring to pass away from the body through the natural channels, but meet mechanical obstructions that are caused by kinks, folds, twists, and knots of the bowels, the result of heavy strains, lifts, and falls that have forced the bowels to abnormal positions in the abdomen, deranging the mesentery at various points. The osteopath feels that he is not justified in administering either purgatives or injections into the bowels until he has straightened out the viscera so that no resisting obstruction is liable to block the passing fecal matter. He proceeds as a mechanic.

Question of Intelligence.

Osteopathy is not so much a question of books as it is of intelligence. A successful osteopath is in all cases, or should be, a person of individuality, with a mechanical eye behind all motions or efforts to re-adjust any part of the body to its original normality, because unguided force is dangerous, often doing harm and failing in giving the relief that should be the reward of well-directed skill. A knowledge of anatomy is only a dead weight if we do not know how to apply that knowledge with successful skill. That is all there is to the question why our knowledge of anatomy should be more perfect than it is with any other school of the healing art. The osteopath should be thoroughly educated by books and by drill, and in my reference to books I mean those that are essential to a complete knowledge of anatomy.

February, 1904

"TO YOUR TENTS, OH, ISRAEL."

Dr. A. T. Still.

LIFE with all its attributes that are as numerous as the sands of the sea is the exhibit that we see every day in the show cases of the mineral, the vegetable, and the animal kingdoms. Each case has a different showing. The mineral exhibits all its beauties to the eye. Under the microscope we see the various minerals, all have some earthly clothing and we only see them dimly. But we do see enough to know that there is a substance of greater or less value enveloped. We proceed by heat and other methods to separate the specimen under consideration from its outer covering which prepares it for another microscopic examination. We discover that we have by the first process separated the mineral from its materal covering, and the birth of the real substance is by this process completed. The child is born, the delivery is complete. We have a something and we do not know what name to give it. We call in the wise men from the East. They proceed now to analyze this substance. On crucial examination they report platinum, gold, aluminum, silver, copper, iron, tin, sulphur and numerous earthy substances. They separate all and report the exact amount that is in each division, without which knowledge their judgment would simply be a confusing blank, and the report would be unsatisfactory to the man who explores the mountains for their valuable substances. We expect by the chemist's analysis a report that is worthy of the amount exacted for such services. We know just what we have in each separate division, and by this report and the value of each substance, we can approximate the value of our discovery. You go the chemist in full confidence that he can analyze and give the results of his investigation. Suppose in your anxiety the chemist would take the specimen and say, "Great is the mystery of godliness! The secrets of God are past finding out," and charge a dollar for his wisdom. How would you feel under such circumstances? Would you call him a fake who would take your money without giving you value received?

Here I wish to make the application of my allegory. We find another substance with whose attributes we desire some acquaintance. These substances come in organized bundles, generally five to six feet in length, with a head, a neck and a cylindrical trunk with arms and legs attached. We place it in the hot sunshine, or throw it into a pool of water, and it begins to perform laughable antics.

We take this to the chemist for anyalysis. He reports all the chemical substances found in earthy matter, but fails to offer a satisfactory explanation of its powers of motion. He says, "You must go to a chemist that is prepared to go further in his analysis. The subject of motion or action is out of the reach of my methods. I am sure there is a substance in that specimen, man, that neither fire or chemicals can unfold, which contains motion, mind and all the attributes of both." I enquire, "To whom shall I go, Mr. Chemist?" He kindly replies, "I have heard there are men who give such thought to life, the soul of man. You will find them in all villages and cities." I ask how I may know when I come to one of their chemical laboratories. He replies, "You will know a great number of them by noting the cross surmounting them. Others are marked 'M. E. Church,' 'Baptist Church,' 'Presbyterian Church,' all claiming to be able to give you all necessary information. They are the men to give a proper analysis of your specimen, and set your mind at ease."

I saddled up mine ass and journeyed with my specimen, man, to many cities and called upon these chemists to analyze what I had found. I have been traveling from office to office for many years in search of the chemist who-could analyze the human body and tell me whether life is a substance or a principle. Thus far I have received no satisfactory answer to the great question, "Is the soul of man a substance?" If so, what is the degree of purity, the height of perfection to which the undiscovered chemist did make his compound known as the soul of man, whose attributes are as innumerable as the stars of heaven. From my youth I have listened to the rantings and unsatisfactory assertions of the theologians. They have contributed nothing to my store of knowledge on this one question, "What is the soul of man?" Patiently, yet with intense desire, I await the answer for which I have paid all charges, and I'm frank to say, have received nothing in reply to this momentous question.

LET US PRAY.

O Lord, Thou knowest Thy book says, "Ask and ye shall receive." Thou knowest that man is mentally far below an ass or Thou wouldst not have sent an ass to counsel and advise Thy chosen people. Wilt Thou please send us an up-to-date ass quick, one of pedigree. We want no Clydesdale. We want a live, wide-awake ass, that will tell us some facts about life, whether it is a substance or a principle. If a substance, how fine that chemical compound had to be made before life, motion, and mind, with their attributes were the absolute results of that chemical effort? O Lord, we do cry piteously from morn 'till night. Canst Thou not hear our groans? Please dip our heads deeper into the rivers of reason. Let all the wrinkles of stupidity be soaked out. Push our heads far under; hold us there 'till we blubber, O Lord. Let Thine ass bray hot blasts of steam in both of our ears, fresh from his compassionate lungs. Send him forth from Thy stable, stir him up soul and body, fill him full of energy, for Thou knowest he has a big job before him, so warm him up and send him on fire into the camp. He will have a Jericho job with us. He will have to go around us more than seven times before our wall of superstition gives way.

O Lord, grease our heels with the oil of energy. Put it on strong so that we may slip forward a little. Keep Thou all grease from off our toes; we want them dry and sharp, so they will hold fast to every inch of progress that our greasy heels have gained for us. O Lord, don't forget our dear professors. Oil their spines with Thy most precious oil, of Thy sunflower of light, and spank them with the paddle of energy.

May that oil run down both arms and purify their hands to that degree that they will not accept anything whatsoever that is handed down by tradition, unless it be the chemically pure gurglings from Thy great jug of wisdom.

Show them the cecum, the vermiform appendix; give them their uses, and speak to them as Thou didst to Abraham, "Put up your knife and let Isaac go; he has no appendicitis."

Now, Lord, we beseech Thee once in a great while to pummel our heads with the hailstones of reason. Make our eyes snap with knowledge like a toad's in a hailstorm. Be merciful to the beginners, for Thou knowest their feet of reason are tender and flat as the negroes' were before Abe Lincoln set them free. O Lord, the instep of the negro did rise with freedom, and Thou knowest the instep of the young osteopath will rise with his freedom from old theories. Amen.

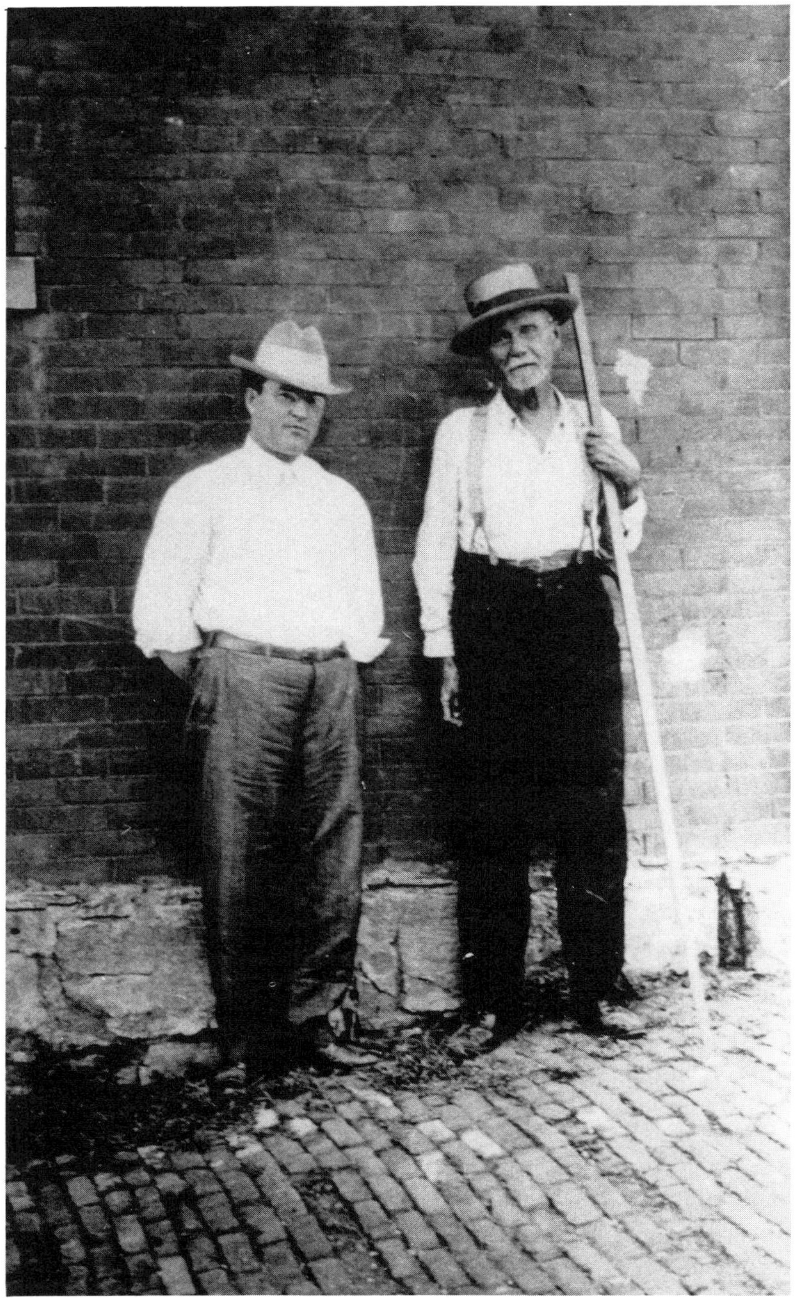

A. T. Still and A. D. Becker, c. 1910

JOHN A. THOMPSON,

Graduate American School of Osteopathy, Kirksville, Mo.

Wheeling, - - - W. Va.

February, 1904

Never send a patient to the office of an osteopath who uses electricity, vibrators and all the adjuncts that he can find. Tell the enquirer of doctors who do not use anything but the straight genius of a doctor who cures by his knowledge of anatomy and physiology which is the sum total of all cures. I say to my clerks, never say yes in answer to a letter of inquiry when you know that the D. O. has his office filled with adjuncts, send such prospective patients to D. O.'s who can and who do cure their patients with the up-to-date skill of the osteopath who knows that a well adjusted system will cure and that adjuncts are only used by feeble-minded persons who never did nor never can reason. I am tired of getting letters asking if I can recommend such as good osteopathic doctors. I say *no* now and forever, keep away from them. A. T. STILL.

May, 1904

THE HEART.

Dr. A. T. Still.

THE heart, not the brain, is the center and source of an intelligence that constructs each division of the body, and combines all parts into one common personage or being. There, we find the first movement of life in the embryo, and the questions arise, "What is life? What is the heart?"

As we commonly speak of the heart we mean the organ of life, the fountain of blood, the engine of blood supply, and so on. We know that it supplies the whole system after building the arteries to carry it. Organs appear, all wisely formed and located to suit their different uses, and connected to the heart by arteries, veins and nerves; when finished all parts are working in harmony. We try to reason how and why this lonely being, the heart, has done so much and shown through all its work such perfect wisdom. Is it the source of this constructive wisdom? Is wisdom an attribute of the heart? If not, what makes the plan by which it does the work and sets it out for inspection where it never fails to get the highest award on its exhibit? So far all evidence points to its individual perfection, its oneness in power to take charge and do all that could possible be asked of a builder, from the first stroke to the perfected structure. It has not only to make the foundation faultless but to prepare the apparatus for the manufacture of the perfectly pure chemicals used and to deliver and adjust all atoms to suit the design of the part under construction; as, some atoms are prepared to form bone, some blood vessels, some nerves, and others the different viscera, each perfect and adapted to the part it helps to form. Thus we reason, that wisdom rules in animal chemistry, otherwise confusion and failure would result. Through all from start to finish we find perfection absolute.

It is not enough to consider the heart a pump or an organ distributing blood to all parts of the body. Let us give the heart credit for all that it does; give it credit for native wisdom, the wisdom it proves by its work to possess.

It builds its own workshop and works without assistance seeming to know its needs. If it makes a turtle, it decides a shell is necessary and constructs one for the protection of the being within. It builds and guards according to kind—man, beast, bird, fish and reptile; all by its native mental and physical powers.

If the foetal heart begins as an atom and can build all around and over itself walls of protection, limbs of motion, and all that is of use to its personal demands, why not give it credit for wisdom to govern all its attributes and say, "You are substance refined to the power of union between life and matter."

If the heart is the center of force and constructive intelligence in the body, why not go to it for repair? Let the osteopath follow the course of the blood from the heart to its destination and return, and remove all obstructions, open all doors, for on it we depend for all the joys of perfect form and functioning, which is health. Be the watchman of the tower to cry, "All is well."

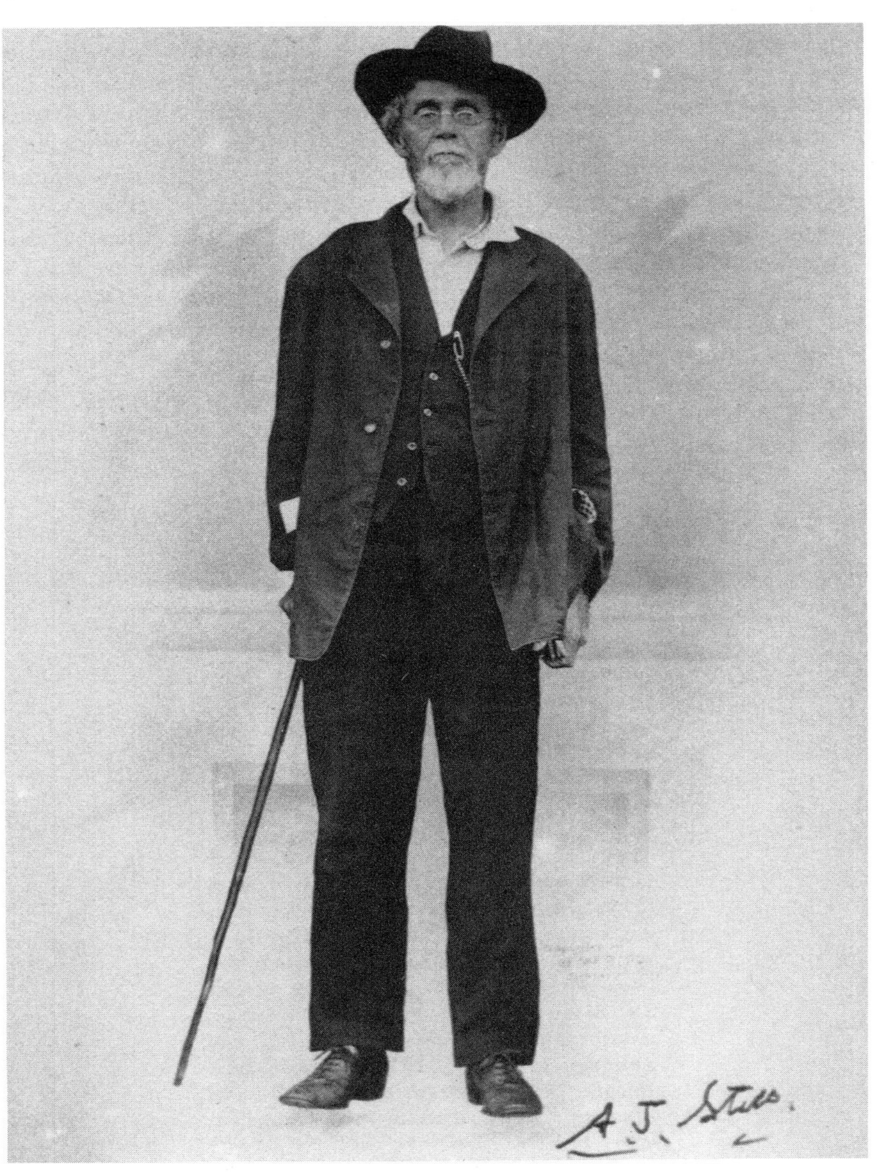

A. T. Still, 1914

May, 1904

Be Original.

When the A. S. O. sends forth a graduate with his diploma under his arm, it is a token. of our respect for him and of our confidence in his ability. It is also a commission to explore new fields and report the truth for the advancement of osteopathy. And I wish it emphatically understood to be in order, without an "if" or a "but," that we will be glad to receive his report and give it place in the Journal of Osteopathy as useful literature, provided it be the result of his personal investigation. It must come without the quotation from the books of any medical school. It must be a discovery either from his own experiments, or the experiments of other graduates of this or some other reputable osteopathic school. The time has come when we cannot give space in the Journal for any prosy compilation of old theories that are without a vestige of the principles of osteopathy. Our time is too precious to spend reading quotations from Flint, Donglison, Osler or any other author whose writings are lacking in the first principles of our science. For the future the Journal is open for osteopathic literature only; we have a large waste basket into which old theories must go. I extend a warm, a very warm invitation to all osteopaths to send us the results of their experiments. The human body, if properly understood, anatomically, physiologically, obstetrically, surgically, in the treatment of diseases generally, chronic or acute, in different seasons and localities, offers enough to be discovered and proven to give your pen exercise much and often. Let the reports give results obtained by osteopaths; not a combination of the sacred tenets of osteopathy with the abortive system of drug slushing. Now, wake up! and please remember this: we cannot give space and fill our columns with a lot of old medical theories from which we get nothing of benefit to our school of practice. We need wideawake, up-to-date osteopaths.

A. T. STILL, President A. S. O.

June, 1904

In answer to the question "What is osteopathy"? I will say it is a knowledge of anatomy applied to the healing of diseases. It is the surgical adjustment of all parts of the body by the anatomist who knows all its bones, their forms, places and how they are held together, where each joint is, where the muscles are attached and how they act when in their normal places, how a normal limb looks, how it feels to the hand, and how an abnormal limb, hand, foot, spine or neck feels to the fingers in which the sense of touch is developed to a very high degree; an essential qualification of a successful osteopathic physician. His successes and failures are the results which show the extent of his knowledge of anatomy and physiology. By his good or bad results he shows his worth. If he is wise in anatomy and physiology, he will at a glance detect any abnormality in form, and can easily prove the cause of any failure in functioning. He fears neither the diseases of climate nor of season. He meets the chronic and the acute with the same confidence of success, because he knows why his patient has failed to keep his normal health. He knows just how to adjust every bone and muscle in his patient's body. He also knows that when all is normal that every organ in the body, beginning with the heart, will go to work and force the blood to all feeble points, carry off the waste, and repair the wound found, thus establishing the normal functioning which is the all of health. If the physician does not know the normal man, he cannot give relief to the sick man, because he does not know the cause of the disease he fails to conquer in the combat. It has triumphed over his generalship and scored a shameful victory from his ignorance of the normal man. Disease and death have won the victory over the would-be osteo-medico doctor, with his thermometer, hypodermic syringe and germ incubator and his ignorance of anatomy and the physical powers of the body to keep and maintain life with all its joys.

The body asks only a little help from the anatomical machinist when a bone or muscle "jumps the track"; this he is able to give if is not an ignoramus or a hopeless theorist.

A. T. STILL.

July, 1904

THE OSTEOPATH AS A SURGEON.

DR. A. T. STILL.

Notwithstanding the fact that osteopathy is just thirty years old, it has proven itself to be a science worthy of commendation.

The question is being asked almost hourly, "What is Osteopathy?" In answer to that, I will say, "It is a system of surgery." And if I should undertake to give a definition of the duties of an osteopath, I would say, "The duties are those of a surgeon, for an osteopath is no more nor less than a surgeon."

I will give a short definition of the term surgery by such authorities as Webster, Dunglison and Chambers. They all agree that surgery is one of the healing arts that gives relief from suffering, deformities, abnormal growths and so on, by manipulations to adjust and correct the bony system when any dislocations appear by accident or other causes. Use the knife and saw or any other appliances necessary to obtain results and relief required in extreme cases. This is something of the crude definition of the word "surgery." The osteopath is a surgeon who relieves the system of deformities, inflammation, rheumatism, neuralgia, or any other painful suffering or irritation of the nervous system. His diagnosis is made by comparing the normal to the abnormal body. He notes the variations from the normal that he finds in his patient. If the suffering be that of a limb, the head, neck, spine, abdomen or pelvis, he seeks to know at what particular place or point in the bony skeleton an abnormal fulness or depression exists which by that partial or complete dislocation, would produce a pressure upon a nerve, a blood vessel, or any organ of the system. On this foundation, he proceeds to obtain a knowledge of variations from the normal, by which he can give a correct diagnosis and relieve his patient by adjusting to the normal. By this method of exploration, he is enabled to find and know the cause of the disease which he is expected to relieve. He has a foundation in truth to give a correct diagnosis and prove by his work that his diagnosis is correct. This system of surgery is just as good and reliable in diagnosing and treating diseases of climate, season and contagion as it is in limb dislocation, because an irritation from over-heat or cold will produce contraction of muscles strong enough to hold the spine, ribs, and other bones upon the nerves as they leave the brain and spinal cord. This causes a stoppage of the fluids of the body long enough to permit of fermentation usually resulting in fever which appears as a result of such abnormal irritation and pressure.

Again as a surgeon in bloody flux, he finds contractures and abnormalties of the spine which he can easily relieve by adjustment and give relief from all suffering from the bowels and the whole system. Thus by his knowledge of surgery, as an osteopath, he is able to know the cause that produced the effect known as flux and give instantaneous relief by surgically adjusting the lower spine. The same process will take him to the cause of pneumonia. He explores the body as a machinist, and never fails, if he carefully examines, to find the cause of pneumonia to be luxation or sub-luxation of the ribs on the suffering side of the spine, and his remedy is to readjust as a surgeon, giving relief from either pleuro or lobar pneumonia. All this he does as a machinist by manipulation guided by his knowledge of the normal body.

Thus you see in every step in his efforts to give relief from disease he is guided by his knowledge of anatomy, physiology, cause and effect.

He is a surgeon and his work is that of a surgeon in all diseases peculiar to the human family that he is called to relieve by his knowledge of normal anatomy.

He knows the abnormal and by his adjustment he gives the relief sought, and he gives it as a surgeon who understands the form and function of the body and all its organs.

The Greater Osteopath.

It is to be hoped that the latest and best truth of the science of healing without drugs and without any imaginary assistance from adjuncts of all kinds will appear in our Journal from time to time as truths that have and can be demonstrated to be such. In contagions, diseases of climate and seasons, the acute as well as the chronic, all submit to the inherent power of life that does the healing in all diseases of man or beast.

The pen of the greater osteopath never can afford to publish his ignorance of anatomy, physiology, cause and effect. If he is an up-to-date osteopath he has no use for a tool to tell how hot his patient is each day, or whether the blood has microbes or hyenas in it. His business is to knew the plumbing of the house of life and turn the water on all force and stop the blaze before "Mark Hanna" is burned up by the fires of death, that should, and would have been put out by a greater osteopath, who is up-to-date and thorough-bred, who guides his engine as nature intended.

The greater osteopath cannot afford to be a bullet-head. He must be a penetrating projectile of finest steel, his mental cannon must be of the long range kind, and of the most obdurate mettle or he will fall an easy prey to the enemy of progress. All his shells must be filled with nitroglycerine of truth truth that has often been tried, never denied and willing to be tried again and again, ad infinitum, or keep out of all combats in which truth is the aggressor and theories the possessor. He must remember that the human mind seldom explores in foreign seas for truth. The masses have their idols; they are taught to love and to defend their gods, governments and their doctors. Thus, the greater osteopath is on "Sacred Grounds" when he enters the territory of the Gods of Tradition.

The feeble-minded, weak-kneed osteopath, like the converted Indian, feels better with a breech-clout than in an up-to-date suit of civilization. So he is not to be blamed but pitied when a greater osteopath finds in his office electric machines, hot air apparatus, alcohol baths, hyperdermic syringes, thermometers, bottles of morphine and on to the whole bill of adjuncts and sees him treat a patient one-half hour to an hour by rubs and pulls. The greater osteopath hates to tell him he is a raving blank. He bites his lips with internal rage and leaves the office disgusted and says, "I am disgusted that man has eyes and he sees not; that he has ears and he hears not." Then he soliloquizes and says, "Man's days are few and full of sorrow. How often I would have gathered you together, as a hen gathers her chickens but ye would not."

Then he consoles himself as the boy did who said when he tried to stop a calf on a down hill run by a pull at the calf's tail, "Go, I had a poor hold anyhow."

✦ ✦

Dr. Gerdine: What is the pathology of Broncho Pneumonia, Mitchell?
Mitchell: A bronco in the lung, isn't it?

Dr. Hamilton: Oglesby, name five methods of examination.
Oglesby: Inspection, Palpation, Ausculation.

Dr. Smith: Groenwood, what are the openings of the left ventricle?
Groenwood: There aren't any, they are all outlets.

HOW OSTEOPATHY WAS EVOLVED.

DR. A. T. STILL.

During the early years of my career as a physician, I had many obstacles to meet and to overcome under the conditions then existing. I was always seeking a better method, and thirty years ago I took as my subject the form and functioning of the human body. Although I was about as well posted in anatomy as the ordinary physician I found that in reality my knowledge of the subject was limited. I knew that there were about 206 bones in man's framework. Each bone had two ends and as many articulations. I knew something about how one bone articulated with another. I looked upon man as the perfect machine which was run by a force we call life. I knew that if a hip was dislocated and the femur kept out of its articulating socket, that a man would have an unnatural, wobbling gait. I knew that the way to correct this was to put the thigh bone back into its socket. So long as it staid out of its socket, just so long the man would not walk properly and would present an unnatural appearance while in motion.

I began to reason that if a dislocated hip would derange the appearance of a man while in the act of walking, what might we expect in the functioning process with the head of a humerous dropped down upon the axillary vessels and nerves? Could a normal action or a normal physical condition of that arm be expected? What would be the effect of pushing a clavicle at its sternal articulation against the nerves and blood vessels of the anterior part of the neck? Would it produce an enlargement of the thyroid gland by pressure on the thyroid veins, causing what is commonly known as goiter? Is that the cause of blood and other fluids being detained in the thyroid gland and is the enlargement caused by venous blood failing to pass back to the heart?

I proceeded to examine the bony relations in a few cases of goiter—both simple and exophthalmic.

In every case I found almost complete dislocation of the clavicle, the inner end onto the blood vessels of the neck and the outer end forward and off the acromion process; also there was usually one or both of the first ribs pushed far back and off their spinal articulations. I adjusted ribs and clavicle to their normal positions, stagnation of fluids stopped and enlargement of the thyroid gland disappeared. I did not stop with one experiment, but tried others. In exophthalmic goiter I proceeded to adjust the bony framework of the upper dorsal, and to my surprise, in a few days or weeks, when the work was properly done, the eyes became natural in appearance, the heaving of the heart stopped and the goiter disappeared. I was proud to know that my philosophy could be demonstrated in all cases of goiter by reduction of the tumor and the disappearance of the distressing symptoms.

In sciatic rheumatism, I found obstruction to blood circulation to be the cause of the pain and suffering in the lower spine and limbs. In every case I found a sub-luxation or dislocation of the head of the femur; or one or both innominates off their articulation with the sacrum. This reduced the subject of sciatic rheumatism to a demonstrable fact of variations in bones and muscles.

Proceeding with my experiments, I found variations in ribs to be the cause of asthma. I adjusted the ribs, the asthma vanished. It was simply an effect of abnormal articulation of the ribs with the transverse processes of the vertebræ.

I found the cause of sick headache and fascial neuralgia to be equally simple. They could both be traced to a slip of one or more of the cervical vertebræ or a subluxation of the heads of the first ribs, shutting off the ascending vertebral artery and the venous drainage from the brain. I continued my explorations of the human body. I dissected to acquaint myself with the forms and function of every organ, its supply and drainage. I tried to acquaint myself with the mechanical and physiological processes of the whole body and I am happy to say I have found and repeatedly demonstrated that the body is a machine and can vindicate all its claims for health in the hands of a man or woman who knows the normal and the abnormal. With me it is no longer a debatable question; if I fail to get the results desired, I am frank to say that my ignorance is responsible for the failure and not the ability of the body to vindicate the intelligence of its architect and builder.

✦

LENGTH OF TIME NECESSARY TO ACQUIRE THE FOUNDATION PRINCIPLES OF OSTEOPATHY.

DR. A. T. STILL.

The question is often asked, "How long will it take a person to learn to do this work successfully?" In reply I will say that with a man or woman of ordinary intelligence, my observation has been that by close application under competent instructors, he will have obtained a comprehensive and practical knowledge of anatomy, physiology and the workings of the body in two years' time. He is then qualified and well prepared to take charge of and do successful work, provided he has been properly taught or is not a mental blank. I have been advised to make our school course longer than two years; to add another year and make it three.

I have been constantly in this service for the past thirty years. I think I know all the requirements of a competent osteopathic physician. My best operators have completed the school course and gone to work at the end of two years. They use no adjuncts and are unqualified successes. My opinion is, that after two years of constant application to his studies in my school, if he can show good grades, he is then as well qualified to begin practicing as he ever will be. He must learn much by experience.

Another point that I would make is that I think my opinion should be as well worth your consideration, after thirty years experience, as that of any man or boy who has gone out from our schools and has only devoted two or three years to the study and practice.

And as the discoverer and unfolder of the science of osteopathy, I will emphatically state that I consider a two years' course sufficient, if the work is confined to the essentials and all obsolete theories carefully excluded, the student attends strictly to his business, keeps out of billiard saloons and is well versed in all branches taught in the schools of our science which are to prepare him for the higher school of experience. The graduate should go to work at the end of the two years or he will lose many of the valuable principles that have been taught him before he has gotten hands and head to practice them until they became second nature, and he finds a proof in the results obtained. Thus I consider every day wasted to the serious detriment of the student, that he delays putting his knowledge into practice, after he completes his two years' course. If he begins on a third year the work assumes a monotonous routine and he begins to unlearn that which should have become a part of himself from frequent practice. At the end of the two years he should be master of the knowledge of the form and functioning of the human body and should be able to assume full charge of the engine of life and wisely direct it along its course. Again the average man or woman does not have the means to spend for an additional year. If I thought a student could not master the science in two years, I would tell him so and refuse his money. We need in our ranks only those qualified to do good work as osteopaths.

Let us stand by our flag or quit!

✦

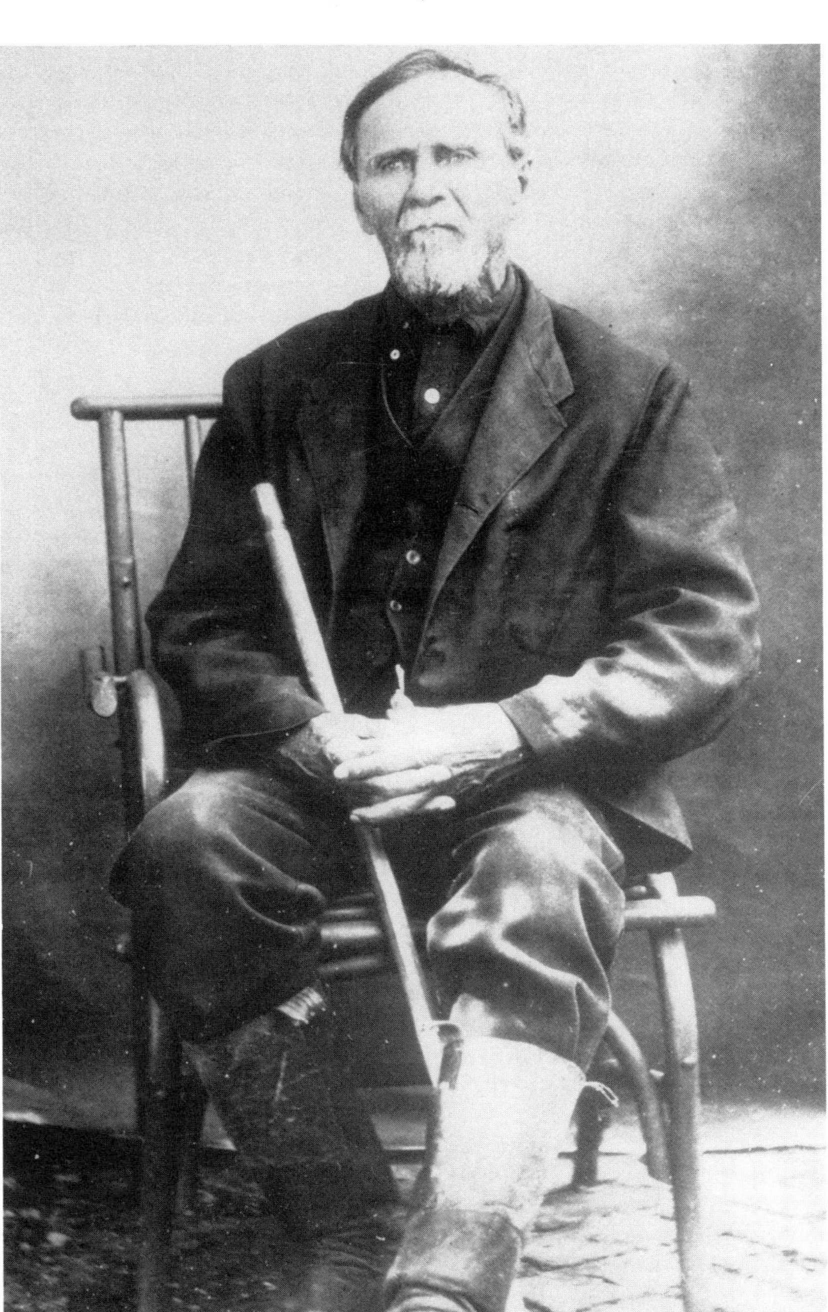

A. T. Still, c. 1914

A Time for all Things.

We should eat when we are hungry, drink when we are thirsty, sleep when we are tired, sit close to the fire when we are cold, and wear spectacles when we are old; we should use such adjuncts as vibrators, electricity, hot bags and ice packs when we are ill, if there is is no osteopath present who understands the the form and functioning of every part of the human body.

The true osteopath does not need such assistance; and the would-be osteopath who adopts such devices should be very careful to avoid talking to a well informed anatomist, one who understands the normal physiological action of the human body, of the "wonderful power of his vibrator." I say he should speak very guardedly of the action of his machine on the human body to the anatomist who is thoroughly acquainted with all parts of the human body and their functioning as he is very apt to make mental notes of the speaker's wisdom or ignorance of his subject.

When the vibrator man tells of the wonderful exploits of his machine, then the anatomist may ask him to prove his statements by demonstration. Let him prove that the architect who formed the plan and wrote the specifications of life, failed to place in the body the necessary machinery with ample force to execute all its functions; to keep every muscle, nerve, vein, artery, bone and viscus in perfect order, and capable of all the action that the wisdom of Diety Himself considered necessary to the preparation, distribution and appropriation of all its fluids.

I will say to the users of vibrators that when you have proven by your vibrating machine the ignorance of God as an architect and builder, then I will cheerfully admit that you have discovered an improvement that is worthy the respect of God and man, and should be adopted by both. You will have succeeded in proving what has never before been proven—God's ignorance and incompetency when he planned and constructed man, the temple of life. It is not for me to say that God has fallen short in constructing your mental vibrator, but will leave your acts to vindicate or condemn your mental superiority in the court of public opinion.

Just one word to the graduates of my school: when a patient first comes into your office, use nothing but the skill of the hand and head of the successful osteopath. The patient does not come to your office to be shaken up by vibrators, shocked by electric batteries or treated by anything but the hand guided by the tenets of osteopathy.

Remember that the intelligent people of the world have long since lost confidence in the ability of adjuncts to assist nature in constructing and repairing from its own laboratories of power and motion. I will say further that I am constantly receiving letters inquiring who are my best operators. I never will knowingly recommend an "adjunctor," because his adjuncts are the strongest evidence of his incompetency as an osteopath. He is a "fallen angel" and I cannot recommend him.

A. T. Still.

* * *

Dentistry From an Osteopathic Standpoint.

BY A. T. STILL.

The work of the dental surgeon has not received the attention of osteopaths that its importance to the health of the body merits.

As a matter of fact, dental surgery ranks ahead of operative surgery as the operative surgeon only removes defects, while the dental surgeon's work is to care for the mouth and keep it in the best possible condition for speech and mastication.

Proper mastication of food is essential to the health of the body, as digestion, assimilation and nutrition are dependent upon it.

This calls for a thorough knowledge of the muscles of the face and jaws, with their nerve and blood supply, as well as a knowledge of the teeth and maxillary bones.

The neck should also receive the careful attention of the dentist, for in the neck the track of life is laid. Here pass the nerves that supply every part of the body the head

The neck should also receive the careful attention of the dentist, for the in neck the track of life is laid. Here pass the nerves that supply every part of the body below the head, furnishing the force necessary to the proper functioning of every organ in the body, thus accomplishing their duty of supplying sensation, motion and nutrition to the organism.

To the student of anatomy and physiology it is undebatable that the health of the body depends upon a perfectly normal neck; thus the importance of a knowledge of the bones, their form, position and how they support the head. With this as a foundation, it is but reasonable and just that we insist that our dental surgeons know the anatomy of the whole body and the ill effects of displacements in the neck and how to correct any injuries he may accidentally inflict in his work of extracting teeth.

In extracting a large tooth, the dentist gets his left arm about the patient's head to steady it, while his right hand holds the forceps which give an additional leverage to the arm of from four to six inches. He pries and pulls until the tooth comes out, when there is an abrupt disconnection between the tooth and the jaw. At that instant occurs the danger of dislocating the neck at some point. The patient feels no pain only at the tooth, so pays the fee and goes away happy, thinking his sufferings are permanently relieved.

But the next morning, all is changed. He gets up with a headache and dizziness; or he tries to read and finds the letters blurred. Occasionally, a patient finds one side of his face drawn out of shape. The family doctor is called in, who says, "You have had a stroke of paralysis." The doctor does not know enough of anatomy to tell his patient that the dentist has dislocated his neck. The dentist is also blissfully ignorant of what he has done. His school has not demanded a thorough knowledge of the anatomy of the human body, neither has the public realized his need of it.

It is the purpose of this brief article to call the attention of the student of osteopathy to the dangers to the patient from employing an ignorant dentist and the possibility of injury to the nerves of the face, neck, lungs, heart and abdominal viscera,. causing disease, either local or constitutional

Can you slip an atlas to the right or to the left, backward or forward and not compress a nerve or blood vessel going to or from the brain? Can you slip any bone of the neck and not compress an important nerve? If not, then you have the cause of enlarged tonsils, goitre, tumors of the neck, diseases of the tongue, mouth, trachea, œsophagus, heart, lungs, and the more common effects of enlarged lymphatics, eruptions on the face and loss of hair. For example, a slip in the neck might put a pressure on the cardiac nerves producing a confusion, manifested by increased, intermittent or decreased heart action. Or the displacement might disturb the nerve to the respiratory system resulting in stagnation of fluids in the lungs.

Should we continue our investigations, we would find that there is no part of the body but would be effected by a cervical displacement. Then how important it is, that any one having anything to do with the care of the body, be he an osteopath or a dentist, should know when the neck is normal and how to correct it when it is abnormal.

But it must not be inferred that I consider the dentist responsible for all neck dislocations. I am only emphasizing the fact that he has unwillingly had a part in their production; a part that has too long been unnoted by osteopaths. In other cases of dislocations of the neck, osteopaths are accustomed to get a history of falls, sudden jerks, running against wires or slips on ice. But I have found that in addition to these accidental causes, a great per cent. of the cases can date the beginning of their illness from the time they required a dentist's services. I have had many cases of facial neuralgia, loss of sight or hearing, facial paralysis and dislocations of the inferior mixillary and cervical bones, that could be traced to the dentist. And how frequently do we hear of a broken drill being left in the cavity of a tooth which is afterward covered up with a filling and left to torture the patient and cause abscesses, or a necrosis of the bone?

In conclusion, I wish to say a few words further in regard to the mechanical duties of a dentist. Of all mechanics, he should be the most accurate; but it seems he too often thinks more of the polish and the appearance of a set of teeth, than he does of the fit, comfort and use. Should the sufferer complain, he is told to be patient, that the mouth will soon become accustomed to the use of the plate.

What would we think of a carpenter, who was called to fit a board in an opening in the floor and should leave one end of the board above the level of the floor and should say, "Never mind; the floor will adjust itself to the board in the course of a few months?" The dentist would discharge any carpenter that would do such imperfect work on his floor.

But the carpenter's course would be just as rational as that too often pursued by the dentist in making a plate for a patient that fits imperfectly and when asked to improve on it, says, "Just keep right on wearing it and your mouth will soon get accustomed to it." Is he unreasonable enough to suppose that the jaw will change to fit the plate? On the contrary, I affirm from over thirty years experience with crippled jaws, that a plate should be so well fitted that a patient may go home and at once be able to eat his dinner, comfortably instead of living on broths for six months. But all too frequently, the patient goes on suffering month in and month out from the ill-fitting plate, the result of the unpardonable ignorance and stupidity of the dentist. At last, his patience is exhausted and he puts the plate away in the bureau drawer; and it is only after he is dead that he is able to wear it permanently.

In this day of scientific investigation, the dentist should remember that he is before the grand jury of progressive intelligence, which may report a true bill of indictment for anatomical and physiological ignorance as the cause of an unlimited number of diseases following injuries received in his office.

* * *

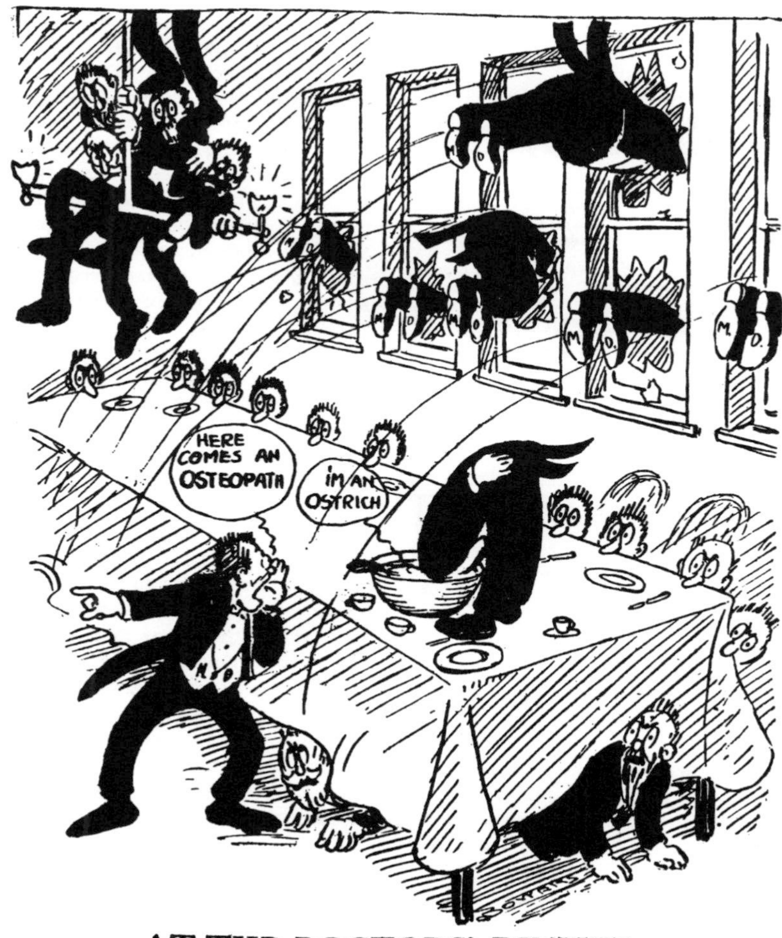

AT THE DOCTORS' DINNER

January, 1905

The Use of the Knowledge of Chemistry to the Osteopath.

A knowledge of chemistry gives the student of osteopathy to understand that by chemical union all substances that appear in the body have been compounded and are prepared by the laboratory of the body from crude substances taken into the body when the work begins with the food and proceeds to atomize, separate, combine and form a compound of all elements that enter into the structure of man's body. That compound, blood, contains bone, muscle, nerve, hair and teeth. The how and why is beyond man's power of rearon and he fails to be able to make any compounds that make a tooth, bone, muscle or hair, a drop of blood, nerve or fat. The laboratory of life makes and uses all but we cannot even imitate an atom of that great manufactory of blood and flesh. One says, why study chemistry if we cannot use it? We teach chemistry in our school hoping that the knowledge the student gets by studying chemical affinity and action will help him to know that living man is only a chemical laboratory in action, from birth to déath, and its good work is life and health and its bad work is sickness and death, and if the doctor keeps the laboratory in good shape to do its work, then he can hope for good results. But if he has no knowledge of elementry chemistry, he fails to be successful as a manager of the machinery of the physiological laboratory. Thus he fails to be able to relieve many cases that would be easily cured if he knew how the body formed blood and other substances and how the blood was taken to and from each part of the body. Some would tell you that you must learn chemistry in order to pass state examinations. That is not why we teach chemistry, but to make successful thinkers, so you can get the good of the machinery that the body has in it for its preservation and repair. You are not supposed to be the makers of blood, bone and flesh any more than a locomotive engineer is supposed to make wood and coal. Your job is to put wood or coal in the furnace, open the supply and drainage pipes, fire up, light your pipes, stand back and look and listen. If it runs right you can do no more than to feed and water.

A. T. Still.

* * *

December, 1907

PNEUMONIA.

A. T. STILL.

Dr. Still has been in better health than for some time, and desires to present a message to the osteopaths. He says that in winter is the time to talk about winter diseases and presents the following talk on one of the most dreaded of the maladies of this season.—Ed.

I think it is well enough to offer a few thoughts on pneumonia, notwithstanding millions of pens have been worn out in trying to say something pertaining to this subject; thoughts that would make one advance step towards combating such a deadly enemy as it has proved to be during all the years of the past as the records show. The reader who desires to obtain some knowledge of what it is and what has produced it finds nothing satisfactory whatever from any author up to the present date.

Pneumonia, enlarged tonsils, inflammation of the trachea, or of the whole pulmonary system, according to any author that I can find, is just as little understood, if their pens have recorded their best knowledge, as their treatment is and it proves itself to be deficient as though nothing had been written, in fact the methods of treatment are just as unreliable as the landing of a vessel would be without a compass to guide it. The medical doctor proves his inability to combat successfully any of these diseases by the percentage of his patients who die, compared with those who do not. He has brought in all the remedies known, and used them with the hope that some accidental dose might give him a compass that would guide him in future successful combats with lung diseases. He has labored and sweated in the laboratory wherein he thinks he has found some ray of light which would give him a better comprehension how to proceed, subdue the disease and save his patient, but alas, his patient dies in spite of all his efforts. He has tried the old, the new, the hot, the cold, the sedative, the stimulant, and the various kinds of gases, but the result is just the same, and I think it always will be until a competent engineer comes who is acquainted with all the parts of the human body. This one realizes that the constriction is generally caused by atmospheric changes and proceeds to take down or remove any pressure from the nervous system at any point from the base of the skull to coccyx that would produce any constricture of the nervous system and stop the flow of venous blood to the heart, which delay would be followed by stagnation, fermentation and destructive decomposition. You must remember that a chemical process soon begins in the venous blood, while not in motion is far from being pure, and continues until the blood becomes poisonous in quality and overplus in quantity, engorging the lungs with such impure blood that it is impossible for them to separate the impure from the pure and return a sufficient quantity of arterial blood, which shall have all the constructive ability that should belong to a healthy circulation. Thus you see the engineer must look at pneumonia as an effect, the cause being a tightening of all parts of the whole system, by the constriction which begins with variation in the atmosphere. To the engineer who understands his engine as an osteopath should, all the mysteries disappear, the law of cause and effect is understood, and he governs himself accordingly and his patient will get well if he has taken the case reasonably early.

When we shall have proved that the competent engineer of the human body is a failure in diseases of the lungs, the pluræ, the tonsils, and all the organs of the respiratory tract, then we will run up the white flag of defeat and join the medical world and cry aloud that we know nothing of the cause or cure of disease of the lungs.

This talk is intended for the consideration of the student or practitioner of osteopathy; the philosophy that health is the result of a perfectly adjusted body and that disease (with contagions and infections excepted) follows and is the result of the failure of the osteopathic engineer to know and to obtain the normal position of every bone, muscle and nerve. My experience for thirty years has been "Yes" and I hope every osteopath will go deep enough into the science to say "Yes" also, and let his work stand as a voucher.

* * *

DEPARTMENT OF DR. STILL.

Tumors—When this subject is brought before the anatomical mechanic's eye, he takes a look, makes a mental note of the size, location, appearance and color of all unnatural growths found in the human body. He knows just what each tumor is called because he reads the label which is attached to each one. By the marks of discrimination one is called malignant, another benign, another cancer, another fibrinous, another rose cancer, another cystic tumor, etc.

Right here the anatomist or physiologist who reasons as a life preserver says to the bloody host of surgeons, "I am president and legally empowered to demand of and accept nothing from nor tolerate any interference by any one's knife who cannot give a demonstrable reason why this abnormal growth has been produced; what important nerve of vaso-constriction or vaso-dilation has been prohibited from executing its work of normal construction and renovation to the degree of normal health."

Tremblingly this engineer approaches the human body under the penalty of pain and death for spilling a single drop of blood or removing an atom of flesh before he, the repairing engineer, shows and demonstrates that he has found and pointed out the absolute cause that has produced this abnormally constructed thing or tumor. Knowing his duty, and the penalty for a hasty conclusion and malpractice is death, he becomes an earnest seeker and a safe man to turn loose in the abdomen as an explorer who can find and demonstrate that he knows the cause of cancers or tumefactions of any or all of the organs of the human body. The order under which he explores, demands wisdom and honesty, or death is the penalty.

Thus saith the Czar of the government under which this mechanic labors, and there is no appeal from the edict. And as Christ did, so shall he work without money or price.

If such were the law of our land, speculative murder would soon be abolished and no longer cause the hundreds of thousands of funerals and millions of yards of mourning crape which is hung at the door of almost every city and village in North America and other countries. I want to insist that the time is fully ripe for legislative interference to stop the unwarranted use of the knife. I want to emphasize with vehemence that he who cannot demonstrate that he has found and that he knows the cause producing such malady, and that the hasty surgeon who is wasting human life simply for the dollar that he can extort from the unfortunate sufferer or his friends by pretending to know the cause and use the knife of death, should hang. Send a few such to the gallows and to the State prison for life, for murder, and this world will soon have surgery take its meritorious place. Give the surgeon of merit a reasonable reward fixed by law for his services, then we will have honest dealing with human life and not before.

It is horrifying to think that we are living in a day and generation that sees nothing sacred in human life. I think it is time for legislation and legal interference to take command and regulate our system of surgery or we will soon become an extinct race. If others think differently you will please use the pen and ink and tell us something better than that which I have written on this subject.

Following this prelude we think we can give you something that will assist the osteopath in leaving the old rut of antiquated customs and learn to hunt for and know the cause of causes, producing tumors of the head, neck, thorax, abd men, mammary glands and all organs and limbs of the human body. I care nothing for analyzing the fluids of the body which are perverted by prohibitory and stagnant action of the circulatory and purifying system of the organs of the human body. My question is, what is the remote cause? How do you know your conclusion is true, and demonstrate that what you say is a truth. You should study until you can do this or quit. Right here I will draw the attention of the reader to the blood supply of the abdomen and its organs, with the accompanying nerve forces and see if we cannot arrive at a satisfactory knowledge of the cause of such effects, tumors.—A. T. S.

PLAIN TALK ON OSTEOPATHY TO ALL RANKS, FROM THE FRESHMAN TO THE DEAN OF THE FACULTY AND PRESIDENT OF THE CORPORATION.

I want the lamp light of reason to be before your eyes in all steps and places while you sojourn with me from the day you enter the school as a student, a professor, president or trustee. I want you to remember that this school is not intended to receive and treat with respect anything but truth with the fact of demonstration as its voucher. I want it definitely understood that undemonstrated talk from any professor in this school of engineers from the president down to the sexton, is an illegitimate child, and is not welcome in the engine room of this institution. You must show the practical ability in all your lectures in chemistry, physiology, anatomy, theory and practice, obstetrics and surgeryy. You must demonstrate as a chemist while talking to the class and supplying them with chemical knowledge, that the human body has a class and teaches it, proving that in the human body is a chemical laboratory also. I want the anatomist to teach and demonstrate to his class that a knowledge of aatomy prepares them to show the skill of a mechanic in adjusting the human body from the abnormal to the normal, and that without a good knowledge of all the parts of the body no engineer has any claim above a pretender for he will be a failure when called upon to inspect and adjust the human body or to tell what has produced an abnormal growth whether in the body, head or limbs. If he knows his business he will tell where the obstruction is that has produced paralysis or excitement of the nervous system, and show you why abnormal growth is the result. If he does not do this he is not worthy of the place he claims to fill.

The mid-wife or obstetrician must know the part that he is dealing with. The "hows" and "whys" of all vital action that is necessary to construct and deliver the child which is a completed engine to be given to the world for the use and purpose for which it was designed. He has no business here without this knowledge.

The osteopathic surgeon, when dealing with tumors, must not spend his time analyzing blood,urine and other fluids taken from a diseased system until he has found and demonstrated that he knows the producing cause of atrophy, over-growth or any failure in the motor system from the crown of the head to the sole of the foot. He might might as well analyze the fluids of a slop barrel, or from the vaults of a privy in order to know what was eaten a week before as to spend his time in this way. His duty is to know the cause of this confusion in the chemical laboratory of life and adjust from the abnormal to the truly normal. If he knows his business and proceeds as an engineer, he will, if called to a patient in reasonable time, soon find that the mud valves will open and conduct the overplus from the body and leave the patient without a tumor. I want to say in conclusion, that if you know your business the world will not call you an unworthy blank as an engineer and say that osteopathy is not the truth and its advocates are liars.

* * *

TRIBULATION.

Let us pray! O, Lord, Thou knowest that the highest aspiration of an osteopath is heaven and an automobile. Thou knowest their daily prayer is that their professional hours will not intrude on their devotional hours in the West as they have in the East. When thou didst make man and endow him with reason thou didst know that he would soon learn that Thy work was so perfectly well done that all the days of mortality would be too short for man to get anything like a comprehensive knowledge of the laws of life in the plan, specification, construction and work of man who is the result of union of human life with matter, in form. Now Lord Thou knowest that our days are few and full of sorrow. Thou knowest just as well that when we try to get some knowledge of life and its attributes that we fall to pieces in disgust when we read from fifteen to fifty pages on tumors, the production, the cause and cure, written and published in the A. O. A., or any other periodical; and after carefully perusinge very page, every paragraph, sentence and word, only find that it is nothing but a school boy's little piece written and compiled from various authors, ancient and modern, both in Europe and America. I say, as a mechanical osteopath, I am disgusted to know that so many of our writers think that such compilations show to us the scholarly ability of the writer, when he has before his eyes all the parts of the human body constituting the most perfect machine for the production and delivery of blood and for sustaining life. O, Lord, Thou knowest that a few of us seek knowledge that we can use; that we can prove what we say is the truth by demonstrating that we know friction in the machinery of life produces a perversion of the normal action of the nervous system on raw material from the mouth to the living blood which is sent forth by the arterial system. Thou knowest that we know that a day's talk falls to the ground from the hand of the philosopher who reasons from effect to cause and substantiates his philosophy by the fact of demonstration. O, Lord, we know that Thou quotest no authority from any American or foreign writer. When Thou talkest, Thou speakest in plain English and talked to the point when Thou workest, Thou quietly proceedeth to plan, specify and construct the machinery that testifies to Thy ability as a wise and correct architect without which no theory is worth the paper it is written on. Thou knowest that the osteopath who has brains enough to reason, if he acquaints himself with the normal machine of life will then and there know the abnormal that has caused the tumor. It matters not what guise they come under, malignant or benign. Thou knowest that if we wish to be acquainted with Thy work we must go into the human body and acquaint ourselves with the plan, specification, and the object of the superstructure. Then when we write if we dip our pens into the red ink of demonstrable truth we will be respected for what we know, not what we say was the opinion of some writer who always winds up the story with a "however," or "possibly so." Thou knowest, O Lord, that our osteopathic periodicals, some of them, make more fuss than all of Pharoh's frogs, and the next day music comes from the same old stagnant pond. O, Lord, Thou knowest that it is very hard work to find a trustworthy professor to teach and demonstrate the truths of osteopathy in our schools. Thou knowest that the professor who talks must do and demonstrate, or he is not worthy of the position of the surgeon, the obstetrician, the physiologist, and the healer. All of which he should demonstrate by doing the work. O, Lord, Thou knowest we have some registered stock, mentally sharp, that will both talk and do before the eyes of the spectator that which will demonstrate to the world that osteopathy is a trustworthy science.—Amen.

* * *

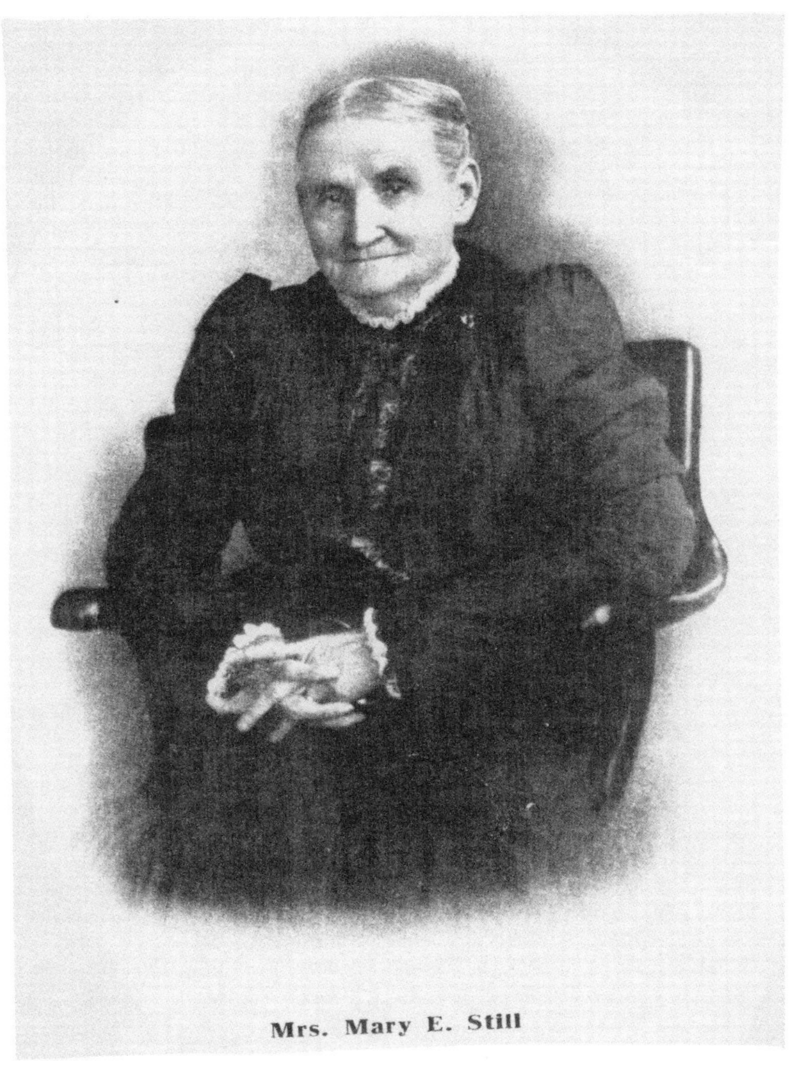

Mrs. Mary E. Still

July, 1908

A PARALLEL.

BY WM. HANNA THOMPSON., M. D. LL. D., Physician to Roosevelt Hospital, Consulting Physician to N. Y. State Manhatten Hospital for the Insane, Formerly Professor of the Practice of Medicine and Diseases of the Nervous system, New York University Medical College, Ex-President of the New York Academy of Medicine, etc., author of "Brain and Personality." In July Everybody's, page 102.

"A specimen of these additions to our knowledge is a fact that among many other things the sympathetic (one division of the nervous system—Ed.) ACTUALLY MAKES DRUGS or true medicine, whose presence in the blood is essential to life. ***It is now generally agreed among physiological chemists that we daily manufacture enough in our alimentary canal to kill us before the day is over were it not that these poisons are neutralized by the liver and other organs before they can enter the blood, and thus reach the brain and other vital parts of the nervous system***extirpating the solar plexus the animal then dying with symptoms closely resembling those of Asiatic Cholera with its profuse rice water discharges. As the micro-organism of cholera never enters the blood, but instead goes in the intestines where it secretes its deadly poison to be then absorbed and thus quickly reach the solar plexus it seems to be a fair inference that it kills chiefly by paralizing that important nerve center with a resultant intestinal flow which drains the blood of its water.

BY ANDREW T. STILL, M. D., Founder of Osteopathy. In the January Ladies' Home Journal.

"I believe that God has placed a remedy for every disease within the material house in which the spirit of life dwells. I believe that the maker of man has deposited in some part or throughout the whole system of the human body drugs in abundance to cure all infirmities; that all the remedies necessary to health are compounded within the human body. They can be administered by adjusting the body in such manner that the remedies will naturally associate themselves together. ***I do not believe that there are such diseases as fever,—typhoid, typhus, or lung—rheumatism, sciatica, gout, colic, liver disease, croup, or any of the present so called diseases, they do not exist as diseases. I hold that separate or combined they are only effects of cause, and that in each case the cause can be found and does exist. In the limited or excited action of the nerves which control the fluid or a part of or of the entire body. My position is, that the living blood swarms with health corpuscles which are carried to all parts of the body.***The result would be a restoration of physiological functioning from disease to health."

DEPARTMENT OF A. T. STILL.

BONES.

The Normal Articulation: The Abnormal Position and Its Effects on General Health.

If the normal position and relation of every bone from the crown of the head to the sole of the foot is a condition necessary to good health, what variations from a socket, facet, or any joint, will be the cause of some progressive disease, such as the fever, tuberculosis, or inflammation of any joint of the neck, back, loin, hip, legs or arms? Can not you, as an engineer with your knowledge, see that a twist of a bone from its normal position, would carry a muscle that is fastened at both ends, backwards and forwards sufficiently far to produce an unnatural crossing of those fibrous strands, muscles or tendons, that unite a rib with the spinous process and other points? Don't you see that there is a great strain, and irritation at the point where one muscle crosses another? Don't you reason that normal vital action is suspended from this point back to the spinal cord or ganglion from which the nerve of this muscle is sent off, and beyond this point this vital action is a failure? As an engineer you see friction, as a philosopher you conclude there is an obstruction, and as a mechanic you remove the obstruction by so adjusting the bone that no strain is on the muscle causing it to press on another muscle, blood vessel, ligament or nerve.

When you are combating effects, such as diseases of the scalp, brain, eye, ear, tongue, throat, lung, heart, liver, spleen, pancreas, stomach, bowels, kidneys, bladder, womb, or limbs, you will arise at a trustworthy, conclusion as to cause, if you use the method of reasoning just outlined. There is no part that I have named but which if affected by disease does not present a philosophical question to be answered by the engineer, and not by the imitator or masseur. The friction or cause that has produced the disease must be removed, and normality established, an honest, thoroughbred, well qualified engineer knows from his experience and qualification that all variations from normal action in an engine have different causes, and the friction of a pulley should never be treated at the steam chest. He must have the power of brain to hold perpetually a perfectly normal image of any part of the human system before his eyes, then he can judge just what is the cause of the malady he has to contend with. Here is a list of leading questions to ask the mechanical critic, the philosopher, and the engineer who can trace from the effect or friction to the cause producing such effects: Why do one person's eyes become, by congestion, abnormally large and a constant stream of tears pass from them? Where is the friction responsible for this unnatural appearance of the eye? Would you go to nerve and blood supply of the eye for the cause, or would you cut those eyes out, and throw them away? If you have polypus, or adenoid, tumors of the nose, would you take the prongs and pull out some nose this month and some more nose every other month, or would you go to the nerve and blood supply and the drainage, and regulate them? If you were consulted on a case of enlarged tonsils would you take your knife out of your belt, whack them off, and throw them away, or would you go to the atlas and axis as a sensible engineer, and give nature a chance to reduce the tonsil to its normal condition? You must know first, last, and all the time that if the blood could have passed to and from the head without obstruction there would be no tumor. Suppose there should be inflammation and soreness of the trachea and esophagus, would an engineer account for the friction by imperfect blood and nerve action, or would he swab the throat with destructive caustic and other poisonings? Would an osteopath accept such conclusion or action as the truth, or would he book such proceedure as ignorance and malpractice? Suppose an engineer who knows his business is consulted on what is known as pleuro-pneumonia, and the lungs are laboring under much excitement and congestion, would that engineer fire up with hot water bags, administer morphine, whiskey, digitalis, strychnine, or would he explore the spine, and ribs from the diaphragm to the head for slips, strains, and partial dislocations of the bones of the neck to know why this shut off from the blood and nerve supply and to know why the pneumogastric could not do its normal work and allow the blood to pass to and from the brain, pleurae and lungs? An engineer that knows his business does not hesitate to proceed at once to adjust all parts of the neck, and passing down from the head and neck he adjusts all parts to the dorsal. Would he be satisfied to stop his work knowing to a certainty that the clavicular articulation is absolutely correct, or would he leave it sufficiently far back of the acromion process to shut off the jugular vein so that it could not deliver venous blood to the heart? He knows that he is dealing with a train that is running very fast, and from the condition of the road it will soon be ditched if he does not adjust his engine, and do it very quickly. His object is perfect drainage from the head, face, neck, pleuræ, lungs, intercostals, and all parts of the thoracic division. He knows that if all pressure is removed from the pneumogastric harmony will follow in its action; that when the resistance caused by closure at the point where the internal carotid enters the head is taken off the unnecessary labors of the arterial system will stop because the veins, or mud valves, or doing trustworthy work. Then breathing and heart action becomes normal. Relief and recovery is sure to follow if the engineer knows and does his business.

Mr. Engineer, allow me to ask you in conclusion a few more questions that I think are of the greatest importance to the success of the Science of Osteopathy. I have asked you questions in reference to the head, face, eyes, neck and organs of the thorax, and I think you are worthy and well qualified to take charge and safely run this engine so far as the organs above the diaphragm are concerned. Now a few hasty questions in reference to the liver: When the nerve and blood supply to this important organ is good, is that all that is necessary for it to do good work? You say, Yes. Give me nerve force blood supply, drainage, and plenty of nourishing diet, and I will guarantee the results to be good and satisfactory. Suppose there should be enlargements of the liver, what conclusion would you come to? I would say at once, if there is no mechanical injury to contend with, that a failure of the venous drainage causes this congestion and overgrowth; would you suggest purgatives, stimulants, dietetics, going to the mountain, pukes, blisters, and hot bags? I would not, I would explore all nerve and blood supply and drainage of the whole hepatic system. I would correct all bony abnormalities, give my partients rest, plenty of good wholesome food, and expect soon to have a liver normal in all particulars, provided I am called in reasonable time, and the patient is not exhausted, and disabled from poisonous drugs. The same rule is just as good and trustworthy in diseases of the spleen, pancreas, stomach, bowels, kidneys, uterus, bladder and limbs. The whole of this discourse has been with an engineer, first water, and no superficial conglomerate of unqualified maybe-so's.

* * *

THE HORROR OF HORRORS.

Pap Ate Bacon and Beans for Dinner—This Dream is the Result.

I dreamed that my spirit was about to bid farewell to my old frame, and take its flight to that world of eternal joy. I thought I soon would see all my friends, and dance with them in the great halls of the New Jerusalem, and when I had left my body and looked upon it for the last time I said, "Well done thou good and faithful old carcas, rest in peace for all ages." Then as I thought of meeting Father and Mother and the countless host of millions of great and good persons from my boyhood to my old age my heart leaped with joy, my eyes gushed forth rivers of hopeful tears. Oh, how happy was that moment. I was handed a compass by some angelic friend, stating that this would take me to my heavenly abode, and I would meet Peter at the Golden Gate that would open to joys immortal. After resting awhile from the labors from my spirit getting out of the old body I picked up the compass that was to guide me to the gates of Heaven. I have no language to describe the emotional feeling of my heart. It seemed that I was heart all over, and that it was full of gladness without any further description of the emotional. I examined my compass for a minute and it pointed to a place that was inscribed "Paradise." In the twinkle of an eye I was at the gate, halted by a guard. He asked my business. I told him I wanted to enter the heavenly city, and would like to see Peter. He conducted me to Peter, who said, "Who are you?" I gave him my name, birth, religion and politics. He asked me what my profession was. I told him I was a doctor. He pointed his finger to a dark room. O! the horror, and said, That room belongs to medical doctors and other feeble minded people. I told him I had nothing to do with medicine, except the drugs manufactured in the laboratory constructed by the infinite. He said, What drugs do you use as a remedy in diseases? I told him that arterial blood was the remedy of the God of the Universe, that Great Architect, whose plan and building was perfection in all particulars, and that I was a mechanic and had studied and treated the human body as a mechanic should, and for forty years I had used the blood of life in all cases and under all circumstances. He says, "Are you an allopath doctor?" I said, "No, verily I make no drunkards, no morphine eaters. I take no human life as an experimenter with the knife of surgery and pretended wisdom. I believe the God of the Universe has the best knife to remove obstructions, and reconstruct from the abnormal to the truly normal living man, and the laboratory of nature to me is wonderful in its preparation, its method of construction, its power and motion, both in mind and body, and the ability of that architect to show the head, arm and hand of intelligence." He said, "What school are you from?" I told him the Amercan School of Osteopathy. He says, "Are you the founder to that school?" I told him, "Yea, verily, I am." He said, "By what name is that school known, and what are the names of the doctors that are educated in that school?" I told him osteopaths. I told him the School of Osteopathy is the place where we teach the structure of the normal man and show the abnormal man also. He says, "A few osteopaths have come, and all had been admitted, and as you are the originator, teacher and practitioner of that great and truthful science, I want you to be seated in my room. I am proud to know that one man has given the Great Architect of the Universe some credit for his ability as an architect and builder of man with perfection in health, in disease and all other particulars that is absolute and says, 'Well done thou good and faithful servant.' I am so proud to know that one doctor is able and willing to give God some credit for intelligence in all places."

* * *

July, 1908

THE TOOLS OF A MECHANICAL INSPECTOR.

It is expected that the mechanic will give a critical examination, and a trustworthy report of such examination. He has a square, a plumb, and a level. By the square he ascertains the fact that all parts are in line, and any variation is told at once when the square is applied to a journal. With a level he ascertains whether all corners are on a level, and equal; so far his foundation is square, and level, he has one more witness, the plumb, that tells whether the superstructure stands perfectly erect, or leans to one side or the other. He squares, plumbs, and levels all foundations, journals, and boxings. Then he plumbs his machineryand all that holds it in place, then he examines all pulleys to know that they are in place and in position, then he examines the belts to know if one side of the belt is longer than the other. He corrects and goes on. When he has finished all parts by the square, the level and the plumb, he then goes to the engine with the same instruments in his hand, inspects, squares, and levels the foundation that supports the engine, then with the square and plumb he adjusts drive wheels, pulleys and journals, he inspects all pipes conducting water to his boiler and all pipes conducting steam to the chest. He is just as particular to square, plumb and level all parts in this department. He proceeds to examine safety and mud valves to know that they are ready to do normal work. Then he inspects the furnace to know that all is in proper order here, and in condition to throw the greatest amount of heat to the boiler. After having corrected all parts by the square, the plumb, and the level, he fires up, starts the engine, and if the answer is perfect work he knows that he has done his duty. and for fear that something may give away such as a pulley slipping on a journal and not doing good work he keeps his eye on the machinery for a few hours or days, that he may feel satisfied to leave it in the hands of a local engineer. He would tell you at once that no inspector can afford to take charge of any machinery and not square, plumb and level his work when he expects good or normal work. He knows where and how power is generated, how applied, and the uses of all parts of the machinery. Can an osteopath afford to ignore this sacred truth when called upon to inspect and find and correct the cause of such friction as will result in imperfect action of the powers and principles of the human body? As a mechanic I say "No." His talk and work will prove him to be a dangerous personage to intrust with the sacred work of life in all departments of the human body. This subject is too serious not to come under the most crucial and exact requirements that human skill is master of. If a mechanic is so particular as to inspect every part and principle belonging to a steam engine which you see he doesi n detaill, for the purpose of getting good results, can you as an engineer, omit any bone in the body, hand or arm, and claim to be a trustworthy engineer, and say this has no importance in a philosophical demand of the greatest engines ever produced—the engine of human life? The student is to remember the responsibility hanging over his head when he is in the sick room. * * *

September, 1908

ADDRESS OF WELCOME.

A. T. Still

While for years I fought the battles of osteopathy alone, meeting great opposition and villification, I knew I had the truth, and that truth was immortal, and that some day the principles of osteopathy would be hailed with gladness throughout the earth. Those principles are in harmony with the great laws of God as seen in nature, that is, proper adjustment and freedom to act. Osteopathy deals with the body as a perfect machine which if kept in proper adjustment, nourished and cared for, will run smoothly into ripe and useful old age. As long as the human machine is in order, like the locomotive or any other mechanical product, it will perform the function which it should. When every part of the machine is correctly adjusted and in perfect harmony, health will hold dominion over the human organism by laws as natural and immutable as the laws of gravity. Every living organism has within it the power to manufacture and prepare all chemicals, and forces needed to build and rebuild itself. No material other than nutritious food taken into the system in proper quantity and quality can be introduced from the outside without deteriment. A proper adjustment of the bony framework and the soft structures of man's anatomical mechanism means good digestion, nutrition and fluid circulation, health and happiness.

Osteopathy is not a theory but a demonstrated fact. You say there are some failures. Yes, who would not expect it. You are called to treat people who have been poisoned and diseased beyond the possibility of anything except a little temporary relief, or perhaps the osteopath is not able properly to apply the knowledge he should have before being granted a diploma from an osteopathic school. This reflects no more upon the science of osteopathy than the farmer who fails does upon the science of farming. Again many are looking for miracles and are disappointed when a few treatments fail to bring wonted strength and vigor.

I hope no speaker, upon this or any other occasion will refer to me as a martyr. I don't belong to that exalted class. I have simply been permitted to grasp a great truth and have been favored with opportunity to develop it and give it to the world. It has been a pleasure and I do not consider that I have been a martyr.

* * *

June, 1909

REMARKS BY DR. A. T. STILL.

Ladies, gentlemen, visitors, friends, and enemies, simple and wise, theorists and practitioners:—All I want to say is that I am glad to see you and a little sorry that I don't feel as well to-day as I have sometimes, but I never was so sick that I could not think. Thirty-five years ago, I had seen so much of nature's work vindicating the perfection of the unknown Architect of the universe, that I concluded that I would criticise the work. For thirty-five years I have inspected as a critic, as an educated mechanic, which I claim to be, as a man of age and experience in all parts of the human body. I have tried all my life to find one single mark of convicting evidence that the God of nature was a failure. I have failed. On that foundation that God as we understand Him is an Architect, He is a Mechanic, He is a Builder, He is an Engineer, and His work is done on the machinery of the universe as an Engineer. It runs on time, no jumping of tracks ever appears in the motion of any planet. It is on time and in place. And I would also repeat to you, that, that Architect in all of His book of healing is absolutely true and trustworthy, and does His work to perfection on all organs and divisions of the whole body and thus we have a Drugless Healer.

Coming to the human body, the question was if he was also a doctor, but not such as we have to-day. I idolized the doctor, because I had been taught to reason that the pill doctor was a product of God's intelligence. I found that he used poisons and the products of chemical laboratories in place of the human laboratory itself, the living chemist. I began to reason, what is the human body, the human laboratory, can it make its own drugs. I saw that the baby was healthy if you gave it just milk. I reasoned again, and found that all disease except in infectious and in contagious diseases, could be managed very easily by mere mechanics and directed by a qualified head. I found that pneumonia, that dread disease would yield and stop in a few minutes, and the question came up, what is responsible for this condition called pneumonia? The respiration must be without oppression, the respiratory nerve and blood vessels, must be without impingement at any point. What is responsible for heart trouble? It is the oppression of some obstruction on the cardiac nerves. When we find lameness in a man's walk—what is wrong? What is re-sponsi ble for the limp; is the hip from the socket? I say yes, in the majority of cases.

Is stammering an effect? Is it a cause? Can you remove the cause, the doctor says? I said yes. Verily, I say unto you. Bring me a stuttering boy, and I will show you, here is one (example of stuttering). Now John I will stop that. I want you to say the words directly after me. Fill your lungs full as you can, get more, more, more, "Hoorah," say that, John, "Hoorah." Don't you see you can shoot better with a loaded gun than an empty one. The respiratory and vocal nerves fail together when there is no air in the lungs. The doctors came in and all examined to see what I had done with John. I said, "John, load up and shoot. Now fill up, John, when did you come here?" "Last month, say that." "John can you speak any other language but the English language?" "Yes." Give us some talk then, load up now and follow me, "Hic non est morator—decede." Without a quiver John said "Hic non est morator—decede." I said, "What is that in English?" He said, "This is no place for loafers." So ended the trouble of stuttering with John.

This same thing is true in asthma, in nerve disturbances, and I am going to tell you we are now after tuberculosis. We have found that paralysis of the pneumogastric is responsible for tuberculosis, because of the bony obstructions, which result in paralysis of the nerves of the pulmonary system, and allow the blood that should pass on and off, to stagnate, ferment and deposit its cheesy matter in the cells of the lungs. Thus the mechanic can give you a reason why tuberculosis is produced and save the life of his patient.

I have talked before this class often. I feel that they are now capable of listening and knowing what I say and know whether what I say is true or false! Now we used to have an old cow bell and I remember I got tired of hearing it,—You have listened to this bell for three years, and I think that is long enough. I will proceed to give you your tickets to pass out, and I want to tell you all goodbye and shake hands—hands up—all together—shake. Good Bye.

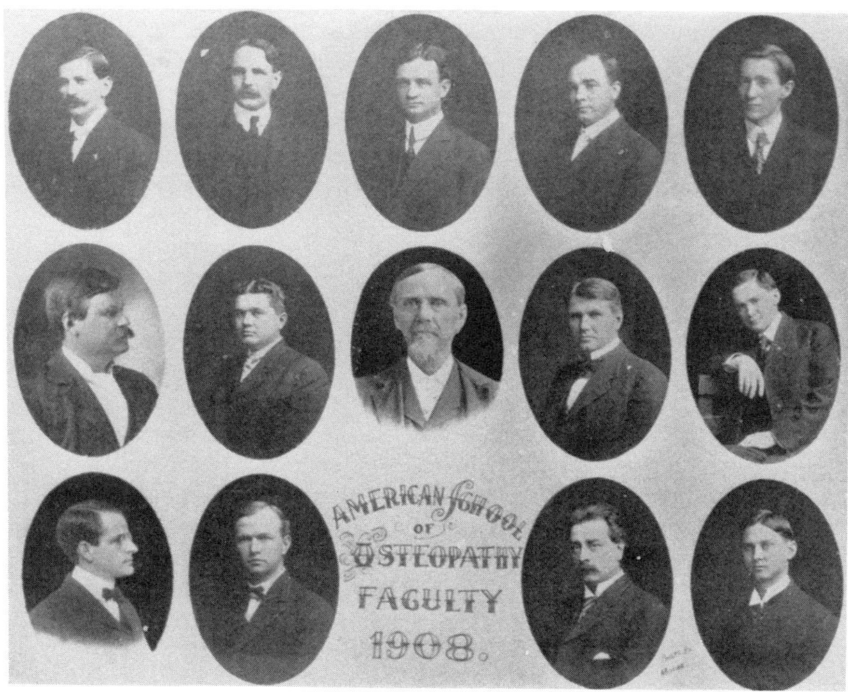

An Open Letter to the Profession.

Dear Boys and Girls:—

It should be the intention of all up-to-date physicians, regardless of School to keep abreast of the times. Most of the States at present are requiring the equal of a four year high school certificate before one can make application for an examination to practice their profession. Under such a rule and without an endowment it is only through the combined efforts of their friends that Schools young as the Osteopathic can exist. It is the intention of the Management of the A. S. O. to undertake this, hence this letter.

We hope to have the co-operation of all our graduates and friends. We appreciate the fact that some of the best men in our profession, as in all professions, have not had the advantage in school that the States are demanding at the present time, but be that as it may, it is up to us to meet the demands.

The January Class of 1910 will probably be the last class that will matriculate at the A. S. O. where the student is not required to have a four year high school education, or the equivalent, so if you have any friends that are contemplating taking up the study of osteopathy, not having the above requirements, we will be very much pleased to have them enroll with our coming January Class.

To say we appreciate everything in the way of encouragement and endorsement that we have received from our graduates in the field is putting it very mildly. I know I cannot always be with you, but I want to see the boys that are left at the helm encouraged, and to call your attention to the fact is all that is necessary.

I have been informed that one of the old graduates, my nephew, C. M. T. Hulett, or Turner as we call him, made the statement at the Minneapolis Meeting that the profession had not supported the Schools as it should. Now this may be true with some, but we feel that the majority have been very loyal. However, we would like to have you feel that the statement made by Turner applies to you so you will make an extra effort to make the January Class the banner class in the way of numbers that has yet matriculated.

From the start it has been my object to have the qualifications of an osteopath up-to-date in every particular, so he will be qualified to represent and defend the philosophy. I believe all Osteopathic Schools should work for intellectual perfection.

Wishing all a Merry Christmas and a Happy New Year, I am

Yours fraternally, A. T. Still.

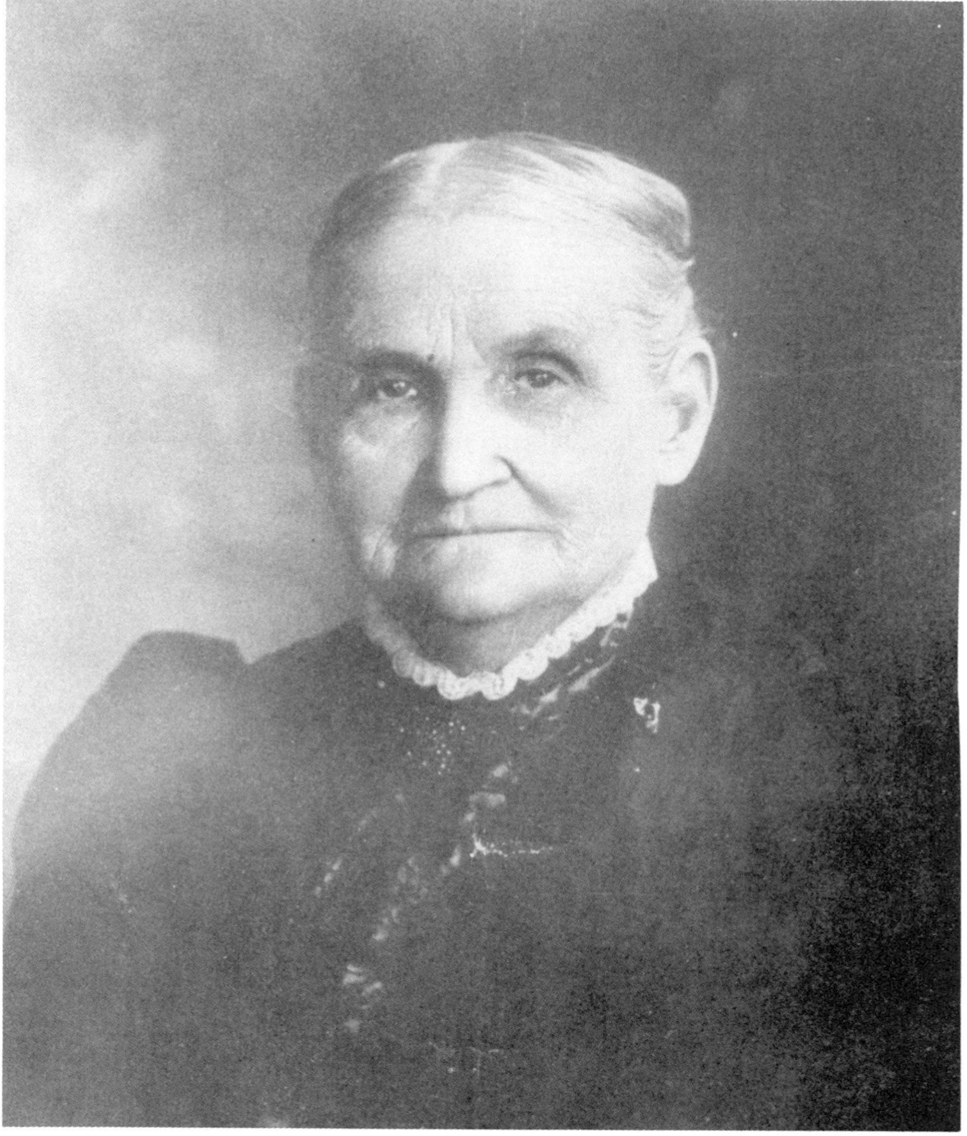

Mary Elvira Turner Still

To Our Friends.

To our friends, who have so kindly remembered us in our time of bereavement in the loss of our dear wife and mother, we wish to take this opportunity of extending our heartfelt thanks. The words of sympathy, and the expressions of high regard for a noble character contained in the numerous messages, have touched our hearts. The beautiful floral tribute, and the kind attentions of friends and neighbors have made us feel the bond of sympathy so freely expressed in other ways.

DR. A. T. STILL AND FAMILY.

January, 1911

Forum

Advocates Whipping Post.

The following letter shows the uncompromising attitude of Dr. Andrew Taylor Still, Founder of Osteopathy, towards a type of brutes which the law does not seem to be able to effectually reach:

E. G. Lewis, Editor Woman's National Daily,
St. Louis, Mo.

Dear Sir:—Missouri and probably many other states need a severe law dealing with wife-beaters. I feel that a man who will beat his wife or his mother should himself suffer a beating, and it should not be in private but in public. The public whipping-post, such as I understand the law provides in Oregon, in extreme instances, seems to me the only cure for these degenerate creatures.

We have good laws against cruelty to animals, and we should just as stringently protect wives from inhuman brutes who, under the cloak of husband, cruelly abuse those they pledge themselves to love and protect.

The osteopathic profession stands with me in the cause of humanity.

Respectfully,
A. T. Still, M. D.,
Founder of Osteopathy.

Kirksville, Mo., Feb. 7, 1911.

* * *

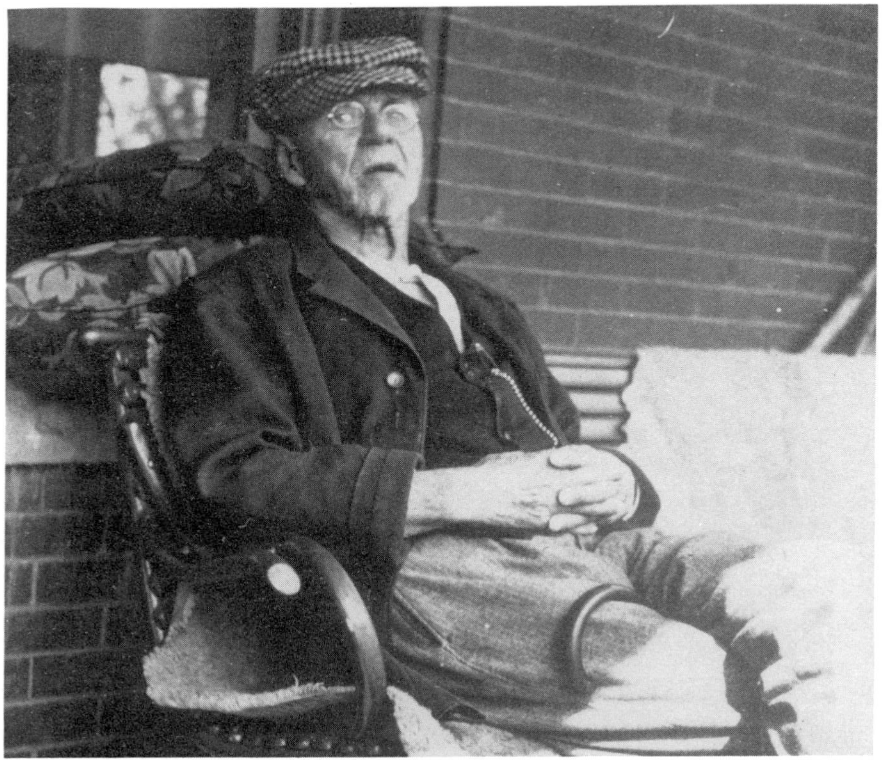

A. T. Still, c. 1915

June, 1912

Dr. A. T. Still's Philosophy of Immortality

In a speech before the Missouri State and Mississippi Valley Osteopathic Associations, at Kirksville, Missouri, May twenty-fourth, nineteen hundred and twelve, Doctor Andrew Taylor Still, the founder of the science of Osteopathy, said the following:

I do not know that I can make the Philosophy of Life and Death that I will present to you at all interesting.

For fifty years I have sought for some kind of gun or artillery that would slay the Black Wolf of Death, or fear, that is in all the pens of the lambs of God. I mean by the pens all the churches,—Catholics, Protestants, Mohammedans and all others.

When the priest or minister comes to the dying hour and you as his physician tell him that he is on the brink of the River of Death, that he cannot live twenty-four hours and tomorrow will be a corpse,—you know how he has lived, devoted all his time to the service of the living God,—even the pope, if you should tell him that tomorrow he would be a corpse and ask him what he sees beyond the river,—the answer of the priest and minister invariably is and I think the pope's answer would also be, "It is all a leap in the dark."

As a physicain I have stood by the bedsides of all of them, both in war and peace, and I am now eighty three years of age. I have stood by the bedsides of ministers who were devoted and who tried to spend their days in preparing to cross that river, and when they asked me to be honest with them, saying, "Do you think I can possibly recover?"—and I told them they could not live, that they would be a corpse tomorrow, and asked them what they saw beyond the River of Death, their answer was, "It is all a leap in the dark."

I will begin with my father. From eighteen years old to seventy-one years he was a devout servant of God and practiced his religion. When he was very low with pneumonia I went to him and he said, "Andrew, be honest with me, don't be afraid,—tell me, is there any chance for my recovery?" I said, "Father, you have asked me a serious question,—tomorrow you will be a corpse. Now I know how you have lived, you are devout, and if there is anything in religion you have been a faithful servant of God,—tell me, what do you see beyond the River of Death, you are on the brink of it." He answered, "Andrew, it is all a leap in the dark, I hope I am in the hands of a merciful God and that all will be right." I said, "I had hoped you would say, 'Beyond thar river I see a brilliant light,' but it is a leap in the dark." I thought it was poor pay for his lifetime's religious service. His name was Abram Still, aged seventy-one, a Methodist preacher.

Abram Roffrock, a Dunker, was one of the most devout and religious men I ever knew. Peculiarly, he and my father both died at seventy-one. He had flux and asked me if he could live through it. I told him tomorrow he would be a corpse. Then I said to him, "What do you see beyond the River of Death, you are on the edge of it." He answered, "It is all a leap in the dark, I hope I am in the hands of a merciful God."

That wolf of dread is in all the pens or churches of all the lambs of God. The pope, bishops, elders and leaders of all the churches dread that wolf and will run into a corner and hide just as quickly as any sheep in the flock. They fear the wolf of death just as much as anyone. I know what I say.

For fifty years I have hunted in all the theological armories to find the gun and ammunition which would shoot that wolf of torture which the theologians all teach from this text,—

"Be ye therefore always ready for at such an hour as ye think not behold the Son of Man cometh."

I have at last found a gun that has driven that wolf of dread from me. Today I have no more fear of death than life. I have a choice for death. Why? Because when I am ripe and been in the body long enough I wish to come out, being confident that it will be a higher step, which is necessary to man's spiritual perfection.

After going to all the theologians for demonstratable truth I went to my henhouse, to my stable, to animal shows and I found that all animate nature, but man, came to the world qualified with perfect knowledge to know and do that which was necessary for their comfort and happiness. When two hours old the calf, colt and lamb got up, went to the mothers and to the right place on the mothers' body, took hold of the teat and sucked the milk of nourishment and every motion showed absolute mental perfection in their orbit.

When a chicken comes out of the shell and is two days old he proves the perfection of the knowledge that is in him, that is according to the orbit or sphere of a bird. You put a spider and a fly down on the ground together and he will eat the fly, leaving the spider. He will eat dry bread which he never saw before, and with a portion of this dry bread in his mouth walk right over to a saucer of water, moisten it and continue his meal in that way. Should a hawk fly over a chicken which has been developed in an incubator it will hide until the hawk has gone. These examples of nature are ample evidence of the perfect intelligence and provision of God for all animate beings at birth, but man, in their various departments of life.

But alas, when I came to man he was both a physical and a mental dependent. He comes into the world a mental blank and when he dies he knows but little more, notwithstanding the days and years that he has spent in theological and scientific schools. By observation he has learned enough only to make a living for himself and those dependent upon him,—so he will have very little to carry away with him. You may go to all the schools you wish but when you come out you are still an immitator.

I learned more from an old hen than all the theologians have ever taught me. I learned the great lesson, which is, that our lives are in a body which could be called an incubator, developing the spiritual man to make the step from mortality to immortality. That hen sat on her eggs and kept them at a temperature between 96° and 108°. Had the temperature varied a few degrees either way the chicken would have died in the shell. When man's temperature goes below 90° or above 110° he is out of the shell and dead and the union of the spiritual with the physical stops. I thought these things over. What do they mean? We know an egg is a substance that will produce a chicken if it is kept in the incubator at the proper temperature. As sure as you run that above 108° the chicken dies.

My eyes have been opened by demonstration to the true philosophy of incubation in man and all animate beings and satisfied me that the union of matter and life is for the purpose of developing man to the degree of perfection which the God of Nature designed.

Man's life here represents the link in the ring which is connected to the ring of eteranl life. I had no difficulty in satisfying myself that the link represents the human body, and that when we come out after the period of incubation we are prepared to fill the sphere of perfect life for which Nature designed us. After the separation of the physcal and spiritual, the spiritual leaves the body, or incubator, prepared to receive and use all the attributes of perfect intelligence which belong to his sphere, man.

This philosophy has driven from me everything like the fear of death when I leave the body and has made me a happy man. That philosophy has made me hope that at the mature hour of my development I will come out with that perfection which the Architect of all nature intended. Every evidence that I have found in all nature is that the God of Life is an architect, a builder an engineer and no imperfection can be found,—and there is no perfection short of completion, for which I think the spiritual man is retained in the physical body until Nature says it is finished, having absolute perfect knowledge of all requirements for his comfort and happiness.

With me it has changed fear and dread to rejoicing at the perfect work of the Great Architect of the Universe, and I am ready to receive all changes that the Architect thinks are necessary to complete the work for which man was designed.

I will close by saying, "Know thyself and be at peace with God."

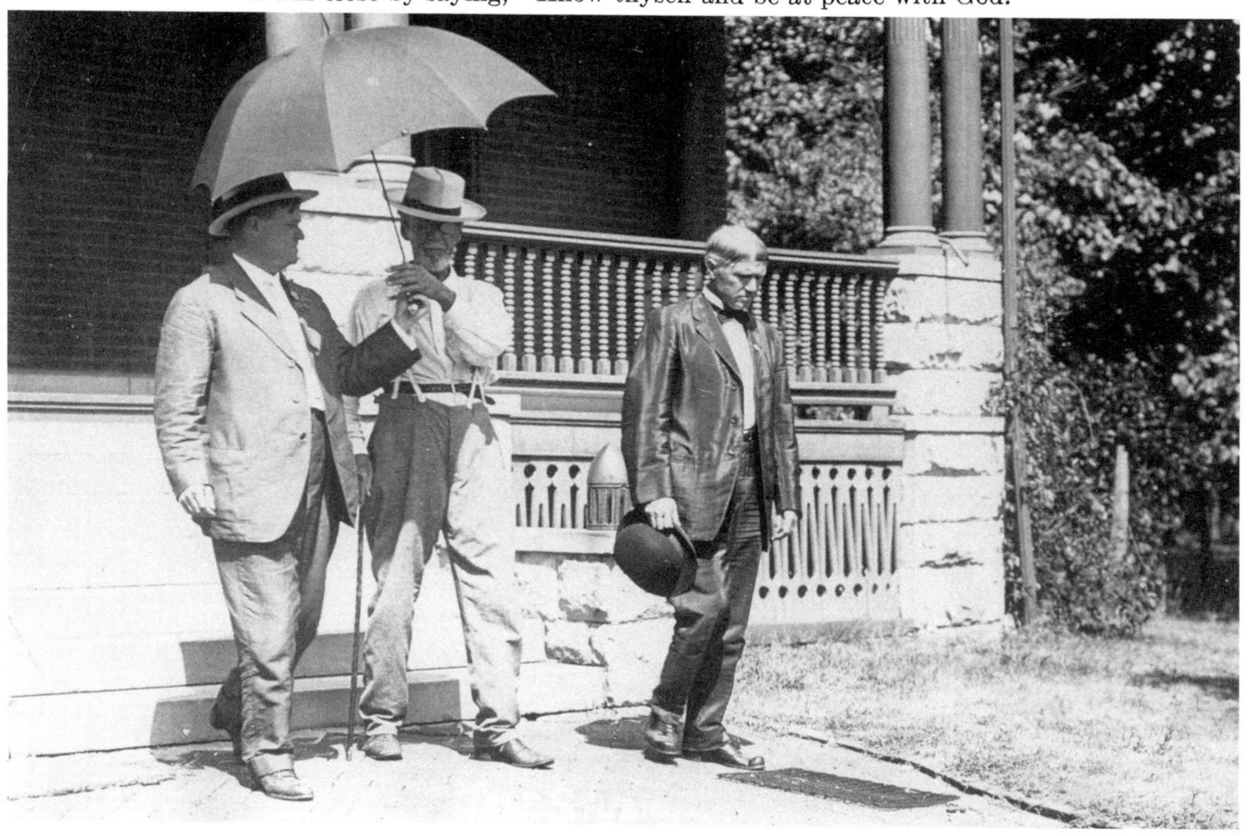

Harry M. Still, A. T. Still, Charles E. Still, c. 1915

Gems from the Old Doctor

INSANITY

(See cut opposite.)

My object is to bring up the subject of insanity and what produces it. For that reason, I give the reader a front and a back view of the spine of one of many insane subjects that we have dissected, in order to show you the abnormal condition found in most of the spines that have been sent to us from the insane asylum. The pill doctor says, "hereditary;" the mechanic says, "a wheel off, a bent axle, a spoke out; fix it, get in your buggy, and go on your journey." More to follow this in other Journals.—July 24, 1913.

* * *

Thirty-nine years ago I raised the flag and swore by the eternal that I would stand for the works of the Divine Architect of the Universe. —August 5, 1913.

* * *

God is an architect, He is a builder, He is an engineer, and all nature comes under the orders of that architect.—August 5, 1913.

* * *

To the osteopath, his first and last duty is to look well to a healthy blood and nerve supply. He should let his eye camp day and night on the spinal column, and he must never rest day or night until he knows that the spine is true and in line from atlas to sacrum, with all the ribs known to be in perfect union with the processes of the spine.—From the Philosophy of Osteopathy.

* * *

Osteopathy believes that all parts of the human body do work on chemical compounds and from the general supply manufacture for local wants; thus the liver builds for itself of the material that is prepared in its own division laboratory. The same of heart and brain. No disturbing or hindering causes will be tolerated to stay if the osteopath can find and remove them.—From the Philosophy of Osteopathy.

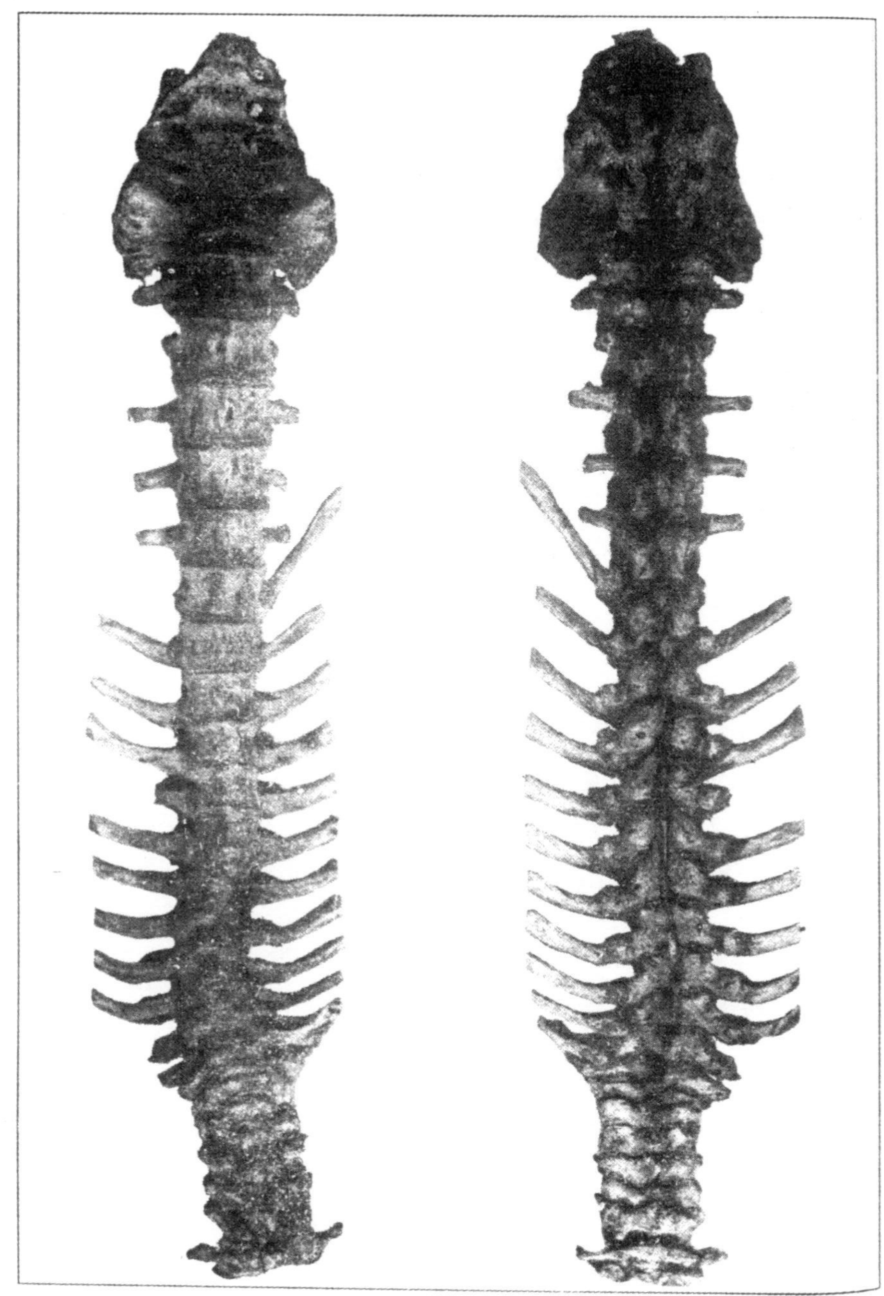

August, 1915

The Old Doctor's Message

High tide of enthusiasm in the meeting was reached when Dr. Hildreth, who is probably closer to the Old Doctor who founded Osteopathy than any other man in the profession, read the personal message of Dr. A. T. Still, which had been sent from Kirksville, Mo., urging them to stand firmly together to hold the principles of their profession free from entanglements and influences of other schools of healing.

"Millions of lives can be saved annually," he said. "Osteopathy is yet in its infancy. I have brought forth the principle and the truth, which I have turned over to the profession which has wisdom and enough moral backbone not to offer any compromise with the enemy.

Stand for Schools Urged

"Stand behind all legitimate research institutes. Give them your support.

"The treatments for insanity and the results obtained at Macon in the past year seem to be nothing more than natural. I have always said that at least 25 per cent of all insane cases could be cured by osteopathic treatment, and I am thankful to be able to live to see this truth demonstrated.

"There are other fields of research. May the grand army march on. If we can't have the pure osteopathic principles taught in our schools, I hope the faithful will rally around the flag and we will build an international school that will offer no compromise unless it is the golden truth.

"D. O.—Means Dig On."

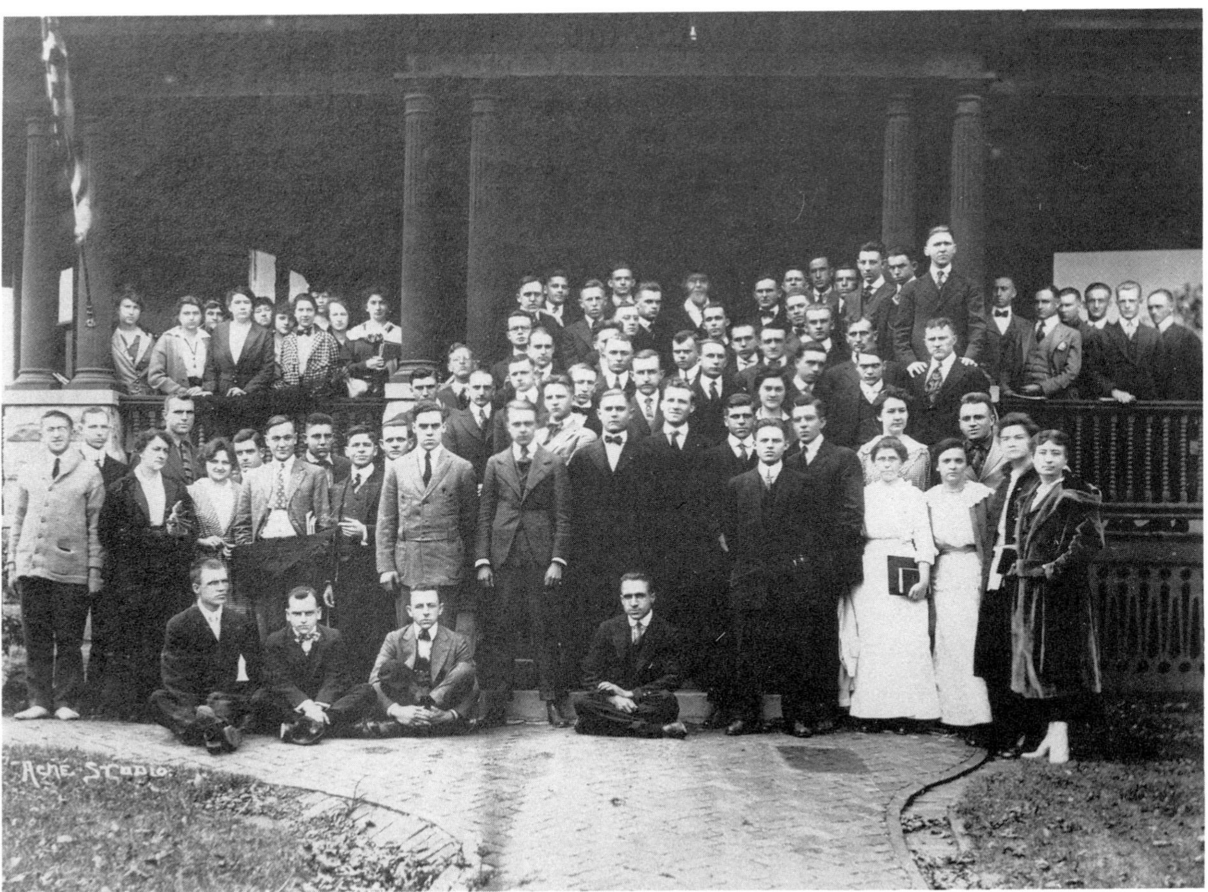

Class of 1917, last class picture containing A. T. Still

March, 1917

"All organs and parts of the human body are the subjects of one general law of demand, supply, construction and renovation in order to keep up normal functioning. Our work as engineers is to keep the engine so adjusted as to perform its functioning perfectly. Osteopathic adjusting means to so adjust the body that normal action will be sufficient to supply nerve force equal to the demand for construction."—A. T. Still.

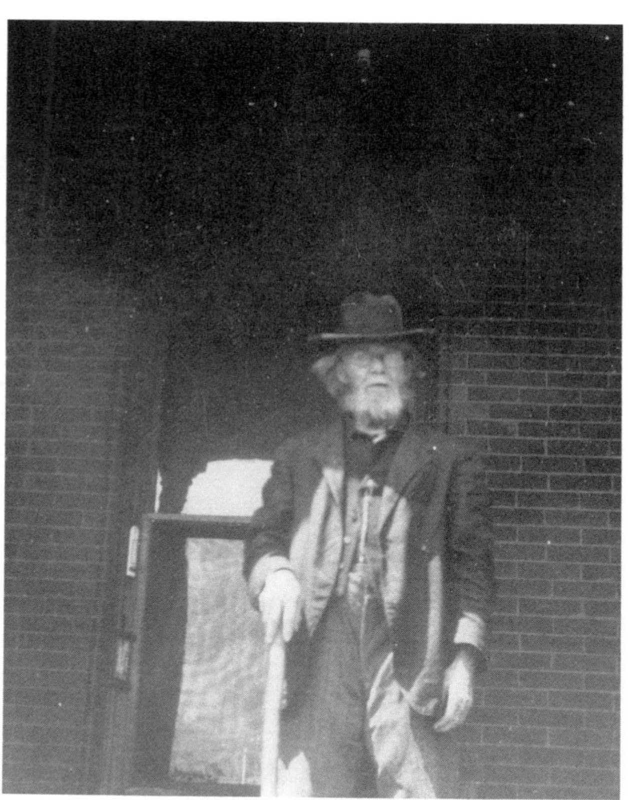

"Life proves its perfection by its work".

A. T. Still.

October 15th, 1916. Kirksville, Mo.

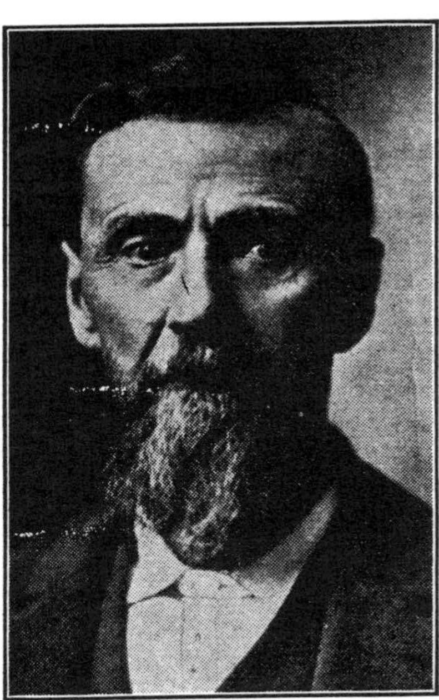

They Never Die

KIND words, like rivers of life, are the odors of thought, the dews and muscles of durability, the stay and comfort of the worrying man or woman who tries to reason or travel a road that runs through the forest of darkness, that must be crossed by all who see the lights beyond the brush of the untrodden paths of faith and logical truth. A kind word lightens the weighted and sinking heart until it can run to the harbor of rest. One kind word is water to the fast wilting tree of hope. There are a few in my heart whose duration has been many years, and are cherished today as rivers of joy, on whose surface float great streams loaded with unspeakable thanks for him, or her, or whoever gave me a smile and held even a lamp on shore to guide my boat to the stoneless channels of safe delivery. Those mites from a friend dropped in my cup which I drank as a famishing being, relished, as none other could, but he who had cruised in seas great and small for truth. I think of those smiles and cheering words as the brightest stars and gems of all my days. Our great word "love" fails to express my feelings to those that said, "Merit is the choicest jewel of all lives," and will attend all funerals of opposition because it cannot die, no never! Give me your kind words and keep all else; and when I am dead and my tongue loses its power, I will ask the bones of my tomb to thank you for them.—A. T. Still.

The Journal of Osteopathy

Vol. XXV JANUARY, 1918 No. 1

YOU AND YOUR PROFESSION

HERITAGE

J. A. van Brakle, D. O., Portland, Oregon

The Old Doctor is gone. The kindly voice, the shrewd, twinkling eye, the keen comment and the sharp-lined truth of thought, all are gone.

The staff-borne tread, the wayside demonstration, the sudden descent upon class-room with message all unconventional; these too have passed away with him.

The Old Doctor dies a poor man—but he leaves a world enriched. Differing from many others who have led the way, he did not die before recognition came to him. Now dead, the recognition of this generation and of all those to come will be his meed. Little by little this will extend as the world realizes that he gave to it a new truth of healing.

But to you and me who have been within the shadow of his teaching, he leaves an even greater heritage. All that we profess to be—he first brought into being. All that we may give to the world—he first gave. He came as a man with a living message and now that he is gone, you and I have become that message.

We will slowly learn to think that he is indeed gone, but the truth that was in him will be our very great inheritance. His message, through the turmoil of time, has begotten a profession and that profession now stands before the world, in his place. And our eternal heritage is this: IN US HE NOW LIVES.

True Osteopathy

THE osteopath who has not confidence enough in the science to implicitly rely upon it under all circumstances, is not entitled to the respect and patronage of his patients, and should blush with very shame when he accepts the money from his patrons. In the hands of the qualified and experienced practitioner it can be depended upon in all diseases incident to this climate. Osteopathy will never be found united with saloons nor combined with drugs.

—A. T. Still.